Springer Series in Statistics

More information about this series at http://www.springer.com/series/692

Grace Y. Yi

Statistical Analysis with Measurement Error or Misclassification

Strategy, Method and Application

Springer

Grace Y. Yi
Department of Statistics and Actuarial Science
University of Waterloo
Waterloo, Canada

ISSN 0172-7397 ISSN 2197-568X (electronic)
Springer Series in Statistics
ISBN 978-1-4939-6638-7 ISBN 978-1-4939-6640-0 (eBook)
DOI 10.1007/978-1-4939-6640-0

Library of Congress Control Number: 2016951935

Printed on acid-free paper

This Springer imprint is published by Springer Nature
The registered company is Springer Science+Business Media LLC
The registered company address is: 233 Spring Street, New York, NY 10013, U.S.A.

To my husband, Wenqing, my children, Morgan and Joy,
and my parents, Liangyu and Zhizhen

Foreword

This book is an authoritative addition to the literature on measurement error and misclassification. I like to think of the field more broadly as statistical analysis when variables are subject to uncertainty of measurement, although the context of measurement error and misclassification is different from the context of uncertainty quantification in applied mathematics and computer modeling.

This book differs considerably from previous books by Fuller (1987), Carroll et al. (1995, 2006), Gustafson (2004), and Buonaccorsi (2010) because of its comprehensive overview of topics in lifetime data analysis, often called survival analysis. If they touch at all on this important topic, which has quite a large literature, they touch it only very lightly. Grace Yi's book covers proportional hazard/Cox regression, additive hazard survival models, and recurrent event data and is the first text to cover these important topics in detail. Of course, the fact that the author is an expert on these topics is very important, and anyone wanting to know about uncertainty of measurement in lifetime data analysis will want this text as their guide.

Three other chapters are also unique: (a) longitudinal data analysis, (b) multistate and Markov models, and (c) case–control studies. Again, these topics are touched upon only lightly by the other books, but Grace Yi has given us a terrific overview of the literature, one not available elsewhere. I happen to know quite a lot about case–control and other retrospective studies, and I am impressed by the book's coverage of the area, and the important warnings that go with this form of sampling.

Not only are new topics covered in this book, but in addition they are covered extremely well. Not just authoritatively, but also Grace Yi has made great efforts to communicate the important ideas well. The book can be used in teaching courses, at all levels ranging all the way up to advanced seminars. I though treasure the book because I know that I have a resource for understanding issues in lifetime data analysis, not an area I am comfortable with, but one I confront on a regular basis.

Department of Statistics
Texas A&M University
College Station, TX 77843-3143, USA
and
School of Mathematical and Physical Sciences
University of Technology Sydney
Broadway, NSW 2007, Australia

Raymond J. Carroll

Preface

Measurement error and misclassification arise ubiquitously and have been a long-standing concern in statistical analysis. The effects of measurement error and misclassification have been well documented for many settings such as linear regression and nonlinear regression models. Consequences of ignoring measurement error or misclassification vary from problem to problem; sometimes the effects are negligible while other times they can be drastic. A general consensus is to conduct a case-by-case examination in order to reach a valid statistical analysis for error-contaminated data.

Over the past few decades, extensive research has been directed to various fields concerning such problems. Research interest in measurement error and misclassification problems has been rapidly spurred in a wide spectrum of data, including event history data (such as survival data and recurrent event data), correlated data (such as longitudinal data and clustered data), multi-state event data, and data arising from case–control studies. The literature on this topic is enormous with many methods scattered diversely. The goal of this monograph is to bring together assorted methods under the same umbrella and to provide an update on the recent development for a variety of settings. Measurement error effects and strategies of handling mismeasurement for different models are to be closely examined in combination with applications to specific problems.

A number of books concerning measurement error and misclassification have been published with distinct focuses. An early book by Fuller (1987) summarizes the development of linear regression models with errors-in-variables. Focusing on nonlinear measurement error models, Carroll, Ruppert and Stefanski (1995) provide analysis strategies for regression problems in which covariates are measured with error; the second edition, Carroll et al. (2006), further documents up-to-date methods with a comprehensive discussion on many topics on nonlinear measurement error models, including Bayesian analysis methods. With the emphasis on the use of relatively simple methods, Buonaccorsi (2010) describes methods to correct for measurement error and misclassification effects for regression models. Under the Bayesian paradigm, Gustafson (2004) provides a dual treatment of mismeasurement in both continuous and categorical variables. Other relevant books on this topic include Biemer et al. (1991), Cheng and Van Ness (1999), Wansbeek and Meijer (2000), and Dunn (2004).

This monograph covers the material that complements those books, although there is overlap in some of the topics. While general principles and strategies may share certain similarities, this book emphasizes unique features in modeling and analyzing measurement error and misclassification problems arising from medical research and epidemiological studies. The emphasis is on gaining insight into problems coming from a wide range of fields. This book aims to present both statistical theory and applications in a self-contained and coherent manner. To increase readability and ease the access for the readers, necessary background and basic inference frameworks for error-free contexts are presented at the beginning of Chapters 3–8, in addition to the discussion in Chapter 1. Each chapter is concluded with bibliographic notes and discussion, supplemented with exercise problems which may be used for graduate course teaching. Extensive references to recent development are given for the readers interested in research on various measurement error and misclassification problems. Applications and numerical illustrations are supplied.

This monograph is designed for multiple purposes. It can serve as a reference book for researchers who are interested in statistical methodology for handling data with measurement error or misclassification. It may be used as a textbook for graduate students, especially for those majoring in Statistics and Biostatistics. This book may also be used by applied statisticians whose interest focuses on analysis of error-contaminated data.

This monograph is intended to be read by readers with diverse backgrounds. Familiarity with inference methods (such as likelihood and estimating function theory) or modeling schemes in varying settings (such as survival analysis and longitudinal data analysis) can result in a full appreciation of the text, but this is not essential. Readers who are not familiar with those topics may enjoy reading the book by going through relevant topics. Chapters 1–2 and the first section of each following chapter provide basic inference frameworks and background material which are useful for unfamiliar readers. The book does not have to be read according to the sequential order of the chapters. Readers may directly read a chapter of interest by skipping prior chapters. The exercises at the end of each chapter supplement the development in the text. Some problems are organized to provide justification of the results discussed in the text; some problems are modified from research papers or monographs to serve as applications of the methods discussed in the text; and some problems are designed to be potential research topics which are worth further explorations. References at the end of the problems indicate the sources from which the problems are modified.

The book is laid out as three parts: Chapters 1 and 2, Chapters 3–8, and Chapter 9. Chapter 1 provides a broad overview of general statistical theory on modeling and inferences for the error-free context, followed by an introductory chapter, Chapter 2, on measurement error and misclassification. Chapter 2 introduces examples and issues on mismeasurement, and outlines a number of measurement error models. This chapter also describes the scope of the coverage of this book and lays out general strategies of handling measurement error models.

The second part is the central body of the book with six chapters, each devoted to a particular field. Chapter 3 concerns the basic ideas and methods for survival analysis with covariate measurement error, where proportional hazards models and additive hazards models are the main emphases. Chapter 4 shares some similarity in theme, but focuses on recurrent event data analysis with error-prone covariates. Chapter 5 discusses various strategies for handling longitudinal data with covariate measurement error. In particular, methods of dealing with covariate measurement error in combination with other features of longitudinal data, such as missing observations and joint modeling with survival data, are described in detail. Chapter 6 concerns multi-state models with error-contaminated variables where Markov models are particularly considered in many cases. Unlike the previous chapters which pertain to prospective studies, Chapter 7 considers issues on measurement error and misclassification which arise from retrospective studies. In this chapter, measurement error effects and inference techniques of accounting for mismeasurement are specifically given for case–control studies. Most of the discussion in Chapters 2–7 addresses measurement error and misclassification related to covariate variables, although some sections in Chapter 7 touch on error-prone response variables (i.e., state misclassification). To complement those topics, Chapter 8 takes up the topic on mismeasurement in response variables. Both univariate and multivariate response variables are considered for settings where measurement error or misclassification may arise. Finally, Chapter 9 is designed to supply an outline of miscellaneous topics which are not touched on in the previous chapters.

I aim to include the main themes and typical methods that have emerged on the subject of measurement error and misclassification. However, just like any other monograph, this book is impossible to comprehensively include all relevant research. The selection of topics, methods, and references is a reflection of my own research interest. I apologize to those authors whose work was missed being cited or should have been better presented in this book. Incompleteness in citations is not a sign of under-appreciation of relevant work but is just an outcome of limited space and inexhaustive access to the daunting amount of the literature on this subject.

I am indebted to many people who, directly or indirectly, helped with the birth of this book. I greatly acknowledge collaboration with Wenqing He, Raymond Carroll, Yanyuan Ma, Donna Spiegelman, Jerry Lawless, Richard Cook, and Lang Wu on measurement error problems. I thank my students, Ying Yan, Zhijian Chen, Feng He, and Di Shu, for their interest in working in this direction for their Ph.D. thesis research. I am extremely thankful to Raymond Carroll, Donna Spiegelman, Nancy

Reid, and Len Stefanski for their useful comments and discussion during the course of the book writing. In particular, I would like to thank Raymond Carroll for reading the manuscript and writing a foreword to this book. I am deeply grateful to Jerry Lawless, Mary Thompson, Ross Prentice, and J.N.K. Rao for reading through the manuscript; I can't thank them enough for providing detailed and constructive suggestions. This book came as an outcome of teaching a research topic course for graduate students in the Department of Statistics and Actuarial Science at the University of Waterloo over the past 10 years, and the students who took this course deserve thanks as well. I would also like to acknowledge the Department of Statistics and Actuarial Science at the University of Waterloo for providing a stimulating research environment and the Natural Sciences and Engineering Research Council of Canada (NSERC) for funding my research.

Above all, I owe my family big thanks for their tremendous support. My parents have been maintaining a great interest in seeing a hard copy of this book at its earliest date. I am particularly grateful to my husband, Wenqing He, my son, Morgan He, and my daughter, Joy He, for their strongest ever-lasting support during the long process of this book writing as well as my career. My husband, who deserves the most credit and has been my close collaborator on many research projects, is always critical and has carefully read through this book by providing numerous constructive suggestions, criticisms, and corrections. My son, who just entered a Master's program in Engineering, has always been supportive and has offered his best to help. He assisted me with typing and formatting the material to comply with the required template, reading through the book draft as an amateur reader with little background in Statistics, and providing comments as a general reader. The development of this book also accompanies my daughter's growth from Grade 4 to her current year in Grade 10. She started constantly asking me why I was so slow in my book writing and then became eager to learn to edit with LaTeX in order to help me with some exercise problem typing. My family is my inspiration and momentum that constantly push me forward to many new exciting destinations. Without their support, criticism, encouragement, and appreciation, this book would not have been possible.

University of Waterloo
Waterloo, Canada
June 8, 2016

Grace Y. Yi

Guide to Notation and Terminology

- Parameters are represented by Greek letters. Random variables and their realizations are usually denoted by upper case letters and the corresponding lower case letters, respectively, except that T_i and t_i represent different quantities in Chapter 3.
- Usually we differentiate random variables and their realizations by respectively using upper and lower case letters, but sometimes we simply use upper case letters to highlight the presence of the variables, especially when discussing the probability behavior of estimators.
- A binary random variable assumes value 0 or 1 unless otherwise stated.
- In the context of mismeasurement in covariates *alone*, the response variable is *often* denoted by Y; X and Z are used to differentiate error-prone and error-free covariates, respectively. The surrogate measurement of X is denoted by X^*.
- In the context of measurement error in response *alone*, covariates are simply expressed as Z; the true response variable is denoted by Y and its surrogate version is written as Y^*.
- In the case where both response and covariate variables are subject to mismeasurement, Y and X represent the true, error-prone response and covariate variables, respectively; and Y^* and X^* represent the corresponding surrogate measurements. Error-free covariates are denoted by Z.
- The subscript i is often used with random variables to label measurements for individuals or units; occasionally, we dispense with the subscript from the notation for ease of exposition. For example, if Y_i represents the response variable for the ith subject, then Y would represent the same type of random variable whose distribution is identical to that of Y_i.
- The dependence on time of a random variable may be indicated by the attached argument of t or a subscript. For example, $Y(t)$ represents the response measurement at time t and Y_{ij} may stand for the response measurement for subject i at time point j.
- Vectors are written in column form; the superscript ^{T} is used to denote the transpose of a vector or matrix.
- The terms "distribution", "conditional distribution", and "marginal distribution" are liberally used to refer to "probability density or mass function", "conditional probability density or mass function", "marginal probability density or mass function", respectively.
- When referring to "estimating function(s)", "parameter(s)", and "random variable (vector)", we usually describe them in the *singular* form for simplicity.
- Notation $E_U\{g(U)\}$ or $E\{g(U)\}$ represents the expectation of $g(U)$ taken with respect to the model for the distribution of U; $E_{U|V}\{g(U)\}$ or $E\{g(U)|V\}$ stands for the conditional expectation of $g(U)$ taken with respect to the model of the conditional distribution of U given V. Similar usage of notation applies to the variance or conditional variance of $g(U)$.

The following list provides quick access to the key notation used in the book. Precise definitions should be referred to the text.

Key Notation Throughout the Book

Symbol	Description
$\mathbb{R}$	The set of all real numbers
1_r	$r \times 1$ unit vector
I_r	$r \times r$ unit matrix
0_r	$r \times 1$ zero vector
$0_{r\times q}$	$r \times q$ zero matrix
0 (or zero)	Depending on the context, it may represent real number zero, a zero vector, or a zero matrix without confusion
$a^{\otimes 2}$	$a^{\otimes 2} = aa^{\mathrm{T}}$ for column vector a
$h(\cdot)$ or $h(\cdot\|\cdot)$	True (conditional) probability mechanism for the random variable(s) indicated by the argument(s)
$f(\cdot)$ or $f(\cdot\|\cdot)$	Statistical (conditional) model that represents a (conditional) probability density or mass function for the random variable(s) indicated by the argument(s)
$I(\cdot)$	Indicator function
$M(\cdot)$	Moment generating function
$\Phi(\cdot)$	Cumulative distribution function of distribution $N(0, 1)$
$d\eta(\cdot)$	Lebesque or counting measure featuring a continuous or discrete variable (vector)
$g^{-1}(\cdot)$	Inverse function of $g(\cdot)$
J^{-1}	Inverse matrix of nonsingular matrix J
X	Error-prone covariate (vector) of dimension p_x
X^*	Surrogate version of X
Z	Precisely measured covariate (vector) of dimension p_z
β_x	Effects of error-prone covariates X
β_z	Effects of precisely measured covaraites Z
β	Parameter (vector) of interest which includes β_x and β_z
σ_e^2 or Σ_e	Variance or covariance matrix for measurement error terms
n	Sample size
u_i	Random effects for $i = 1, \ldots, n$
$\mathcal{M}$	Subject index set for the main study
$\mathcal{V}$	Subject index set for the validation sample
t^- or t^+	A timc that is infinitesimally smaller or larger than t
$\xrightarrow{p}$	Convergence in probability
$\xrightarrow{d}$	Convergence in distribution

Chapter 1

Symbol	Description
Y	Random variable (or vector)
θ	Parameter (vector) that takes values in the parameter space
Θ	Parameter space which is a subset of Euclidean space $\mathbb{R}^p$; p is the dimension of θ
θ_0	True value of parameter θ
$\theta = (\alpha^{\mathrm{T}}, \beta^{\mathrm{T}})^{\mathrm{T}}$	α is a nuisance parameter subvector; β is a subvector of interest
$\mathbb{Y}$	Random sample $\{Y_1, \ldots, Y_n\}$ with each Y_i independently chosen from the same population
$y(n)$	Measurements $\{y_1, \ldots, y_n\}$ of $\mathbb{Y}$
$\widehat{\theta}$ or $\widehat{\theta}_n$	Estimator (or estimate) of θ
$L(\theta)$	Likelihood function
$S(\theta)$	Likelihood score function
$U(\theta; y)$	Estimating function (or a vector of estimating functions) for parameter θ

Chapter 2

Symbol	Description
Y	Response variable (or vector)
e	Measurement error variable (vector)
$\mathcal{O}$	Observed data $\{(y_i, x_i, z_i) : i = 1, \ldots, n\}$
$L_{\mathrm{O}}(\theta)$	Likelihood for the observed data
$L_{\mathrm{C}}(\theta)$	Likelihood for the complete data
$U(\cdot)$	Estimating function (or a vector of estimating functions) expressed in terms of $\{Y, X, Z\}$ or their realizations
$U^*(\cdot)$	Estimating function (or a vector of estimating functions) expressed in terms of $\{Y, X^*, Z\}$ or their realizations
π_{jk}	(Mis)classification probabilities $P(X^* = k \mid X = j, Z)$ for $j, k = 0, 1$

Chapter 3

Symbol	Description
T_i	Survival time for subject i
C_i	Censoring time for subject i
t_i	Observed time $\min(T_i, C_i)$
δ_i	Censoring indicator for subject i
$\lambda(t)$ or $\lambda(t\|X, Z)$	(Conditional) hazard function
$\lambda_0(t)$	Baseline hazard function
$S(t)$ or $S(t\|X, Z)$	(Conditional) survivor function
$\mathcal{H}_{it}^{\mathrm{X}}$	History $\{X_i(v) : 0 \leq v \leq t\}$ for subject i up to time t
$dN_i(t)$	Indicator variable $I\{T_i \in [t, t + \Delta t); \delta_i = 1\}$
$R_i(t)$	At risk indicator $I(t_i \geq t)$
η_i	Indicator variable $I(i \in \mathcal{V})$
$\mathcal{O}$	Observed data $\{(t_i, \delta_i, x_i^*, z_i) : i = 1, \ldots, n\}$
$\mathbb{T}$	Collection of $\{T_1, \ldots, T_n\}$
$\mathbb{C}$	Collection of $\{C_1, \ldots, C_n\}$
$\mathbb{X}$	Collection of $\{X_1, \ldots, X_n\}$
$\mathbb{X}^*$	Collection of $\{X_1^*, \ldots, X_n^*\}$
$\mathbb{Z}$	Collection of $\{Z_1, \ldots, Z_n\}$

Chapter 4

Symbol	Description
T_{ij}	Time of the jth event for individual i
W_{ij}	Waiting (or gap) time between events $(j - 1)$ and j for individual i
$N_i(t)$	Number of events over $[0, t]$ experienced by subject i
$\mathcal{H}_{it}^{\mathrm{N}}$	Event history $\{N_i(v) : 0 \leq v < t\}$ until (not including) time t for subject i
$\mathcal{H}_{it}^{\mathrm{XZ}}$	Covariate history $\{(X_i(v), Z_i(v)) : 0 \leq v \leq t\}$ up to and including time t for subject i
$\mu_i(t)$ or $\mu(t\|X_i, Z_i)$	(Conditional) mean function $E\{N_i(t)\|X_i, Z_i\}$ at time t
τ_i	Stopping time for individual i
$R_i(t)$	At risk indicator $I(t \leq \tau_i)$
π_{jk}^*	(Mis)classification probabilities $P(X = k\|X^* = j, Z)$ for $j, k = 0, 1$

Chapter 5

Symbol	Description
Y_{ij}	Response variable at time j for individual i (or for subject j in cluster i)
X_{ij}	Error-prone covariates at time j for individual i (or for subject j in cluster i)
X^*_{ij}	Surrorage measurement for X_{ij}
Z_{ij}	Precisely measured covariates at time j for individual i (or for subject j in cluster i)
m_i or m	The number of repeated measurements for subject i (or the number of subjects in cluster i)
μ_{ij}	Conditional mean response given covariates
R_{ij}	Missing data indicator for subject i at time j

Chapter 6

Symbol	Description
$Y(t)$	State occupied at time t
Y^*_{ij}	Surrogate measurement of $Y_{ij} = Y_i(t_{ij})$
K	The number of states
X^*_{ij}	Surrogate measurement of X_{ij}
$\mathcal{H}^{\mathrm{Y}}_t$	History of states $\{Y(v) : 0 < v < t\}$ up to but not including time t
$\mathcal{H}^{\mathrm{X}}_t$	History of covariates X, $\{X(v) : 0 \le v \le t\}$, up to and including time t
$\mathcal{H}^{\mathrm{Z}}_t$	History of covariates Z, $\{Z(v) : 0 \le v \le t\}$, up to and including time t
$\mathcal{H}^{\mathrm{XZ}}_t$	Union of $\mathcal{H}^{\mathrm{X}}_t$ and $\mathcal{H}^{\mathrm{Z}}_t$
$\mathcal{H}^{\mathrm{Y}*}_t$	History of surrogate measurements $\{Y^*(v) : 0 \le v < t\}$
$p_{jk}(s, t \mid \mathcal{H}^{\mathrm{Y}}_s)$	Transition probability $P(Y(t) = k \mid Y(s) = j, \mathcal{H}^{\mathrm{Y}}_s)$
$\lambda_{jk}(t \mid \mathcal{H}^{\mathrm{Y}}_t)$	Transition intensity at time t from state j to state k
γ_{iljk}	(Mis)classification probability for subject i at time point l $P(Y^*_{il} = k \mid Y_{il} = j, \mathcal{H}^{\mathrm{Y}*}_{il}, \mathcal{H}^{\mathrm{Z}}_{il})$

Chapter 7

Symbol	Description
Y	Binary response variable for disease status
ψ	Odds ratio
π^*_{ijk}	(Mis)classification probability $P(X = k\|Y = i, X^* = j)$
π_{ijk}	(Mis)classification probability $P(X^* = k\|Y = i, X = j)$
p^*_{ij}	Conditional probability $P(X^* = j\|Y = i)$
p_{ij}	Conditional probability $P(Z = j\|Y = i)$ or $P(X = j\|Y = i)$
q_{ij}	Conditional probability $P(Y = j\|Z = i)$ or $P(Y = j\|X = i)$
$f_{\cdot\|\cdot}(\cdot\|\cdot)$	Conditional model for the random variables indicated by the arguments
$f^{(v)}_{\cdot\|\cdot}(\cdot\|\cdot)$	Conditional model of the random variables indicated by the arguments for subjects in the validation sample or the main study (i.e., $v = 1$ or 0)

Chapter 8

Symbol	Description
Y	Random variable (or vector)
Y^*	Proxy version of Y
$\gamma_{j,1-j}(Z_i)$	(Mis)classification probability $P(Y^*_i = 1 - j\|Y_i = j, Z_i)$ for $j = 0, 1$
$\gamma_{j,1-j}(X^*_i, Z_i)$	(Mis)classification probability $P(Y^*_i = 1 - j\|Y_i = j, X^*_i, Z_i)$ for $j = 0, 1$
γ	Parameter (vector) for the model of the response misclassification process
R_{ij}	Misclassification indicator $I(Y^*_{ij} = Y_{ij})$

Key Acronyms Throughout the Book

Symbol	Description
AFT	Accelerated failure time (model)
AH	Additive hazards (model)
CI	Confidence interval
CR	Coverage rate (of 95% CIs)
EEE	Expected estimating equation(s)
EM	Expectation-maximization
EST	Estimate
EV	Empirical variance
GEE	Generalized estimating equations
GLM(s)	Generalized linear model(s)
GLMM(s)	Generalized linear mixed model(s)
GMM	Generalized method of moments
i.i.d.	Independently and identically distributed
IPTW	Inverse probability-of-treatment weighting
IPWGEE	Inverse probability weighted generalized estimating equation(s)
KLIC	Kullback-Leibler information criterion
MAR	Missing at random
MCAR	Missing completely at random
MCEM	Monte Carlo EM
MLE	Maximum likelihood estimator (estimate)
MM	Method of moments
MNAR	Missing not at random
MSE	Mean squared error
MVE	Model-based variance estimate
PH	Proportional hazards (model)
PO	Proportional odds (model)
RC	Regression calibration
ROC	Receiver operating characteristic
SE	Standard error
SIMEX	Simulation-extrapolation
UMVU	Uniformly minimum variance unbiased

About the Author

Grace Y. Yi is Professor of Statistics and University Research Chair at the University of Waterloo. Her broad research interests include measurement error models, missing data problems, high dimensional data analysis, survival data and longitudinal data analysis, estimating function and likelihood methods, and statistical applications. Professor Yi received her Ph.D. in Statistics from the University of Toronto in 2000. She is the 2010 winner of the CRM-SSC Prize, an honor awarded in recognition of a statistical scientist's professional accomplishments in research during the first 15 years after having received a doctorate. She was a recipient of the prestigious University Faculty Award granted by the Natural Sciences and Engineering Research Council of Canada (NSERC). She serves as an associate editor for several statistical journals and is the editor of *The Canadian Journal of Statistics* (2016–2018). She is a Fellow of the American Statistical Association and an Elected Member of the International Statistical Institute. She was President of the Biostatistics Section of the Statistical Society of Canada in 2016 and the Founder and Chair of the first chapter (Canada Chapter) of the International Chinese Statistical Association (ICSA).

Contents

1

Inference Framework and Method

This chapter sets the stage for the development of the book. The discussion in this chapter concerns the standard context in which mismeasurement is absent. This chapter lays out a broad framework for parametric inferences where estimation is of central interest. §1.1 outlines the inference framework and the objectives. Important issues concerning modeling and inferences are discussed in §1.2. Representative and useful estimation methodology is reviewed in §1.3. Strategies of handling model misspecification are described in §1.4, and the extension to the regression setting is included in §1.5. Brief bibliographic notes are presented in §1.6.

1.1 Framework and Objective

Statistical inference draws conclusions from data about the mechanism giving rise to the data. As data are often obtained from planned experiments and observational studies, a typical feature in conducting inference is to address the uncertainty that is induced from sampling variability, observational error, and chance variation or randomness. To this end, *statistical models* are employed to portray the data as realizations of certain random variables through probability distributions.

Throughout the book, we do not try to distinguish between a *scalar* random variable or a *multidimensional* random vector, but liberally use the term "*a random variable*" to refer to both cases unless otherwise stated. We use capital letters (e.g., Y) to represent random variables and corresponding lower case letters (e.g., y) for their realizations. Suppose we have the data, or a set of measurements $\{y_1, \ldots, y_n\}$ of a random variable Y whose probability density or mass function, denoted as $h(y)$, is unknown, where n is the size of the data. We want to gain an understanding of $h(y)$ using the measurements $\{y_1, \ldots, y_n\}$. A strategy is to specify a family of probability

G. Y. Yi, *Statistical Analysis with Measurement Error or Misclassification*, Springer Series in Statistics, DOI 10.1007/978-1-4939-6640-0_1

density or mass functions and hope this family would capture $h(y)$, or at least, contain a function which reasonably approximates $h(y)$. That is, we specify a family of models, written as

$$f(y;\theta),$$

where $f(\cdot)$ is called the *model function*, or *model* as a short form; it is a function of y and θ. The argument y represents a realization of random variable Y whose values fall in a *sample space*, denoted by $\mathcal{Y}$; and θ is called a *parameter* which takes values in the *parameter space*, denoted by Θ, where $\mathcal{Y} \subset \mathbb{R}^m$ with m representing the dimension of Y and $\mathbb{R}$ being the set of all real numbers. In parametric modeling, θ usually involves only a vector of *finite* number, say p, of unknown parameters $\theta = (\theta_1, \ldots, \theta_p)^{\mathrm{T}}$, and Θ is a subset of the Euclidean space $\mathbb{R}^p$. In a semiparametric setting, the dimension of θ may be infinite, and may depend on the sample size n. In this book, we do not attempt to precisely differentiate a parameter vector or a scalar parameter, and loosely use "*a parameter*" to refer to both situations. It is our hope that one of the functions in the class $\{f(y;\theta) : \theta \in \Theta\}$ would catch $h(y)$, i.e., there exists $\theta_0 \in \Theta$ such that $f(y;\theta_0) = h(y)$. This θ_0 is called the *true value* of θ.

Our aim in performing inferences is to use the data *inductively* to narrow down which distribution is likely to occur and obtain information about the true value of θ. This is the opposite of the *deductive* approach of probability theory where we are often interested in evaluating the chance of observing particular outcomes based on a *specified* distribution. In the probability theory, parameter θ in the model $f(y;\theta)$ is treated as known, and we stress that $f(y;\theta)$ is a function of the variable Y. On the contrary, in conducting statistical inference, we emphasize that data are given and view $f(y;\theta)$ as a function of parameter θ. Throughout the book, for convenience, we loosely use the terms "probability density function", "probability distribution", "distribution", or "probability mass function" interchangeably for function $f(\cdot)$ or $h(\cdot)$.

In *parametric statistical inference*, $f(\cdot)$ is completely specified as a known analytic form, such as a probability density or mass function from the *exponential family* (e.g., Lehmann and Casella 1998, §1.5). When $f(\cdot)$ is partially specified, resulting inferential procedures are usually termed as *semiparametric inference*. A third type of inference pertains to *nonparametric inference* for which data are not described by a parametric or semiparametric representation.

In this book, we are mostly concerned with parametric or semiparametric inference. Our objective is, on the basis of the observed data

$$\{y_1, \ldots, y_n\},$$

to make inference about the entire parameter vector θ, or a subvector of θ that is of particular interest. In this regard, several types of inference procedures may proceed: (i) *estimation*, (ii) *hypothesis testing*, (iii) *prediction*, and (iv) *model assessment*. While these topics are related, in this book, we mainly concentrate on the estimation problem. Our central goal is to develop various estimation methods and establish asymptotic distributions for the resulting estimators. Statistical inference, such as constructing confidence intervals or performing hypothesis testing, may be carried out using those asymptotic results.

1.2 Modeling and Estimator

1.2.1 Parameter and Identifiability

Statistical modeling is the basis for parametric or semiparametric inference. In reality, it is rare or almost impossible that the distribution $h(y)$ for the true data generation mechanism can be pinned down exactly. In parametric modeling, a viable routine is to specify a class of distributions, or a *model*, $\{f(y;\theta) : \theta \in \Theta\}$, so that one of the distributions identifies or well approximates the true distribution $h(y)$. By the term "model", we mean a specification of the variables and parameters of interest, the relationships among the variables, and the assumptions about the stochastic properties of the random variables (e.g., Thompson and Carter 2007).

A function $f(\cdot)$ is specified or partially specified to feature basic structures of the data. It may be chosen as a particular model form, such as a generalized linear model, or may be given by a distributional form with certain assumptions, such as independently and identically normally distributed. A feasible functional form of $f(\cdot)$ may be suggested by the data, while in some situations, the selection of the function form $f(\cdot)$ may be driven by the mathematical flexibility and tractability. On the other hand, an appropriate value of θ is unknown and needs to be estimated. The introduction of parameter θ in a statistical model initially serves to index probability distributions, and we wish to find the one that best approximates the true data generation mechanism $h(y)$ (e.g., Draper 1995). Mathematically, any one-to-one transformation of θ would serve equally well for this purpose. But in application, the parameter form often comes together with the specification of the analytic form of $f(\cdot)$. In some circumstances, a reparameterization of θ is useful to simplify inferential procedures (e.g., Problem 1.22). In settings including regression analysis, model parameters usually have a practically meaningful interpretation (e.g., Bickel and Doksum 1977; Cox 2006).

Although there may not be a unique principle to specify a suitable model, a fundamental requirement applies universally. To make inferences meaningful, a specified model $f(y;\theta)$ must be *identifiable*. Specifically, if there are two parameter values θ_1 and $\theta_2 \in \Theta$ such that

$$f(y;\theta_1) = f(y;\theta_2) \text{ for all possibly observed } y \text{ (in a set of probability 1)},$$

then

$$\theta_1 = \theta_2.$$

This identifiability requirement ensures that each parameter value would uniquely correspond to a distribution of a random variable. It implies that the true value θ_0 defined in §1.1 is *unique*.

Sometimes, one may simply say the model parameter θ is identifiable (or unidentifiable) if the model $f(y;\theta)$ is identifiable (or unidentifiable). The following example gives a quick illustration of the identifiability or nonidentifiability of models.

Example 1.1. Let $f(y;\theta)$ denote a probability density function for the random vector $Y = (Y_1, Y_2)^{\mathrm{T}}$, where $\theta = (\theta_1, \theta_2)^{\mathrm{T}}$ is a vector of parameters taking values in the parameter space $\Theta = (0, \infty) \times (0, \infty)$. If the probability density function of Y takes the form

$$f(y;\theta) = \exp\left(-\frac{\theta_1}{\theta_2}y_1 - \frac{\theta_2}{\theta_1}y_2\right) \text{ for } y_1 > 0 \text{ and } y_2 > 0,$$

then $\theta = (\theta_1, \theta_2)^{\mathrm{T}}$ is not identifiable. However, if the probability density function of Y is given by

$$f(y;\theta) = \frac{\theta_1^2}{\theta_2}\exp\left(-\frac{\theta_1}{\theta_2}y_1 - \theta_1 y_2\right) \text{ for } y_1 > 0 \text{ and } y_2 > 0,$$

then $\theta = (\theta_1, \theta_2)^{\mathrm{T}}$ is identifiable.

While nonidentifiability may arise from ill-specified model structures or parameter forms, it can also occur from a well-defined model that has a practical meaning. In this case, a common strategy is to impose additional constraints or assumptions on either the model structure or the parameters to achieve the model identifiability. In other situations, an identifiable model may become unidentifiable due to the degrading quality of the data. For example, a linear regression model can be well-defined when the response and covariate variables are precisely measured, but in the presence of measurement error, nonidentifiability may become an issue because of the lack of precise measurements for the variables involved in the model. This issue is to be further discussed in subsequent chapters.

1.2.2 Parameter Estimator

We wish to use measurements $\{y_1, \ldots, y_n\}$ of a random variable Y to infer the true data generation mechanism $h(y)$. Suppose we have a well defined model $\{f(y;\theta) : \theta \in \Theta\}$ and this model fortunately includes $h(y)$ as a member with $f(y;\theta_0) = h(y)$ for some $\theta_0 \in \Theta$. Our objective is to estimate θ_0 using the collected measurements $\{y_1, \ldots, y_n\}$.

To this end, we use a function, say $\widehat{\theta}(\cdot)$, of the observations to summarize the information carried by the data. We develop an estimation procedure in order to come up with a sensible function $\widehat{\theta}(\cdot)$ and then guess the true value of θ by applying the function $\widehat{\theta}(\cdot)$ to the data $\{y_1, \ldots, y_n\}$. In many applications, data $\{y_1, \ldots, y_n\}$ are independently collected as n replicated measurements of Y; equivalently, they are regarded as a realization of a sequence of *independently and identically distributed* (i.i.d) random variables $Y_1, \ldots, Y_n$, each having the same distribution as Y. We write $\mathbb{Y} = \{Y_1, \ldots, Y_n\}$ and simply say that $\mathbb{Y} = \{Y_1, \ldots, Y_n\}$ is a *random sample* from the distribution $h(y)$.

To derive a sensible function $\widehat{\theta}(\cdot)$, it is important to understand the probability behavior of the random variable $\widehat{\theta}(\mathbb{Y})$, called an estimator of θ_0, which is obtained by applying function $\widehat{\theta}(\cdot)$ to *hypothetical repetitions* $\mathbb{Y}$ of the data generation under the same conditions (Young and Smith 2005).

Given the data, there are many ways to form an estimator of θ_0. How does one select a good or even the best estimator? What criteria are useful for this purpose? Because the true value θ_0 is unknown, it is not possible to evaluate $\widehat{\theta}(\mathbb{Y})$ relative to the true underlying distribution $h(y)$, or $f(y;\theta_0)$. Instead, we extend our attention from evaluating $\widehat{\theta}(\mathbb{Y})$ for *a single* sequence $\mathbb{Y}$ to assessing $\widehat{\theta}(\mathbb{Y}_\theta)$ for *a class* $\{\mathbb{Y}_\theta : \theta \in \Theta\}$ of all possible sequences, where $\mathbb{Y}_\theta = \{Y_{\theta 1}, \ldots, Y_{\theta n}\}$ is a *random sample* drawn from model $f(y;\theta)$ for *all* $\theta \in \Theta$. To adequately assess the performance of an estimation procedure, we thus evaluate the probability behavior of the random variable $\widehat{\theta}(\mathbb{Y}_\theta)$ for *all* $\theta \in \Theta$ (rather than a single value or some values of θ).

In the following development, unless otherwise stated, all the discussion is intended for *all* the parameter values in the parameter space even though this is not explicitly pointed out everywhere. Thus, we do not emphasize the difference in notation but just use $\mathbb{Y} = \{Y_1, \ldots, Y_n\}$ to refer to all possible sequences $\mathbb{Y}_\theta = \{Y_{\theta 1}, \ldots, Y_{\theta n}\}$, and let $y(n) = \{y_1, \ldots, y_n\}$ denote the corresponding realizations or *sample measurements* of $\mathbb{Y}$. Estimation of the true parameter value θ_0 is liberally phrased as "*estimation of parameter* θ".

In contrast to $\widehat{\theta}(\mathbb{Y})$ being called an *estimator* of θ, $\widehat{\theta}(y(n))$ is called an *estimate* of θ. Sometimes, $\widehat{\theta}(\mathbb{Y})$ and $\widehat{\theta}(y(n))$ are simply denoted as $\widehat{\theta}$ for ease of exposition. In the rest of this section, our discussion is directed to the case where θ is a scalar unless otherwise stated; extensions to multidimensional parameter θ are straightforward with proper notation of matrices or vectors required.

To describe the probability behavior of an estimator $\widehat{\theta}$ of θ, one often uses the *mean squared error* (MSE) of $\widehat{\theta}$ which is defined as

$$\text{MSE}(\theta;\widehat{\theta}) = E\{(\widehat{\theta} - \theta)^2\},$$

where the expectation is evaluated with respect to the joint distribution of the associated variables $\mathbb{Y}$ which typically depends on θ; in the case where $Y_1, \ldots, Y_n$ are i.i.d random variables having the distribution $f(y;\theta)$, the joint distribution of $\mathbb{Y}$ is given by $\prod_{i=1}^n f(y_i;\theta)$.

The MSE measure is a function of parameter θ and is well-defined if the first two moments of the estimator $\widehat{\theta}$ exist. This measure emphasizes joint evaluation of the first two moments of an estimator, as suggested by its alternative expression

$$\text{MSE}(\theta;\widehat{\theta}) = \text{BIAS}^2(\theta;\widehat{\theta}) + \text{var}(\widehat{\theta}),$$

where

$$\text{BIAS}(\theta;\widehat{\theta}) = E(\widehat{\theta}) - \theta$$

is the *bias* of the estimator $\widehat{\theta}$, which quantifies how far and in what direction the expected value of $\widehat{\theta}$ is away from the target θ. The variance $\text{var}(\widehat{\theta})$ of $\widehat{\theta}$ is evaluated with respect to the joint distribution of $\mathbb{Y}$; it measures how tightly the distribution of $\widehat{\theta}$ clusters about its expectation, or the variability of $\widehat{\theta}$. The dependence of $E(\widehat{\theta})$ and $\text{var}(\widehat{\theta})$ on θ is suppressed in the notation.

Ideally, we wish to have an estimator which has the smallest bias and the smallest variance. However, this is rarely possible except for trivial cases. One strategy to get around this difficulty is to minimize one aspect of the estimator with the other held to be the smallest (such as zero). Dually, one may look at either the class of estimators with zero variance or the class of estimators with zero bias, and then try to find an estimator with the smallest bias or the smallest variance from each class.

It is not feasible, however, to focus on the class of estimators with zero variance because useless estimators would arise. For instance, if we set an estimator $\widehat{\theta}$ to be a constant θ_1 for some $\theta_1 \in \Theta$, then this estimator has variance zero, but its bias could be substantial when θ is not close to θ_1. On the other hand, it is possible to find useful estimators by confining attention to the family of the estimators whose bias is zero, and then from this class we choose an estimator with the smallest variance.

Requiring an estimator $\widehat{\theta}$ to have zero bias in estimating θ is the same as requiring

$$E(\widehat{\theta}) = \theta \text{ for all } \theta \in \Theta, \tag{1.1}$$

where the expectation is evaluated with respect to the joint distribution of $\mathbb{Y}$. An *estimator* satisfying the requirement (1.1) is called an *unbiased estimator* of θ. In contrast, if there exists an estimator $\widehat{\theta}$ satisfying (1.1) for a model $\{f(y;\theta) : \theta \in \Theta\}$, then *parameter* θ is called *U-estimable* (Lehmann and Casella 1998). Some authors call such a parameter θ *estimable* (e.g., Freedman 2009; Shao 2003), but we do not use this term in this book to avoid a possibly misleading indication that any θ not possessing this property cannot be well estimated. If model parameters are U-estimable, they are identifiable (e.g., Problem 1.2); but the converse is not true: a parameter can be identifiable without being U-estimable (e.g., Problem 1.1).

For some models, for instance, a model coming from the exponential family, it is possible to restrict attention to the class of all unbiased estimators and then to identify the best estimator such that its MSE is the smallest. This is equivalent to finding an unbiased estimator with the smallest variance. An estimator $\widehat{\theta}$ for θ is called *uniformly minimum variance unbiased* (UMVU), if it is an unbiased estimator with $E(\widehat{\theta}) = \theta$ and $\text{var}(\widehat{\theta}^*) - \text{var}(\widehat{\theta})$ is nonnegative for *any* unbiased estimator $\widehat{\theta}^*$ of θ. In general, a UMVU estimator does not necessarily exist; but if it does, then it is unique. A detailed discussion on UMVU estimators can be found in Bickel and Doksum (1977), Lehmann and Casella (1998) and Shao (2003), among many others.

Although unbiased estimators are useful for some models, several limitations prevent their universal applicability. Unbiased estimators do not always exist for *any* statistical model. Unbiasedness is not invariant under a one-to-one transformation. In other words, a parameter θ can be U-estimable, but its reparameterization, say $q(\theta)$, may not be U-estimable for a one-to-one function $q(\cdot)$ (e.g., Problem 1.1). Moreover, many estimation methods, such as the method of moments or the maximum likelihood method, do not necessarily produce unbiased estimators (e.g., Problem 1.3).

Even in the situation where the parameter θ is U-estimable, there is no guarantee that any of its unbiased estimators are always desirable; an estimator with some bias might be preferred due to its minimum MSE (e.g., Problem 1.3). This does not, of course, suggest that one should not care about the magnitude of bias. A large bias is usually considered as a drawback; bias reduction may be considered. See, for example, the *jackknife* method which is outlined in Problem 1.4.

Given the foregoing discussion, one might then attempt to discard the requirement of unbiasedness of an estimator, but directly to compare MSE for two estimators in order to decide which estimator is better. However, there is a difficulty in doing so. Because the MSE depends on the value of θ, the ratio between the MSE of any two estimators may not be uniformly smaller or greater than 1 for all $\theta \in \Theta$, hence failing to provide a clear indication of which estimator is better. This difficulty is present if we stick to finding a preferable estimator by treating the size of data, n, as fixed. If we are, however, willing to allow n to vary, meaningful criteria for selecting a sensible estimator may be developed for a much wider class of practical models. In the next subsection, we discuss this in detail.

1.2.3 Concepts in Asymptotic Sense

To emphasize the dependence of an estimator $\widehat{\theta} = \widehat{\theta}(\mathbb{Y})$ on the sample size n, in this subsection we write $\widehat{\theta}$ as $\widehat{\theta}_n$. An estimator $\widehat{\theta}_n$ is called a *consistent* estimator of θ if $\widehat{\theta}_n$ converges to θ in probability as n approaches infinity. Mathematically, this requires that for any $\epsilon > 0$,

$$P\{|\widehat{\theta}_n - \theta| > \epsilon\} \to 0 \quad \text{as } n \to \infty,$$

where the probability is evaluated with respect to the joint distribution of $\mathbb{Y}$. Intuitively, a consistent estimator is close to θ with probability tending to 1 as the size of the data is getting large (e.g., Bickel and Doksum 1977).

The notion of consistency is not defined for an estimator with a fixed data size n. It is only meaningful for a sequence of estimators $\{\widehat{\theta}_n : n = 1, 2, \ldots\}$, obtained from applying a common method to a sequence of data that are usually indexed by the sample size n. This definition is more used to describe an estimation method in terms of its long run probability behavior than to describe a concrete estimate calculated for a particular data set itself. For simplicity, however, we often liberally say an estimator $\widehat{\theta}_n$ is consistent, although we actually mean that a sequence of estimators, produced by the same method, has this property.

Consistency is a very important requirement for finding a sensible estimator (strictly speaking, a sensible estimation method). It becomes essential in many applications so that any *inconsistent* estimators are not even considered. The consistency property of estimators pertains to the nature of model parameters as well. Unidentifiable model parameters cannot be consistently estimated (see Problem 1.6; Gabrielsen 1978).

A consistent estimator is not necessarily unbiased. In application, a naturally constructed estimator may not even have a well-defined expectation. The measure of BIAS or MSE would thereby become meaningless for such an estimator. To get around this issue, we introduce *asymptotic measures*, parallel to the measures of BIAS and MSE which are defined for estimators with a fixed size of data (Shao 2003, Ch. 2).

Definition 1.2. *Let* $\{\widehat{\theta}_n : n = 1, 2, \ldots\}$ *be a sequence of random variables, and* $\{a_n : n = 1, 2, \ldots\}$ *be a sequence of positive numbers satisfying* $a_n \to \infty$ *or* $a_n \to a$ *for some* $a > 0$*, as* $n \to \infty$.

(a) If there exists a random variable V *with* $E(|V|) < \infty$ *such that*

$$a_n \widehat{\theta}_n \stackrel{d}{\longrightarrow} V \text{ as } n \to \infty,$$

then $E(V)/a_n$ *is called an "asymptotic expectation" of* $\widehat{\theta}_n$.

(b) If $\widehat{\theta}_n$ *is an estimator of* θ *for every* n*, then an asymptotic expectation of* $\widehat{\theta}_n - \theta$ *is called an "asymptotic bias" of* $\widehat{\theta}_n$*, provided it exists.*

Let $\mathrm{ABIAS}(\theta; \widehat{\theta}_n)$ *denote this asymptotic bias. If* $\mathrm{ABIAS}(\theta; \widehat{\theta}_n)$ *approaches* 0 *as* $n \to \infty$*, then the sequence of estimators* $\widehat{\theta}_n$ *is said "asymptotically unbiased", or* $\widehat{\theta}_n$ *is "asymptotically unbiased" for simplicity.*

At first sight, this definition is flawed because combinations of different scale factors a_n with a different sequence of random variables $\widehat{\theta}_n$ might yield different ratios $E(V)/a_n$. However, the results in Problem 1.7 essentially show the uniqueness of the asymptotic expectation of $\widehat{\theta}_n$, thus the notion of *asymptotic expectation* is well defined. It is immediate that a consistent estimator is asymptotically unbiased. The following definition extends the discussion of the usual second moment of $\widehat{\theta}_n$ to the asymptotic context (Shao 2003, Ch. 2).

Definition 1.3. *Let* $\{\widehat{\theta}_n : n = 1, 2, \ldots\}$ *be a sequence of estimators of* θ*,* V *be a random variable, and* $\{a_n : n = 1, 2, \ldots\}$ *be a sequence of positive numbers satisfying* $a_n \to \infty$ *or* $a_n \to a$ *for some* $a > 0$*, as* $n \to \infty$*. Assume that* $a_n(\widehat{\theta}_n - \theta) \stackrel{d}{\longrightarrow} V$ *as* $n \to \infty$ *and* $E(V^2) < \infty$.

(a) The asymptotic expectation of $(\widehat{\theta}_n - \theta)^2$ *is defined as the "asymptotic mean squared error" of* $\widehat{\theta}_n$:

$$\mathrm{AMSE}(\theta; \widehat{\theta}_n) = \frac{E(V^2)}{a_n^2},$$

and the "asymptotic variance" of $\widehat{\theta}_n$ *is defined to be*

$$\mathrm{Avar}(\widehat{\theta}_n) = \frac{\mathrm{var}(V)}{a_n^2}.$$

(b) Suppose $\{\widehat{\theta}_n^* : n = 1, 2, \ldots\}$ *is another sequence of estimators of* θ*. "The asymptotic relative efficiency" of* $\widehat{\theta}_n^*$ *to* $\widehat{\theta}_n$ *is defined to be*

$$\mathrm{ARE}(\widehat{\theta}_n^*, \widehat{\theta}_n) = \frac{\mathrm{AMSE}(\theta; \widehat{\theta}_n)}{\mathrm{AMSE}(\theta; \widehat{\theta}_n^*)}.$$

$\widehat{\theta}_n^*$ *is said to be "asymptotically more efficient" than* $\widehat{\theta}_n$ *if*

$$\text{ARE}(\widehat{\theta}_n^*, \widehat{\theta}_n) \geq 1 \textit{ for all } \theta,$$

and

$$\text{ARE}(\widehat{\theta}_n^*, \widehat{\theta}_n) > 1 \textit{ for some } \theta.$$

These asymptotic measures are basically introduced to delineate the limiting behavior in the probability sense for those estimators whose moments are not well defined or difficult to calculate. A natural concern is: what if an estimator has the moments, do its asymptotic measures differ from its usual measures defined for a given size of data? The answer is yes. When the MSE of $\widehat{\theta}_n$ exists, MSE$(\theta; \widehat{\theta}_n)$ is not smaller than AMSE $(\theta; \widehat{\theta}_n)$; under certain conditions, these two measures may be equal (see Problem 1.8).

As discussed previously, consistency is often imposed as a basic condition for finding a sensible estimator. The consistency property of $\widehat{\theta}_n$ yields that the difference between $\widehat{\theta}_n$ and the parameter θ converges in distribution to zero. If solely looking at such a difference, we are not able to differentiate different types of consistent estimators in their asymptotic distributions, because they all degenerate to zero. To compare these differences, we need to view them more closely using a "magnifier". For this purpose, we *scale* the differences between estimators and the parameter θ by a sequence of positive numbers $\{a_n : n = 1, 2, \ldots\}$ so that the resulting variables have nondegenerate asymptotic distributions. For most applications, we are interested in finding those estimators $\widehat{\theta}_n$ such that the limiting distribution of their transformed versions, $a_n(\widehat{\theta}_n - \theta)$, is a normal distribution, i.e., V is a random variable with a normal distribution with mean zero if using the symbols in Definition 1.3. Often, the sequence $\{a_n : n = 1, 2, \ldots\}$ is of an order of the sample size, such as $a_n = O(n^c)$ for a positive constant c. In parametric inference, a_n is often taken as $\sqrt{n}$, and the corresponding consistent estimator $\widehat{\theta}_n$ is sometimes called $\sqrt{n}$*–consistent* (Newey and McFadden 1994, p. 2114).

In some applications, we are not only interested in estimating the parameter θ itself but also a function, say $q(\theta)$, of the parameter θ. The following theorem offers a convenient tool to calculate asymptotic measures of the estimator for $q(\theta)$ using the measures for the original estimator of θ.

Theorem 1.4. *Let* $\{\widehat{\theta}_n : n = 1, 2, \ldots\}$ *be a sequence of estimators for* θ *satisfying*

$$a_n(\widehat{\theta}_n - \theta) \xrightarrow{d} V \textit{ as } n \to \infty,$$

where V *is a random variable with* $0 < E(V^2) < \infty$ *and* $\{a_n : n = 1, 2, \ldots\}$ *is a sequence of positive numbers satisfying* $a_n \to \infty$ *or* $a_n \to a$ *for some* $a > 0$ *as* $n \to \infty$.

Suppose $q(\theta)$ *is differentiable with the derivative* $q'(\theta)$, *and let* $\widehat{\vartheta}_n = q(\widehat{\theta}_n)$ *be an estimator of* $q(\theta)$, *where* $n = 1, 2, \ldots$. *Then the asymptotic mean squared error of* $\widehat{\vartheta}_n$ *is*

$$\text{AMSE}(q(\theta); \widehat{\vartheta}_n) = \frac{E[\{q'(\theta)V\}^2]}{a_n^2},$$

and the asymptotic variance of $\widehat{\vartheta}_n$ *is*

$$\text{Avar}(\widehat{\vartheta}_n) = \frac{\{q'(\theta)\}^2 \text{var}(V)}{a_n^2}.$$

The asymptotic analysis (i.e., with a varying sample size approaching infinity) provides a useful tool to handle problems for which an exact analysis method is unavailable for a given sample size. Often, the asymptotic method requires less stringent mathematical assumptions than the exact approach does, and it has a broader range of applicability. A major drawback of the asymptotic method is the lack of a good sense of what specific value of the sample size is adequate for reasonable inference results, although in principle, the larger the better. Due to this difficulty, in application of asymptotic theory it is a common routine to perform numerical studies, such as simulations, to assess the *finite sample performance* of a method that is theoretically justified using asymptotic properties. Discussion on this can be found in Shao (2003), among others.

1.3 Estimation Methods

In this section, we describe estimation methods which are commonly used to produce estimators with desirable properties from the large sample viewpoint. Typically, these estimators are consistent and have asymptotically normal distributions under suitable regularity conditions.

1.3.1 Likelihood Method

We start with the *maximum likelihood* method, a method that has become a centerpiece of statistical inference since it was advocated by Fisher (1922). To illustrate the idea, we begin with a simple case where Y is a discrete variable and $f(y;\theta)$ is the probability mass function $P(Y = y)$ with parameter θ. If the data generation mechanism were known (i.e., the true value of parameter θ is known), then the probability of obtaining a given sample $y(n)$ is determined by the joint probability mass function

$$f(y(n);\theta) = \prod_{i=1}^{n} f(y_i;\theta).$$

This function, although dependent on the input from both the data and the parameter value, can be stressed as a function of data *alone* with parameter θ fixed, and can be, hence, used to evaluate the probability of generating *any* specific sample of interest.

From the opposite perspective, if a particular sample is given but we do not know which model $f(y;\theta)$ generates such data, we treat $f(y(n);\theta)$ as a function of θ while holding $y(n)$ fixed at the observed sample measurements. In this case, we use an *inductive* approach to find a value of θ so that the probability of obtaining the given sample is the highest. With $y(n)$ fixed at the observed sample values, we maximize the function $f(y(n);\theta)$ with respect to θ where θ varies in the parameter space Θ. For this purpose, we define the *likelihood function* of θ, given the data $y(n)$, to be

$$L(\theta) = \prod_{i=1}^{n} f(y_i;\theta).$$

This function is basically viewed as a function of θ for the fixed $y(n)$, so its dependence on $y(n)$ is often suppressed in the notation $L(\theta)$. This definition extends to the case with a continuous random variable Y, where $f(y_i;\theta)$ represents a probability density function evaluated at measurement y_i for $i = 1, \ldots, n$.

If there is a value of θ which maximizes $L(\theta)$, this value is called a *maximum likelihood estimate* (MLE), usually denoted by $\widehat{\theta} = \widehat{\theta}(y(n))$, or $\widehat{\theta}$ for simplicity. Unlike explicitly expressing the dependence on the sample size of the estimators in §1.2.3, in the rest of the book, we suppress the dependence on n in the notation of estimators. A maximum likelihood estimate does not necessarily exist for every model parameter nor is necessarily unique (e.g., Problems 1.10 and 1.11). However, in many regular applications, it exists and is unique. In this case, we use "the" to describe such an estimate.

It is known that applying any strictly increasing transformation to the likelihood function does not change its maximizer. Since many distributions we work with come from the exponential family, it is mathematically simpler to work with the log-likelihood than the likelihood itself to find the MLE:

$$\ell(\theta) = \log L(\theta).$$

In situations where $\ell(\theta)$ is differentiable, finding the MLE is frequently proceeded by solving the *likelihood equation*

$$S(\theta; y(n)) = 0, \tag{1.2}$$

where $S(\theta; y(n)) = \partial\ell(\theta)/\partial\theta$, called the vector of *score functions*, or simply the score function (e.g., Young and Smith 2005).

Generally speaking, the solutions to the likelihood equation (1.2) are not necessarily the maximizers of $L(\theta)$; they can be *local* maximizers, local minimizers, global minimizers, or even just stationary points of $L(\theta)$. But under the circumstances where the MLE exists and is unique, solving the likelihood equation gives us the MLE.

The likelihood method is conceptually clear, especially for handling irregular problems, such as multiple solutions that arise from solving equations (e.g., Heyde and Morton 1998) and the boundary issue when the equations have no interior solutions (e.g., Self and Liang 1987). The MLE enjoys the *parameterization invariance* (or *invariance property*): for a one-to-one function $q(\cdot)$, the MLE of $q(\theta)$ is given by $q(\widehat{\theta})$, where $\widehat{\theta}$ is the MLE of θ. The invariance principle is valuable and may be used to choose one inferential procedure over another; it ensures that the conclusions of a statistical analysis do not change with reparameterization of θ.

To study the performance of the MLE, it is useful to position ourselves in the sampling framework. We replace the concrete observations $y(n)$ in $\widehat{\theta} = \widehat{\theta}(y(n))$ with random vector $\mathbb{Y}$ and form a random vector $\widehat{\theta} = \widehat{\theta}(\mathbb{Y})$. We call $\widehat{\theta} = \widehat{\theta}(\mathbb{Y})$ the *maximum likelihood estimator* (MLE) of θ. Without confusion, we use the same symbol $\widehat{\theta}$ to denote both the maximum likelihood *estimator* and the maximum likelihood *estimate*. In the same manner, we view the likelihood function and score functions as random variables by replacing the concrete observations $y(n)$ with random vector $\mathbb{Y}$, and write

$$L(\theta; \mathbb{Y}) = \prod_{i=1}^{n} f(Y_i; \theta) \text{ and } S(\theta; \mathbb{Y}) = \frac{\partial \log L(\theta; \mathbb{Y})}{\partial \theta},$$

where the definition of the derivatives of a function with respect to a vector is given in Appendix A.1.

With regular problems where the order of differentiation with respect to θ and integration over the sample space can be exchanged, we obtain that the mean of the score functions is zero:

$$E\{S(\theta; \mathbb{Y})\} = 0,$$

and the covariance matrix of $S(\theta; \mathbb{Y})$ is

$$\text{var}\{S(\theta; \mathbb{Y})\} = E\left\{ - \frac{\partial^2 \ell(\theta; \mathbb{Y})}{\partial \theta \partial \theta^{\mathrm{T}}} \right\}, \tag{1.3}$$

where the expectations are evaluated under the distribution of $\mathbb{Y}$. Matrix (1.3), defined in Appendix A.1, is called the *expected* (or *Fisher*) *information matrix* and is denoted by $J(\theta)$.

For an i.i.d. sequence of random variables $\{Y_1, \ldots, Y_n\}$, it is often convenient to use entries for a *single* random variable to express the corresponding entries for the *entire* sequence of random variables. Let $\ell_i(\theta; y_i) = \log f(y_i; \theta)$. Then based on a single random variable Y_i, we define

$$S_i(\theta; y_i) = \frac{\partial \ell_i(\theta; y_i)}{\partial \theta} \text{ and } J_1(\theta) = E\left\{ -\frac{\partial S_i(\theta; Y_i)}{\partial \theta^{\mathrm{T}}} \right\},$$

where the expectation is evaluated with respect to the distribution of Y_i. Then the score function and the expected information matrix based on the sequence of random variables are

$$S(\theta; y(n)) = \sum_{i=1}^{n} S_i(\theta; y_i) \text{ and } J(\theta) = nJ_1(\theta),$$

respectively.

Although the MLE does not necessarily exist nor is unique for every parametric model, the maximum likelihood method has proven useful for many settings due to its nice asymptotic properties, given in the following theorem.

Theorem 1.5. *Under regularity conditions, the following results hold for the MLE* $\widehat{\theta}$*:*

(a) $\widehat{\theta} \xrightarrow{p} \theta$ *as* $n \to \infty$*;*

(b) $\sqrt{n}(\widehat{\theta} - \theta) \xrightarrow{d} N(0, J_1^{-1}(\theta))$ *as* $n \to \infty$*.*

This theorem has important implications. Regardless of any specific model form which derives the MLE $\widehat{\theta}$, a normal distribution can serve, in the asymptotic sense, as a basis for statistical inference, such as constructing confidence intervals or hypothesis testing. The precision of this procedure, however, depends on the size of the sample as well as the underlying distribution which generates the data. The theorem says that the MLE $\widehat{\theta}$ is a consistent estimator for parameter θ and is approximately normally distributed with mean θ and covariance matrix $[nJ_1(\theta)]^{-1}$. The asymptotic covariance matrix $[nJ_1(\theta)]^{-1}$ is identical to the *Cramér–Rao Lower Bound* (see Problem 1.13), a quantity which is not necessarily attained by any estimator with a given sample size. The MLE is thereby taken to be *asymptotically efficient* (e.g., Young and Smith 2005; van der Vaart 1998, Ch. 8).

The proof of Theorem 1.5 is available in many references; for instance, see Lehmann and Casella (1998, §6.3) and Serfling (1980, §4.2.2). With the establishment of Theorem 1.5 (a), a key idea of showing Theorem 1.5 (b) is to apply the Taylor series expansion to the score function around the MLE to spell out the difference $\widehat{\theta} - \theta$ and then scale this difference with the factor $\sqrt{n}$; the result of Theorem 1.5 (b) can then be derived using the Weak Law of Large Numbers and the Central Limit Theorem in combination with suitable regularity conditions. Basically, with regularity conditions, the consistency of the MLE is ensured by the zero mean of the score function:

$$E\left\{\frac{\partial \ell_i(\theta; Y_i)}{\partial \theta}\right\} = 0, \tag{1.4}$$

and the asymptotic covariance matrix of the MLE comes as a result of the property

$$E\left\{-\frac{\partial^2 \ell_i(\theta; Y_i)}{\partial \theta\, \partial \theta^{\mathrm{T}}}\right\} = E\left\{\frac{\partial \ell_i(\theta; Y_i)}{\partial \theta} \cdot \frac{\partial \ell_i(\theta; Y_i)}{\partial \theta^{\mathrm{T}}}\right\}. \tag{1.5}$$

Regularity conditions required in Theorem 1.5 are not unique. A set of conditions is listed in Lehmann (1999, pp. 499–501). We comment that suitable regularity conditions are often imposed in order to yield good properties, such as consistency and asymptotic normality, for a derived estimator. These conditions usually vary from problem to problem and are often identified as sufficient, but not necessarily the weakest, conditions which lead to the desired asymptotic properties.

In addition to the basic requirement for the model parameter in $f(y;\theta)$ to be identifiable, regularity conditions commonly include the assumption that the support of $f(y;\theta)$ is parameter free. Regularity conditions are often pertinent to the assumptions about both the parameter space and the model structures, and they can compensate for each other. If more stringent conditions are imposed on the parameter space, then the model form may be subject to fewer requirements, and vice versa. For instance, if the parameter space Θ is assumed to be finite, then the existence and consistency of the MLE can hold even if no strict condition, such as smoothness, is imposed on the model form $f(\cdot)$; see, for example, Corollary 3.5 of Lehmann and Casella (1998, p. 445). On the other hand, if the parameter space is not finite but contains an open set in which the true value of θ is an interior point, the existence and consistency of the MLE can be established if certain conditions, such as smoothness, are imposed on probability models; see, for example, Theorem 3.7 of Lehmann and Casella (1998, p. 447). A comprehensive discussion on regularity conditions can be found in Newey and McFadden (1994), Lehmann and Casella (1998, Ch. 6), Shao (2003, §4.4, §4.5) and the references therein. Problem 1.14 illustrates that the MLE may not possess asymptotic normality if the true parameter is not interior to the parameter space.

1.3.2 Estimating Equations

The likelihood method relies on correct specification of the distribution form, which may be difficult in application. Various methods are developed to relax some requirements of the likelihood method. These approaches include *quasi-likelihood* (Wedderburn 1974; McCullagh 1983), *pseudo-likelihood* (Gourieroux, Monfort and Trognon 1984) and *composite likelihood* methods (Lindsay 1988; Lindsay, Yi and Sun 2011; Varin, Reid and Firth 2011). All these methods can be umbrellaed under a broad framework of estimating functions (Godambe 1991).

In this section, we outline some basics of estimating function theory, originating from Godambe (1960) and Durbin (1960). The idea is to find a set of functions that link the parameter θ and the data so that the functions mimic certain properties of the score functions. In particular, the zero mean property (1.4) is critical to be preserved when developing estimating function theory. The following theorem provides the theoretical basis for this.

Suppose that random variable Y has a probability model $f(y;\theta)$ where the dimension of θ is p, and that $U(\theta;y)$ is a $p \times 1$ vector of functions of parameter θ for a given y. Define

$$\Gamma_U(\theta) = E\left\{\frac{\partial U(\theta;Y)}{\partial \theta^{\mathrm{T}}}\right\}, \quad \Sigma_U(\theta) = E\left\{U(\theta;Y)U^{\mathrm{T}}(\theta;Y)\right\}, \tag{1.6}$$

and

$$J_U^{-1}(\theta) = \Gamma_U^{-1}(\theta)\Sigma_U(\theta)\Gamma_U^{-1\mathrm{T}}(\theta),$$

where the expectations are taken with respect to $f(y;\theta)$ and the inverse matrices are assumed to exist.

Theorem 1.6. *Assume that*

$$E\{U(\theta;Y)\} = 0, \tag{1.7}$$

where the expectation is taken with respect to $f(y;\theta)$.

Suppose $\{Y_1,\ldots,Y_n\}$ is a random sample having the same distribution as Y. If

$$\sum_{i=1}^{n} U(\theta;Y_i) = 0 \tag{1.8}$$

has a unique solution, say $\widehat{\theta}$, for θ, then under regularity conditions, the following results hold:

(a) $\widehat{\theta} \xrightarrow{p} \theta$ *as* $n \to \infty$;

(b) $\sqrt{n}(\widehat{\theta} - \theta) \xrightarrow{d} N(0, J_U^{-1}(\theta))$ *as* $n \to \infty$.

We call $U(\theta; y)$ an *estimating function* for θ (or more precisely, a vector of estimating functions when θ is multidimensional), and (1.8) *estimating equations*. Sometimes, the *sum* of the estimating functions in (1.8) is equivalently written as a *sample average*, $n^{-1} \sum_{i=1}^{n} U(\theta; Y_i)$, to indicate its connection with (1.7). When estimating function $U(\theta; y)$ is applied to random sample $\mathbb{Y}$ or sample measurements $y(n)$, the solution to (1.8) is, respectively, called an *estimator* or an *estimate* of θ; without confusion we use the same notation, $\widehat{\theta}$, to denote them.

Theorem 1.6 (a) says that $\widehat{\theta}$ is a consistent estimator of θ, while Theorem 1.6 (b) can be used to perform inferences such as calculating confidence intervals. Condition (1.7), or its approximate version for some settings, is important for ensuring the consistency of the estimator $\widehat{\theta}$, and is often used as a prerequisite for finding useful estimating functions (e.g., Liang 1987). If estimating function $U(\theta; y)$ satisfies

$$E\{U(\theta; Y)\} = 0 \text{ for all } \theta \in \Theta,$$

where the expectation is evaluated with respect to $f(y; \theta)$, then $U(\theta; y)$ is called *unbiased*. The role of unbiasedness of estimating functions was discussed by Yanagimoto and Yamamoto (1991) who related it to conditional likelihood inference for the exponential family. More discussion on estimating functions can be found in Heyde (1997) and Shao (2003, §5.4).

The asymptotic covariance matrix $J_U^{-1}(\theta)$ is called the *sandwich covariance matrix*, and matrix $J_U(\theta)$ is called the *Godambe information matrix* of estimating function $U(\theta; y)$. The asymptotic covariance matrix may be used to compare the performance of different estimating functions. In particular, for two unbiased estimating functions $U(\theta; y)$ and $U^*(\theta; y)$, if $J_{U^*}^{-1}(\theta) - J_U^{-1}(\theta)$ is nonnegative definite for *all* $\theta \in \Theta$, then $U(\theta; y)$ is said to be *more efficient* than $U^*(\theta; y)$, or more precisely, *at least as efficient as* $U^*(\theta; y)$ (Heyde 1997, p. 12).

A rigorous proof of Theorem 1.6 and discussion on required regularity conditions were presented in Chapter 12 of Heyde (1997). The following theorem provides the connection between the likelihood method and general estimating function theory (Godambe 1960; Bhapkar 1972).

Theorem 1.7. *Let $S(\theta; y) = \partial \log f(y; \theta)/\partial\theta$. Under regularity conditions, the following results hold:*

(a) Score function $S(\theta; y)$ is unbiased;

(b) $J_S(\theta) = J_1(\theta)$. That is, the Godambe information is identical to the Fisher information for the score function;

(c) For any unbiased estimating function $U(\theta; y)$, $J_U^{-1}(\theta) - J_S^{-1}(\theta)$ is nonnegative definite for all $\theta \in \Theta$. That is, the score function is the most efficient.

This theorem says that the score functions are optimal among regular unbiased estimating functions. In application, however, it is often impossible or insensible to consider the class of *all* regular unbiased estimating functions. Commonly, we confine our attention to a class of estimating functions which does not include the score function; optimal estimating functions are then searched within this class, which turn out to be closely related to the score function (see Problem 1.16). A strategy of formulating a useful class is to identify elementary estimating functions which are unbiased and readily constructed, and then combine them linearly. The following theorem provides the detail on this scheme and the formulation of optimal estimating functions (Morton 1981).

Theorem 1.8. *Suppose there is a class of elementary unbiased estimating functions for* θ, $\{U_j(\theta; y) : j = 1, \ldots, d\}$, *where* $U_j(\theta; y)$ *is a* $p \times 1$ *vector of estimating functions,* p *is the dimension of* θ, *and* d *is a positive integer. Define* $U(\theta; y) = (U_1^{\mathrm{T}}(\theta; y) \ldots U_d^{\mathrm{T}}(\theta; y))^{\mathrm{T}}$. *Let*

$$\mathcal{L} = \{C(\theta)U(\theta; y) : C(\theta) \text{ is a } p \times pd \text{ matrix consisting of constants that may depend on } \theta \text{ but not on variable } y\}$$

be the collection of linear combinations of $\{U_1(\theta; y), \ldots, U_d(\theta; y)\}$. *Let* $\Gamma_U(\theta)$ *and* $\Sigma_U(\theta)$ *be defined as in (1.6). If* $\Sigma_U(\theta)$ *is nonsingular, define*

$$U^*(\theta; y) = \Gamma_U^{\mathrm{T}}(\theta)\Sigma_U^{-1}(\theta)U(\theta; y).$$

Then $U^*(\theta; y)$ *is an optimal estimating function for* θ *in* $\mathcal{L}$, *i.e.,* $U^*(\theta; y)$ *is more efficient than any estimating function in* $\mathcal{L}$.

The following example is an application of Theorem 1.8 and presents two estimation methods that are widely used in practice.

Example 1.9. Suppose Y is a univariate random variable with mean $\mu(\theta) = E(Y)$ and variance $v(\theta) = \mathrm{var}(Y)$, where θ is the associated parameter. Then, by Theorem 1.8, setting $d = 1$ and $U(\theta; y) = y - \mu(\theta)$ leads to an estimating function:

$$U^*(\theta; y) = \left(\frac{\partial \mu(\theta)}{\partial \theta}\right) \frac{y - \mu(\theta)}{v(\theta)}.$$

We apply this result to a sequence of univariate random variable $\{Y_i : i = 1, \ldots, n\}$, each Y_i having mean $\mu_i(\theta) = E(Y_i)$ and variance $v_i(\theta) = \mathrm{var}(Y_i)$. For each observation, y_i, of Y_i, we define

$$U^*(\theta; y_i) = \left(\frac{\partial \mu_i}{\partial \theta}\right) \frac{y_i - \mu_i(\theta)}{v_i(\theta)}.$$

Then estimating equations

$$\sum_{i=1}^{n} U^*(\theta; y_i) = 0$$

may be used to estimate θ. This approach is called a *quasi-likelihood method* (Shao 2003, p. 361).

If Y_i is a random vector with $Y_i = (Y_{i1}, \ldots, Y_{im})^{\mathrm{T}}$ where m is a positive integer, then the preceding formulation is generalized as follows. Let $\mu_i(\theta) = E(Y_i)$ and $V_i(\theta) = \mathrm{var}(Y_i)$ be the mean vector and covariance matrix of Y_i, respectively. Then estimation of θ can proceed with solving

$$\sum_{i=1}^{n} \left(\frac{\partial \mu_i^{\mathrm{T}}(\theta)}{\partial \theta} \right) V_i^{-1}(\theta) \{y_i - \mu_i(\theta)\} = 0 \tag{1.9}$$

for θ, where $\{y_1, \ldots, y_n\}$ are sample measurements and the inverse matrices are assumed to exist. Such equations are called *generalized estimating equations* (GEE) (Liang and Zeger 1986).

We conclude this subsection with a comment on roots of estimating functions. The existence and uniqueness of solutions to estimating equations are not automatic without conditions. A well-defined estimating function may have multiple roots. When multiple roots occur for likelihood score functions, evaluation of the likelihood function at those multiple roots allows us to identify the maximum likelihood estimator. However, when multiple roots arise from solving estimating equations, it is not obvious how to choose a suitable estimator from those roots. In such a situation, one may follow the criteria by Heyde and Morton (1998) to discriminate a consistent estimator from multiple roots of estimating functions. More discussion on this issue can be found in Hanfelt and Liang (1995) and (Heyde 1997, §13.2, §13.3).

1.3.3 Generalized Method of Moments

Estimating function theory generalizes the likelihood method and provides a useful and flexible estimation method that covers a wide class of applications. Unbiasedness (of estimating functions) is frequently imposed when using this method (e.g. Liang 1987). As discussed in §1.3.2 for the quasi-likelihood or GEE methods, unbiased estimating functions may be constructed based on using the assumed mean and variance structures for the outcome variables. More generally, higher order moments (if existing) may be invoked to meet the unbiasedness requirement for constructing useful estimating functions. This route is related to the *method of moments* (MM), a method that is intuitive and easy to implement for many problems.

The method of moments is basically to equate the *sample* moments to the corresponding *population* moments and then solve them for the associated parameters. To be specific, suppose random variable Y has the probability density or mass function $f(y; \theta)$ where θ is the parameter vector of dimension p. Suppose that the population moment $\mu_k = E(Y^k)$ exists (or $E(|Y^k|) < \infty$) for $k = 1, \ldots, p$, and that the μ_k are functions of parameter θ, so we write $\mu_k = g_k(\theta)$ for some functions $g_k(\cdot)$ defined on $\mathbb{R}^p$.

Let $\mathbb{Y} = \{Y_1, \ldots, Y_n\}$ be a random sample drawn from $f(y; \theta)$. Define

$$\widehat{\mu}_k = \frac{1}{n} \sum_{i=1}^{n} Y_i^k$$

to be the kth *sample moment*, which is an unbiased estimator of the *population moment* μ_k, i.e., $E(\widehat{\mu}_k) = \mu_k$ for $k = 1, \ldots, p$, where the expectation is evaluated with respect to the joint distribution of $\mathbb{Y}$. Then we use the sample moments to estimate the population moments and obtain estimating equations for θ, given by

$$\frac{1}{n}\sum_{i=1}^{n} Y_i^k = g_k(\theta) \text{ for } k = 1, \ldots, p. \tag{1.10}$$

Under suitable conditions, solving these equations leads to a *moment estimator*, $\widehat{\theta}$, of θ.

Example 1.10. Suppose random variable Y has the $N(\mu, \sigma^2)$ distribution with mean μ and variance σ^2. Let $\mathbb{Y} = \{Y_1, \ldots, Y_n\}$ be a random sample chosen from $N(\mu, \sigma^2)$. Then the first two moments $\mu_1 = E(Y)$ and $\mu_2 = E(Y^2)$ of Y are given by

$$\mu_1 = \mu;$$
$$\mu_2 = \sigma^2 + \mu^2.$$

Equating the first two population and sample moments gives

$$\frac{1}{n}\sum_{i=1}^{n} Y_i = \mu;$$
$$\frac{1}{n}\sum_{i=1}^{n} Y_i^2 = \sigma^2 + \mu^2;$$

leading to the moment estimator of $\theta = (\mu, \sigma^2)^{\mathrm{T}}$:

$$\widehat{\mu} = \overline{Y}$$

and

$$\widehat{\sigma}^2 = \frac{1}{n}\sum_{i=1}^{n} Y_i^2 - \overline{Y}^2 = \frac{1}{n}\sum_{i=1}^{n}(Y_i - \overline{Y})^2,$$

where $\overline{Y} = n^{-1}\sum_{i=1}^{n} Y_i$. This estimator is identical to the MLE of θ under the normality assumption for random variable Y, but its derivation does not require the normality assumption of Y.

The method of moments is easy to implement but has a weakness. The choice of order of moments is not unique, which generates somewhat ambiguity. In the preceding example, any higher moments depend on both mean μ and variance σ^2, and the method of moments may be equally applied to any two moments of the normal distribution, thus leading to different estimators of θ. A question then arises: which set of moments should be used? Such a question always comes up in situations where a number of moments are available but there are no apparent reasons to choose one set of moments over others. To address this issue, it is convenient to position us within a broader framework and develop the so-called *generalized method of moments.*

The generalized method of moments was first introduced into the econometrics literature by Hansen (1982). This method may be regarded as a general estimation principle which derives estimators from the *(population) moment conditions*. A moment condition is broadly defined in terms of a zero expectation statement for functions of the data and parameters. Specifically, suppose $U(\theta; y)$ is a $q \times 1$ vector of functions (simply said a function) satisfying a moment condition:

$$E\{U(\theta_0; Y)\} = 0,$$

where q is a positive integer, and θ_0 is the true value of θ. Then under suitable conditions for function $U(\theta; y)$, we can produce sensible estimators by applying function $U(\theta; y)$ to sample measurements.

To ensure function $U(\theta; y)$ to be useful, it is important that model parameter θ must be identified from using such a function. If function $U(\theta; y)$ satisfies

$$E\{U(\theta; Y)\} = 0 \text{ if and only if } \theta = \theta_0,$$

then θ is identified by using function $U(\theta; y)$. Because it is difficult to find necessary and sufficient conditions for checking the identification property for any function, one has to examine the suitability of estimating functions case by case.

As a quick start, checking the dimensionality may give us an immediate indication of the feasibility of function $U(\theta; y)$. If q is smaller than p, then function $U(\theta; y)$ cannot yield a consistent estimator of θ since θ is not identifiable from $U(\theta; y)$. When q equals p, then solving the equation based on the sample moment

$$\frac{1}{n}\sum_{i=1}^{n} U(\theta; Y_i) = 0 \tag{1.11}$$

may give us a sensible estimator of θ, provided suitable regularity conditions; such an estimator is broadly called the *method of moments* estimator, extending the discussion on (1.10).

In situations with $q > p$, trying to solve (1.11) may be fruitless because the equation number is bigger than the parameter dimension; solutions may not even exist. In this case, instead of attempting to find a parameter value to make the sample moment $n^{-1}\sum_{i=1}^{n} U(\theta; Y_i)$ *equal* zero, we look for the parameter value that would *minimize* a certain type of distance of the sample moment from its mean, zero. A sensible way of expressing such a distance defines a quadratic measure

$$Q_n(\theta) = \left\{\frac{1}{n}\sum_{i=1}^{n} U(\theta; Y_i)\right\}^{\mathrm{T}} W_n \left\{\frac{1}{n}\sum_{i=1}^{n} U(\theta; Y_i)\right\},$$

where W_n is a $q \times q$ weight matrix that is symmetric and nonnegative definite, and may depend on size n as well as the random sample $\mathbb{Y}$. Then the minimizer of $Q_n(\theta)$ with respect to θ, given the data, is called the *generalized method of moments* (GMM) estimator:

$$\widehat{\theta} = \text{argmin}_{\theta \in \Theta} Q_n(\theta).$$

GMM estimators are useful in conducting inferences; their asymptotic properties are summarized in the following theorem.

Theorem 1.11. *With the preceding setup, assume that* $W_n \xrightarrow{p} W$ *as* $n \to \infty$, *where* W *is a nonnegative definite matrix. Let*

$$G = E\left\{ \left. \frac{\partial U^{\mathrm{T}}(\theta; Y)}{\partial \theta} \right|_{\theta=\theta_0} \right\} WE \left\{ \left. \frac{\partial U(\theta; Y)}{\partial \theta^{\mathrm{T}}} \right|_{\theta=\theta_0} \right\},$$

and

$$H = E\left\{ \left. \frac{\partial U^{\mathrm{T}}(\theta; Y)}{\partial \theta} \right|_{\theta=\theta_0} \right\} WE\left\{U(\theta_0; Y)U^{\mathrm{T}}(\theta_0; Y)\right\} WE \left\{ \left. \frac{\partial U(\theta; Y)}{\partial \theta^{\mathrm{T}}} \right|_{\theta=\theta_0} \right\}.$$

Then under regularity conditions, the following results hold for the GMM estimator $\widehat{\theta}$:

(a) $\widehat{\theta} \xrightarrow{p} \theta_0$ *as* $n \to \infty$;

(b) $\sqrt{n}(\widehat{\theta} - \theta_0) \xrightarrow{d} N(0, G^{-1}HG^{-1\mathrm{T}})$ *as* $n \to \infty$.

Regularity conditions required by Theorem 1.11, the existence and the uniqueness of the GMM estimator are discussed by Newey and McFadden (1994) in detail. When using the GMM, one needs to specify a proper weight matrix W_n. Ideally, W_n should be set as a matrix so that the resulting GMM estimator is the most efficient. When W is the inverse matrix of the covariance matrix $E\{U(\theta_0; Y)U^{\mathrm{T}}(\theta_0; Y)\}$, we have $H = G$ and that the GMM estimator with the corresponding asymptotic covariance matrix is asymptotically most efficient (Hansen 1982). As the evaluation of the covariance matrix $E\{U(\theta_0; Y)U^{\mathrm{T}}(\theta_0; Y)\}$ is not possible in many circumstances, approximate algorithms are often introduced in actual implementation. For example, a two-stage procedure is used in practice. At the first step, set W_n to be a unit matrix and obtain an estimate $\widetilde{\theta}$ by minimizing $Q_n(\theta)$; at the second step, set W_n to be the empirical counterpart $n^{-1} \sum_{i=1}^{n} U(\widetilde{\theta}; y_i)U^{\mathrm{T}}(\widetilde{\theta}; y_i)$, and then find the estimate $\widehat{\theta}$ that minimizes $Q_n(\theta)$.

We conclude this subsection with brief comments on the foregoing estimation methods. The GMM may be viewed as a generalization of the likelihood method in that the score functions, derived from the likelihood functions, satisfy the moment condition required by the GMM. The GMM also generalizes the estimating equations method as well as the MM. The GMM differs from the estimating equations approach in that the dimension of function

$U(\theta; y)$ may be equal or larger than that of parameter θ, whereas the estimating equations approach requires the equality for the dimension of $U(\theta; y)$ and of parameter θ. The GMM extends the MM in that function $U(\theta; y)$ does not have to be constructed from the difference between the population and sample moments, and the dimension of $U(\theta; y)$ does not have to equal the dimension of the parameter either.

1.3.4 Profiling Method

The foregoing estimation methods are directed to the entire parameter vector where all components are of the same interest and, thus, treated equally. In application, however, this is not always the case. To reflect this, we write $\theta = (\alpha^{\mathrm{T}}, \beta^{\mathrm{T}})^{\mathrm{T}}$, where β denotes the subvector of parameters at which our inference aims, and α denotes the subvector of those parameters which are not of interest but necessary to be coupled with β in order to make the model complete or meaningful. Often, components of α are called *nuisance* parameters. In this subsection, we discuss estimation procedures which handle parameters β and α differently.

Profile Likelihood

As discussed in §1.3.1, maximizing the likelihood function $L(\theta)$ with respect to θ gives estimates of both β and α. Sometimes, it is difficult to do so simultaneously with respect to both β and α. An alternative strategy is to break the one-step maximization into two steps, each relative to one type of parameters of a smaller dimension. To show the idea clearly, we now refer $L(\theta)$ as to $L(\alpha, \beta)$. At the first step, we fix a value for β and maximize $L(\alpha, \beta)$ with respect to α, yielding an estimate $\widehat{\alpha}_\beta$ for parameter α; at the second step, we fix α as $\widehat{\alpha}_\beta$ and then maximize $L(\widehat{\alpha}_\beta, \beta)$ with respect to β, producing an estimate of β.

Specifically, for any given β, let $\Omega_\beta = \{\alpha : (\alpha^{\mathrm{T}}, \beta^{\mathrm{T}})^{\mathrm{T}} \in \Theta\}$ be the collection of all values of α so that $\theta = (\alpha^{\mathrm{T}}, \beta^{\mathrm{T}})^{\mathrm{T}}$ falls in the parameter space Θ. For a fixed value of β, maximizing $L(\alpha, \beta)$ with respect to α over Ω_β gives an estimate of α. The resulting estimator, denoted by $\widehat{\alpha}_\beta$, is called a *restricted maximum likelihood estimator* (restricted MLE) of α. Define

$$L_{\mathrm{P}}(\beta) = \sup_{\alpha \in \Omega_\beta} L(\alpha, \beta),$$

or identically,

$$L_{\mathrm{P}}(\beta) = L(\widehat{\alpha}_\beta, \beta),$$

to be the *profile likelihood* function of β. Then maximizing the profile likelihood $L_{\mathrm{P}}(\beta)$ with respect to β gives an estimate of β. The resulting estimator, denoted by $\widehat{\beta}_{\mathrm{P}}$, is called the *profile likelihood estimator* of β.

The profile likelihood is not a genuine likelihood because it does not necessarily represent the probability density or mass function for a random variable. However, when α is treated as a nuisance, using the profile likelihood to infer β seems natural and tempting. The profile likelihood $L_P(\beta)$ has some properties similar to those of the likelihood function. For example, the maximum profile likelihood estimator $\widehat{\beta}_P$ of β equals $\widehat{\beta}$, the component of the MLE $\widehat{\theta} = (\widehat{\alpha}^T, \widehat{\beta}^T)^T$ corresponding to parameter β. The log profile likelihood ratio statistic $2\{\ell_P(\widehat{\beta}) - \ell_P(\beta_T)\}$ equals the log-likelihood ratio statistic for the hypothesis $H_o : \beta = \beta_T$, where β_T is a given value to be tested. Namely,

$$2\{\ell_P(\widehat{\beta}) - \ell_P(\beta_T)\} = 2\{\ell(\widehat{\alpha}, \widehat{\beta}) - \ell(\widehat{\alpha}_{\beta_T}, \beta_T)\}.$$

While the profile likelihood function is sometimes used as if it were a true likelihood (Young and Smith 2005, p. 135), it may give misleading inference for parameter β in certain situations, especially when the dimension of α is of the same magnitude as the sample size. A profile likelihood estimator may not be consistent, as illustrated in the following example.

Example 1.12. Suppose that $Y_1, \ldots, Y_n$ are independent, and that for $i = 1, \ldots, n$, $Y_i = (Y_{i1}, \ldots, Y_{im})^T$ where m is a given positive integer, and the Y_{ij} are independent random variables, each following the normal distribution $N(\alpha_i, \beta)$ with $\beta > 0$ and $-\infty < \alpha_i < \infty$.

Let $\alpha = (\alpha_1, \ldots, \alpha_n)^T$ and $\theta = (\alpha^T, \beta^T)^T$. The log-likelihood of θ is then given by $\ell(\theta) = \sum_{i,j} \ell_{ij}(\theta)$ where with a constant omitted,

$$\ell_{ij}(\theta) = -\frac{1}{2}\log\beta - \frac{(Y_{ij} - \alpha_i)^2}{2\beta}.$$

Calculation shows that the restricted MLE of α_i is $\widehat{\alpha}_{i\beta} = \overline{Y}_{i+}$, and thus, the log profile likelihood for β is

$$\ell_P(\beta) = \sum_{i,j}\left\{-\frac{1}{2}\log\beta - \frac{(Y_{ij} - \overline{Y}_{i+})^2}{2\beta}\right\},$$

where $\overline{Y}_{i+} = m^{-1}\sum_j Y_{ij}$. Maximizing $\ell_P(\beta)$ with respect to β gives the profile likelihood estimator of β:

$$\widehat{\beta}_P = \frac{1}{nm}\sum_{i,j}(Y_{ij} - \overline{Y}_{i+})^2.$$

This estimator converges in probability to $(m-1)\beta/m$ as $n \to \infty$, suggesting that $\widehat{\beta}_P$ is not a consistent estimator for β.

This is the well-known Neyman–Scott problem (Neyman and Scott 1948) which concerns the maximum likelihood estimator for the situation where only a parameter subvector is of interest while the dimension of nuisance parameters has the same magnitude as the sample size. The inconsistency of $\widehat{\beta}_P$ is pertinent to the inconsistency of the estimators of nuisance parameters α_i.

In addition, inconsistency of $\widehat{\beta}_{\mathrm{P}}$ may be explained by the lack of unbiasedness of the profile likelihood score function:

$$S_{\mathrm{P}}(\beta; \mathbb{Y}) = \frac{\partial \ell_{\mathrm{P}}(\beta)}{\partial \beta} = \sum_{i,j} \left\{ -\frac{1}{2\beta} + \frac{(Y_{ij} - \overline{Y}_{i+})^2}{2\beta^2} \right\},$$

where $\mathbb{Y} = \{Y_1, \ldots, Y_n\}$. In fact, the expectation of $S_{\mathrm{P}}(\beta; \mathbb{Y})$ is $-n/(2\beta)$.

A direct way of modifying the profile likelihood score functions is to work with the difference

$$U(\beta; \mathbb{Y}) = S_{\mathrm{P}}(\beta; \mathbb{Y}) - E\{S_{\mathrm{P}}(\beta; \mathbb{Y})\},$$

which is unbiased, where the expectation is evaluated with respect to the distribution of $\mathbb{Y}$. Thus, under regularity conditions, solving $U(\beta; \mathbb{Y}) = 0$ for β gives a consistent estimator of β. For Example 1.12, this approach gives a consistent estimator

$$\widehat{\beta} = \frac{1}{n(m-1)} \sum_{i,j} (Y_{ij} - \overline{Y}_{i+})^2.$$

In the literature, various modifications to profile likelihood functions have been proposed. For instance, Cox and Reid (1987) suggested a modified profile likelihood function for settings where the nuisance parameter α is orthogonal to β in the sense that the expectation of the mixed second partial derivatives of the log-likelihood with respect to α and β is zero:

$$E\left\{ \frac{\partial^2 \log f(Y_i; \theta)}{\partial \alpha_j \partial \beta_k} \right\} = 0$$

for any elements α_j of α and β_k of β. Other modifications were discussed by Barndorff-Nielsen (1983, 1986), Liang (1987), and McCullagh and Tibshirani (1990), among others.

In the presence of nuisance parameters, inference about the parameters of interest may also be carried out using other strategies, including methods based on conditional or marginal likelihoods. Succinct discussion on this can be found in Kalbfleisch and Sprott (1970), McCullagh and Nelder (1989, §7.2), and Ferguson, Reid and Cox (1991).

Joint Estimation

In many settings, the likelihood function for parameter $\theta = (\alpha^{\mathrm{T}}, \beta^{\mathrm{T}})^{\mathrm{T}}$ is not available, but suitable estimating functions may be constructed for estimating θ, where θ is of a finite dimension. Suppose $U_\alpha(\theta; y)$ and $U_\beta(\theta; y)$ are two *unbiased* estimating functions, where $U_\alpha(\theta; y)$ is used to estimate α if β were known, and $U_\beta(\theta; y)$ is used to estimate β if the value of α were given. Define

$$U(\theta; y) = \{U_\alpha^{\mathrm{T}}(\theta; y), U_\beta^{\mathrm{T}}(\theta; y)\}^{\mathrm{T}}.$$

As discussed in §1.3.2, for given sample measurements $y(n) = \{y_1, \ldots, y_n\}$, solving

$$\frac{1}{n}\sum_{i=1}^{n} U(\theta; y_i) = 0 \tag{1.12}$$

for θ yields an estimate of θ.

Let $\widehat{\theta} = (\widehat{\alpha}^{\mathrm{T}}, \widehat{\beta}^{\mathrm{T}})^{\mathrm{T}}$ denote the resultant estimator of θ. Under regularity conditions (e.g., those of Theorem 3.4 of Newey and McFadden 1994) and the assumption of a unique solution for (1.12), $\widehat{\theta}$ is consistent, and its asymptotic distribution is derived as follows.

For a given random sample $\mathbb{Y} = \{Y_1, \ldots, Y_n\}$, we expand $n^{-1}\sum_{i=1}^{n} U(\widehat{\theta}; Y_i)$ around θ using the Taylor series expansion:

$$\frac{1}{n}\sum_{i=1}^{n} U(\widehat{\theta}; Y_i) = \frac{1}{n}\sum_{i=1}^{n} U(\theta; Y_i) + \frac{1}{n}\left\{\sum_{i=1}^{n} \frac{\partial U(\theta; Y_i)}{\partial \theta^{\mathrm{T}}}\right\}(\widehat{\theta} - \theta) + o_p(1).$$

By definition of $\widehat{\theta}$ and the identity

$$\frac{1}{n}\sum_{i=1}^{n} \frac{\partial U(\theta; Y_i)}{\partial \theta^{\mathrm{T}}} = E\left\{\frac{\partial U(\theta; Y)}{\partial \theta^{\mathrm{T}}}\right\} + o_p(1),$$

where Y is a random variable having the same distribution as Y_i, we obtain

$$\sqrt{n}(\widehat{\theta} - \theta) = -\left\{E\left[\frac{\partial U(\theta; Y)}{\partial \theta^{\mathrm{T}}}\right]\right\}^{-1} \frac{1}{\sqrt{n}}\sum_{i=1}^{n} U(\theta; Y_i) + o_p(1). \tag{1.13}$$

Applying the Central Limit Theorem to the right-hand side of (1.13) establishes the asymptotic distribution of $\sqrt{n}(\widehat{\theta} - \theta)$, as stated in Theorem 1.6 (b).

In circumstances where β is of interest while α is a nuisance, it is desirable to *explicitly* express the asymptotic distribution of the estimator $\widehat{\beta}$ which is immediate by calculating the product of the corresponding block matrices. Let

$$A_{\alpha\alpha} = \left(E\left\{\frac{\partial U_\alpha(\theta; Y)}{\partial \alpha^{\mathrm{T}}}\right\} - E\left\{\frac{\partial U_\alpha(\theta; Y)}{\partial \beta^{\mathrm{T}}}\right\}\left[E\left\{\frac{\partial U_\beta(\theta; Y)}{\partial \beta^{\mathrm{T}}}\right\}\right]^{-1} E\left\{\frac{\partial U_\beta(\theta; Y)}{\partial \alpha^{\mathrm{T}}}\right\}\right)^{-1},$$

$$A_{\beta\alpha} = -E\left\{\frac{\partial U_\beta(\theta; Y)}{\partial \beta^{\mathrm{T}}}\right\}^{-1} E\left\{\frac{\partial U_\beta(\theta; Y)}{\partial \alpha^{\mathrm{T}}}\right\} A_{\alpha\alpha},$$

$$A_{\beta\beta} = \left(E\left\{\frac{\partial U_\beta(\theta; Y)}{\partial \beta^{\mathrm{T}}}\right\} - E\left\{\frac{\partial U_\beta(\theta; Y)}{\partial \alpha^{\mathrm{T}}}\right\}\left[E\left\{\frac{\partial U_\alpha(\theta; Y)}{\partial \alpha^{\mathrm{T}}}\right\}\right]^{-1} E\left\{\frac{\partial U_\alpha(\theta; Y)}{\partial \beta^{\mathrm{T}}}\right\}\right)^{-1},$$

and

$$G(y; \theta) = A_{\beta\beta} U_\beta(\theta; y) + A_{\beta\alpha} U_\alpha(\theta; y).$$

Then under regularity conditions,

$$\sqrt{n}(\widehat{\beta} - \beta) \xrightarrow{d} N(0, \Sigma_G) \text{ as } n \to \infty, \tag{1.14}$$

where $\Sigma_G = E\{G(Y;\theta)G^{\mathrm{T}}(Y;\theta)\}$.

Profiling Estimating Equations/Two-Stage Estimation

Simultaneously estimating β and α by solving (1.12) may be computationally intensive sometimes. An alternative is to divide the estimation procedure into two stages. At the first stage, we fix β at a given value and then calculate an estimate of α by solving the equation

$$\frac{1}{n}\sum_{i=1}^{n} U_\alpha(\alpha, \beta; y_i) = 0$$

for α using the Newton–Raphson algorithm. At the second stage, we solve

$$\frac{1}{n}\sum_{i=1}^{n} U_\beta(\widehat{\alpha}_\beta, \beta; y_i) = 0$$

for β, where $\widehat{\alpha}_\beta$ is the estimate of α obtained at the first stage. Keep iterating these steps until convergence of the estimates. We call the resulting estimator of β the *two-stage* or the *profile* estimator of β, and $U_\beta(\widehat{\alpha}_\beta, \beta; y)$ the *profile estimating function* for β.

The two-stage estimation algorithm has been widely used, especially when $U_\alpha(\theta; y)$ is free of β and dependent on α only. Specifically, suppose $U_\alpha(\alpha; y)$ is an unbiased estimating function of α, and $U_\beta(\alpha, \beta; y)$ is an unbiased estimating function of β if α were known. With given sample measurements $y(n) = \{y_1, \ldots, y_n\}$, at the first stage, we solve

$$\frac{1}{n}\sum_{i=1}^{n} U_\alpha(\alpha; y_i) = 0$$

for α, and obtain an estimate of α, say $\widehat{\alpha}$. At the second stage, we solve

$$\frac{1}{n}\sum_{i=1}^{n} U_\beta(\widehat{\alpha}, \beta; y_i) = 0$$

for β.

Let $\widehat{\beta}$ denote the resulting estimator of β. This two-stage estimator $\widehat{\beta}$ is identical to the estimator of β obtained from joint estimation by solving (1.12) for θ. The asymptotic distribution of $\widehat{\beta}$, given by (1.14), becomes

$$\sqrt{n}(\widehat{\beta} - \beta) \xrightarrow{d} N(0, \Gamma^{-1}\Sigma\Gamma^{-1\mathrm{T}}) \text{ as } n \to \infty, \tag{1.15}$$

where

$$\Gamma = E\left\{\frac{\partial U_\beta(\theta; Y)}{\partial \beta^{\mathrm{T}}}\right\}, \ \Sigma = E\{Q(\theta; Y)Q^{\mathrm{T}}(\theta; Y)\},$$

and

$$Q(\theta; y) = U_\beta(\theta; y) - E\left\{\frac{\partial U_\beta(\theta; Y)}{\partial \alpha^{\mathrm{T}}}\right\}\left[E\left\{\frac{\partial U_\alpha(\alpha; Y)}{\partial \alpha^{\mathrm{T}}}\right\}\right]^{-1} U_\alpha(\alpha; y).$$

Inference about β can be conducted by using the asymptotic distribution (1.15) with Γ and Σ replaced by their empirical estimates, respectively, given by

$$\widehat{\Gamma} = \frac{1}{n}\sum_{i=1}^{n} \left.\frac{\partial U_\beta(\theta; y_i)}{\partial \beta^{\mathrm{T}}}\right|_{\theta=\widehat{\theta}} \quad \text{and } \widehat{\Sigma} = \frac{1}{n}\sum_{i=1}^{n} \widehat{Q}(\widehat{\theta}; y_i)\widehat{Q}^{\mathrm{T}}(\widehat{\theta}; y_i),$$

where $\widehat{\theta} = (\widehat{\theta}^{\mathrm{T}}, \widehat{\beta}^{\mathrm{T}})^{\mathrm{T}}$ and

$$\widehat{Q}(\widehat{\theta}; y) = U_\beta(\widehat{\theta}; y) - \left\{\frac{1}{n}\sum_{i=1}^{n} \left.\frac{\partial U_\beta(\theta; y_i)}{\partial \alpha^{\mathrm{T}}}\right|_{\theta=\widehat{\theta}}\right\}\left\{\frac{1}{n}\sum_{i=1}^{n} \left.\frac{\partial U_\alpha(\alpha; y_i)}{\partial \alpha^{\mathrm{T}}}\right|_{\theta=\widehat{\alpha}}\right\}^{-1} U_\alpha(\widehat{\alpha}; y).$$

The formulation of Σ in (1.15) reflects how estimation of nuisance parameter α at the first stage affects the asymptotic covariance of the estimator $\widehat{\beta}$ obtained from the second stage. Ignoring variability induced from the first stage often distorts the variance estimate of the estimator $\widehat{\beta}$, hence leading to invalid inference results for β. To see this more clearly, we consider a hypothetical situation where the true value α_0 of α is known and we estimate β by solving

$$\frac{1}{n}\sum_{i=1}^{n} U_\beta(\alpha_0, \beta; y_i) = 0$$

for β; let $\widetilde{\beta}$ denote the resultant estimator of β.

The performance of $\widehat{\beta}$ and $\widetilde{\beta}$ is generally different, which is suggested by their covariance estimates. The covariance estimate of $\widehat{\beta}$ is given by $n^{-1}\widehat{\Gamma}^{-1}\widehat{\Sigma}\widehat{\Gamma}^{-1\mathrm{T}}$, while by Theorem 1.6 (b), the covariance estimate of $\widetilde{\beta}$ is $n^{-1}\widetilde{\Gamma}^{-1}\widetilde{\Sigma}\widetilde{\Gamma}^{-1\mathrm{T}}$, where

$$\widetilde{\Gamma} = \frac{1}{n}\sum_{i=1}^{n} \left.\frac{\partial U_\beta(\alpha_0, \beta; y_i)}{\partial \beta^{\mathrm{T}}}\right|_{\beta=\widetilde{\beta}}; \tag{1.16}$$

$$\widetilde{\Sigma} = \frac{1}{n}\sum_{i=1}^{n} \widehat{U}_\beta(\alpha_0, \widetilde{\beta}; y_i)\widehat{U}_\beta^{\mathrm{T}}(\alpha_0, \widetilde{\beta}; y_i). \tag{1.17}$$

In the instance where α must be estimated, ignoring variability induced from estimating α at the first stage but just replacing α_0 with its estimate for (1.16) and (1.17) would usually give rise to invalid variance estimate for the estimator of β, unless in special situations, such as $E\{\partial U_\beta(\theta; Y)/\partial\alpha^{\mathrm{T}}\} = 0$, or equivalently, estimating function $U_\beta(\alpha, \beta; Y)$ is uncorrelated with the score function for the nuisance parameter α (see Problem 1.15).

It is interesting and counterintuitive that ignoring variability induced from the estimation of α can sometimes produce a larger variance estimate for the estimator of β than taking into account of the variation caused from the first stage estimation of α. This phenomenon was observed by many authors, including Robins, Rotnitzky and Zhao (1994) and Ning, Yi and Reid (2017), among many others. This paradox does not appear when estimation is based on a likelihood method but may occur when using estimating functions to conduct parameter estimation. A geometric explanation was provided by Henmi and Eguchi (2004). Newey and McFadden (1994, §6) discussed this issue in detail.

1.4 Model Misspecification

In parametric modeling, we specify a working model $\{f(y; \theta) : \theta \in \Theta\}$ with the hope to capture or well approximate the true data generation mechanism $h(y)$. In reality, however, there is no way to know whether or not a specified working model can reach this goal. It is, therefore, important to understand the consequences when a working model deviates from the true data generation mechanism, a scenario that is called *model misspecification*. In this section, we describe some principal strategies for characterizing asymptotic biases caused from model misspecification. We begin with the likelihood framework for which a number of authors, including Huber (1967), White (1982), Kent (1982), and Royall (1986), have contributed basic setup and tools for handling misspecification issues. Extensions to handling model misspecification with marginal analysis then follow with the discussion concentrated on relevant asymptotic properties.

Let $y(n) = \{y_1, \ldots, y_n\}$ be the measurements of a random sample $\mathbb{Y} = \{Y_1, \ldots, Y_n\}$ generated by the true mechanism $h(y)$, where $h(y)$ is defined on a measurable Euclidean space. Suppose $f^*(y; \theta)$ is a *working* probability density or mass function that is user-specified and is measurable in y for every $\theta \in \Theta$, where Θ is the parameter space. Here we use $f^*(\cdot)$ rather than $f(\cdot)$ for the model form to indicate the possibility of model misspecification. We write the working log-likelihood of the sample as

$$\ell^*(\theta; y(n)) = \sum_{i=1}^{n} \log f^*(y_i; \theta).$$

With certain conditions on the working model, as given in the following theorem, there exists a value of θ that maximizes the working log-likelihood, and we let $\widehat{\theta}^*$ denote this "working" estimator of θ.

Theorem 1.13. *Assume that Θ is a compact subset of a Euclidean space, and $f^*(y; \theta)$ is continuous in θ for every y in the sample space. Then for all n and the given sample measurements $y(n)$, there exists a value $\widehat{\theta} \in \Theta$ that maximizes $\ell^*(\theta; y(n))$:*

$$\widehat{\theta} = \arg\max_{\theta \in \Theta} \ell^*(\theta; y(n)).$$

To describe the discrepancy of the working model from the true data generation mechanism, we define the *Kullback–Leibler Information Criterion* (KLIC):

$$I(h : f^*; \theta) = E\left[\log\left\{\frac{h(Y)}{f^*(Y;\theta)}\right\}\right],$$

where the expectation is taken with respect to the true distribution $h(y)$, and Y represents a random variable with distribution $h(y)$.

When $h(y)$ falls in the class $\{f^*(y;\theta) : \theta \in \Theta\}$, there exists $\theta_0 \in \Theta$ such that $h(y) = f^*(y;\theta_0)$, hence $I(h : f^*;\theta_0) = 0$. The magnitude of $I(h : f^*;\theta)$ reflects the ignorance about the true distribution structure $h(\cdot)$ when using a working distribution $f^*(\cdot)$.

Theorem 1.14. *Assume that the conditions of Theorem 1.13 hold and that*

(a) *$E\{\log h(Y)\}$ exists and $|\log f^*(y;\theta)| \le m(y)$ for all $\theta \in \Theta$, where $m(y)$ is integrable with respect to $h(y)$ and the expectation is taken with respect to the distribution $h(y)$;*
(b) *$I(h : f^*;\theta)$ has a unique minimum at θ^* in Θ.*

Then we have that

$$\widehat{\theta} \xrightarrow{p} \theta^* \quad \text{as } n \to \infty.$$

In the case where the probability model is correctly specified with $h(y) = f^*(y;\theta_0)$ for some $\theta_0 \in \Theta$, then $I(h : f^*;\theta)$ attains its unique minimum (i.e., zero) at $\theta^* = \theta_0$. Therefore, the resulting working estimator $\widehat{\theta}$ is consistent for the true parameter value θ_0.

Theorem 1.15. *Under regularity conditions on $f^*(y;\theta)$ presented by White (1982), including the assumptions in Theorems 1.13 and 1.14, we have that as $n \to \infty$,*

$$\sqrt{n}(\widehat{\theta} - \theta^*) \xrightarrow{d} N(0, \Gamma^{*-1}(\theta^*)\Sigma^*(\theta^*)\Gamma^{*-1\mathrm{T}}(\theta^*)),$$

where

$$\Gamma^*(\theta) = E\left\{\frac{\partial^2 \log f^*(Y;\theta)}{\partial\theta\partial\theta^T}\right\}, \ \Sigma^*(\theta) = E\left\{\frac{\partial \log f^*(Y;\theta)}{\partial\theta} \cdot \frac{\partial \log f^*(Y;\theta)}{\partial\theta^T}\right\},$$

and the expectations are taken with respect to the true distribution $h(y)$.

Theorems 1.13 and 1.15 suggest the existence and the asymptotic distribution for the estimator obtained from a working model while Theorem 1.14 can be used to characterize the asymptotic bias induced from using a working model. The induced asymptotic bias may be quantified by the difference $\theta - \theta^*$. By definition, it is readily seen that under regularity conditions, θ^* may be found by solving the equation

$$E\left\{\frac{\partial \log f^*(Y;\theta)}{\partial\theta}\right\} = 0, \tag{1.18}$$

where the expectation is under the true distribution $h(y)$.

These results were discussed in detail by White (1982). They are useful for studying the effects of various types of model misspecification under the likelihood framework. In many applications, however, we do not work with a full distributional setup but rather focus on marginal structures such as mean and variance of the distribution. In this case, working with estimating functions may be a useful and necessary alternative. As discussed in §1.3.2, to result in consistent estimators, unbiasedness of estimating functions is often a prerequisite. This condition cannot, however, always be satisfied. Many naturally and easily constructed estimating functions are not unbiased. Yi and Reid (2010) investigated asymptotic biases resulted from using *biased* estimating functions and established associated asymptotic properties.

Theorem 1.16. *Suppose that $U(\theta; y)$ is a vector of estimating functions for a p-dimensional parameter θ which may not be unbiased. Suppose that Y is a random variable having the cumulative distribution $F = F(y;\theta_0)$ or the probability density or mass function $f(y;\theta_0)$ for a value $\theta_0 \in \Theta$. Assume that Θ is a convex compact set and that*

$$|U_j(\theta; y)| \le m_j(y)$$

for all y and θ, where $m_j(\cdot)$ is integrable with respect to F, and $U_j(\theta; y)$ is the jth element of $U(\theta; y)$ for $j = 1, \ldots, p$. Assume that

$$E_{\theta_0}\{U(\theta; Y)\} = 0$$

has a unique solution θ_0^*, where the expectation E_{θ_0} is evaluated with respect to $f(y;\theta_0)$. For a sequence of independent random variables $\mathbb{Y} = \{Y_1, \ldots, Y_n\}$ each having distribution F, suppose that

$$\frac{1}{n}\sum_{i=1}^{n} U(\theta; Y_i) = 0$$

has a solution $\widehat{\theta}^*$. Then under regularity conditions,

$$\widehat{\theta}^* \xrightarrow{p} \theta_0^* \quad \text{as } n \to \infty.$$

This theorem characterizes the convergence of the estimator $\widehat{\theta}^*$ obtained from a *working* estimating function $U(\theta; y)$ that is not necessarily unbiased. The difference $\theta_0^* - \theta_0$ is the asymptotic bias induced from using a biased estimating function to estimate θ_0. If function $U(\theta; y)$ is unbiased, then $\theta_0^* = \theta_0$ and $\widehat{\theta}^*$ is consistent for θ_0. Theorem 1.16 can be used for some applications to find consistent estimators by adjusting for inconsistent working estimators. The idea is illustrated as follows.

Suppose that $h(y)$ is correctly or reasonably modeled by $\{f(y;\theta) : \theta \in \Theta\}$, and $U(y;\theta)$ is a vector of estimating functions of θ which may be biased. Assume that for any $\theta \in \Theta$, there exists a $\theta^* \in \Theta$ such that

$$E_\theta\{U(\theta^*; Y)\} = 0, \tag{1.19}$$

where the expectation E_θ is taken with respect to the model $f(y;\theta)$. That is, θ^* is defined as a function of θ, say, $\theta^* = \widetilde{k}(\theta)$ for a $p \times 1$ vector of functions $\widetilde{k}(\cdot)$. Assuming the inverse function vector

$$\theta = k(\theta^*) \tag{1.20}$$

exists, then we use this to define an estimator of θ_0 as

$$\widehat{\theta} = k(\widehat{\theta}^*).$$

If $k(\cdot)$ is continuous, then $k(\widehat{\theta}^*)$ converges to $k(\theta_0^*)$ in probability, thus, the adjusted estimator $\widehat{\theta}$ is consistent for θ_0.

Inference on θ may be carried out based on the asymptotic distribution of $\widehat{\theta}$, established as follows. Let

$$\Gamma^*(\theta) = E_{\theta_0}\left\{\frac{1}{n}\sum_{i=1}^{n}\frac{\partial U(\theta;Y_i)}{\partial\theta^{\mathrm{T}}}\right\},\ \Sigma^*(\theta) = E_{\theta_0}\left\{\frac{1}{n}\sum_{i=1}^{n}U(\theta;Y_i)U^{\mathrm{T}}(\theta;Y_i)\right\},$$

and

$$C^*(\theta) = \Gamma^{*-1}(\theta)\Sigma^*(\theta)\Gamma^{*-1\mathrm{T}}(\theta),$$

where $\Gamma^*(\theta)$ is assumed to be nonsingular.

Theorem 1.17. *Suppose that the conditions in Theorem 1.16 are satisfied and that $U_j(\theta;y)$ is a continuously differentiable function of θ for each y, where $j = 1,\ldots,p$. Under regularity conditions on $U_j(\theta;y)$ and the model F, the following results hold as $n \to \infty$,*

(a) $\sqrt{n}(\widehat{\theta}^* - \theta_0^*) \xrightarrow{d} N\{0, C^*(\theta_0^*)\}$;
(b) assuming $k(\cdot)$, defined at (1.20), exists and is differentiable,

$$\sqrt{n}(\widehat{\theta} - \theta_0) \xrightarrow{d} N\left(0, \left\{\frac{\partial k(\theta_0^*)}{\partial\theta^{\mathrm{T}}}\right\} C^*(\theta_0^*)\left\{\frac{\partial k(\theta_0^*)}{\partial\theta^{\mathrm{T}}}\right\}^{\mathrm{T}}\right). \tag{1.21}$$

Result (1.21) provides us a means to conduct inference on θ, such as constructing confidence intervals or testing hypotheses. In doing so, one replaces the relevant quantities with their empirical counterparts to obtain a consistent estimate for the asymptotic covariance matrix of $\widehat{\theta}$. The regularity conditions for Theorems 1.16 and 1.17 are similar to those outlined in Ch. 5 of van der Vaart (1998); see in particular the discussion following his Theorems 5.9 and 5.21 and the discussion by Yi and Reid (2010).

Finally, we comment that (1.18) or (1.19) is sometimes called the *bridge function*; this function is commonly used to characterize the asymptotic bias induced from a working model (e.g., Jiang and Turnbull 2004). See discussions in §4.3 and §7.3 for details.

1.5 Covariates and Regression Models

Our discussion in the previous sections is laid out for a single random variable. Examining a single variable is rarely the case in application. Measurements for multiple variables from either planned experiments or observational studies are usually collected. To formulate viable models for statistical inference, we often split data into two parts: y, and $\{x, z\}$, where y is the observed measurement of a random variable Y, regarded as the *outcome, response*, or *dependent* variable; and $\{x, z\}$ are the measurements of variables $\{X, Z\}$, called *covariates, predictors, risk factors, explanatory variables* or *independent variables*, in application. In this book, we use the terms *response* and *covariate* variables for Y and $\{X, Z\}$, respectively.

The book focuses on delineating the relationship between a response variable and covariates using various modeling techniques that are tailored for individual applications. We are interested in describing the distribution of a response variable conditional on covariates, often denoted by a conditional probability density or mass function $h(y|x, z)$. However, it is barely the case that the form $h(y|x, z)$ can be identified exactly.

In *parametric statistical inference*, we consider a family of conditional probability density or mass functions and hope $h(y|x, z)$ would be contained by this family. In other words, statistical modeling is commonly done by specifying a model, called a *regression model*,

$$f(y|x, z; \beta),$$

where $f(\cdot|\cdot)$ represents structural assumptions and is usually specified (or partially specified) as a known analytic form but involves a vector of unknown parameters $\beta = (\beta_1, \ldots, \beta_p)^{\mathrm{T}}$ with a finite dimension, say p; the dimension of β can be infinite in semiparametric regression models. All possible values of β form a subset of the Euclidean space $\mathbb{R}^p$, and we call this the *parameter space* and denote it by Θ_β. Having β vary in Θ_β reflects the lack of knowledge to pin down which $f(y|x, z; \beta)$ would actually capture or well approximate the true conditional probability density or mass function $h(y|x, z)$. It is our hope that one of the functions in the class $\{f(y|x, z; \beta) : \beta \in \Theta_\beta\}$ would catch $h(y|x, z)$, i.e., there exists $\beta_0 \in \Theta_\beta$ such that $f(y|x, z; \beta_0) = h(y|x, z)$. This β_0 is called the *true value* of β.

The function $f(\cdot|\cdot)$ is called the *model function* or *regression model*. Specifying the function form of $f(\cdot|\cdot)$, together with associated assumptions, is called *modeling*. Statistical modeling is, to some extent, an art. There are no definite rules on how to determine a suitable model rigorously, although certain principles may be useful. The general consensus is that no models are correct, but some may be useful (Box 1979). Sometimes, the form of $f(\cdot|\cdot)$ is merely chosen due to its mathematically convenient properties. For example, generalized linear models (GLMs) are popularly used for independent univariate data (McCullagh and Nelder 1989), while in contrast, generalized linear mixed models (GLMMs) are often employed for clustered or longitudinal data where random effects are introduced to feature association structures (e.g., Fitzmaurice et al. 2009). Sometimes, the nature of response variables or the research interest suggests a modeling scheme. But often, the combination of these considerations drives us to choose a model form.

Selecting a regression model is usually not separable from the way we use data. When modeling, we commonly face a number of questions, such as, do we need to include all the covariates in the model? In what form should the covariates appear? Do we need to include interaction terms among the covariates? In the presence of multiple candidate models, *model selection* may be invoked to choose a suitable one. In principle, good model selection methods are struck to balance between *goodness-of-fit* and *parsimony*. Adding an extra term to the model may improve the fit to the observed data, but this would usually induce additional estimation variability and degrade the inference results. In addition, this would make the model more complex and reduce the interpretability of model parameters. Normally, it is recommended to assess the adequacy of a model form using the goodness-of-fit or *model diagnosis* techniques whenever possible. Some model checking techniques were discussed by McCullagh and Nelder (1989, Ch. 12) and the references therein.

With a regression model, the treatment of the model function $f(\cdot|\cdot)$ and parameter β may, in principle, follow the same lines outlined as in §1.2 for model parameter θ. Estimation and inference methods described in the previous sections may carry over with proper modifications, which require our care of covariate variables. For example, issues concerning model misspecification can be more subtle in the presence of covariates. In particular, we need to recognize that with model misspecification, the limit, say β^*, to which $\widehat{\beta}$ converges in probability, depends on the joint distribution of $\{Y, X, Z\}$. In this situation, investigation of model misspecification may be carried out by conditioning on $\{X, Z\}$, which allows us to not consider the joint distribution of $\{Y, X, Z\}$ but just the conditional distribution of Y given $\{X, Z\}$.

In standard regression analysis, the conditional analysis is commonly employed with covariates $\{X, Z\}$ kept fixed. For instance, in planned experiments, covariate variables are frequently used to specify certain aspects of the system or design features, and it is often plausible to take them as fixed without being assigned a distribution. In some observational studies, however, it may be more feasible and convenient to treat covariate measurements or some of them as the observed values of certain random variables. To allow for a flexible presentation, in this book we use X to denote covariates that may be a random vector with a certain distribution, and Z is reserved for covariates that are taken as fixed without being assigned a distribution.

1.6 Bibliographic Notes and Discussion

This note does not attempt to provide a comprehensive discussion (in fact, it is far from that) of the research and history of statistical inference. Only a few points are highlighted here. Model identifiability is a fundamental requirement to ensure meaningful inferences. Discussion on this aspect was provided by Koopmans (1949), Koopmans and Reiersøl (1950), Rothenberg (1971), Roehrig (1988), Rao (1992), Gustafson (2005), Allman, Matias and Rhodes (2009), Chen (2011), and the references therein, among many others. Because the distribution of a useful estimator for the model parameter is often difficult to derive, large sample theory plays a cornerstone role in conducting inferences for which examining the consistency and asymptotic normality is usually the focus.

The consistency of estimators is often a result of making suitable conditions for objective functions or estimating functions. A general set of conditions can be found in Newey and McFadden (1994, Theorems 2.1 and 2.7) and specific conditions for the consistency of the MLE and the GMM estimator are, respectively, given in Theorems 2.5 and 2.6 of Newey and McFadden (1994). Establishment of the asymptotic normality of an estimator may be carried out according to the smoothness of the objective functions or estimating functions. Discussion on this was given by Bickel and Doksum (1977), Pollard (1985), Pakes and Pollard (1989), Newey and McFadden (1994), Lehmann and Casella (1998), van der Vaart (1998), Shao (2003) and the references therein.

The asymptotic distribution of an estimator provides the basis for performing inferences, where a consistent estimate of the asymptotic covariance matrix is required. A common way for doing so is to substitute the point estimate into the asymptotic covariance matrix. Newey and McFadden (1994) provided a detailed discussion on this method. For complex models, this strategy may become computationally cumbersome. The bootstrap technique or the jackknife method may be employed by using repeated sampling procedures to work out an asymptotic covariance estimate. Discussion on these algorithms is available in Efron and Tibshirani (1993) and sketched in Appendix A.4.

Two-stage estimators, discussed in §1.3.4, may be generalized to the case where the finite-dimensional parameter α is replaced by a function or an infinite-dimensional parameter. Resulting estimators for β may be termed as *semiparametric two-stage estimators*. Discussion on such estimators was given by Serfling (1980), Härdle and Linton (1994), and Newey and McFadden (1994, §8), among others.

1.7 Supplementary Problems

1.1. Suppose Y is a binomial random variable with the probability mass function

$$P(Y = 1) = \theta \text{ and } P(Y = 0) = 1 - \theta, \tag{1.22}$$

where θ is a parameter with $0 < \theta < 1$.

(a) (i) Write $f(y;\theta) = \theta^y(1-\theta)^{1-y}$ with $y = 0, 1$. Is θ identifiable? U-estimable?

(ii) Consider a reparameterization $\vartheta = \sqrt{\theta}$, then the model becomes $f(y;\vartheta) = \vartheta^{2y}(1-\vartheta^2)^{1-y}$ with $y = 0, 1$. Show that ϑ is identifiable but not U-estimable.

(iii) Consider a reparameterization $\vartheta = \theta^3$ for model (1.22). Is ϑ identifiable? U-estimable?

(b) Suppose $Y_1, \ldots, Y_n$ are independently and identically distributed with the same distribution as Y.

(i) Let $\overline{Y} = n^{-1}\sum_{i=1}^n Y_i$. Show that $\overline{Y}$ is a UMVU estimator of θ.

(ii) Let $q(\theta) = \theta/(1-\theta)$ be the *odds ratio*. Show that the *odds ratio* $q(\theta)$ is not U-estimable whatever n is.

(Freedman 2009, §7.2; Bickel and Doksum 1977, Ch. 4)

1.2.

(a) Prove the results of Example 1.1 in §1.2.1.
(b) Prove that if model parameters are U-estimable, then they are identifiable.

(Freedman 2009, §7.2)

1.3. Suppose $\{Y_1, \ldots, Y_n\}$ is a random sample chosen from the $N(\mu, \sigma^2)$ distribution, where μ is a real number and σ is a positive constant. Let

$$V = \frac{1}{n-1} \sum_{i=1}^{n} (Y_i - \overline{Y})^2$$

be the sample variance, where $\overline{Y} = n^{-1} \sum_{i=1}^{n} Y_i$. Let $\theta = (\mu, \sigma^2)$ and $q(\theta)$ be a function of θ given by $q(\theta) = \sigma^2$.

(a) Find the maximum likelihood estimator of $q(\theta)$. Is this estimator unbiased?
(b) Show that V is an unbiased estimator $q(\theta)$.
(c) Show that the MSE of $(n-1)n^{-1}V$ is smaller than the MSE of V.
(d) Can you find an estimator of the form cV with a constant c such that its MSE is smaller than that of $(n-1)n^{-1}V$?

(Shao 2003, §2.6)

1.4. (The *jackknife method* for bias reduction). Suppose $\mathbb{Y} = \{Y_1, \ldots, Y_n\}$ is a random sample chosen from the probability model $f(y; \theta)$. Let

$$\widehat{\theta} = \widehat{\theta}(Y_1, \ldots, Y_n)$$

be an estimator of parameter θ based on the sample $\mathbb{Y}$. For $i = 1, \ldots, n$, let $\mathbb{Y}_{(-i)}$ be the subset of $\mathbb{Y} = \{Y_1, \ldots, Y_n\}$ with Y_i excluded, and $\widehat{\theta}_{(-i)}$ be the corresponding estimator of θ based on the subsample $\mathbb{Y}_{(-i)}$. Define the *jackknife version* of $\widehat{\theta}$ to be

$$\widehat{\theta}_J = n\widehat{\theta} - \frac{n-1}{n} \sum_{i=1}^{n} \widehat{\theta}_{(-i)}.$$

Suppose that the expectation of $\widehat{\theta}$ can be written as

$$E(\widehat{\theta}) = \theta + \sum_{k=1}^{\infty} \frac{a_k}{n^k},$$

where for $k = 1, 2, \ldots$, constants a_k may depend on θ but not on n. Hence, $E(\widehat{\theta}) = \theta + O(1/n)$.

(a) Show that the expectation of the jackknife estimator $\widehat{\theta}_J$ is

$$E(\widehat{\theta}_J) = \theta - \frac{a_2}{n^2} + O\left(\frac{1}{n^3}\right).$$

(b) Show that if $\mathrm{var}(\widehat{\theta}) = O(1/n)$, then $\mathrm{var}(\widehat{\theta}_J) = O(1/n)$. Thus, the jackknife reduces bias but not increases variance.

(Lehmann and Casella 1998, Ch. 2)

1.5.

(a) Show that a UMVU estimator is always consistent.
(b) Is an unbiased estimator always consistent?
(c) Is a consistent estimator always unbiased?

(Bickel and Doksum 1977, §4.4)

1.6. Suppose Y is a random variable following distribution $N(\theta, 1)$, where θ is a parameter taking values in $\mathbb{R}$. Let $Y_1, \ldots, Y_n$ be independently and identically distributed having the same distribution as Y. Define $V = |Y|$, and $V_i = |Y_i|$ for $i = 1, \ldots, n$.

(a) Find the distribution of V.
(b) Show that θ is unidentifiable in the distribution of V in (a).
(c) Show that θ cannot be estimated consistently if we have only the observations of the V_i.

(Lehmann 1999, §7.1)

1.7. Let $\{Y_n : n = 1, 2, \ldots\}$ be a sequence of random variables, and $\{a_n : n = 1, 2, \ldots,\}$ and $\{b_n : n = 1, 2, \ldots,\}$ be two sequences of positive constants, respectively, satisfying that as $n \to \infty$,

$$a_n \to \infty \text{ or } a_n \to a \text{ for some } a > 0$$

and

$$b_n \to \infty \text{ or } b_n \to b \text{ for some } b > 0.$$

If there exist random variables Y_a and Y_b with $E(|Y_a|) < \infty$ and $E(|Y_b|) < \infty$ such that

$$a_n Y_n \xrightarrow{d} Y_a \text{ and } b_n Y_n \xrightarrow{d} Y_b \text{ as } n \to \infty,$$

then one of the following four statements must hold:

(a) $E(Y_a) = E(Y_b) = 0$;
(b) $E(Y_a) \neq 0$, $E(Y_b) = 0$, and $b_n/a_n \to 0$ as $n \to \infty$;
(c) $E(Y_a) = 0$, $E(Y_b) \neq 0$, and $a_n/b_n \to 0$ as $n \to \infty$;
(d) $E(Y_a) \neq 0$, $E(Y_b) \neq 0$, and $\{E(Y_a)/a_n\}/\{E(Y_b)/b_n\} \to 1$ as $n \to \infty$.

(Shao 2003, §2.5)

1.8. Let $\{\widehat{\theta}_n : n = 1, 2, \ldots\}$ be a sequence of estimators of θ, V be a random variable, and $\{a_n : n = 1, 2, \ldots\}$ be a sequence of positive numbers satisfying that as $n \to \infty$,

$$a_n \to \infty \text{ or } a_n \to a \text{ for some } a > 0.$$

Assume that $a_n(\widehat{\theta}_n - \theta) \xrightarrow{d} V$ as $n \to \infty$, and $E(V^2) < \infty$. Show the following results:

(a) $E(V^2) \le \liminf_{n\to\infty} E\{a_n^2(\widehat{\theta}_n - \theta)^2\}$;
(b) $E(V^2) = \lim_{n\to\infty} E\{a_n^2(\widehat{\theta}_n - \theta)^2\}$ if and only if $\{a_n^2(\widehat{\theta}_n - \theta)^2 : n = 1, 2, \cdots\}$ is uniformly integrable.

(Shao 2003, §2.5)

1.9. Let $\{Y_1, \ldots, Y_n\}$ be a random sample chosen from the Poisson distribution with the probability mass function

$$f(y;\theta) = \frac{\theta^y \exp(-\theta)}{y!} \quad \text{for } y = 0, 1, \ldots, \tag{1.23}$$

where θ is a positive constant. Consider the reparameterization

$$\vartheta = \exp(-\theta)$$

which represents $P(Y_i = 0)$ for $i = 1, 2, \ldots$.
(a) Define

$$V_n = \frac{1}{n}\sum_{i=1}^{n} I\{Y_i \in (-\infty, 0]\},$$

where $I(\cdot)$ is the indicator function.
(i) Show that V_n is an unbiased estimator of ϑ.
(ii) Find $\text{MSE}(\vartheta; V_n)$.
(iii) Show that the MSE and asymptotic MSE of V_n are equal.
(b) Define

$$V_n^* = \exp\left(-\frac{1}{n}\sum_{i=1}^{n} Y_i\right).$$

(i) Find the MSE of V_n^*.
(ii) Find the asymptotic MSE of V_n^*.
(iii) Show that V_n^* is asymptotically more efficient than V_n.

(Shao 2003, §2.5)

1.10. Suppose $y(n) = \{y_1, \ldots, y_n\}$ are measurements of a random sample chosen from the Cauchy probability density function

$$f(y;\theta) = \frac{1}{\pi\{1 + (y-\theta)^2\}} \quad \text{for } -\infty < y < \infty,$$

where θ is a real number.
(a) Find the likelihood equation.
(b) With $n = 2$, discuss the existence and uniqueness of the maximizers of the likelihood function.
(c) As $n \to \infty$, discuss the problems in (b).

(Ferguson 1978; Bai and Fu 1987; Lehmann 1999, §7.3)

1.11. Let $\{X_i : i = 1, \ldots, n\}$ and $\{Y_i : i = 1, \ldots, n\}$ be independently and normally distributed random variables with means

$$E(X_i) = \mu_i \text{ and } E(Y_i) = \beta\mu_i,$$

and variances σ_x^2 and σ_y^2, respectively. Let $\theta = (\beta, \sigma_x^2, \sigma_y^2, \mu_1, \ldots, \mu_n)^{\mathrm{T}}$ be the vector of parameters, where the first three components are called *structural* parameters and the μ_i are called *incidental* parameters.

(a) Construct the likelihood function for θ.
(b) Show that the likelihood is unbounded.
(c) Show that an MLE of θ does not exist.
(d) If the constraint $\sigma_x^2 = \sigma_y^2$ is imposed, show that the MLE of β exists and is consistent.

(Lehmann and Casella 1998, §6.7)

1.12. Suppose that $\{Y_1, \ldots, Y_n\}$ is a random sample chosen from the uniform distribution UNIF $[0, \theta]$ with the probability density function

$$f(y; \theta) = \frac{1}{\theta} I(0 \leq y \leq \theta) \text{ for } -\infty < y < \infty,$$

where θ is a positive parameter.

(a) Find the MLE $\widehat{\theta}$ of θ.
(b) Is $\widehat{\theta}$ unbiased? consistent?
(c) Is $\sqrt{n}(\widehat{\theta} - \theta)$ asymptotically normal?

(Lehmann 1999, §7.2)

1.13. Suppose that Y is a random variable having a probability density or mass function $f(y; \theta)$.

(a) Show that

$$E\left\{\frac{\partial^2 \log f(Y;\theta)}{\partial\theta\partial\theta^{\mathrm{T}}}\right\} - E\left[\left\{\frac{\partial \log f(Y;\theta)}{\partial\theta}\right\}\left\{\frac{\partial \log f(Y;\theta)}{\partial\theta}\right\}^{\mathrm{T}}\right],$$

provided certain regularity conditions. What conditions do you need?

(b) Suppose $V = V(Y)$ is a function of Y that is used as an estimator of θ. Let $m(\theta) = E(V)$ and $J(\theta) = E\{-\frac{\partial^2 \log f(Y;\theta)}{\partial\theta\partial\theta^{\mathrm{T}}}\}$. If θ is a scalar, show that

$$\mathrm{var}(V) \geq \frac{\{m'(\theta)\}^2}{J(\theta)}.$$

The right-hand side is known as the *Cramér–Rao Lower Bound.*

(c) Show that any unbiased estimator which attains the Cramér–Rao Lower Bound is a UMVU estimator, but there is no guarantee the Cramér–Rao Lower Bound would be achieved exactly by any estimator.
(d) Can the inequality in (b) be generalized to the case where θ is a vector?

(Young and Smith 2005, §8.2)

1.14. Suppose that $\{Y_1, \ldots, Y_n\}$ is a random sample chosen from the distribution with the probability density function

$$f(y;\theta) = \frac{1}{\sqrt{2\pi}\sigma} \exp\left\{ -\frac{(y-\mu)^2}{2\sigma^2} \right\} \quad \text{for } -\infty < y < \infty,$$

where $\theta = (\mu, \sigma^2)^{\mathrm{T}} \in \Theta$ and $\Theta = [0, \infty) \times (0, \infty)$.

(a) Find the MLE $\widehat{\theta} = (\widehat{\mu}, \widehat{\sigma}^2)^{\mathrm{T}}$ of θ.

(b) If the true value of μ is $\mu_0 = 0$, show that $\sqrt{n}(\widehat{\mu} - \mu_0)$ does not have an asymptotic normal distribution.

(Newey and McFadden 1994, §3)

1.15. Suppose Y is a random variable having a probability density or mass function $f(y;\theta)$, where $\theta = (\alpha^{\mathrm{T}}, \beta^{\mathrm{T}})^{\mathrm{T}}$ is the parameter vector. Let $S_\alpha(\theta; y) = \partial \log f(y;\theta)/\partial\alpha$ be the score function corresponding to α. Suppose $U(\alpha, \beta; y)$ is a vector of functions whose partial derivatives with respect to α exist.

(a) Assume that the operations of expectation and differentiation are exchangeable. Show that if $E\{U(\alpha, \beta; Y)\} = 0$, then

$$E\left\{ \frac{\partial U(\alpha, \beta; Y)}{\partial \alpha^{\mathrm{T}}} \right\} = -E\{U(\alpha, \beta; Y) S_\alpha^{\mathrm{T}}(\theta; Y)\}.$$

(b) Is the converse statement of (a) true?

1.16. Let Y be a random variable with a probability density or mass function $f(y;\theta)$, and $S(\theta; y) = \partial \log f(y;\theta)/\partial\theta$ be the score function, where θ is a scalar parameter. Suppose $U(\theta; y)$ is an unbiased estimating function for θ, and $\mathcal{U}$ is a class of estimating functions which contains $U(\theta; y)$.

(a) Show that if $U(\theta; y)$ is an optimal estimating function in $\mathcal{U}$, then $U(\theta; Y)$ has maximal correlation (in absolute value) with the score function $S(\theta; Y)$. That is, for *any* $U^*(\theta; y) \in \mathcal{U}$, we have

$$|\mathrm{corr}\{U^*(\theta; Y), S(\theta; Y)\}| \leq |\mathrm{corr}\{U(\theta; Y), S(\theta; Y)\}|.$$

(b) Is the converse statement of (a) true? Can you identify a useful class $\mathcal{U}$?

1.17. Let $y(n) = \{y_1, \ldots, y_n\}$ be the measurements of a random sample $\mathbb{Y} = \{Y_1, \ldots, Y_n\}$ drawn from the probability density or mass function $f(y;\theta)$ with the support of all nonnegative real values, where $\theta = (\mu, \sigma)$, μ is the mean, and σ is the standard deviation of the distribution. Let $\vartheta = q(\theta)$, given by $q(\theta) = (\sigma/\mu)^2$. This is called the *squared coefficient of variation*. Define

$$\overline{y} = \frac{1}{n}\sum_{i=1}^{n} y_i, \; s^2 = \frac{1}{n-1}\sum_{i=1}^{n}(y_i - \overline{y})^2, \text{ and } U(\vartheta; y(n)) = s^2 - \vartheta \bar{y}^2.$$

(a) Show that the conventional moment estimate of ϑ is obtained by solving

$$U(\vartheta; y(n)) = 0.$$

(b) Show that $U(\vartheta; y(n))$ is not an unbiased estimating function for ϑ.
(c) Define

$$U^*(\vartheta; y(n)) = s^2 - \vartheta(\bar{y}^2 - s^2/n).$$

Show that $U^*(\vartheta; y(n))$ is an unbiased estimating function for ϑ, and the resulting estimate of ϑ is:

$$\widehat{\vartheta} = \frac{s^2}{\bar{y}^2 - s^2/n}.$$

(d) Compare the estimators obtained from (a) and (c).

(Yanagimoto and Yamamoto 1991)

1.18. Suppose $\{Y_1, \ldots, Y_n\}$ is a random sample chosen from a Poisson distribution with the probability mass function (1.23).
(a) Find the MLE of θ.
(b) Find a moment estimator of θ using the first moment of Y_i, where $i = 1, \ldots, n$.
(c) Find a moment estimator of θ using the second moment of Y_i, where $i = 1, \ldots, n$.
(d) Derive a GMM estimator of θ by combining the estimating functions in (b) and (c).
(e) Compare the estimators obtained from (a), (b) and (c).

1.19. Suppose $\{Y_1, \ldots, Y_n\}$ is a random sample chosen from the normal distribution $N(\mu, \sigma^2)$ with mean μ and variance σ^2. Let $\theta = (\mu, \sigma^2)$ and $\overline{Y} = n^{-1} \sum_{i=1}^{n} Y_i$.
(a) Find the MLE $\widehat{\theta}$ of θ.
(b) Let $q(\theta) = \sigma/\mu$ denote the *coefficient of variation*. Show that $q(\widehat{\theta}) = \sqrt{n^{-1} \sum_{i=1}^{n} (Y_i - \overline{Y})^2} / \overline{Y}$, and that $q(\widehat{\theta})$ is a consistent estimator of $q(\theta)$.
(c) Find the asymptotic distribution of $\sqrt{n}\{q(\widehat{\theta}) - q(\theta)\}$. Can you find the exact distribution of $q(\widehat{\theta})$?

1.20. Suppose $\mathbb{Y} = \{Y_1, \ldots, Y_n\}$ is a random sample chosen from the probability density or mass function $f(y; \theta)$, and $U(\theta; y)$ is an unbiased estimating function for θ which is of the same dimension as θ. Suppose that for given $\mathbb{Y}$,

$$\sum_{i=1}^{n} U(\theta; Y_i) = 0$$

has a unique solution $\widehat{\theta}$.
(a) Under certain regularity conditions, show that

$$\widehat{\theta} \xrightarrow{p} \theta \quad \text{as } n \to \infty.$$

(b) Discuss regularity conditions in (a).
(c) Do unbiased estimating functions always give unbiased estimators?

(Newey and McFadden 1994, §2)

1.21.

(a) Suppose $y(n) = \{y_1, \ldots, y_n\}$ are the measurements of a random sample $\{Y_1, \ldots, Y_n\}$ chosen from the probability density or mass function $f(y; \theta)$, where $\theta = (\alpha^{\mathrm{T}}, \beta^{\mathrm{T}})^{\mathrm{T}}$. Let

$$L(\theta; y(n)) = \prod_{i=1}^{n} f(y_i; \theta) \text{ and } S_\beta(\beta, \alpha; y(n)) = \frac{\partial \log L(\theta; y(n))}{\partial \beta^{\mathrm{T}}}.$$

Suppose that there exists a unique MLE $\widehat{\theta} = (\widehat{\alpha}^{\mathrm{T}}, \widehat{\beta}^{\mathrm{T}})^{\mathrm{T}}$ and that for each β there is a unique *restricted MLE* $\widehat{\alpha}_\beta$ of α. Assume certain regularity conditions.

(i) Show that $\widehat{\beta}$ is the solution of $S_\beta(\widehat{\alpha}_\beta, \beta; y(n)) = 0$.
(ii) Show that $\widehat{\alpha} = \widehat{\alpha}_{\widehat{\beta}}$.
(iii) Discuss what regularity conditions are required for (i) and (ii).

(b) Let $f(y; \alpha, \beta)$ be the probability density function of a Weibull distribution:

$$f(y; \alpha, \beta) = \beta \alpha y^{\beta - 1} \exp(-\alpha y^\beta) \text{ for } y > 0,$$

where parameters α and β are positive.

(i) Verify the conclusions in (a).
(ii) Show that the profile likelihood score function for β is not unbiased.

(Liang and Zeger 1995)

1.22. Suppose the Y_{ij} are independent each following a Poisson distribution Poisson(μ_{ij}), where μ_{ij} is the mean of Y_{ij} for $j = 1, \ldots, m_i$ and $i = 1, \ldots, n$. Consider the log-linear regression model

$$\log \mu_{ij} = \alpha_i + \beta X_{ij},$$

where X_{ij} is a fixed covariate, and β and α_i are regression coefficients. Let $\alpha = (\alpha_1, \ldots, \alpha_n)$, and $\theta = (\alpha^{\mathrm{T}}, \beta)^{\mathrm{T}}$. Here β is the parameter of interest, and α is a nuisance.

(a) Find the profile likelihood $L_{\mathrm{P}}(\beta)$ for parameter β.
(b) Let $\widehat{\beta}_{\mathrm{P}}$ be the maximizer of the profile likelihood $L_{\mathrm{P}}(\beta)$. Is $\widehat{\beta}_{\mathrm{P}}$ a consistent estimator of β?
(c) Define $W = \sum_{i,j} X_{ij} Y_{ij}$, $V_i = \sum_j Y_{ij}$, and $V = (V_1, \ldots, V_n)^{\mathrm{T}}$. Consider a reparameterization of θ, given by $\vartheta = (\xi^{\mathrm{T}}, \beta)^{\mathrm{T}}$, where $\xi = (\xi_1, \ldots, \xi_n)^{\mathrm{T}}$, and $\xi_i = \exp(\alpha_i) \sum_j \exp(\beta X_{ij})$ for $i = 1, \ldots, n$.

(i) Find the joint probability mass function for W and V indexed by parameter ϑ.
(ii) Find the conditional probability mass function of W, given V.
(iii) Find an estimator of β using the result in (c)(ii).

1.23. Suppose the Y_{ij} are independent following a Bernoulli distribution $\text{Ber}(\mu_{ij})$ for $j = 1, \ldots, m_i$ and $i = 1, \ldots, n$, where μ_{ij} is the mean of Y_{ij}. We consider a logistic regression model

$$\text{logit}\,\mu_{ij} = \alpha_i + \beta X_{ij},$$

where X_{ij} is a fixed covariate, and β and α_i are regression coefficients. Can the development in Problem 1.22 be repeated?

(Cox and Hinkley 1974, §5.7)

1.24. Verify the expressions in (1.14) and (1.15).

2

Measurement Error and Misclassification: Introduction

In Chapter 1, we provide an overview of statistical modeling and inference methods. There is a critical condition underlying the development: variables included in the models must be measured precisely. This condition is, however, frequently violated. Imprecise measurements, or mismeasurements, have long been a concern in various fields, including medical, health and epidemiological studies. They arise commonly in a broad range of applications including analysis of survival data, longitudinal studies, case–control studies and survey sampling. Measurement error and misclassification often degrade the quality of inference and should be avoided whenever possible. However, these features are inevitable in practice.

This chapter provides an overview of issues concerning measurement error and misclassification. Preliminary discussion on the impact of ignoring measurement error is presented. Inference objectives and the scope of analysis of error-prone data are outlined. General strategies of accounting for mismeasurement effects are discussed. Models which are often used to characterize measurement error or misclassification are described. The chapter is concluded with examples of measurement error or misclassification under different settings. This layout serves as a prelude of the book to introduce the problems to be considered in subsequent chapters.

2.1 Measurement Error and Misclassification

The terminology "*measurement error*" may not be consistently used in the literature. By name, it may be used for situations of an incorrect recording of a precise measurement of a variable, for circumstances of the correct recording of an inaccurate measurement of a variable, or even for both. Sometimes this term is used to contrast *systematic error* to *random error*, while other times it may be used to refer to *sampling error* as opposed to *nonsampling error*. Systematic error, also called *statistical bias* by some researchers, may occur from imperfections in measuring instruments or measuring procedures; it is usually viewed as repeatable and does not

G. Y. Yi, *Statistical Analysis with Measurement Error or Misclassification*, Springer Series in Statistics, DOI 10.1007/978-1-4939-6640-0_2

change over time. Systematic error may be controlled or reduced by carefully planning the measurement procedure and using a better measurement device. Random error, or random variation, on the other hand, is an inherent feature associated with the variables being measured for which we cannot control; it is unreproducible and varies from observation to observation and/or from time to time. Sampling error, sometimes called *estimation error*, is caused by the uncertainty or variability of using only a portion (i.e., a sample) of measurements from a population rather than the measurements from the whole population to estimate the target values.

Regardless of varying definitions of *"measurement error"* by different authors, in this book we use the term *"measurement error"* or *"mismeasurement"* to refer broadly to any setting where the ideal measurement (if available) of a variable in the model may *differ* from the actual value obtained by a data collection procedure.

Measurement error may arise with different reasons and from various sources (e.g., Yi and Cook 2005; Carroll et al. 2006). In addition to the *reading error* induced from machine and reader variability, a variable may be difficult to be observed precisely due to physical location or cost. For example, the degree of narrowing of coronary arteries may reflect the risk of heart failure, but physicians may measure the degree of narrowing in carotid arteries instead, due to the less invasive nature of this assessment method. Sometimes it is impossible to measure a variable accurately due to the nature of the variable. For example, the level of exposure to potential risk factors for cancer, such as radiation, can never be measured accurately. A variable may represent an average of a certain quantity over time, and any practical way of measuring such a quantity necessarily involves biological variability and temporal variation. In certain situations, data may be intentionally manipulated for ethical reasons. For instance, to preserve confidentiality of participants in survey studies, we may alter the measurements of those variables X which may reveal the identity of the participants and report only their surrogate measurements X^*, where X^* is generated from X with a known mechanism, such as $X^* = Xe$ for a random value e simulated from a given distribution (e.g., Hwang 1986).

In application, *measurement error* in a variable may include any of these variabilities or be a mix of them. Although the reasons and sources for imprecise measurements are diverse, there are common features that may be sorted out to form valid statistical inference. Measurement error problems may be phrased as *covariate measurement error* or *response measurement error* according to error-prone variables being covariates or responses. Sometimes, one may distinguish *misclassification* from *measurement error* where the former term is used for *discrete* error-prone variables and the latter for *continuous* error-prone variables.

In this and subsequent chapters (except for Chapters 3 and 4), we reserve symbol Y for the true response variable that may be subject to measurement error or misclassification, and the letter X for the vector of the true covariates that are subject to measurement error or misclassification. We add the asterisk to the variables to indicate their corresponding measurements, Y^* and X^*, which are imprecisely measured, and we call Y^* and X^* *surrogate* versions of Y and X, respectively. The terminology "*surrogacy*" has been used differently by other authors (e.g., Buzas, Stefanski and Tosteson 2007; Prentice 1989) with certain conditions imposed. Here we loosely use this term to show that the actual measurement of a variable may differ from the measurement of the variable we intend to put in the model. Some authors call Y^* and X^* *proxy variables*. The notation Z is reserved for the vector of error-free covariates.

2.2 An Illustration of Measurement Error Effects

We consider a simple but illustrative example to demonstrate measurement error effects. Let $\{(Y_i, X_i) : i = 1, \ldots, n\}$ be a sequence of i.i.d random variables, where Y_i is a response variable, and X_i is a covariate for $i = 1, \ldots, n$. Consider simple linear regression

$$Y_i = \beta_0 + \beta_x X_i + \epsilon_i \tag{2.1}$$

for $i = 1, \ldots, n$, where β_0 and β_x are regression parameters, and ϵ_i is independent of X_i with mean zero and a constant variance σ^2.

Without a full distributional assumption for ϵ_i, the estimating function approach outlined in Example 1.9 or the least squares regression method is a natural option for estimation of the regression parameter $\beta = (\beta_0, \beta_x)^{\mathrm{T}}$ if covariate X_i were precisely measured. The resulting estimator $\widehat{\beta}_x$ of β_x is given by

$$\widehat{\beta}_x = \frac{\sum_{i=1}^n (X_i - \overline{X})(Y_i - \overline{Y})}{\sum_{i=1}^n (X_i - \overline{X})^2},$$

where $\overline{X} = n^{-1} \sum_{i=1}^n X_i$, and $\overline{Y} = n^{-1} \sum_{i=1}^n Y_i$.

In the presence of covariate measurement error, X_i is often not observed, but a surrogate measurement X_i^* is available for $i = 1, \ldots, n$. One may attempt to replace X_i with X_i^* in estimation procedures. Let $\widehat{\beta}_x^*$ denote the resulting estimator of the slope β_x, given by

$$\widehat{\beta}_x^* = \frac{\sum_{i=1}^n (X_i^* - \overline{X}^*)(Y_i - \overline{Y})}{\sum_{i=1}^n (X_i^* - \overline{X}^*)^2},$$

where $\overline{X}^* = n^{-1} \sum_{i=1}^n X_i^*$; this estimator is called a *naive* estimator of β_x. The naive estimator $\widehat{\beta}^*$ may be a consistent or inconsistent estimator of β_x, depending on the relationship between X_i and X_i^*.

If X_i and X_i^* are linked through the model

$$X_i = X_i^* + e_i \tag{2.2}$$

for $i = 1, \ldots, n$, where e_i is independent of $\{X_i^*, \epsilon_i\}$ and has mean zero and a constant variance σ_e^2, then the naive estimator $\widehat{\beta}_x^*$ for the slope is consistent, i.e., $\widehat{\beta}_x^*$ converges to β_x in probability as $n \to \infty$.

On the other hand, if X_i and X_i^* are connected via the model

$$X_i^* = X_i + e_i \tag{2.3}$$

for $i = 1, \ldots, n$, where e_i is independent of $\{X_i, \epsilon_i\}$ and has zero mean and a constant variance σ_e^2, then the naive estimator $\widehat{\beta}_x^*$ is not a consistent estimator for the slope β_x (Fuller 1987). In fact,

$$\widehat{\beta}_x^* \xrightarrow{p} \beta_x^* \text{ as } n \to \infty, \tag{2.4}$$

where $\beta_x^* = \omega\beta_x$ with $\omega = \sigma_x^2/(\sigma_x^2+\sigma_e^2)$ and σ_x^2 is the variance of X_i. The factor ω, called the *reliability ratio*, may be alternatively viewed as the ratio of the variability of X_i to that of X_i^*:

$$\omega = \frac{\text{var}(X_i)}{\text{var}(X_i^*)}.$$

Since ω is no greater than 1, covariate measurement error, in this case, has an *attenuated* effect on the estimation of covariate effect β_x.

Now we explain why naive estimators behave differently under different measurement error models. If expressing (2.3) as $X_i = X_i^* - e_i$ and plugging it into (2.1), we obtain

$$Y_i = \beta_0 + \beta_x X_i^* + \epsilon_i^*, \tag{2.5}$$

where $\epsilon_i^* = \epsilon_i - \beta_x e_i$. At first sight, model (2.5) seems to suggest that the naive analysis using model (2.1) with X_i replaced by X_i^* is valid, because such an analysis adopts the same model structure as (2.5) where the mean of ϵ_i^* is identical to the mean of ϵ_i in (2.1) (i.e., both are zero). However, routine methods, such as the least squares method, cannot be blindly applied to model (2.5) for the estimation of β, even though the mean of ϵ_i^* is zero. The reason is that the error term ϵ_i^* in (2.5) is *not uncorrelated* with the predictor X_i^*. In addition to different predictors, (2.5) differs from (2.1) in two aspects: (1) ϵ_i^* and X_i^* are correlated in (2.5) while ϵ_i and X_i are uncorrelated in (2.1); (2) the variance of ϵ_i^* in (2.5) is $\sigma^2 + \beta_x^2\sigma_e^2$, greater than the variance of ϵ_i in (2.1) (unless $\beta_x = 0$ or $\sigma_e^2 = 0$).

On the other hand, if the measurement error model is given by (2.2), then plugging (2.2) into (2.1) gives an expression similar to (2.5):

$$Y_i = \beta_0 + \beta_x X_i^* + \epsilon_i^{**}, \tag{2.6}$$

where $\epsilon_i^{**} = \epsilon_i + \beta_x e_i$. It is noted that error term ϵ_i^{**} does not only have mean zero but also is uncorrelated with the predictor X_i^*. In this instance, the model employed by the naive analysis differs from (2.6) only in the variance of the noise term. Thus, the least squares method can still legitimately apply to the model adopted by the naive analysis, yielding a consistent estimator of β.

Next, we comment on the variability associated with $\widehat{\beta}_x$ and $\widehat{\beta}_x^*$ where the measurement error model is given by (2.3). Because the data $\{(Y_i, X_i^*) : i = 1, \ldots, n\}$ are more scattered than the data $\{(Y_i, X_i) : i = 1, \ldots, n\}$ (if X_i were observed), one might intuitively expect that the naive estimator $\widehat{\beta}_x^*$ would incur more variation than $\widehat{\beta}_x$ does. However, this surmise is not necessarily true. Buzas, Stefanski and Tosteson (2007) identified circumstances where a naive estimator of the slope can asymptotically have less variability than the true data estimator does.

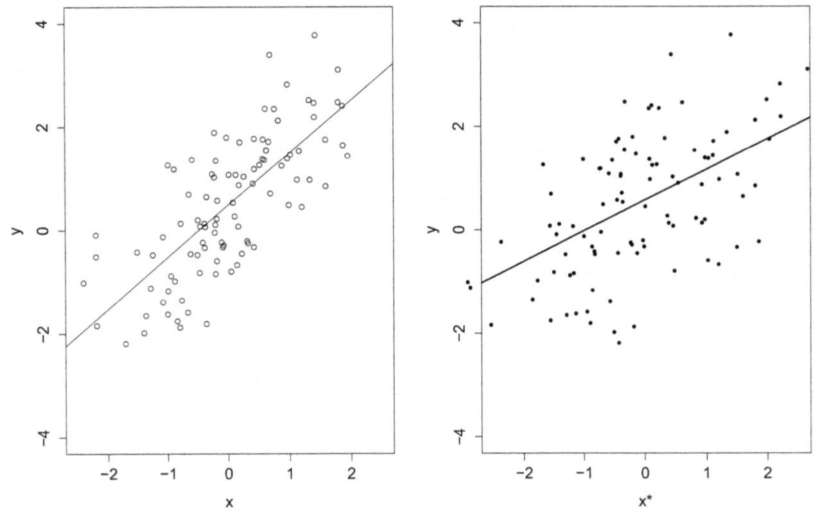

Fig. 2.1. *Effects of Measurement Error Model (2.3) on Simple Linear Regression*

Example 2.1. We conduct a simulation study to demonstrate measurement error effects on fitting linear regression models, where two measurement error models are considered. Set $n = 100$ and generate response measurements independently from model (2.1) for $i = 1, \ldots, n$, where we set $\beta_0 = 0.5, \beta_x = 1.0$, and $\epsilon_i \sim N(0, 1)$.

In the first case, generate the true covariate X_i from the standard normal distribution $N(0, 1)$ and then surrogate measurements X_i^* from model (2.3) independently for $i = 1, \ldots, n$, where $e_i \sim N(0, 1)$. In the second case, generate surrogate measurements X_i^* from distribution $N(0, 1)$ and then the true covariate X_i from model (2.2) independently for $i = 1, \ldots, n$, where $e_i \sim N(0, 1)$.

The results for the first and second cases are displayed in Figs. 2.1 and 2.2, respectively, where the scatter plots of $\{(X_i, Y_i) : i = 1, \ldots, n\}$ and $\{(X_i^*, Y_i) : i = 1, \ldots, n\}$ and fitted least squares regression lines are included.

In Fig. 2.1, the slope on the right panel is smaller than that of the left panel, and this confirms the attenuation effect established in (2.4). The variability difference for the data is also visualized in Fig. 2.1. On the other hand, the consistency of the naive estimator is demonstrated from the parallel lines of Fig. 2.2 if the measurement error model is given by (2.2).

In terms of evaluating the joint effect of covariate measurement error on the point estimator and the associated variance, one may examine how hypothesis testing procedures may be affected. Some details are included in Problem 2.4 and discussed by Fuller (1987, §1.3). Here we make a quick observation for a special test for no covariate effect under measurement error model (2.3). Because "$H_o : \beta_x = 0$" is the same as "$H_o : \omega\beta_x = 0$", the naive test for $H_o : \beta_x = 0$, based on the observed measurements on $\{(Y_i, X_i^*) : i = 1, \ldots, n\}$, can still lead to a correct calculation of the Type I error rate when measurement error in X_i is ignored. However, the power would decrease due to the increased residual variance. Measurement error effects are more complex when the null value of the hypothesis is nonzero.

A typical phenomenon occurring in many applications, although not universal, is that naive estimators incur larger biases than estimators obtained from valid methods but the latter ones entail more variation than naive estimators do. This naturally prompts a concern: is it worthwhile to make efforts to develop new analysis methods in order to correct for biases contained in naive estimators? There might be cases where an estimator with a smaller variance, even though incurring some biases, is preferred to a consistent estimator that involves a larger variability; attempting to adjust for measurement error effects might end up with worse inference results than ignoring measurement error. To look into these issues, Carroll et al. (2006, §3.5) used the mean squared error criterion and illustrated that in sufficiently large samples, it is beneficial to correct for measurement error effects. This aspect is also discussed in §9.1.

The discussion here is merely based on a simple linear regression model for the response variable Y_i and the true covariate X_i, but sheds some light on measurement error effects on inference results. When the response model is complex with multiple covariates or nonlinear structures, measurement error effects become more dimensional and complicated. Measurement error may not only attenuate point estimates, but also inflate or even reverse signs of the estimates as well.

Generally speaking, the nature and degree of measurement error effects are governed by many factors, including the form of the response and measurement error models, the variability of the variables, and their association structures. It is generally agreed that a problem by problem study needs to be invoked if measurement error or misclassification is a concern in the analysis. In the following chapters, we explore a variety of problems with measurement error or misclassification in detail.

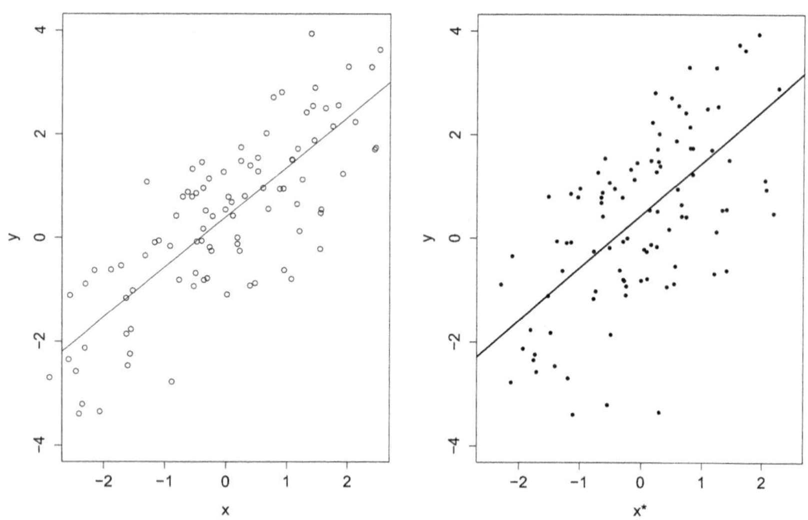

Fig. 2.2. *Effects of Measurement Error Model (2.2) on Simple Linear Regression*

2.3 The Scope of Analysis with Mismeasured Data

Although the reasons for imprecise measurement are diverse and measurement error effects are complex, inference objectives and scopes for error-present settings are not different than those for error-free contexts. *Estimation*, *hypothesis testing*, *prediction*, and *model selection* are often of central interest. Many inference methods for addressing measurement error share common principles and strategies. In this book, we focus on estimation procedures for a variety of models arising from different fields.

Based on the observed data, our goal is to understand the relationship between a response variable, Y, and associated covariates, $\{X, Z\}$. Suppose the true probability density or mass function of $\{Y, X, Z\}$ is $h(y, x, z)$. This function is unknown but can be written as

$$h(y, x, z) = h(y|x, z)h(x, z), \tag{2.7}$$

where $h(y|x, z)$ is the conditional probability density or mass function of Y given $\{X, Z\}$, and $h(x, z)$ is the probability density or mass function of X and Z. Factorization (2.7) provides a convenient framework to show specific features of many studies, such as cohort or observational studies, for which response measurements are collected when or after covariates are measured.

Although factorization (2.7) does not really help us gain knowledge of the true data generation mechanism $h(y, x, z)$ (because both $h(y|x, z)$ and $h(x, z)$ are equally unknown), (2.7) offers us a way of modeling and developing inference methods. In the absence of measurement error, we usually leave $h(x, z)$ unattended to and solely modulate $h(y|x, z)$ using a model, say $\{f(y|x, z; \beta) : \beta \in \Theta_\beta\}$, where model function $f(\cdot|\cdot)$ is fully or partially specified, and parameter β is unknown, taking values in the parameter space Θ_β. The conditional analysis is commonly employed for inference about parameter β.

However, in the presence of measurement error, do we still stand at the same point? Do we need to concern ourselves about the distributional form of covariates? To highlight the ideas, we consider the case where only covariates are subject to measurement error; discussion on measurement error in response is deferred to Chapter 8.

Suppose X is subject to mismeasurement. An additional variable, X^*, comes along to represent the actual measurement of X. In principle, valid inference comes from jointly evaluating the stochastic changes in all the relevant variables. Unlike the error-free context which involves $h(y, x, z)$, the joint probability density or mass function $h(y, x, z, x^*)$ for $\{Y, X, Z\}$ and X^* serves as the basis for inferences in the presence of measurement error in X. Because it is difficult to come up with a meaningful and transparent model to describe *simultaneous* stochastic changes in $\{Y, X, Z\}$ and X^*, we often take a viable means by factorizing the joint distribution $h(y, x, z, x^*)$ into the product of a sequence of conditional distributions (and a marginal distribution), each for a single type of variables. This factorization allows us to examine those conditional distributions separately, each distribution being handled with a usual modeling scheme.

Technically, there is no unique way to factorize the joint distribution $h(y, x, z, x^*)$, hence different modeling strategies may be used to facilitate different applications. Broadly speaking, modeling and inference should be carried out in light of the study objectives and the nature of the data. We elaborate on this in the next section. Here and elsewhere, we use $h(\cdot)$ and $h(\cdot|\cdot)$, respectively, to represent the true marginal and conditional probability density or mass functions for the random variables indicated by the arguments and $f(\cdot)$ and $f(\cdot|\cdot)$ for the corresponding models.

2.4 Issues in the Presence of Measurement Error

In this section, we outline several basic issues concerning analysis for settings with covariate measurement error or misclassification.

Measurement Error/Misclassification Mechanism

Measurement error mechanisms are classified according to the relationship between Y and X^*: whether or not Y and X^* are conditionally independent, given the true covariates $\{X, Z\}$. If

$$h(y|x^*, x, z) = h(y|x, z), \tag{2.8}$$

then the measurement error process is called to possess the *nondifferential measurement error mechanism* (if X is continuous) or the *nondifferential misclassification mechanism* (if X is discrete). Sometimes, the term "*nondifferential (measurement) error mechanism*" is loosely used for both cases. This mechanism says that Y and X^* are conditionally independent, given the true covariates X and Z; the surrogate X^* carries no information on inference about the response process if the true covariates are given. Assumption (2.8) is ubiquitously adopted, explicitly or implicitly, for analysis of error-contaminated data arising from observational studies, or prospective studies, where covariate measurements occur at a fixed point in time, and a response is measured at a later time.

In retrospective studies, such as case–control studies, the nondifferential error mechanism may be infeasible. In such studies, the response variable is obtained first, then antecedent exposures and other covariates are measured. In this case, controlling the true covariates may not completely remove the dependence between X^* and Y. For example, in nutrition studies, a true predictor is taken as long-term dietary intake before diagnosis, but the dietary interview data are obtained only after diagnosis. A woman who was diagnosed having breast cancer may tend to exaggerate her estimated fat intake. In such circumstances, estimated fat intake may still be associated with disease status even after conditioning on the true long-term diet intake (Carroll et al. 2006, p. 36).

If

$$h(y|x^*, x, z) \neq h(y|x, z), \tag{2.9}$$

then the corresponding mechanism is called the *differential measurement error mechanism* (if X is continuous) or the *differential misclassification mechanism* (if X is discrete). Occasionally, one may simply use the *differential (measurement) error mechanism* to refer to both scenarios.

Classification of measurement error using (2.8) and (2.9) is meaningful only for settings with *covariate* measurement error alone. If other features are present in the data, such a classification may become useless. In §5.5, we discuss this issue for settings with co-existing missing observations and covariate measurement error. With censored data, we describe a modified definition of measurement error mechanisms in §3.2.2. In contrast to error-prone responses, to be discussed in §8.1, one may refer to (2.8) and (2.9) as nondifferential *covariate* measurement error and differential *covariate* measurement error, respectively, to stress that only covariates are subject to error.

Inference and Modeling

Different measurement error mechanisms may suggest different modeling strategies. Under the nondifferential error mechanism, it is natural to conduct inference based on the factorization

$$\begin{aligned} h(y, x, x^*, z) &= h(y|x, x^*, z)h(x, x^*, z) \\ &= h(y|x, z)h(x, x^*, z), \end{aligned}$$

whereas, with a differential error mechanism, one may alternatively proceed with

$$h(y, x, x^*, z) = h(x^*|x, y, z)h(y|x, z)h(x, z).$$

These decompositions offer us convenient ways to explicitly spell out the distribution $h(y|x, z)$, a quantity of prime interest. The distribution $h(y|x, z)$ is then characterized by standard modeling techniques that are developed for error-free settings. In particular, we assume a model $\{f(y|x, z; \beta) : \beta \in \Theta_\beta\}$ and hope there exists $\beta_0 \in \Theta_\beta$ such that $h(y|x, z) = f(y|x, z; \beta_0)$.

Distinguished from the usual statistical analysis for error-free contexts, additional modeling is the unique feature for the analysis of data with measurement error. Under a differential error mechanism, modeling $h(x^*|y, x, z)$ and $h(x, z)$ is generally needed unless certain assumptions are imposed. For settings with nondifferential measurement error, we need to examine $h(x, x^*, z)$ by further factorizing it as

$$h(x, x^*, z) = h(x^*|x, z)h(x, z) \tag{2.10}$$

or

$$h(x, x^*, z) = h(x|x^*, z)h(x^*, z) \tag{2.11}$$

to accommodate different modeling schemes for the measurement error process.

In error-free contexts, covariates $\{X, Z\}$ are usually treated as fixed or are regarded as random but their distributions are left unspecified. In contrast, in the presence of covariate error in X, covariates $\{X, Z\}$ can be handled with two methods. In some circumstances, we treat $\{X, Z\}$ as fixed and base inference on conditioning on $\{X, Z\}$, thus the distribution $h(x, z)$ of $\{X, Z\}$ is left unmodeled. This strategy is called a *functional method*. In other situations, we regard $\{X, Z\}$ as random variables whose distribution (i.e., $h(x, z)$) is needed, and this leads to the so-called *structural modeling strategy*. When using this strategy, modeling $h(x, z)$ is often realized using the factorization

$$h(x, z) = h(x|z)h(z),$$

where the conditional probability density or mass function $h(x|z)$ for X given Z is modeled, but the marginal probability density or mass function $h(z)$ for Z is left unmodeled.

There are no definite rules on deciding which strategy should be used. Generally speaking, functional modeling is distribution-robust while structural modeling can be more efficient when there is good knowledge about the distribution of the true covariates. In addition, structural modeling is basically required when inference is conducted within the Bayesian paradigm.

A tacit assumption is commonly made in parametric modeling: parameters governing different models are assumed to be *distinct*. With the full distributional assumptions available for modeling all the relevant processes, inference about the response parameter β may be conducted by applying the maximum likelihood method in a straightforward manner. In situations where a full distributional model is difficult to specify or is not of primary interest, we often confine our attention to certain aspects of the associated variables and focus on modeling those features only. In this case, the principle of breaking a joint model for all the relevant variables into several "smaller" models, each being a conditional model for a single variable, can still guide us to develop marginal or semiparametric inferential procedures for various settings.

Identifiability and Additional Data

As discussed previously, analysis of error-prone data often requires additional modeling of measurement error and/or covariate processes, besides modeling the response process which links Y and $\{X, Z\}$. This extra layer of modeling adds complications to inferential procedures. Parameter *identifiability* becomes a particular concern. This pertains to the enlargement of the initial parameter space Θ_β to a new parameter space which also includes the parameters arising from additional modeling of measurement error and/or covariate processes. Although the initial sample space for the variables $\{Y, X, Z\}$ is expanded to include an extra variable X^*, the sample space for the *observed* data may not be rich enough to differentiate the joint model for $h(y, x, z, x^*)$ (e.g., Problem 2.12).

A strategy to overcome model nonidentifiability is, as described briefly in §1.2.1, to impose suitable constraints on the parameter space to make it smaller. However, it is often unclear what constraints should be used so that the resultant smaller parameter space can work equally well as the original parameter space in order to capture or well approximate the true distribution $h(y, x, z, x^*)$. This strategy basically reduces our choices of possible models, which is unappealing in that we are more likely to be placed in a situation of model misspecification.

An alternative approach is to call for additional data to help us delineate the measurement error process. Depending on the measurement error mechanism, the requirement of additional data may be different. With nondifferential measurement error, it is possible to estimate parameter β in the response model $f(y|x, z; \beta)$ even when the true covariates X are not observable. This is, however, usually not true for differential measurement error (except for special cases, such as with linear models). In this case, measurements of X are often required for a subsample of subjects.

Here we describe several types of data sources that are used in the analysis of error-contaminated data. In many applications, our analysis is directed to the data collected from the main study which consists of measurements of Y, Z and X^*. We let $\mathcal{M}$ denote the index set of subjects who are in the main study. The measurements $\{Y_i, X_i^*, Z_i\}$ are available if $i \in \mathcal{M}$. For an additional data set, let $\mathcal{V}$ denote the set of subject indices, and $\mathcal{D} = \{W_i : i \in \mathcal{V}\}$ be the collection of various types of measurements W_i we now describe. The data $\mathcal{D}$ are called *internal* if $\mathcal{V}$ is a subset of $\mathcal{M}$, while the data $\mathcal{D}$ are called *external* if $\mathcal{V}$ has no overlap with $\mathcal{M}$. Three types of data $\mathcal{D}$ commonly arise from applications (Carroll et al. 2006, Ch. 2).

- *Validation Subsample*

  A validation subsample often contains measurements for both the true and surrogate covariate variables. Response measurements may or may not be available for those subjects in $\mathcal{V}$. Often, in an *internal validation* subsample, W_i contains $\{Y_i, X_i, X_i^*, Z_i\}$ while for an *external validation* subsample, W_i may include only $\{X_i, X_i^*, Z_i\}$.

  An internal validation data set permits direct examination of the measurement error structure and usually leads to a good precision of estimation and inference. When external validation data are used to assess the measurement error model, it is assumed that the measurement error model, based on the external data, is *transportable* to the data for the main study (Carroll et al. 2006, §2.3; Yi et al. 2015).

- *Repeated Measurements*

  In settings where replicate surrogate measurements of X_i are available, W_i may have the form (X_{ij}^*, Z_i) or (Y_i, X_{ij}^*, Z_i), where the X_{ij}^* are repeated measurements of X_i for $j = 1, \ldots, n_i$ and n_i is an integer greater than 1. In this case, index set $\mathcal{V}$ may be a subset of $\mathcal{M}$, or has no overlap with $\mathcal{M}$. Usually, one would make replicate measurements of X_i if there were good reasons to believe that the average of replicates is a better estimate of X_i than a single observation. If a classical additive error model is assumed (to be discussed in §2.6), then replication data can be used to estimate the variance of the measurement error model.

- *Instrumental Data*

  In addition to the primary surrogate measurement X_i^* of X_i, a second measurement V_i is available sometimes. Variable V_i is correlated with X_i with a weaker relationship than that of X_i^* to X_i, and is often called an *instrumental variable*. In this case, $W_i = \{X_i^*, Z_i, V_i\}$ or $W_i = \{Y_i, X_i^*, Z_i, V_i\}$. If V_i is external (i.e., $\mathcal{V}$ has no overlap with $\mathcal{M}$), it can be useful if it is unbiased for X_i in the sense that $E(V_i|X_i) = X_i$; in this case, V_i may be used in a regression calibration analysis (to be discussed in §2.5.2). If V_i is internal (i.e., $\mathcal{V}$ is a subset of $\mathcal{M}$), it does not need to be unbiased to be useful (Carroll et al. 2006, §2.3). A discussion of instrumental variables was provided by Carroll et al. (2006, Ch. 6) and Buonaccorsi (2010, Ch. 5).

  Choosing an instrumental variable may be somewhat subjective, although the mathematical definition is possible. For instance, Fuller (1987, §1.4) provided a formal definition of an instrumental variable under simple regression models. An overview of the role of instrumental variables in epidemiological studies was provided by Greenland (2000).

In situations where model identifiability is an issue and no additional data $\mathcal{D}$ are available to facilitate estimation of parameters associated with the measurement error process, conducting *sensitivity analyses* is a viable way to address measurement error effects. We take a number of candidate models for the measurement error process together with representative values specified for the model parameters, and then apply a valid method which accommodates measurement error effects to perform inference about the response parameters. It is then interesting to assess how sensitive the results are to different degrees of measurement error or misclassification.

2.5 General Strategy of Handling Measurement Error

In the presence of measurement error, several strategies are commonly invoked to correct for measurement error effects for various applications. In this section, we outline those schemes in broad terms; elaboration on genuine application to specific problems is to be presented in subsequent chapters.

Suppose response variable Y and covariates $\{X, Z\}$ are linked by the conditional probability density or mass function $h(y|x,z)$, and the class $\{f(y|x,z;\beta) : \beta \in \Theta_\beta\}$ of conditional probability density or mass functions is specified in the hopes of capturing or well approximating $h(y|x,z)$. Assume that the precise value of X is not observed, but its surrogate version X^* is measured. Suppose the available data, denoted by $\mathcal{O} = \{(y_i, x_i^*, z_i) : i = 1, \ldots, n\}$, are realizations of a random sample $\{(Y_i, X_i^*, Z_i) : i = 1, \ldots, n\}$ drawn from the distribution of $\{Y, X^*, Z\}$. Our objective is to infer parameter β (of dimension p) using the observed data $\mathcal{O}$.

Many strategies may be developed for this purpose. These strategies are generally classified into three categories, according to the way of introducing adjustments for the measurement error effects. The first category contains likelihood-based correction methods; the second category includes adjustment methods based on unbiased estimating functions; and the third class of methods focuses on directly correcting estimators obtained from usual analysis with the difference between X and X^* ignored.

In the formulation of the first strategy, parameter β is paired with the nuisance parameter so notation θ for the full vector of model parameters appears in the expressions; in the second and third strategies, only parameter β appears explicitly with the nuisance parameters suppressed in the relevant notation.

2.5.1 Likelihood-Based Correction Methods

A likelihood-based method is viewed as a structural modeling strategy which requires the specification of the distribution of the true covariate X. For illustrations, we examine the case where nondifferential measurement error is assumed and the true covariate X is not available.

Induced Model Method/Observed Likelihood Method

An analysis method for error-contaminated data is to directly work on *the induced model* for the observed data. First, we derive the relationship between the response Y and the observed covariates $\{X^*, Z\}$ using the given response model for $h(y|x, z)$ and the measurement error model which links the variables $\{X^*, X, Z\}$. Secondly, we apply a standard analysis method to the induced model which associates Y and $\{X^*, Z\}$. We call this strategy the *induced model method*, or the *observed likelihood method.*

Depending on the way of modeling the relationship between the true covariate X and its surrogate version X^*, the model for the conditional distribution of the outcome variable given the observed covariate variables may be formulated as

$$f(y|x^*, z; \theta) \propto \int f(y|x, z; \beta) f(x^*|x, z) f(x|z) d\eta(x)$$

or

$$f(y|x^*, z; \theta) \propto \int f(y|x, z; \beta) f(x|x^*, z) d\eta(x),$$

where $d\eta(x)$ represents the dominating measure which is either Lebesgue or the counting measure, corresponding to continuous or discrete random variables; $\theta = (\alpha^{\mathrm{T}}, \beta^{\mathrm{T}})^{\mathrm{T}}$ is the vector of all associated model parameters; and α is the parameter associated with the measurement error and/or covariate processes which is suppressed in the notation. Parameter β is of prime interest whereas α is regarded as a nuisance; β and α are often assumed to be functionally independent.

With the available data $\mathcal{O}$, the likelihood for the observed data is given by

$$L_{\mathrm{o}}(\theta) = \prod_{i=1}^{n} f(y_i|x_i^*, z_i; \theta). \tag{2.12}$$

Maximizing the observed likelihood function $L_{\mathrm{o}}(\theta)$ with respect to θ gives the MLE of θ.

Likelihood-based methods are conceptually simple and efficient in dealing with error-prone problems. However, model robustness is a major concern. Typically, the specification of the distribution of X is difficult since X is often not observable. Due to the integrals involved, likelihood methods are often computationally demanding. To ease these issues, modified versions, often phrased as *pseudo-likelihood methods*, are developed for various contexts.

The induced model methods and their modified versions are discussed in §3.4, §5.4.1, §5.4.2, §5.6.1, §6.2, §6.3, §6.4, §6.5, §6.6, §7.3, §7.4, §8.3, §8.4, and §8.6.

Expectation-Maximization Algorithm

In some applications, the observed likelihood (2.12) based on the measurements of $\{(Y_i, Z_i, X_i^*) : i = 1, \ldots, n\}$ may be difficult to maximize whereas the complete likelihood based on all the variables $\{(Y_i, X_i, Z_i, X_i^*) : i = 1, \ldots, n\}$ may be relatively easy to maximize. In such instances, the *expectation-maximization* (EM) algorithm comes into play.

We decompose the model for the joint distribution of $\{Y, X, X^*\}$ given Z as:

$$f(y, x, x^*|z; \theta) = f(x|y, x^*, z; \theta) f(y, x^*|z; \theta).$$

Then taking the logarithm and applying the result to random variables $\{Y, X, Z, X^*\}$ gives

$$\log f(Y, X^*|Z; \theta) = \log f(Y, X, X^*|Z; \theta) - \log f(X|Y, X^*, Z; \theta).$$

For a given value θ^* of the parameter, taking conditional expectation on both sides with respect to $f(x|y, x^*, z; \theta^*)$, we obtain

$$\begin{aligned} &\int \log f(y, x^*|z; \theta) f(x|y, x^*, z; \theta^*) d\eta(x) \\ &= \int \log f(y, x, x^*|z; \theta) f(x|y, x^*, z; \theta^*) d\eta(x) \\ &\quad - \int \log f(x|y, x^*, z; \theta) f(x|y, x^*, z; \theta^*) d\eta(x). \end{aligned}$$

Applying this identity to the random sample $\{(Y_i, X_i, Z_i, X_i^*) : i = 1, \ldots, n\}$ and its measurements, we obtain

$$\ell_o(\theta) = Q(\theta; \theta^*) - H(\theta; \theta^*), \tag{2.13}$$

where

$$\ell_o(\theta) = \sum_{i=1}^{n} \log f(y_i, x_i^*|z_i; \theta);$$

$$Q(\theta; \theta^*) = \sum_{i=1}^{n} E_{X_i|(Y_i, X_i^*, Z_i; \theta^*)} \{\log f(Y_i, X_i, X_i^*|Z_i; \theta)\}; \tag{2.14}$$

$$H(\theta;\theta^*) = \sum_{i=1}^{n} E_{X_i|(Y_i,X_i^*,Z_i;\theta^*)}\{\log f(X_i|Y_i,X_i^*,Z_i;\theta)\}; \qquad (2.15)$$

with the expectations evaluated with respect to $f(x_i|y_i,x_i^*,z_i;\theta^*)$ and $\{Y_i,X_i^*,Z_i\}$ in $Q(\theta;\theta^*)$ and $H(\theta;\theta^*)$ assuming their observations $\{y_i,x_i^*,z_i\}$.

Interestingly, for the given data $\mathcal{O}$, formulation (2.13) expresses a function of θ (i.e., $\ell_o(\theta)$) as the difference of two functions which depend not only on θ but also on an additional parameter θ^*. The introduction of this additional parameter θ^* offers us an extra dimension to examine $\ell_o(\theta)$. Specifically, considering two possible values of θ, say $\theta^{(k)}$ and $\theta^{(k+1)}$, we set θ^* as $\theta^{(k)}$ for the right-hand side of (2.13) and then evaluate the difference of $\ell_o(\theta)$ at those two values:

$$\begin{aligned}&\ell_o(\theta^{(k+1)}) - \ell_o(\theta^{(k)})\\ &= \{Q(\theta^{(k+1)};\theta^{(k)}) - Q(\theta^{(k)};\theta^{(k)})\} - \{H(\theta^{(k+1)};\theta^{(k)}) - H(\theta^{(k)};\theta^{(k)})\}.\end{aligned}$$

By that $H(\theta_1;\theta_2) \le H(\theta_2;\theta_2)$ for any θ_1,θ_2 in Θ, we obtain that

$$-\{H(\theta^{(k+1)};\theta^{(k)}) - H(\theta^{(k)};\theta^{(k)})\} \ge 0.$$

Thus, if we can choose $\theta^{(k+1)}$ such that

$$Q(\theta^{(k+1)};\theta^{(k)}) - Q(\theta^{(k)};\theta^{(k)}) \ge 0,$$

then we can ensure the increment of $\ell_o(\theta)$ from $\theta^{(k)}$ to $\theta^{(k+1)}$ to be nonnegative, leading to

$$\ell_o(\theta^{(k+1)}) \ge \ell_o(\theta^{(k)}).$$

This argument prompts an algorithm of finding the maximizer of the observed log-likelihood (2.13). For the given data $\mathcal{O}$, the algorithm essentially iterates among the two operations of expectation and maximization, respectively called the *E-step* and *M-step*, until convergence of $\theta^{(k)}$, where $\theta^{(k)}$ stands for the estimate of θ obtained at the kth iteration for $k = 0, 1, 2, \ldots$.

This procedure is called the *EM algorithm*. To be more specific, let

$$L_C(\theta) = \prod_{i=1}^{n} f(Y_i, X_i, X_i^*|Z_i;\theta) \qquad (2.16)$$

be the *complete data likelihood* formulated for $\{(Y_i,X_i,X_i^*,Z_i) : i = 1,\ldots,n\}$. At iteration $(k+1)$ of the E-step, using (2.14) we calculate $Q(\theta;\theta^{(k)})$ for the conditional expectation of the logarithm of the complete data likelihood (2.16), where the expectation is evaluated with respect to the model for the conditional distribution of the unobserved variable X given the observed variables $\{Y, X^*, Z\}$ with θ taken as $\theta^{(k)}$, and the variables $\{Y_i, X_i^*, Z_i\}$ in $Q(\theta;\theta^{(k)})$ are assessed at their observations $\{y_i, x_i^*, z_i\}$. At the M-Step, we maximize $Q(\theta;\theta^{(k)})$ with respect to θ and obtain the estimate $\theta^{(k+1)}$. Cycle through these steps until convergence of $\{\theta^{(k)} : k = 0, 1, \ldots\}$ as $k \to \infty$.

The EM algorithm was initially developed by Dempster, Laird and Rubin (1977) to perform likelihood analysis with missing data. It has been remarkably used for a wide variety of situations which are pertinent to incomplete data problems. Modifications and extensions of the EM algorithm have been extensively proposed in the literature (e.g., Meng and Van Dyk 1998; Booth and Hobert 1999). Comprehensive explorations of this algorithm may be found in McLachlan and Krishnan (1997) and the references therein.

Application of the EM algorithm to handle measurement error problems is discussed in §3.8.3, §5.4.3, §5.5.4, §5.6.1, §6.3, §6.6, and §8.6.

We note that both the EM algorithm and the induced likelihood method base the estimation of θ on the observed data $\mathcal{O}$. The formulation of the observed likelihood, however, is somewhat different. The EM algorithm works with $f(y_i, x_i^*|z_i;\theta)$, suggested by (2.13), while the induced likelihood method focuses on using $f(y_i|x_i^*, z_i;\theta)$, as shown in (2.12).

Conditional Score Method

At the E-step of the EM algorithm, calculating the conditional expectation of the logarithm of $L_C(\theta)$ allows us to have a function (i.e., the $Q(\cdot)$ function) free of the unobserved X_i variables, thus giving us a computable function for the next step (i.e., the M-step). To have a computable function, one might alternatively attempt to view the complete data likelihood $L_C(\theta)$ with the X_i regarded as parameters, and then maximize the complete data likelihood $L_C(\theta)$ with respect to parameter θ together with "parameters" $\{X_1, \ldots, X_n\}$. This method is conceptually straightforward. However, this procedure does not necessarily ensure the resulting estimator for β to be consistent due to the infinite dimension of parameters $\{X_1, \ldots, X_n\}$, as discussed in §1.3.4.

A modified scheme is to treat nuisance "parameters" $\{X_1, \ldots, X_n\}$ differently from θ in the complete data likelihood $L_C(\theta)$. First, we examine $L_C(\theta)$ to find a "sufficient statistic", say $\Omega(\theta)$, for $\{X_1, \ldots, X_n\}$ by taking θ as fixed. Secondly, we use such a statistic to construct a conditional distribution of $\mathbb{Y} = \{Y_1, \ldots, Y_n\}$, given $\Omega(\theta)$, such that this distribution depends only on the observed data and θ and not on $\{X_1, \ldots, X_n\}$. Thirdly, using this conditional distribution we carry out inference about β. For certain problems, this method yields valid inference results about β.

This strategy, related to Lindsay (1982), was elaborated by Stefanski and Carroll (1987) for generalized linear measurement error models. It is called the *conditional score method*. This method is implemented in §5.6.2, §6.5, and §7.5.

2.5.2 Unbiased Estimating Functions Methods

The preceding strategies basically apply to settings where a full distributional form for the response process is assumed. In application, specifying the full distribution of the response variable may be difficult, or our interest is merely in marginal features of the response process. In such instances, inferences are often based on estimating functions. Suppose $U(\beta; y, x, z)$ is a user-specified estimating function for β;

it can be the score function $(\partial/\partial\beta)\log f(y|x,z;\beta)$ when a full distributional model $f(y|x,z;\beta)$ is available. Such a function is usually required to be *unbiased* (more precisely, *conditionally unbiased*) in the sense that

$$E\{U(\beta;Y,X,Z)|X,Z\}=0, \tag{2.17}$$

where the expectation is taken with respect to the conditional model $f(y|x,z;\beta)$ for all $\beta \in \Theta_\beta$.

In this subsection, we describe several schemes of accommodating measurement error effects using estimating function theory. The basic idea is to construct a *valid* estimating function for parameter β which is of principal interest. Being valid, this estimating function needs to have two basic properties: (1) the function should be computable in a sense of being expressed in terms of X^*, rather than X, along with other observable variables and the model parameters; and (2) this function should be able to produce an estimator of β which has good statistical properties such as consistency and asymptotic normality, provided suitable regularity conditions. By the discussion in §1.3.2, the unbiasedness is commonly imposed when constructing an estimating function to meet the requirement (2).

Subtraction Correction Method

Replacing X with X^* in $U(\beta;Y,X,Z)$ and calculating the conditional expectation $E\{U(\beta;Y,X^*,Z)\}$, we define

$$U^*(\beta;y,x^*,z)=U(\beta;y,x^*,z)-E\{U(\beta;Y,X^*,Z)\},$$

where the expectation is evaluated with respect to the model for the joint distribution of $\{Y,Z,X^*\}$. Such an estimating function is unbiased and computable in the sense that the arguments (y,x^*,z) can be evaluated with the availability of the observed data $\mathcal{O}$.

This scheme is called the *subtraction correction strategy*. It is implemented to obtain (3.54) in §3.6.3 and was discussed by Yi and Reid (2010), Yan and Yi (2016b), and Yi et al. (2016). If $E\{U(\beta;Y,X^*,Z)\}$ cannot be computed exactly, then some approximation may be used. For example, one may employ the bootstrap algorithm to approximate $E\{U(\beta;Y,X^*,Z)\}$ by adapting the idea of McCullagh and Tibshirani (1990) who used a bootstrap estimate of the mean to correct the bias of score functions derived from the log profile likelihood.

Expectation Correction Method

Another approach is called the *expectation correction strategy*. Define

$$U^*(\beta;Y,X^*,Z)=E\{U(\beta;Y,X,Z)|Y,X^*,Z\},$$

where the expectation is taken with respect to the model for the conditional distribution of X given $\{Y,X^*,Z\}$.

Function $U^*(\beta; Y, X^*, Z)$ is workable due to its noninvolvement of the unobserved X, and its unbiasedness follows from that of $U(\beta; Y, X, Z)$, as indicated below:

$$
\begin{aligned}
&E_{(Y,X,X^*,Z)}\{U^*(\beta; Y, X^*, Z)\} \\
&= E_{(Y,X,X^*,Z)}\left[E\{U(\beta; Y, X, Z)|Y, X^*, Z\}\right] \\
&= E_{(Y,X^*,Z)}\left(E_{X|(Y,X^*,Z)}\left[E\{U(\beta; Y, X, Z)|Y, X^*, Z\}\right]\right) \\
&= E_{(Y,X^*,Z)}\left[E_{X|(Y,X^*,Z)}\{U(\beta; Y, X, Z)\}\right] \\
&= E_{(Y,X,X^*,Z)}\{U(\beta; Y, X, Z)\} \\
&= E_{(Y,X,Z)}\{U(\beta; Y, X, Z)\} \\
&= 0,
\end{aligned}
$$

where the expectations are evaluated with respect to the models for the corresponding distributions indicated by the associated random variables. Here and throughout the book, for ease of exposition, we interchangeably use $E\{g(U, V)|V\}$ and $E_{U|V}\{g(U, V)\}$ to refer to the conditional expectation of $g(U, V)$ taken with respect to the model for the conditional distribution of U given V, where $g(U, V)$ is a function of any random variables U and V.

The expectation correction strategy has some similarities to the EM algorithm in that the operation of the conditional expectation of the unobserved quantities given the observed variables is needed, but these two methods are not the same. The EM algorithm centers around the likelihood formulation while the expectation correction approach applies to estimating functions. The EM algorithm requires the evaluation of the conditional expectation of the log-likelihood for the complete data $\{Y, X, X^*, Z\}$, but the expectation correction method needs an evaluation of estimating functions involving $\{Y, X, Z\}$ but not X^*. The expectation correction strategy is relevant to the *expected estimating equation* (EEE) method exploited by Wang and Pepe (2000), where the nondifferential measurement error mechanism is assumed and estimation of nuisance parameters is coupled with that of β.

Modified versions of the expectation correction strategy are available in the literature. For instance, instead of evaluating the conditional expectation $E\{U(\beta; Y, X, Z)|Y, X^*, Z\}$ for a function $U(\beta; Y, X, Z)$ in order to produce a computable estimating function, one may directly replace X in $U(\beta; Y, X, Z)$ with a workable version $E(X|X^*, Z)$. This is the widely used *regression calibration* (RC) method (Prentice 1982; Thurston, Spiegelman and Ruppert 2003; Carroll et al. 2006). If estimating function $U(\beta; Y, X, Z)$ is linear in X, then the regression calibration and the expectation correction strategies yield the same unbiased estimating function; otherwise, the regression calibration method often produces *inconsistent* estimators, because estimating function $U\{\beta; Y, E(X|X^*, Z), Z\}$ is not necessarily unbiased. Consequently, the expectation correction method may be regarded as a valid extension to nonlinear models of the regression calibration algorithm (which is valid for linear models).

To reduce the bias for the estimator obtained from the regression calibration method for nonlinear models, Freedman et al. (2004) proposed the *moment reconstruction* method, which replaces X with a variance-preserving estimate X^*_{MR}, where, under the condition $E(X^*|Y, Z) = E(X|Y, Z)$, X^*_{MR} is given by

$$X^*_{\text{MR}} = E(X|Y,Z)(I_{p_x} - G) + X^*G \tag{2.18}$$

with $G = \{\text{var}(X^*|Y,Z)\}^{-1/2}\{\text{var}(X|Y,Z)\}^{1/2}$. Here notation $A^{1/2}$ represents the Cholesky decomposition of matrix A, defined by $(A^{1/2})^{\text{T}}A^{1/2} = A$, notation I_{p_x} stands for the $p_x \times p_x$ unit matrix, and p_x is the dimension of X. Conditional on $\{Y, Z\}$, X^*_{MR} has the same mean and covariance as the unobserved true covariate X (see Problem 2.9).

The expectation correction method is implemented in §3.3.1, §3.5.2, and §5.3.1.

Insertion Correction Method

As opposed to the expectation correction method, we introduce the *insertion correction method*. The idea is to find a computable estimating function, denoted by $U^*(\beta; y, x^*, z)$, so that its conditional expectation recovers an unbiased estimating function $U(\beta; y, x, z)$ which is derived from the original model for $h(y|x,z)$. As long as

$$E\{U^*(\beta; Y, X^*, Z)|Y, X, Z\} = U(\beta; Y, X, Z) \tag{2.19}$$

where the expectation is evaluated with respect to the model for the conditional distribution of X^*, given $\{Y, X, Z\}$, working with $U^*(\beta; y, x^*, z)$ would produce a consistent estimator for β under regularity conditions.

With generalized linear models, Nakamura (1990) used the insertion correction strategy to develop the so-called *"corrected" likelihood* or *"corrected" score* method. If estimating function $U(\beta; y, x, z)$ is the score function computed from the model for $h(y|x,z)$, then this method is phrased as the *"corrected" score* method. When the insertion correction strategy applies to the log-likelihood function for the model of $h(y|x,z)$, this method is also called the *"corrected" likelihood* method.

These two methods are closely related. Let $\ell(\beta; y, x, z)$ denote the log-likelihood function derived from the model for $h(y|x,z)$. Suppose there is a function $\ell^*(\beta; y, x^*, z)$ of the observed data and the model parameter such that

$$E\{\ell^*(\beta; Y, X^*, Z)|Y, X, Z\} = \ell(\beta; Y, X, Z). \tag{2.20}$$

Let $U^*(\beta; y, x^*, z) = \partial\ell^*(\beta; y, x^*, z)/\partial\beta$. If integration and differentiation are interchangeable, then by identity (2.20), the conditional expectation of $U^*(\beta; Y, X^*, Z)$, given $\{Y, X, Z\}$, recovers the score function for the model of $h(y|x,z)$.

The insertion correction method has been used successfully for regression models, such as Normal, Poisson and Gamma regression models (Carroll et al. 2006, Ch. 7), for which covariates typically appear in a form of exponential, polynomial or their product functions. Extensions of this strategy to various settings were discussed by several authors, including Huang and Wang (2001), Yi (2005), Yi, Ma and Carroll (2012), and Yi and Lawless (2012).

When the form of $U(\beta; y, x, z)$ is complex, it is difficult or even impossible to find functions $U^*(\beta; y, x^*, z)$ to satisfy (2.19). An alternative is to work with a weighted version of $U(\beta; y, x, z)$:

$$U_{\text{w}}(\beta; y, x, z) = w(\beta; x, z)U(\beta; y, x, z),$$

where $w(\beta; x, z)$ is an arbitrary weight function of the parameter and the covariates but free of the response variable. Properly choosing a weight function $w(\beta; x, z)$ may enable us to readily find a computable estimating function, say $U^*(\beta; y, x^*, z)$, which satisfies

$$E\{U^*(\beta; Y, X^*, Z)|Y, X, Z\} = U_{\mathrm{w}}(\beta; Y, X, Z).$$

Such an estimating function is unbiased, justified as follows:

$$\begin{aligned}
&E_{(Y,X,X^*,Z)}\{U^*(\beta; Y, X^*, Z)\} \\
&= E_{(Y,X,Z)}\left[E_{X^*|(Y,X,Z)}\{U^*(\beta; Y, X^*, Z)\}\right] \\
&= E_{(Y,X,Z)}\{U_{\mathrm{w}}(\beta; Y, X, Z)\} \\
&= E_{(X,Z)}\left[E_{Y|(X,Z)}\{w(\beta; X, Z)U(\beta; Y, X, Z)\}\right] \\
&= E_{(X,Z)}\left[w(\beta; X, Z) \cdot E_{Y|(X,Z)}\{U(\beta; Y, X, Z)\}\right] \\
&= 0,
\end{aligned}$$

where the last equation is due to the unbiasedness (2.17) of $U(\beta; y, x, z)$.

The insertion correction method is implemented in §3.5.1, §3.6, §3.7, §4.4, §4.5, §4.6, §5.3.2, §5.5.3, and §8.7.1.

2.5.3 *Methods of Correcting Naive Estimators*

The third class of correction methods for mismeasurement effects is to directly adjust for naive estimators obtained from usual analysis procedures which ignore the difference between X^* and X.

Naive Estimator Correction Method

One scheme starts with producing a working estimator by directly applying estimating function $U(\beta; y, x, z)$ to the data $\mathcal{O}$ with argument (y, x, z) evaluated at (y_i, x_i^*, z_i). Solving

$$\sum_{i=1}^{n} U(\beta; y_i, x_i^*, z_i) = 0$$

for β yields a naive estimate of β. Let $\widehat{\beta}^*$ denote the corresponding estimator of β. At the next step, we examine the relationship between the naive estimator $\widehat{\beta}^*$ and a valid estimator obtained from using $U(\beta; y, x, z)$ by treating X_i as if available. This is often carried out by evaluating the asymptotic bias for $\widehat{\beta}^*$ using the bridge function discussed in §1.4. Finally, we correct the naive estimator $\widehat{\beta}^*$ by using the relationship established in the previous step. We call this three-step procedure the *naive estimator correction* strategy.

This strategy is implemented in §4.3 and §7.3 and was also discussed by Stefanski and Carroll (1985), Yi and Reid (2010), and Yan and Yi (2016a), among others.

Simulation-Extrapolation Method

Another approach for *reducing* bias involved in the naive estimator is simulation based. The basic idea is to first establish the trend of measurement error-induced bias as a function of the variance of the added measurement error, and then extrapolate this trend back to the case without measurement error. This is the *simulation-extrapolation* (SIMEX) approach proposed by Cook and Stefanski (1994) for the measurement error model

$$X_i^* = X_i + e_i \tag{2.21}$$

for $i = 1, \ldots, n$, where e_i is independent of $\{X_i, Z_i\}$ and the response variable, and e_i follows a $N(0, \Sigma_e)$ distribution with known covariance matrix Σ_e.

Given an integer B (say, $B = 200$) and a sequence of increasingly ordered values $\{c_1, \ldots, c_N\}$ taken from $[0, c_N]$ (say, $c_N = 1$ and $N = 20$) with $c_1 = 0$, we carry out the SIMEX method as follows.

- Step 1: Simulation.
  Given $b = 1, \ldots, B$, for each $c = c_1, \ldots, c_N$, generate e_{ib} from the distribution $N(0, \Sigma_e)$ and set
  $$x_{ib}^*(c) = x_i^* + \sqrt{c}e_{ib}. \tag{2.22}$$
- Step 2: Estimation.
  Replace x_i in the estimating function $U(\beta; y_i, x_i, z_i)$ with $x_{ib}^*(c)$ and solve
  $$\sum_{i=1}^{n} U(\beta; y_i, x_{ib}^*(c), z_i) = 0$$
  for β to obtain an estimate $\widehat{\beta}(b, c)$. Define $\widehat{\beta}(c) = B^{-1} \sum_{b=1}^{B} \widehat{\beta}(b, c)$.
- Step 3: Extrapolation.
  For each component $\widehat{\beta}_k(c)$ of $\widehat{\beta}(c)$ where $k = 1, \ldots, p$, fit a regression model to the sequence $\{(c, \widehat{\beta}_k(c)) : c = c_1, \ldots, c_N\}$ and extrapolate it to $c = -1$; let $\widehat{\beta}_k$ denote the corresponding predicted value at $c = -1$. Then $\widehat{\beta} = (\widehat{\beta}_1, \ldots, \widehat{\beta}_p)$ is called the *SIMEX estimate* of β.

The SIMEX method is implemented in §3.3.2 and §5.5.3. Its theoretical justification was given by Carroll et al. (1996) for parametric regression under the assumption that the exact extrapolation function is known together with suitable regularity conditions.

The idea of the SIMEX method can be intuitively illustrated by the discussion in §2.2 for simple linear regression (2.1) with the measurement error model (2.3). If replacing X_i with its observed measurement X_i^*, then the resulting least squares estimator $\widehat{\beta}_x^*$ converges in probability to the limit

$$\left\{ \frac{\text{var}(X_i)}{\text{var}(X_i^*)} \right\} \beta_x = \left(\frac{\sigma_x^2}{\sigma_x^2 + \sigma_e^2} \right) \beta_x \quad \text{as } n \to \infty.$$

Analogously, if replacing X_i with simulated surrogate value $X^*_{ib}(c) = X^*_i + \sqrt{c}e_{ib}$, then the resultant estimator $\widehat{\beta}^*_x(b, c)$, and hence $\widehat{\beta}^*_x(c)$, converges in probability to

$$\left[\frac{\text{var}(X_i)}{\text{var}\{X^*_{ib}(c)\}}\right]\beta_x = \left\{\frac{\sigma^2_x}{\sigma^2_x + (1+c)\sigma^2_e}\right\}\beta_x \text{ as } n \to \infty.$$

If $c = 0$, $\widehat{\beta}^*_x(0)$ is just the naive estimator $\widehat{\beta}^*_x$. However, if we set $c = -1$, the corresponding limit is identical to the true parameter β_x.

The SIMEX approach is attractive because it does not require the modeling of the covariate process, and hence the resultant estimators are robust to possible misspecification of the distribution of the true covariates. Although being time-consuming, implementation of the SIMEX method can be readily realized by adapting existing statistical software.

Implementation of the SIMEX method pertains to several aspects. The specification of B, N and c_N is not unique. Quantity c_N is often set as 1 or 2. In principle, larger values of B and N may improve the performance of a SIMEX estimator in the sense that Monte Carlo sampling error in the simulation step may be reduced. A main source of uncertainty is induced in the selection of a suitable regression function in the extrapolation step. As the exact extrapolation function form is unknown, a user-specified regression function has to be used to approximate the exact extrapolation function. Such an approximation distorts the consistency of the resultant estimators (established by Carroll et al. 1996), therefore, the SIMEX estimators are only *approximately* consistent. Many numerical studies suggest that a quadratic regression function may serve as a fairly reasonable approximation to the extrapolation function. Although the SIMEX method is robust in the sense that the distribution of the true covariates is left unspecified, it is sensitive to the distributional assumption of the measurement error model. SIMEX estimators can incur larger bias than naive estimators do when the measurement error model involves misspecification (Yi and He 2012).

The foregoing SIMEX procedure is described for the scenario where an additive normal error model with known covariance matrix Σ_e is available. In the case where covariance matrix Σ_e is unknown but replicate surrogate measurements are available, a modified version of the SIMEX procedure was described by Devanarayan and Stefanski (2002), and is to be given in §3.3.2. With misclassified covariates in regression models, Küchenhoff et al. (2006) proposed the MC-SIMEX algorithm using the same principle of the SIMEX method. Stefanski and Cook (1995) provided theoretical support for the SIMEX procedure and established a relationship between SIMEX estimation and jackknife estimation. Apanasovich, Carroll and Maity (2009) investigated the basic theory for the SIMEX method in semiparametric problems in which the error-prone variable X_i is modeled parametrically, nonparametrically or a combination of both. Yi et al. (2015) developed the augmented-SIMEX approach to extend the scope of the SIMEX method to handling data with the mix of misclassified discrete covariates and mismeasured continuous covariates.

2.5.4 Discussion

The aforementioned strategies focus on producing a point estimate for the parameter β which associates with the response model and is of interest. Variance estimates may be obtained using the accompanying theory with each specific method. For instance, when using the induced model method in §2.5.1, the inverse of the negative second partial derivatives of the logarithm of the observed likelihood can be used to calculate the variance estimate for the corresponding estimator. The Godambe information matrix, described in §1.3.2, may be applied to derive variance estimates for the estimators of β if schemes outlined in §2.5.2 are invoked. In circumstances where a variance estimate is not easy to produce, the bootstrap method may presumably be used.

The sketched methods require different model assumptions, thus may be used differently. The methods in §2.5.1 are basically derived from jointly examining the response and measurement error models, whereas the approaches in §2.5.2 emphasize on constructing valid estimating functions of the response model parameter β alone. Tacitly, estimating functions described in §2.5.2 involve nuisance parameters associated with measurement error models (and sometimes covariate models as well). To estimate parameter β from those estimating functions, nuisance parameters need to be specified or replaced with their estimates. Often, an extra set of estimating functions is constructed for estimation of the nuisance parameters using additional data sources and then coupled with the estimating functions for β to perform parameter estimation. Discussion in §1.3.4 may be applied for this purpose. Similarly, to use the methods in §2.5.3, we often need the knowledge of the measurement error process.

The procedures described in this section mainly serve as a template to handle problems with mismeasured covariates. It does not mean that those methods can be directly used without being tailored to fit individual situations. Depending on the characteristics of individual problems and the availability of additional data sources, the methods outlined in this section often require proper modifications to reflect meaningful estimation and inference procedures. Furthermore, the methods discussed here are not the only possible tools to handle measurement error problems; other options are available in the literature, see, for example, Carroll and Stefanski (1985), Carroll, Gallo and Gleser (1985), Whittemore and Keller (1988), Carroll and Stefanski (1990), Woodhouse et al. (1996), Nummi (2000), He and Liang (2000), Schafer (2001), Novick and Stefanski (2002), Kuha and Temple (2003), Thoresen and Laake (2003), Pierce and Kellerer (2004), Staudenmayer and Buonaccorsi (2005), Yucel and Zaslavsky (2005), Huang and Wang (2006), Carroll et al. (2006), Carroll and Wang (2008), Thomas, Stefanski and Davidian (2011), and many others.

2.6 Measurement Error and Misclassification Models

In this section, we describe measurement error and misclassification models which are frequently used in the literature. Symbol e or e with a subscript is usually used to represent the error term in a measurement error model. We consider models for scenarios with nondifferential measurement error or misclassification. For settings with differential measurement error or misclassification, a validation sample is often required, which may then suggest a natural way for postulating the measurement error or misclassification process.

In terms of notation in (2.10), to model the probability density or mass function $h(x^*|x, z)$, we specify a family of probability density or mass functions $f(x^*|x, z; \sigma_e)$ with parameter σ_e varying in the parameter space Θ_e, and hope that $h(x^*|x, z) = f(x^*|x, z; \sigma_{e0})$ for some σ_{e0} in Θ_e. A simple scenario is that given the true covariate X, surrogate X^* is independent of error-free covariate Z.

Dually, if using (2.11), we would specify a family $\{f(x|x^*, z; \sigma_e) : \sigma_e \in \Theta_e\}$ of probability density or mass functions, hoping that $h(x|x^*, z) = f(x|x^*, z; \sigma_{e0})$ for some σ_{e0} in Θ_e. A simple scenario corresponds to that, given the surrogate covariate X^*, the true covariate X is independent of error-free covariate Z.

Classical Additive Error Model

A *classical additive error model* is of the form

$$X^* = X + e, \tag{2.23}$$

where the error term e is often assumed to be independent of the true covariates $\{X, Z\}$, and has mean zero and a covariance matrix Σ_e.

This model implies that the observed surrogate X^* is more variable than the true covariates X. When the surrogate X^* is thought of as fluctuating around the true covariate X, this model may be a feasible option to link X^* and X. An equivalent form

$$X^* = X + \Sigma_e^{1/2} e$$

is sometimes used, where e has zero mean and an identity covariance matrix and is independent of the true covariates $\{X, Z\}$. The degree of measurement error is reflected by the magnitude of the elements in covariance matrix Σ_e.

Model (2.23) may be modified to accommodate situations with replicate measurements. Suppose X is being independently measured m times, contributing replicated surrogate measurements X_j^*. A classical additive model is then specified as

$$X_j^* = X + e_j$$

for $j = 1, \ldots, m$, where the e_j are assumed to be independent of each other and of $\{X, Z\}$ and have mean zero and covariance matrix Σ_e. The requirement of mean zero for e_j indicates that the replicates X_j^* are unbiased measurements of X in the sense that $E(X_j^*|X) = X$. The independence assumption for the e_j may be relaxed when the replicates X_j^* are not independently collected. The error structure of e_j may be *homoscedastic* where the covariance matrix Σ_e is the same for all subjects, or *heteroscedastic* where the covariance matrix varies from subject to subject.

Berkson Model

A *Berkson model* takes an opposite perspective to facilitate the relationship between X and X^*. Instead of viewing X^* as a function of X as in (2.23), a Berkson model treats the true covariate X as varying around the surrogate X^*:

$$X = X^* + e, \tag{2.24}$$

where the error term e is often assumed to be independent of the surrogate X^* as well as covariate Z, and has mean zero and covariance matrix Σ_e.

This model delineates a situation where the true covariate X is more variable than the surrogate X^*. For example, in herbicide studies, the amount of herbicide applied to a plant is measurable, denoted by X^*, but the actual amount X absorbed by the plant cannot be precisely measured, and it usually differs from the applied amount X^*. In this case, it is more reasonable to treat X as a function of X^* than to think of X^* varying around X. In radiation epidemiology, the Berkson model is useful to characterize radiation exposure of a patient. It says that the true, absorbed dose is equal to the prescribed or estimated dose plus measurement error, and thereby the true, absorbed dose has more variability than the estimated dose.

Remark

The classical additive error model and the Berkson model are perhaps the most popular models used in the subject of measurement error. When using these models, the error term e is usually assumed to have zero mean so that the surrogate X^* is an unbiased version of the true covariate X, hence $E(X^*) = E(X)$. These two models differ in the perspective of viewing the relationship between X^* and X, where one is treated as a dependent variable and the other is regarded as an independent variable. The choice of a suitable model is largely dependent on specific contexts (Carroll et al. 2006, §2.2). In many applications, the usage of these models is coupled with a specified distributional form for the error term e. Constantly, e is assumed to have a normal distribution $N(0, \Sigma_e)$ where Σ_e is the covariance matrix with possibly unknown parameters, denoted by σ_e. More flexibly, a mixture of normal distributions may be assumed for e, as discussed by Carroll, Roeder and Wasserman (1999).

Latent Variable Model

In some applications, simply using a classical additive error model or a Berkson model may be too restrictive, but a mixture of these two models offers flexibility in modeling measurement error processes. In this case, using a latent variable may be helpful to express the relationship between X and X^*:

$$X = u + e_{\text{C}} \text{ and } X^* = u + e_{\text{B}}, \tag{2.25}$$

where u is a latent variable having mean μ_u and covariance matrix Σ_u, and e_{C} and e_{B} are error terms both having mean zero and respective covariance matrices Σ_{C}

and Σ_{B}. Often, conditional on Z, mutual independence is assumed among u, e_{C} and e_{B} together with a marginal distribution for each variable.

An extreme form of model (2.25) corresponds to a classical additive model or a Berkson model. Setting $\Sigma_{\text{C}} = 0$ for model (2.25) gives model (2.23), and constraining $\Sigma_{\text{B}} = 0$ for model (2.25) yields model (2.24). In situations where Σ_{C} and Σ_{B} are nonzero matrices, model (2.25) is viewed as a mixture of a classical additive model and a Berkson model (Reeves et al. 1998). Model (2.25) may also be used to feature transformed variables. For example, Mallick, Hoffman and Carroll (2002) considered model (2.25) with the logarithm transformation applied to X and X^*.

Other forms of latent variables may be employed to delineate more complex relationship between X and X^*. For example, Li, Shao and Palta (2005) considered a latent model to analyze data arising from a Sleep Cohort Study. The true covariate X represents the severity of sleep-disordered breathing (SDB), and the observed surrogate X^* is the apnea-hypopnea index (AHI) which records the number of breathing pauses per unit time of sleep. If SDB is positive, the observed AHI can be larger or smaller than SDB, but cannot be negative; if SDB is zero, the AHI can only be larger than or equal to the true value of SDB. To feature this kind of measurement error, the following model is adopted:

$$X^* = \max(0, u + e) \text{ and } X = \max(0, u),$$

where u is a latent variable and assumes a normal distribution; e is the measurement error on the latent variable, independent of u, and follows the distribution $N(0, \sigma_e^2)$ with variance σ_e^2.

Multiplicative Model

Classical additive error and Berkson models characterize measurement error by facilitating the *difference* between the surrogate covariate X^* and the true covariate X. The magnitude of measurement error in the true covariate X may also be quantified through other forms; *multiplicative models* are among such instances (Iturria, Carroll and Firth 1999). To illustrate this, we consider the case where X and X^* are scalar; extensions to accommodating multidimensional covariates are straightforward with proper modifications of the presentation.

A multiplicative model is given by

$$X^* = Xe, \tag{2.26}$$

where the error term e is independent of $\{X, Z\}$. To ensure X^* to have the same mean as X, the mean of e is assumed to be 1.

Model (2.26) implies that the observed X^* must be zero if the true covariate X is zero. This feature is, for instance, used by Pierce et al. (1992) to describe the relationship between the true but unobservable radiation dose X and the available estimate X^*.

Another example of using model (2.26) comes from survey sampling. Hwang (1986) discussed a household survey study for which releasing measurements of some variables may reveal the identity of household owners. To preserve the privacy of participants, the measurements for those variables, denoted by X, are artificially manipulated by using model (2.26), where the error term is generated from a specified distribution. Resultant surrogate measurements X^* then replace the actual measurements of the variables X and are being reported.

Transformed Additive Model

Mathematically, a multiplicative model may become an additive error model if applied a logarithm transformation. For positive variables, taking logarithm on both sides of the multiplicative model (2.26) yields an additive error model. More generally, Eckert, Carroll and Wang (1997) proposed a *transformed additive error model*

$$g(X^*) = g(X) + e, \tag{2.27}$$

where $g(\cdot)$ is a monotone transformation function, and error term e is assumed to be independent of $\{X, Z\}$.

Taking $g(v) = \log(v)$ gives a multiplicative error model, while setting $g(v) = v$ recovers an additive error model. To accommodate complex measurement error structures, $g(\cdot)$ may assume a form from the Box–Cox transformations or piecewise-polynomial spline functions. More generally, model (2.27) may be extended by allowing different transformations, say, $g^*(\cdot)$ and $g(\cdot)$ on X^* and X, respectively:

$$g^*(X^*) = g(X) + e.$$

The inclusion of parameters in the specification of function $g(\cdot)$ is also possible. For instance, setting $g^*(v) = v$ and $g(v) = \gamma_0 + \gamma_1 v + \gamma_2 v^2 + \ldots + \gamma_r v^r$ for a positive integer r gives a *polynomial measurement error model* where $\gamma_0, \gamma_1, \gamma_2, \ldots$, and γ_r are parameters.

Regression Model

The foregoing models are often useful for settings where the surrogate X^* is independent of error-free covariate Z, given the error-prone covariate X. In some applications, however, the surrogate covariate X^* depends on not only error-prone covariate X but also error-free covariate Z. A regression model may be used to reflect this dependence:

$$X^* = \alpha_0 + \Gamma_x X + \Gamma_z Z + e, \tag{2.28}$$

where the error term e is independent of $\{X, Z\}$ and has mean zero and covariance matrix Σ_e, α_0 is a $p_x \times 1$ vector, Γ_x is a $p_x \times p_x$ matrix, Γ_z is a $p_x \times p_z$ matrix, and p_z is the dimension of Z. Different specifications of the matrices characterize various measurement error models. For instance, setting $\alpha_0 = 0_{p_x}$, $\Gamma_x = I_{p_x}$ and $\Gamma_z = 0_{p_x \times p_z}$ gives a classical additive model, where 0_d represents a $d \times 1$ zero vector for a positive integer d, and $0_{d_1 \times d_2}$ stands for a $d_1 \times d_2$ zero matrix for positive integers d_1 and d_2.

Dually, switching X and X^* in model (2.28) gives a different model

$$X = \alpha_0 + \Gamma_x X^* + \Gamma_z Z + e, \tag{2.29}$$

where e is assumed to be independent of $\{X^*, Z\}$. This model generalizes the Berkson model and facilitates the correlation between the true covariate X and Z.

The elements of matrices Σ_e, Γ_x and Γ_z in (2.28) and (2.29) are often unknown and need to be estimated. A normal distribution is commonly assumed for the error term e in (2.28) or (2.29).

Misclassification Model

The preceding models concern cases where continuous covariate X is subject to measurement error. In settings where X is a vector of discrete variables subject to *misclassification*, two methods may be employed to characterize misclassification processes. The difference between those two methods is reflected by choosing conditioning variables when modeling; they are somewhat analogous to those differences between a classical additive model and a Berkson model for continuous error-prone covariates. Conditional on error-free covariate Z, one method is to model the conditional probability $P(X^* = x^*|X = x, Z)$ by treating X^* to depend on X while the other approach modulates X to be conditional on X^* via the conditional probability $P(X = x|X^* = x^*, Z)$. Sometimes the probabilities $P(X^* = x^*|X = x, Z)$ are called the *misclassification probabilities* (e.g., Buonaccorsi, Laake and Veierød 2005) to distinguish from the *reclassification probabilities* $P(X = x|X^* = x^*, Z)$ termed by Spiegelman, Rosner and Logan (2000). With a binary variable X, $P(X^* = 1|X = 1)$ and $P(X^* = 0|X = 0)$ are also called *sensitivity* and *specificity*, respectively. In this book, we loosely call these conditional probabilities *(mis)classification probabilities*.

As an example, we consider a special but commonly occurring situation where X is a binary scalar variable. Let $\pi_{10} = P(X^* = 0|X = 1, Z)$ and $\pi_{01} = P(X^* = 1|X = 0, Z)$. Regression models for binary data, such as logistic regression models, are often employed to describe the dependence of (mis)classification probabilities through their dependence on covariates, bearing in mind that other parametric modeling may be employed for individual problems:

$$\text{logit}\, \pi_{10} = \alpha_{00} + \alpha_{0z}^{\mathrm{T}} Z \ \text{ and } \ \text{logit}\, \pi_{01} = \alpha_{10} + \alpha_{1z}^{\mathrm{T}} Z,$$

where $\alpha_{00}, \alpha_{0z}, \alpha_{10}$, and α_{1z} are the regression parameters.

General Modeling Strategy

The aforementioned models portray scenarios of either measurement error or misclassification, but not both. When error-contaminated variables involve both discrete and continuous variables, modeling of measurement error and misclassification processes becomes more complicated. Here we discuss two strategies for handling the conditional probability density or mass function $h(x^*|x, z)$; dealing with $h(x|x^*, z)$ may proceed in the same principle.

The first strategy emphasizes the different nature of continuous and discrete covariates. Write $X = (X_{\mathrm{C}}^{\mathrm{T}}, X_{\mathrm{D}}^{\mathrm{T}})^{\mathrm{T}}$ so that X_{C} and X_{D} represent subvectors containing continuous and discrete covariate components, respectively. Let X_{C}^* and X_{D}^* denote the observed surrogate measurements of X_{C} and X_{D}, respectively, and write $X^* = (X_{\mathrm{C}}^{*\mathrm{T}}, X_{\mathrm{D}}^{*\mathrm{T}})^{\mathrm{T}}$. To model measurement error and misclassification processes, we would not attempt to directly modulate the entire conditional distribution function $h(x_{\mathrm{C}}^*, x_{\mathrm{D}}^*|x, z)$, instead, we *separately* postulate the measurement error process and the misclassification process by using the factorization

$$h(x_{\mathrm{C}}^*, x_{\mathrm{D}}^*|x, z) = h(x_{\mathrm{C}}^*|x_{\mathrm{D}}^*, x, z)h(x_{\mathrm{D}}^*|x, z).$$

It is often reasonable to assume that $h(x_{\mathrm{C}}^*|x_{\mathrm{D}}^*, x, z) = h(x_{\mathrm{C}}^*|x, z)$, saying that the surrogate X_{C}^* is independent of the surrogate X_{D}^*, given the true covariates $\{X, Z\}$. Therefore, to model $h(x_{\mathrm{C}}^*, x_{\mathrm{D}}^*|x, z)$, it suffices to separately model a measurement error process for $h(x_{\mathrm{C}}^*|x, z)$ and a misclassification process for $h(x_{\mathrm{D}}^*|x, z)$, using the foregoing modeling strategies. An example of using this strategy was given by Yi et al. (2015).

Alternatively, one may ignore the nature of discreteness or continuousness of covariates and use the factorization strategy to obtain a sequence of conditional probability density or mass functions for a *univariate* variable. To do so, we spell out all components of X^* individually by writing $X^* = (X_1^*, \ldots, X_{p_x}^*)$. Then the factorization

$$h(x^*|x, z) = h(x_1^*|x, z) \prod_{k=2}^{p_x} h(x_k^*|x_1^*, \ldots, x_{k-1}^*, x, z) \tag{2.30}$$

offers a way to characterize $h(x^*|x, z)$ via modeling a sequence of probability density or mass functions of the right-hand side of (2.30), which is easily implemented by standard model techniques for a univariate variable. An application of this strategy was provided by Spiegelman, Rosner and Logan (2000).

Although a number of measurement error and misclassification models are outlined here, one must be reminded that those models are not exhaustive. In fact, they are far from adequate to handle all practical problems. Other treatments of measurement error and misclassification processes are possible. For instance, to protect us against misspecification of measurement error models, Carroll and Wand (1991) developed an estimation method for logistic regression parameters where the measurement error model is not explicitly specified and is handled with the kernel regression techniques. The nonclassical measurement error model considered by Prentice et al. (2002) is not explicitly discussed in the book, but it may be useful for a range of settings, especially in situations where the "instrument" used in the study involves self-report information. Discussion on this aspect also appears in §9.1.

The preceding discussion is directed towards the case where covariates are subject to measurement error or misclassification. Although the same principles may be broadly applied to other error-contaminated situations, technical details may be quite different from problem to problem. Generally speaking, measurement error and misclassification problems are divided into three categories: (1) only covariates are subject to measurement error, misclassification, or both, (2) only the response variable is subject to measurement error (if it is continuous) or misclassification (if it is discrete), and (3) the response variable and covariates are subject to measurement error or misclassification. In this book, we mainly look at inference methods for problems falling into the first category. Discussion on the second category is deferred to Chapter 8, where a brief discussion on the third category is also provided.

2.7 Measurement Error and Misclassification Examples

In the foregoing sections, we outline the issues on dealing with measurement error and misclassification problems. Modeling and inference strategies are sketched in general terms to reflect common features or similarities for analysis of error-contaminated data. With different application settings, those procedures need to be further elaborated and modified in order to fully incorporate problem-specific characteristics. In subsequent chapters, we present modeling and inference methods for a variety of areas in greater details. We conclude this chapter with several examples of measurement error or misclassification, each related to the development of a chapter followed. More mismeasurement examples were discussed by Carroll et al. (2006, Ch. 1) and the references therein.

2.7.1 Survival Data Example: Busselton Health Study

Survival data concern time to events, which are encountered frequently in medical research, epidemiological studies and industrial application. Survival times may be defined as times to death, times to occurrence of a disease or a complication, or times from changing one condition to another. It is common that survival data contain error-contaminated covariate measurements.

Here we discuss the data arising from the Busselton Health Study which were collected by a repeated cross-sectional survey in the community of Busselton in Western Australia from 1966 to 1981. Health surveys gathered data for couples on demographic variables and general health and lifestyle variables as well as survival information. Detailed descriptions of this study were provided by Knuiman et al. (1994).

Table 2.1 displays a sample data set, where "PAIR" labels the identification number of spouse pairs; "AGE" records the age of a study subject at survey (in year); "SEX" reports the gender of each study subject; "SBP" and "DBP", respectively, refer to systolic blood pressure and diastolic blood pressure (in mmHg); "BMI" displays body mass index (in kg/m^2); "CHOL" is totalcholesterol level (in mmol/l); "DIAB" records the history of diabetes (1 if diabetes, and 0 otherwise); "SURV" stands for survival time from survey date to date last known alive (in year); and "CENS" indexes whether or not a study subject died (1 for death, and 0 otherwise). Variable "SMOKE" shows the smoking status, coded as 1, 2, 3, 4, and 5, to respectively correspond to "never smoked", "ex-smoker", "current smoker with less

Table 2.1. *Sample Data of the Busselton Health Study*

PAIR	AGE	SEX	SBP	DBP	BMI	CHOL	DIAB	SMOKE	DRINK	SURV	CENS
1	50.4	F	127	82	24.61	6.32	0	2	3	25.9	1
1	52.3	M	145	92	27.37	6.13	0	4	1	28.1	0
2	40.3	F	132	98	26.39	5.13	0	1	1	25.1	0
2	40.5	M	156	76	29.54	5.79	0	2	4	25.1	0
3	56.5	F	141	82	39.66	6.92	0	1	2	23.4	1
3	66.8	M	97	56	23.63	7.11	0	4	3	11.7	1
4	38.9	F	169	102	23.10	4.87	0	2	1	17.1	0
4	66.5	M	171	96	20.24	4.16	0	4	1	2.8	1
5	49.7	F	185	90	22.67	7.71	0	1	3	28.1	0
5	52.4	M	131	92	27.16	6.05	0	1	3	28.1	0

than 15 cigarettes/day", "current smoker with no less than 15 cigarettes/day", and "smokes pipe or cigars only"; and variable "DRINK" represents alcohol consumption, coded as 1, 2, 3, 4, and 5, to respectively feature "non-drinker", "ex-drinker", "light drinker", "moderate drinker", and "heavy drinker".

An objective of the study was to evaluate the effect of cardiovascular risk factors on the risk of death due to coronary heart disease (Knuiman et al. 1994). The data set considered by Yi and Lawless (2007) includes survival information for 2306 spouse pairs. Of these, 2266 pairs have at least one censored response (i.e., at least one member of the couple was still alive at the final observation time). It is known that measurements of the risk factors, such as blood pressure and cholesterol level, are subject to measurement error due to the inherent nature of those variables. In the analysis of data with those error-prone covariates, it is important to take the measurement error effects into account.

2.7.2 Recurrent Event Example: rhDNase Data

Recurrent event data arise frequently from biomedical sciences, demographical studies, and industrial research. Examples include seizures of epileptic patients, successive tumors in cancer patients, multiple births in a woman's lifetime, and times to warranty claims for a manufactured item. Mismeasurements may occur in data collection of recurrent events.

As an example, we discuss a data set arising from a study of pulmonary exacerbations and rhDNase. Fuchs et al. (1994) reported on a double-blind randomized multicenter clinical trial designed to assess the effect of rhDNase, a recombinant deoxyribonuclease I enzyme, versus placebo on the occurrence of respiratory exacerbations among patients with cystic fibrosis. The rhDNase operates by digesting the extracellular DNA released by leukocytes that accumulate in the lung as a result of bacterial infection and, thus, aerosol administration of rhDNase would be expected to reduce the incidence of exacerbations (Cook and Lawless 2007, p. 365).

Six hundred and forty-five patients were recruited in this trial. Each subject was followed up for about 169 days. Data on the occurrence and resolution of all exacerbations were recorded. Treatment assignment and two baseline measurements of forced expiratory volume (FEV) reflecting lung capacity were available for each patient. In addition, the number of days from randomization to the beginning of the exacerbations was recorded, as well as the day on which treatment for each exacerbation ended and patients became at risk of a new exacerbation. It is of interest to evaluate whether the treatment has the desired effect on reducing the incidence of exacerbations and how covariate FEV is associated with exacerbations. Here FEV refers to the long-term average of forced expiratory volume for a patient, however, available baseline replicate measurements are bound to be subject to variability from this long-term average.

Table 2.2 displays a sample of the data, where "ID" shows the patient identification number, "TRT" is the treatment indicator (1 if treated and 0 otherwise), "FEV1" and "FEV2" record two baseline measurements of FEV, "EVENT" shows the number of respiratory exacerbations, Column Bj reports on the number of days from randomization to the beginning of the jth exacerbation, and column Ej displays the day on which treatment for the jth exacerbation ended and patients became at risk for a new exacerbation for $j = 1, 2, \ldots$. A complete data set is available from Cook and Lawless (2007).

Table 2.2. *Sample Data of the Study of Pulmonary Exacerbations and rhDNase*

ID	TRT	FEV1	FEV2	EVENT	B1	E1	B2	E2	...
493301	1	28.8	28.1	0					
493305	0	67.2	68.7	1	65	75			
589303	0	112.0	110.7	2	60	74	83	124	
589307	1	96.0	94.5	0					
589310	1	70.4	70.1	2	35	64	71	108	

2.7.3 Longitudinal Data Example: Framingham Heart Study

The Framingham Heart Study is a longitudinal prospective study of risk factors for cardiovascular disease (CVD). The objective of the study was to identify common factors or characteristics that contribute to CVD by following its development over a long period of time. The study followed up a large group of participants who had not yet developed overt symptoms of CVD or suffered a heart attack or stroke (Kannel et al. 1986).

Among potential risk factors, age at the study entry, body mass index, and smoking status are error-free variables, while systolic blood pressure and serum cholesterol are variables measured with error. As discussed by Carroll et al. (2006, p. 12), systolic blood pressure is the main predictor of interest, but its long-term average X is impossible to measure. Instead, a specific measurement X^* at a clinic visit is available. The long-term measurement X and a single-visit measurement X^* are generally different due to daily and seasonal variation, and confounding factors.

2.7.4 Multi-State Model Example: HL Data

Hairy leukoplakia (HL) is an oral lesion that is thought to have prognostic significance for the progression of HIV disease. HL appears as a whitish lesion on the lateral border of the tongue and is usually diagnosed by visual oral examination. Routine oral examinations, however, often overlook HL lesions. For instance, in a study of comparing diagnoses made by oral medicine specialists and trained medical assistants, Hilton et al. (2001) found that the medical assistants detected HL in only 12 of the 40 patients diagnosed with HL by oral medicine clinicians. In the study of Bureau, Shiboski and Hughes (2003), it was estimated that the probability of a positive diagnosis of HL for a HL free individual (i.e., a false positive rate) is 3.4% with standard error 0.006, and the probability of a negative diagnosis of HL for a subject with HL (i.e., a false negative rate) is 24.2% with standard error 0.025.

Misdiagnosis of HL lesions comes from different sources. Although HL lesions tend to be fairly persistent, spontaneous remission and reappearance may occur in some patients. In addition, HL lesions respond to treatment with antiviral drugs (for example, Acyclovir). Other oral lesions may be misdiagnosed as HL or co-occur with HL (for example, oral candidiasis), thus leading to false positive or false negative diagnoses. To study potential risk factors for development and remission of HL, it is important to accommodate misdiagnosis (i.e., misclassified outcome) in the analysis.

Bureau, Shiboski and Hughes (2003) presented a data set of those subjects who were assessed at most 4 times with intervals between visits being approximately 6 months. For subject i let Y_{ik} and Y_{ik}^* represent the true HL status and the diagnostic value at time point t_k, respectively, where taking value 1 or 0, respectively, corresponds to having HL or HL free for $k = 1, 2, 3, 4$; and Z_i represents CD4 counts for subject i that were categorized to assume three values, 1, 2, and 3, respectively, corresponding to the range: CD4 count < 200, $200 <$ CD4 count ≤ 500, and CD4 count > 500.

It is interesting to study how the transition among the Y_{ik} is associated with covariate Z_i. However, the Y_{ik} are not precisely measured, and their observed values Y_{ik}^* may differ from Y_{ik}. Table 2.3 records the frequencies of the observed value of HL for the individuals classified by the CD4 counts, together with the frequencies of the observed diagnostic HL for those individuals whose CD4 counts are unknown.

2.7.5 Case–Control Study Example: HSV Data

The data discussed by Carroll, Gail and Lubin (1993) were collected from a case–control study for which the primary objective was to examine the association between invasive cervical cancer and exposure to herpes simplex virus type 2 (HSV-2). The biological background was provided by Hildesheim et al. (1991).

Exposure to HSV-2 was assessed by a refined western blot procedure, denoted as X, or a less accurate western blot procedure, denoted as X^*, for cases ($Y = 1$) and

Table 2.3. *HL Data (Bureau, Shiboski and Hughes 2003)*

Observed HL				CD4 count			No stratification
Y_{i1}^*	Y_{i2}^*	Y_{i3}^*	Y_{i4}^*	$Z_i = 1$	$Z_i = 2$	$Z_i = 3$	
1	0			10	6	5	18
1	1			17	23	6	39
0	0			45	101	100	207
0	1			7	9	4	18
1	1	0		2	4		6
1	1	1		6	12		26
1	0	0		7			12
1	0	1		2			4
0	1	0					8
0	1	1					6
0	0	0		23	59	76	184
0	0	1		5	2	2	8
1	1	1	0				8
1	1	1	1				18
0	0	0	0				153
0	0	0	1				6

Table 2.4. *HSV Data from a Case–Control Study (Carroll, Gail and Lubin 1993)*

	Y	X	X^*	FREQ
Validation data	1	0	0	13
	1	0	1	3
	1	1	0	5
	1	1	1	18
	0	0	0	33
	0	0	1	11
	0	1	0	16
	0	1	1	16
Main study data	1		0	318
	1		1	375
	0		0	701
	0		1	535

controls ($Y = 0$). Less than 6% of the subjects were observed with the test result X. Measurements X^* based on the less accurate western blot test were available for all subjects. The complete data are reported in Table 2.4, where "FREQ" records the frequency for each category.

To study the relationship between Y and X, one may use the validation data alone, since measurements of both Y and X are available. But this usage of the data would incur considerable efficiency loss as data from about 94% subjects with measurements of (Y, X^*) were thrown away. If also using all the measurements X^* in the main study to examine the relationship between Y and X, misclassification in X needs to be incorporated in inferential procedures.

2.8 Bibliographic Notes and Discussion

Research on measurement error and misclassification problems has not been just restricted to the statistics community; it has also been active in many other fields, including medical, health and epidemiological studies as well as econometrics. Several synonyms for "*measurement error*" or "*misclassification*" are commonly used in the literature, including "*predictors measured with error*", "*errors-in-variables*", "*covariate measurement error*", "*measurement error models*", "*mismeasurement*", "*response error*", "*error-prone data*", and "*error-contaminated data*", etc.

Many researchers examined measurement error effects in varying settings and proposed correction methods to account for these effects. To name a few, see Berkson (1950), Richardson and Wu (1970), Carroll and Gallo (1982), Carroll et al. (1984), Stefanski (1985), Stefanski and Carroll (1985), Selén (1986), Prentice (1986), Gleser, Carroll and Gallo (1987), Chesher (1991), Pepe and Fleming (1991), Carroll and Stefanski (1994), Wang, Carroll and Liang (1996), Carroll and Ruppert (1996), Carroll (1997), Dagenais and Dagenais (1997), Coffin and Sukhatme (1997), Reeves et al. (1998), Cheng, Schneeweiss and Thamerus (2000), Gustafson (2002), Hong and Tamer (2003), Wang (2003, 2007), Kim and Saleh (2005), Thiébaut et al. (2007), Gorfine et al. (2007), Li and Greene (2008), Wei and Carroll (2009), Huang and Tebbs (2009), Carroll, Chen and Hu (2010), Prentice and Huang (2011), and Kipnis et al. (2016), among many others.

It is known that measurement error and misclassification may seriously degrade the quality of inference and should be avoided whenever possible. Improving measurement procedures and designs of data collection may sometimes reduce or eliminate measurement error or misclassification. For example, in designing questionnaires for survey sampling, properly wording the questions and involving more experienced interviewers may help collect more accurate measurements. But in many situations, it is inevitable that collected measurements contain error due to the nature of the variables themselves. It is necessary and important to develop statistical strategies to cope with this issue.

There are instances where ignoring measurement error in data analysis does not really matter, but the problem is that we are not sure when this happens. Understanding measurement error effects and developing valid inference methods to accommodating them enable us to deal with various error-prone data more comprehensively. The study of measurement error problems offers us opportunities to unveil the truth that is obscured by the presence of measurement error or misclassification.

Concerns on measurement error effects date back at least to Adcock (1878). Early work includes the investigations of the effects of mismeasurements on inferences. For instance, Stouffer (1936) observed that estimates of partial correlations can be biased when the variables are measured with error. Aigner (1973) showed that with misclassification in a binary covariate, the least squares estimator is biased downward. Modelling of measurement error has a long history, see, for instance, Wald (1940), Madansky (1959) and the references therein for early work. Research on measurement error models has been increasingly growing over the past few decades. It is difficult to supply a complete list of work in this area (e.g., Yi 2009). Many interesting references on diverse topics can be found in the books by Fuller (1987), Gustafson (2004), Carroll et al. (2006), and Buonaccorsi (2010), as well as the reference list of this book.

As commented by Carroll et al. (2006, pp. 23–24), the lack of conventional notation makes it difficult to read papers in this area. Unfortunately, we are not able to use the notation adopted by Carroll et al. (2006) but have to create a new set of key symbols for a coherent presentation of this book. We use X and Z to represent the true covariate vectors, where X is reserved for error-prone covariates and Z for error-free ones. Following the convention, we let Y denote the response variable in this book except for Chapters 3 and 4 where, instead, we use T to denote the survival time, and $N(t)$ the number of events occurring over time period $[0, t]$. The Greek letter β is reserved for the parameter vector associated with the response process that is of primary interest, and θ is *often* adopted to denote the vector of all associated variables in the model, including nuisance parameters which are often written as $\alpha, \gamma, \vartheta, \sigma_e$, etc. Notation $U(\beta; y, x, z)$ is usually used to denote an unbiased estimating function of β derived from the model for $\{Y, X, Z\}$.

Intending to provide an easy way to match connected quantities, we use superscripts and subscripts as well. To correspond surrogate variables to their true error-prone variables, we add asterisks to the true variables to denote the corresponding surrogate measurements. For example, X^* stands for a surrogate version of X, and Y^* stands for a surrogate version of Y. As opposed to β representing a parameter vector under the model for $\{Y, X, Z\}$, β^* is used to denote a corresponding parameter vector for the naive analysis which disregards the difference between X^* and X, or/and the difference between Y^* and Y. Corresponding to the estimating function $U(\beta; y, x, z)$, we usually use $U^*(\beta; y, x^*, z)$ to represent an unbiased estimating function for β which is expressed in terms of the observable variables $\{Y, X^*, Z\}$.

Superscripts $^{\text{Y}}, ^{\text{X}}$ and ^{Z}, or subscripts y, x and z, are used to indicate the association of certain quantities with the processes, respectively, corresponding to Y, X and Z. Subscripts i and j are used to index subjects and replicated measurements, respectively.

Although great effort is paid to make different quantities be expressed by different symbols, it is unavoidable that the same symbol may be used to refer to different meanings at different places. For precise meaning of each symbol, we should look up the chapter in which the symbol appears.

2.9 Supplementary Problems

2.1. Suppose $\{(Y_i, X_i) : i = 1, \ldots, n\}$ is a sequence of independently and identically distributed random variables. Consider a simple regression model

$$Y_i = \beta_0 + \beta_x X_i + \epsilon_i \tag{2.31}$$

for $i = 1, \ldots, n$, where β_0 and β_x are regression parameters, and the ϵ_i are mutually independent and independent of the X_i and have mean zero and variance σ_ϵ^2. Suppose covariate X_i is subject to measurement error and X_i^* is an observed version of X_i. Assume that X_i has variance σ_x^2.

(a) Assume that the measurement error model is

$$X_i^* = X_i + e_i \tag{2.32}$$

for $i = 1, \ldots, n$, where the e_i are mutually independent and independent of the $\{\epsilon_i, X_i\}$ and have mean zero and variance σ_e^2.

(i) Let $\widehat{\beta}_x^*$ denote the least squares estimator of β_x obtained from fitting model (2.31) with X_i replaced by X_i^*. Show that

$$\widehat{\beta}_x^* \xrightarrow{p} \omega\beta_x \text{ as } n \to \infty,$$

where $\omega = \sigma_x^2/(\sigma_x^2 + \sigma_e^2)$.

(ii) Can you work out the asymptotic variance of $\widehat{\beta}_x^*$? Do you need to make any assumptions?

(iii) Let $\widehat{\beta}_x$ denote the least squares estimator obtained from fitting model (2.31) if X_i were available. Work out the asymptotic variance of $\widehat{\beta}_x$. Do you need to make any assumptions?

(iv) Compare the asymptotic variances of $\widehat{\beta}_x^*$ and $\widehat{\beta}_x$.

(v) Further assume that ϵ_i and e_i follow normal distributions. Can you work out the conditional distribution of Y_i given X_i^*?

(b) Suppose the measurement error model is instead given by

$$X_i = X_i^* + e_i \tag{2.33}$$

for $i = 1, \ldots, n$, where the e_i are mutually independent and independent of the $\{\epsilon_i, X_i^*\}$ and have mean zero and variance σ_e^2. Repeat the discussion on the similar questions in (a). Comment on the differences between the results of (a) and (b).

2.2. Consider model (2.31). Suppose response Y_i is subject to measurement error and Y_i^* is an observed version of Y_i. Let $\widehat{\beta}_x$ denote the least squares estimator of β_x obtained from fitting model (2.31) with Y_i replaced by Y_i^*, and $\widehat{\beta}_x$ be the least squares estimator of β_x obtained from fitting model (2.31) assuming Y_i were available.

(a) Assume that the measurement error model is

$$Y_i^* = Y_i + e_i$$

for $i = 1, \ldots, n$, where the e_i are mutually independent and independent of the $\{Y_i, \epsilon_i\}$ and have mean zero and variance σ_e^2. Repeat the discussion on the similar questions in Problem 2.1 (a).

(b) Suppose the measurement error model is instead given by

$$Y_i = Y_i^* + e_i$$

for $i = 1, \ldots, n$, where the e_i are mutually independent and independent of the $\{Y_i^*, \epsilon_i\}$ and have mean zero and variance σ_e^2. Repeat the discussion on the questions similar to (a). Comment on the differences between the results of (a) and (b).

2.3. Consider model (2.31). Suppose both X_i and Y_i are subject to measurement error and their observed versions are X_i^* and Y_i^*, respectively. Let $\widehat{\beta}_x^*$ denote the least squares estimator obtained from fitting model (2.31) with X_i replaced by X_i^* and Y_i replaced by Y_i^*.

Suppose covariate measurement error is described by model

$$X_i^* = \alpha_{x0} + \alpha_{x1} X_i + e_{xi}$$

with e_{xi} assumed independent of $\{\epsilon_i, X_i\}$, or model

$$X_i = \alpha_{x0} + \alpha_{x1} X_i^* + e_{xi}$$

with e_{xi} assumed independent of $\{\epsilon_i, X_i^*\}$, where $i = 1, \ldots, n$; e_{xi} has mean zero and variance σ_{ex}^2; and α_{x0} and α_{x1} are regression coefficients.

Suppose response error is described by model

$$Y_i^* = \alpha_{y0} + \alpha_{y1} Y_i + e_{yi}$$

with e_{yi} assumed independent of $\{Y_i, e_{xi}\}$, or model

$$Y_i = \alpha_{y0} + \alpha_{y1} Y_i^* + e_{yi}$$

with e_{yi} assumed independent of $\{Y_i^*, e_{xi}\}$, where $i = 1, \ldots, n$; e_{yi} has mean zero and variance σ_{ey}^2; and α_{y0} and α_{y1} are regression coefficients.

For each combination of the measurement error models, work out the following problems.

(a) Repeat the discussion on the similar questions in Problem 2.1 (a).
(b) Discuss identifiability issues for the model parameters.

(c) The measurement error mechanisms discussed in §2.4 are classified for the situation with covariate measurement error only. Are those classification mechanisms still meaningful for the case with measurement error in both response and covariate variables? What modifications may be done in order to feature useful measurement error mechanisms?

2.4. Consider model (2.31). We are interested in testing the null hypothesis H_o : $\beta_x = c$ where c is a given value of interest. Suppose covariate X_i is subject to measurement error and X_i^* is an observed version of X_i. Assume that the measurement error model is given by (2.32) or (2.33).

(a) Construct a test statistic for testing H_o using the observed data $\{(Y_i, X_i^*) : i = 1, \ldots, n\}$.

(b) If the true covariate X_i were available, construct a test statistic for testing H_o using the true measurements $\{(Y_i, X_i) : i = 1, \ldots, n\}$.

(c) Compare the two test procedures in terms of the Type I error and the power for the hypothesis with zero c or nonzero c.

2.5.

(a) Can you repeat the discussion in Problem 2.4 for the case where the response variable Y_i is subject to measurement error?

(b) What if both X_i and Y_i are subject to measurement error? Does the issue of model identifiability become a concern?

2.6. Suppose $\{(Y_i, X_i, Z_i) : i = 1, \ldots, n\}$ is a sequence of independently and identically distributed random variables, where Y_i is the response variable and X_i and Z_i are covariates. Consider a multiple regression model

$$Y_i = \beta_0 + \beta_x^{\mathrm{T}} X_i + \beta_z^{\mathrm{T}} Z_i + \epsilon_i \tag{2.34}$$

for $i = 1, \ldots n$, where the ϵ_i are mutually independent and independent of $\{X_i, Z_i\}$ and have mean zero and variance σ^2.

Suppose covariate X_i is subject to measurement error and X_i^* is an observed version of X_i. Assume that the covariance matrix of $\{X_i, Z_i\}$ is

$$\mathrm{var}\begin{pmatrix} X_i \\ Z_i \end{pmatrix} = \begin{pmatrix} \Sigma_x & \Sigma_{xz} \\ \Sigma_{zx} & \Sigma_z \end{pmatrix}$$

with $\Sigma_{xz} = \Sigma_{zx}^{\mathrm{T}}$.

(a) Assume that the measurement error model is

$$X_i^* = X_i + e_i \tag{2.35}$$

for $i = 1, \ldots, n$, where the e_i are mutually independent and independent of the $\{Y_i, X_i, Z_i\}$ and have mean zero and covariance matrix Σ_e.

(i) Let $\widehat{\beta}^* = (\widehat{\beta}_x^{*\mathrm{T}}, \widehat{\beta}_z^{*\mathrm{T}})^{\mathrm{T}}$ be the least squares estimator obtained from fitting model (2.34) with X_i replaced by X_i^*. When $n \to \infty$, what does $\widehat{\beta}^*$ converge to in probability?

(ii) Can you work out the asymptotic covariance matrix of $\widehat{\beta}_x^*$? Do you need to make any assumptions?

(iii) Let $\widehat{\beta}_x$ denote the least squares estimator obtained from fitting model (2.34) assuming that X_i were available. Can you work out the asymptotic covariance of $\widehat{\beta}_x$? Do you need to make any assumptions?

(iv) Compare the asymptotic covariances of $\widehat{\beta}_x^*$ and $\widehat{\beta}_x$.

(v) Assume that ϵ_i and e_i follow normal distributions. Can you find the conditional distribution of Y_i given $\{X_i^*, Z_i\}$?

(vi) We are interested in testing $H_o : \beta_x = 0$. Construct two test statistics each using variables $\{(Y_i, X_i^*, Z_i) : i = 1, \ldots, n\}$ and $\{(Y_i, X_i, Z_i) : i = 1, \ldots, n\}$. Compare the performance of those two test statistics in terms of the Type I error and the power.

(vii) We are interested in testing $H_o : \beta_z = 0$. Construct two test statistics each using variables $\{(Y_i, X_i^*, Z_i) : i = 1, \ldots, n\}$ and $\{(Y_i, X_i, Z_i) : i = 1, \ldots, n\}$. Compare the performance of those two test statistics in terms of the Type I error and the power.

(b) Suppose the measurement error model is instead given by

$$X_i = X_i^* + e_i \tag{2.36}$$

for $i = 1, \ldots, n$, where the e_i are mutually independent and independent of the $\{X_i^*, Z_i, Y_i\}$ and have mean zero and covariance matrix Σ_e. Repeat the discussion on the questions similar to those in (a).

2.7. Consider a different version of model (2.34) where X_i is a scalar binary covariate subject to misclassification. Suppose X_i^* is an observed version of X_i, and the nondifferential misclassification mechanism holds. Repeat the discussion in Problem 2.6 for the following misclassification models.

(a) The misclassification probabilities are given by

$$\pi_{01} = P(X_i^* = 1|X_i = 0) \text{ and } \pi_{10} = P(X_i^* = 0|X_i = 1).$$

(b) The misclassification probabilities are given by

$$\pi_{01}^* = P(X_i = 1|X_i^* = 0) \text{ and } \pi_{10}^* = P(X_i = 0|X_i^* = 1).$$

(Buonaccorsi, Laake and Veierød 2005)

2.8. Let $H(\theta; \theta^*)$ be defined by (2.15). Show that for any $\theta_1, \theta_2 \in \Theta$,

$$H(\theta_1; \theta_2) \leq H(\theta_2; \theta_2).$$

2.9. Let X_{MR}^* be defined as (2.18). Show that

(a) $E(X_{\text{MR}}^*|Y, Z) = E(X|Y, Z)$;

(b) $\text{var}(X_{\text{MR}}^*|Y, Z) = \text{var}(X|Y, Z)$;

(c) $\text{var}(X_{\text{MR}}^*, Y|Z) = \text{var}(X, Y|Z)$.

(Freedman et al. 2004)

2.10.

(a) Consider a simple case where X is a scalar binary variable with a surrogate measurement X^*. Let

$$\pi_{01} = P(X^* = 1|X = 0) \text{ and } \pi_{10} = P(X^* = 0|X = 1)$$

be the misclassification probabilities. Suppose $g(X;\beta)$ is a real valued function of X and β. Show that function

$$g^*(X^*;\beta) = \frac{g(0;\beta)(1-\pi_{10}) - g(1;\beta)\pi_{01} - X^*\{g(0;\beta) - g(1;\beta)\}}{1-\pi_{01}-\pi_{10}}$$

satisfies the requirement that

$$E\{g^*(X^*;\beta)|X\} = g(X;\beta),$$

where the conditional expectation is evaluated with respect to the conditional probability mass function of X^* given X.

(b) Generalize the result in (a) to the case where X is a categorical variable with more than two levels.

(c) Generalize the result in (a) to the case where X is a vector of binary variables.

2.11. Suppose $\{(Y_i, X_i, Z_i) : i = 1, \ldots, n\}$ is a sequence of independently and identically distributed random variables, where Y_i is the binary response variable and X_i and Z_i are covariates. Consider a logistic regression model

$$\text{logit } P(Y_i = 1|X_i, Z_i) = \beta_0 + \beta_x^{\mathrm{T}} X_i + \beta_z^{\mathrm{T}} Z_i \tag{2.37}$$

for $i = 1, \ldots, n$, where β_0, β_x and β_z are parameters. Suppose covariate X_i is subject to measurement error and X_i^* is an observed version of X_i.

(a) Assume that the measurement error model is (2.35).
   (i) Is the structure of the logistic regression model (2.37) preserved by the conditional probability function $P(Y_i = 1|X_i^*, Z_i)$?
   (ii) We are interested in testing $H_o : \beta_x = 0$. Construct two test statistics each using variables $\{(Y_i, X_i^*, Z_i) : i = 1, \ldots, n\}$ and $\{(Y_i, X_i, Z_i) : i = 1, \ldots, n\}$. Compare the performance of these two test statistics in terms of the Type I error and the power.
   (iii) We are interested in testing $H_o : \beta_z = 0$. Construct two test statistics each using variables $\{(Y_i, X_i^*, Z_i) : i = 1, \ldots, n\}$ and $\{(Y_i, X_i, Z_i) : i = 1, \ldots, n\}$. Compare the performance of these two test statistics in terms of the Type I error and the power.

(b) Suppose the measurement error model is given by (2.36). Repeat the discussion on the questions in (a).

(c) If the link function logit in model (2.37) is replaced by a probit link. How would the discussions for (a) and (b) change?

(Carroll 1989)

2.12. Suppose $\{(Y_i, X_i) : i = 1, \ldots, n\}$ is a sequence of independently and identically distributed random variables, where Y_i is the response variable and X_i is a scalar covariate. Consider a simple regression model

$$Y_i = \beta_0 + \beta_x X_i + \epsilon_i \tag{2.38}$$

for $i = 1, \ldots, n$, where the ϵ_i are mutually independent and have distribution $N(0, \sigma_{\epsilon\epsilon})$ with variance $\sigma_{\epsilon\epsilon}$.

Suppose X_i^* is an observed version of X_i and follows the model

$$X_i^* = X_i + e_i \tag{2.39}$$

for $i = 1, \ldots, n$, where the e_i are mutually independent and have distribution $N(0, \sigma_{ee})$ with variance σ_{ee}.

Assume that the (X_i, ϵ_i, e_i) are independently and identically distributed and follow

$$\begin{pmatrix} X_i \\ \epsilon_i \\ e_i \end{pmatrix} \sim N\left(\begin{pmatrix} \mu_x \\ 0 \\ 0 \end{pmatrix}, \begin{pmatrix} \sigma_{xx} & \sigma_{x\epsilon} & \sigma_{xe} \\ \sigma_{x\epsilon} & \sigma_{\epsilon\epsilon} & \sigma_{\epsilon e} \\ \sigma_{xe} & \sigma_{\epsilon e} & \sigma_{ee} \end{pmatrix} \right), \tag{2.40}$$

where μ_x and σ_{xx} are the mean and variance of X_i, respectively; $\sigma_{x\epsilon}$ is the covariance of X_i and ϵ_i; σ_{xe} is the covariance of X_i and e_i; and $\sigma_{\epsilon e}$ is the covariance of ϵ_i and e_i. Suppose that the nondifferential measurement error mechanism holds.

(a) Assume that $\sigma_{x\epsilon} = \sigma_{xe} = \sigma_{\epsilon e} = 0$ in model (2.40).

(i) Show that (Y_i, X_i^*) follows a bivariate normal distribution

$$N\left(\begin{pmatrix} \mu_y \\ \mu_x \end{pmatrix}, \begin{pmatrix} \sigma_{yy} & \sigma_{x^*y} \\ \sigma_{x^*y} & \sigma_{x^*x^*} \end{pmatrix} \right), \tag{2.41}$$

where

$$\mu_y = \beta_0 + \beta_x \mu_x; \quad \sigma_{yy} = \beta_x^2 \sigma_{xx} + \sigma_{\epsilon\epsilon};$$
$$\sigma_{x^*y} = \beta_x \sigma_{xx}; \quad \sigma_{x^*x^*} = \sigma_{xx} + \sigma_{ee}.$$

(ii) Let $\theta = (\beta_0, \beta_x, \mu_x, \sigma_{xx}, \sigma_{\epsilon\epsilon}, \sigma_{ee})^{\mathrm{T}}$ be the parameter vector associated with models (2.38) and (2.39). Show that parameter θ is not identifiable from model (2.41) for the observed data $\{(Y_i, X_i^*) : i = 1, \ldots, n\}$.

(iii) Model parameters of (2.38) and (2.39) may be identifiable from the observed data $\{(Y_i, X_i^*) : i = 1, \ldots, n\}$ if certain conditions are imposed. Show that if σ_{ee} or the reliability coefficient $\omega = \sigma_{xx}/(\sigma_{xx} + \sigma_{ee})$ is given, then θ is identifiable from the model (2.41) for the observed data $\{(Y_i, X_i^*) : i = 1, \ldots, n\}$.

(b) Assume that there is an instrumental variable V_i that is uncorrelated with $\{\epsilon_i, e_i\}$ but correlated with X_i. In particular, we have a model

$$X_i = \alpha_0 + \alpha_v V_i + r_i,$$

where error r_i is independent of $\{V_i, \epsilon_i, e_i\}$. Assume that both r_i and V_i follow normal distributions with $E(r_i) = 0$, $E(V_i) = \mu_v$ and $\mathrm{var}(V_i) = \sigma_{vv}$.

(i) Show that β_0 and β_x in model (2.38) may be estimated by

$$\widehat{\beta}_0 = \overline{Y} - \widehat{\beta}_x \overline{X}^* \text{ and } \widehat{\beta}_x = \widehat{\sigma}_{x^*v}^{-1} \widehat{\sigma}_{yv},$$

respectively, where

$\widehat{\sigma}_{yv} = (n-1)^{-1} \sum_{i=1}^n (V_i - \overline{V})(Y_i - \overline{Y})$;
$\widehat{\sigma}_{x^*v} = (n-1)^{-1} \sum_{i=1}^n (X_i^* - \overline{X}^*)(V_i - \overline{V})$;
$\overline{V} = n^{-1} \sum_{i=1}^n V_i$; $\overline{Y} = n^{-1} \sum_{i=1}^n Y_i$;
$\overline{X}^* = n^{-1} \sum_{i=1}^n X_i^*$.

(ii) Find the asymptotic distribution of $\sqrt{n}(\widehat{\beta} - \beta)$, where $\widehat{\beta} = (\widehat{\beta}_0, \widehat{\beta}_x)^{\mathrm{T}}$ and $\beta = (\beta_0, \beta_x)^{\mathrm{T}}$.

(iii) Thompson and Carter (2007) discussed the data, presented in Table 2.5, which are measurements of blood glucose taken from three different measurement techniques on 16 "normal" patients. Of the three measurement techniques, one is a manual method and the other two are done by machines, labeled as machine A and machine B.

Let Y_i be the measurement on the ith patient taken by machine B, and X_i^* be the measurement on the ith patient taken by the manual method. Let V_i be the measurement on the ith patient taken by machine A, which is treated as an instrumental variable for the true blood glucose X_i. True blood glucose is a variable contaminated with measurement error.

Perform the naive least squares regression analysis using the data $\{(Y_i, X_i^*) : i = 1, \ldots, n\}$. In contrast, use the instrumental variable, perform estimation of parameter β using the data $\{(Y_i, X_i^*, V_i) : i = 1, \ldots, n\}$ by following the lines of (i) and (ii) in (b).

(Fuller 1987, Ch. 1; Thompson and Carter 2007)

Table 2.5. *Three Measures of Blood Glucose (Thompson and Carter 2007)*

Patient	Manual	Machine A	Machine B	Patient	Manual	Machine A	Machine B
1	99	100	94	9	137	132	127
2	118	118	111	10	99	100	96
3	94	92	90	11	153	150	140
4	98	102	96	12	116	116	112
5	71	70	67	13	74	80	78
6	96	96	92	14	108	108	102
7	133	132	125	15	88	90	85
8	86	88	86	16	117	116	110

3
Survival Data with Measurement Error

Survival analysis is commonly challenged by the presence of covariate measurement error. Biomarkers, such as blood pressure, cholesterol level, and CD4 counts, are subject to measurement error due to biological variability and other sources of variation. It is known that standard inferential procedures often produce seriously biased estimation if measurement error is not properly taken into account. Since the seminal paper by Prentice (1982), there has been a large number of research papers devoted to handling covariate measurement error for survival data.

In this chapter, we direct our attention to this area and discuss analysis methods for dealing with error-contaminated survival data. We begin with an overview of survival analysis in the error-free context. In subsequent sections we explore various inference schemes to account for covariate measurement error and misclassification associated with survival data.

In the discussion of this chapter, we differentiate the notation for the distribution of survival times from its model, but we use the same symbols for the hazard function and its model (i.e., $\lambda(t)$ or $\lambda(t|X, Z)$), and for the survivor function and its model (i.e., $S(t)$ or $S(t|X, Z)$) for ease of exposition. Letters t_i and T_i represent different quantities as defined in §3.1.5. Other variables, such as X_i and Z_i, are loosely used; sometimes we differentiate random variables and their realizations by using upper case and lower case letters, respectively; sometimes we just use upper case letters for both random variables and their realizations to highlight the presence of the variables, especially when discussing the probability behavior of estimators. In addition, in the arguments of the likelihood functions or distributions, we interchangeably use (T_i, C_i) and (t_i, δ_i) to refer to the same quantities.

G. Y. Yi, *Statistical Analysis with Measurement Error or Misclassification*, Springer Series in Statistics, DOI 10.1007/978-1-4939-6640-0_3

3.1 Framework of Survival Analysis: Models and Methods

In survival analysis, the response measurement often concerns time to an event. An event of interest may take on different types, such as death of a patient, occurrence of a disease, or failure of a manufactured product, etc. Terms of *survival time*, *lifetime*, *failure time*, *time-to-event*, or *event time*, are commonly used to refer to a response variable in survival analysis.

Survival analysis deals with the probability behavior of time to an event. With a single population, research interests usually center around characterizing the distribution or marginal features (such as mean or median) of survival times. In the presence of multiple populations, comparing differences among survival distributions may be of primary interest. More generally, understanding the association between survival times and relevant covariates attracts major research efforts.

A comprehensive discussion on survival analysis is available in a number of monographs, including Kalbfleisch and Prentice (2002) and Lawless (2003). In this section, we provide only a brief review of models and methods used for survival analysis in the error-free context. In the first two subsections, we discuss basic concepts and strategies that are useful for characterizing a single survival process. Extensions to accommodating covariates are briefly described in the third subsection. Special features of survival data are discussed in the fourth subsection. This section is ended with discussion on inference methods.

3.1.1 Basic Measures

Let T denote the nonnegative random variable representing the lifetime of an individual. To describe the stochastic change of T, we may directly examine the probability density function, say $h(t)$, of T. An alternative scheme is to specify the *hazard function*, defined as

$$\lambda(t) = \lim_{\Delta t \to 0+} \frac{P(t \le T < t + \Delta t | T \ge t)}{\Delta t} \quad \text{for } t \ge 0.$$

The hazard function $\lambda(t)$ describes the instantaneous failure rate at time t, given that the individual survives up to time t. Roughly, in a tiny time period of length Δt, $\lambda(t)\Delta t$ provides an approximate probability of failure or death during time period $[t, t+\Delta t)$, given that the subject is alive prior to time t. Unlike the probability density function, which must satisfy nonnegativity (i.e., $h(t) \ge 0$) and the unit integral over the interval of all positive real numbers (i.e.,$\int_0^\infty h(v)\, dv = 1$), the hazard function is constrained by a single condition of nonnegativity $\lambda(t) \ge 0$.

In contrast to the cumulative distribution of T, $H(t) = P\,(T \le t)$, we often use a *survivor function* to represent the probability that a subject's survival time exceeds a time point. A survivor function is defined as

$$S(t) = P(T > t) \quad \text{for } t \ge 0.$$

The four measures are uniquely determined each other via

$$H(t) = \int_{-\infty}^{t} h(v)dv,$$

$$S(t) = \int_{t}^{\infty} h(v)dv = \exp\left\{-\int_{0}^{t} \lambda(v)dv\right\},$$

or

$$\lambda(t) = \frac{h(t)}{S(t)}. \tag{3.1}$$

Mathematically, characterization of distributions of survival times may be based on one of those four measures alone. But in application, a particular measure may be preferred because it has the most direct relevance to the questions we want to answer.

In addition to these four measures, the *cumulative hazard function* is sometimes useful. It is defined as

$$\Lambda(t) = \int_{0}^{t} \lambda(v)dv.$$

This measure uniquely determines the distribution of T through, for instance, the relationship $S(t) = \exp\{-\Lambda(t)\}$.

Response variable T is constantly taken as a continuous variable. Occasionally, it is treated as a discrete variable with mass taken at fixed time points. In this chapter, our discussion is directed to continuous response variable T unless stated otherwise.

3.1.2 Some Parametric Modeling Strategies

Parametric modeling is commonly invoked to characterize a survival distribution. This modeling scheme has several advantages. Implementation of inferential procedures is simple and the interpretation of the model parameters is usually transparent. Moreover, the likelihood theory can often be applied directly to characterize the asymptotic properties of the resulting estimators.

One approach for parametrically modeling survival times is to specify a class of distributions for survival times, usually with unknown parameters involved. For instance, a Gamma distribution may be used to describe survival time T where the probability density function of T is modeled as

$$f(t;\beta_1,\beta_2) = \frac{\beta_2^{\beta_1}}{\Gamma(\beta_1)} t^{\beta_1 - 1}\exp(-\beta_2 t) \quad \text{for } t > 0$$

with parameters $\beta_1 > 0$ and $\beta_2 > 0$.

In principle, any distribution of a nonnegative random variable may be employed to model the stochastic process for T. In practice, however, some distributions are more commonly used than others. Exponential, Weibull, log-normal, log-logistic and Gamma distributions are widely used.

More generally, we apply a transformation to survival times to remove their nonnegativity constraint. Any distributions may then be legitimately employed to delineate the transformed survival times. To be specific, let $Y = \log T$, then for the transformed variable Y, assuming a location-scale probability density function

$$f(y;\mu,\sigma) = \frac{1}{\sigma} f_0\left(\frac{y-\mu}{\sigma}\right) \quad \text{for } -\infty < y < \infty$$

gives a model for the distribution of the original survival time T, where $f_0(y)$ is a specified probability density function on $(-\infty, \infty)$, μ is a location parameter with $-\infty < \mu < \infty$, and σ is a scale parameter with $\sigma > 0$.

Varying the form of function $f_0(\cdot)$ characterizes different survival distributions. For example, we write $\widetilde{Y} = (Y - \mu)/\sigma$, then setting the survivor function of $\widetilde{Y}$ to correspond to the standard extreme value, normal and logistic distributions, respectively, given by

$$S_0(\widetilde{y}) = \exp\{-\exp(\widetilde{y})\},$$
$$S_0(\widetilde{y}) = 1 - \Phi(\widetilde{y}),$$
$$S_0(\widetilde{y}) = \{1 + \exp(\widetilde{y})\}^{-1},$$

yields the Weibull, log-normal, and log-logistic distributions for T, respectively, where $\Phi(\cdot)$ is the cumulative distribution for the standard normal distribution. Extensions may also be done, for instance, by letting $f_0(\widetilde{y})$ or $S_0(\widetilde{y})$ include some "shape" parameters (Lawless 2003, p. 27).

An alternative strategy for parametrically modeling survival times is to characterize the hazard function $\lambda(t)$ by specifying its function form. For instance, setting

$$\lambda(t) = \beta_1\beta_2(\beta_1 t)^{\beta_2 - 1}$$

for positive parameters β_1 and β_2 characterizes a survival process which has a Weibull distribution. Further constraining $\beta_2 = 1$ gives an exponential distribution, which corresponds to the simplest scenario of survival processes featured by a constant hazard function.

A more flexible way of describing the hazard function $\lambda(t)$ is to use a sequence of specified functions, instead of a single given function. A simple scheme for this is to use the *piecewise-constant* approach to model $\lambda(t)$. Let

$$\lambda(t) = \rho_k \quad \text{for } t \in A_k, \tag{3.2}$$

where the ρ_k are nonnegative parameters; $A_k = (a_{k-1}, a_k]$; $k = 1, \ldots, K$; and $0 = a_0 < a_1 < \ldots < a_{K-1} < a_K = \infty$ is a sequence of pre-determined constants for a given positive integer K.

For $k = 1, \ldots, K$, let $u_k(t) = \max\{0, \min(a_k, t) - a_{k-1}\}$ be the length of the intersection of interval $(0, t]$ with interval A_k. Then, the hazard function and the cumulative hazard function are, respectively, written as

$$\lambda(t) = \sum_{k=1}^{K} \rho_k I(t \in A_k) \text{ and } \Lambda(t) = \sum_{k=1}^{K} \rho_k u_k(t).$$

Consequently, the probability density function $h(t)$ is piecewise exponential, and the survivor function is given by

$$S(t) = \exp\left\{ -\sum_{k=1}^{K} \rho_k u_k(t) \right\}.$$

With suitable choices of K and cut points a_k, this modeling can provide reasonable approximations to arbitrary shape of lifetime distributions. This approach allows for conducting inferences in a straightforward manner and offers a convenient tool to bridge parametric and nonparametric methods. A somewhat unappealing aspect of this modeling is the discontinuity of $\lambda(t)$ and $S(t)$ at cut points a_k. To get around this, one may model $\lambda(t)$ by using *spline functions*, such as cubic spline functions, which consist of polynomial pieces joined smoothly at cut points a_k (Lawless 2003, §1.3).

While the models we discuss here are frequently used in survival analysis, many other flexible or complex distributions may be employed for individual applications. We refer the readers to Lawless (2003) and Kalbfleisch and Prentice (2002) for more detailed discussion on many other parametric models.

3.1.3 Regression Models

The foregoing discussion applies to settings with a single population or multiple populations that are stratified by certain "obvious" discrete characteristics such as gender or the treatment indicator. When populations are heterogeneous according to different values of covariates, regression analysis provides a useful tool to facilitate the association between survival times and covariates. While there are many ways to formulate regression models, we focus on some models that are in common use.

Let X and Z be the covariates that are associated with survival time T. To understand the dependence of survival time T on covariates $\{X, Z\}$, we may, in principle, apply the same strategies outlined in §3.1.2. However, there is an important difference where the formulation here must be directed to the *conditional probability density function* $h(t|X, Z)$ of the survival time T, given covariates $\{X, Z\}$ while the discussion in §3.1.2 is addressed to the marginal distribution of T. Here we describe two modeling strategies: modeling conditional survivor functions and modeling conditional hazard functions. We use the notation $f(\cdot|\cdot)$ for the model of the conditional probability density function $h(t|X, Z)$ of the survival time T, given covariates $\{X, Z\}$, where model parameters may or may not be explicitly indicated. For ease of exposition, given covariates $\{X, Z\}$, we use the same notation $S(t|X, Z)$ for the conditional survivor function for T and its model and $\lambda(t|X, Z)$ for the conditional hazard function for T and its model.

We first outline the *transformation-location-scale* modeling scheme, a useful technique for modeling conditional survivor functions. To remove the constraint that survival time T must be nonnegative, we apply a monotone transformation on T so that the transformed survival time assumes values in $\mathbb{R}$. Often, a logarithm transformation is applied. Let $Y = \log T$ and $S(y|X, Z) = P(Y > y|X, Z)$.

A class of location-scale models is commonly used to portray the distribution of Y:

$$S(y|X,Z) = S_0\left(\frac{y - m(X,Z;\beta)}{\sigma}\right), \tag{3.3}$$

where $S_0(\cdot)$ is a survivor function and σ is a scale parameter. The dependence of response Y on the covariates is featured in $m(X,Z;\beta)$ via a specified function form $m(\cdot)$ and associated parameter β. In many applications, $m(\cdot)$ assumes a linear structure in X and Z with $m(X,Z;\beta) = \beta_0 + \beta_x^{\mathrm{T}}X + \beta_z^{\mathrm{T}}Z$ and $\beta = (\beta_0, \beta_x^{\mathrm{T}}, \beta_z^{\mathrm{T}})^{\mathrm{T}}$, where β_0, β_x and β_z are regression parameters.

The interpretation of model (3.3) is more transparent if written in terms of the original survival time T:

$$P(T > t|X,Z) = S_0^*\left[\left\{\frac{t}{m^*(X,Z;\beta)}\right\}^{\sigma^{-1}}\right] \tag{3.4}$$

for $t > 0$, where $S_0^*(t) = S_0(\log t)$ and $m^*(X,Z;\beta) = \exp\{m(X,Z;\beta)\}$. Through function $m^*(\cdot)$, covariates $\{X,Z\}$ alter the time scale in an accelerating or decelerating manner. Such a model is called the *accelerated failure time* (AFT) model. Common choices of the survivor function $S_0(\cdot)$ include the standard normal, extreme value and logistic distributions (Lawless 2003, §6.1).

Equivalently, model (3.3) is expressed as an alternative form

$$Y = m(X,Z;\beta) + \sigma\epsilon, \tag{3.5}$$

where ϵ is a random variable with survivor function $S_0(\cdot)$. Model (3.5) may be further extended for greater flexibility. Two ways are apparent. The first one is to leave the survivor function $S_0(\cdot)$ unspecified, yielding semiparametric models in the sense that the dependence of T on $\{X,Z\}$ is parametric in a specified form for function $m(\cdot)$ but the actual distribution of T is left arbitrary.

A second extension is to relax the transformation form applied to T. Instead of applying the decisive logarithm transformation to T, we apply a function $g(\cdot)$ that is increasing but its form is unspecified. Then model (3.5) for $Y = g(T)$ gives a wider class of models than (3.5) with $Y = \log T$. In particular, model (3.5) with $Y = g(T)$ and $m(X,Z;\beta) = \beta_0 + \beta^{\mathrm{T}}X + \beta_z^{\mathrm{T}}Z$ defines the *semiparametric linear transformation model* (Dabrowska and Doksum 1988; Cheng, Wei and Ying 1995). Furthermore, set $\sigma = 1$, then specifying $S_0(\cdot)$ to be the survivor function of the standard logistic distribution gives the *proportional odds* (PO) model, and setting $S_0(\cdot)$ to correspond to the extreme value distribution yields the *proportional hazards* (PH) model.

In contrast to the transformation-location-scale modeling scheme, we discuss another strategy which focuses on directly modeling the conditional hazard function. Given covariates $\{X,Z\}$, let $S(t|X,Z) = P(T > t|X,Z)$ be the (conditional) survivor function of survival time T, and

$$\lambda(t|X,Z) = \lim_{\Delta t \to 0+} \frac{P(t \le T < t + \Delta t | T \ge t, X, Z)}{\Delta t}$$

be the (conditional) hazard function of T.

If, for instance, the hazard function $\lambda(t|X, Z)$ is time-invariant and dependent on covariates only, i.e., $\lambda(t|X, Z) = \lambda(X, Z)$ for a nonnegative function $\lambda(\cdot)$, then the survivor function becomes

$$S(t|X, Z) = \exp\{-\lambda(X, Z)t\},$$

which implies that survival time T follows an exponential distribution with rate $\lambda(X, Z)$.

Often, the hazard function is both covariate dependent and time-varying, so the hazard function $\lambda(t|X, Z)$ should be specified as a function of both covariates and time. Although any nonnegative function may be used for this purpose, a multiplicative or additive form is usually taken. For instance, we may set

$$\lambda(t|X, Z) = \lambda_0(t)g(X, Z)$$

or

$$\lambda(t|X, Z) = \lambda_0(t) + g(X, Z),$$

where $\lambda_0(t)$ is the baseline hazard function that features the temporal effect, and $g(X, Z)$ reflects the covariate effects for a nonnegative function $g(\cdot)$. These models are widely used in survival analysis and are, respectively, called *proportional hazards* (PH) models and *additive hazards* (AH) models.

Equivalently, in terms of survivor functions, these models are, respectively, expressed as

$$S(t|X, Z) = \{S_0(t)\}^{g(X,Z)} \tag{3.6}$$

and

$$S(t|X, Z) = S_0(t)[\exp\{-g(X, Z)\}]^t,$$

where $S_0(t) = \exp\{-\int_0^t \lambda_0(v)dv\}$.

The preceding model formulation enables us to separate the dependence of $\lambda(t|X, Z)$ on time and covariates, which allows a more transparent interpretation of covariate effects. Since it is rarely possible to identify the exact function form for $\lambda_0(\cdot)$ and $g(\cdot)$, common practice is to model these functions, parametrically, semiparametrically or even nonparametrically. When both $\lambda_0(\cdot)$ and $g(\cdot)$ are modeled parametrically, an assumption is constantly made that these two models are governed by distinct parameters.

In many applications, the baseline hazard function $\lambda_0(\cdot)$ is treated nonparametrically and, thus, left unspecified; only function $g(\cdot)$ is modeled with a parametric form. A common specification is

$$g(X, Z; \beta) = \exp(\beta_x^{\mathrm{T}} X + \beta_z^{\mathrm{T}} Z)$$

for the proportional hazards model (Cox 1972, 1975) and

$$g(X, Z; \beta) = \beta_x^{\mathrm{T}} X + \beta_z^{\mathrm{T}} Z$$

for the additive hazards model, where $\beta = (\beta_x^{\mathrm{T}}, \beta_z^{\mathrm{T}})^{\mathrm{T}}$ is the vector of parameters.

The interpretation of the covariate effects is different for these two models. In the proportional hazards model, the relative hazard for different covariate values

$$\frac{\lambda(t|X,Z)}{\lambda(t|\widetilde{X},\widetilde{Z})} = \exp\{\beta_x^{\mathrm{T}}(X-\widetilde{X}) + \beta_z^{\mathrm{T}}(Z-\widetilde{Z})\}$$

is time-free, which suggests the name *proportional hazards* because any two individuals have hazard functions that are constant multiples of one another (Lawless 2003, p. 272). On the other hand, in the additive hazards model, regression parameters are related to the risk difference which represents the expected number of events occurring during a unit time interval caused by a unit change in the covariates. This model was considered by many authors, including Breslow and Day (1980), Cox and Oakes (1984), and Lin and Ying (1994).

The discussion assumes tacitly that covariates X and Z are time-independent. In situations where some covariates vary with time, the involvement of covariates with modeling becomes more complicated. Let $X(t)$ represent a covariate vector at time t and Z be a time-independent covariate vector. Rather than a single measurement at a time point, an entire covariate process $\mathcal{H}^{\mathrm{x}} = \{X(t) : t \geq 0\}$, together with time-invariant covariate Z, may or may not come into play when building a model to facilitate the dependence of survival times on covariates. Kalbfleisch and Prentice (2002, §6.3) discussed this issue in detail.

Modeling with time-varying covariates is constantly carried out via the dependence on the covariate history under the assumption

$$S(t|\mathcal{H}^{\mathrm{x}}, Z) = S(t|\mathcal{H}_t^{\mathrm{x}}, Z),$$

where $\mathcal{H}_t^{\mathrm{x}} = \{X(v) : 0 \leq v \leq t\}$ represents the covariate history up to and including time t. Equivalently, this assumption says that

$$\lambda(t|\mathcal{H}^{\mathrm{x}}, Z) = \lambda(t|\mathcal{H}_t^{\mathrm{x}}, Z),$$

which allows us to model $\lambda(t|\mathcal{H}^{\mathrm{x}}, Z)$, or $\lambda(t|\mathcal{H}_t^{\mathrm{x}}, Z)$, as a function of time t and some specific form of the covariate history $\mathcal{H}_t^{\mathrm{x}}$. For instance, a multiplicative form may be specified for the conditional hazard function

$$\lambda(t|\mathcal{H}_t^{\mathrm{x}}, Z) = \lambda_0(t)\exp\{\beta_x^{\mathrm{T}} W(t) + \beta_z^{\mathrm{T}} Z\},$$

where $W(t)$ is a vector that represents special features of the history $\mathcal{H}_t^{\mathrm{x}}$, $\lambda_0(t)$ is the baseline hazard function, and β_x and β_z are parameters (Lawless 2003, §1.4).

3.1.4 Special Features of Survival Data

A key feature that distinguishes survival analysis from usual regression analysis is *censoring*. Censoring is prevalent with survival data; it occurs when the survival time for an individual is not completely observed. Censoring may be classified as *right censoring*, *left censoring* and *interval censoring*. Right censoring arises if the survival time T of an individual is not observed but is known to be greater than a given time, while left censoring refers to the case where the survival time T is less than a certain duration. When the exact value of T is not observed but we know that T has a value falling in a certain finite time interval, then this is called interval censoring. In survival analysis, right censoring has perhaps received the most attention.

Censoring occurs for many reasons. Censoring may be caused by design. For example, survival times for study subjects cannot be observed if they are still alive when the study terminates. Censoring can happen due to the lost to follow-up by reasons which may be related or unrelated to the study. Sometimes, participants drop out of the study due to the observed effects on survival. For instance, when comparing survival of cancer patients, the control arm may be ineffective, leading to more recurrences and patients becoming too sick to follow-up. On the other hand, patients on the intervention arm may be completely cured by an effective treatment and no longer feel the need to follow-up.

Many studies are designed to *randomly* select individuals from the population. In some studies, however, not every individual can be selected; certain selection conditions are imposed to screen or exclude subjects from the study population: only subjects who experience certain prerequisite events or meet the required conditions are to be observed by the investigator. This creates *truncation* of data, which may be further refined as *left truncation* or *right truncation.*

In standard designs, survival times of individuals are defined to be the duration at selection or the entry of the study to failure, where the lifetime at the entry is set as 0. But in practice, this is not always true. Often, selection of an individual at time w (> 0) requires that $T \geq w$; otherwise, this subject cannot be included in the study. For example, if T represents death times of elderly residents of a retirement community, then only those elderly people can be observed if they live to a certain age (say, w) so they can be admitted to the community. People who died before this age cannot be observed. In this case, we say that the lifetime T is *left truncated* (at w). Left truncation is also called *delayed entry*.

While many studies are designed *prospectively* by following individuals until failure time or censoring time occurs, some observational plans may be *retrospective* to some degree. Such plans are useful when it is not feasible to follow individuals long enough prospectively to obtain desired information. For example, Kalbfleisch and Lawless (1989) discussed the data on people infected with HIV, where the study group consisted of individuals who had a diagnosis of AIDS prior to July 1, 1986, and failure time T is defined to be the duration between HIV infection and AIDS diagnosis for a patient. If v represents the time between an individual's HIV infection and July 1, 1986, then only those individuals with $T \leq v$ can be included in the study. That is, the data were collected *retrospectively* by the condition that $T \leq v$. This creates a scenario of *right truncation* of the lifetime T.

Truncation and censoring are typical features for survival analysis, and they are quite different. Truncation is applied when the study group has not been formed yet; whereas censoring occurs only for those subjects included in the study group, namely, the study group has been formed already. Censoring is addressed at the subject-level and is used to characterize the availability or completeness of a subject's survival time. Truncation is, however, about selection conditions for the formulation of the study group. With certain selection criteria imposed, survival times of the study subjects may be constrained by lower or upper bounds, that is, survival times are truncated by those bounds. Involvement of truncation generally changes the scope of the target population for which we infer analysis results; sampling bias (or selection bias) is often an issue to be addressed via conditional analysis in this case. In this chapter, we do not specifically discuss inference with truncation involved unless otherwise stated. For more details, we refer the readers to Lawless (2003, §2.4).

To develop valid statistical analysis for censored data, we need to, at least in principle, consider the two processes which generate survival times and censoring times in order to feature their possibly complicated association. Different from usual regression analysis, the censoring process generally requires our care although it is not of our interest. Fortunately, for a wide variety of practical settings, convenient censoring mechanisms may be assumed so that only modeling of survival processes is required for conducting inferences. In this case, statistical procedures can be established based on the likelihood for the observed data and the associated model parameters. In the next subsection, we discuss a likelihood formulation.

3.1.5 Likelihood Method

Suppose that n individuals in the study are followed from $t = 0$ until they fail or are right censored. For individual $i = 1, \ldots, n$, let T_i be the lifetime, C_i be the censoring time, δ_i be the censoring indicator variable with $\delta_i = I(T_i \le C_i)$, and $t_i = \min(T_i, C_i)$ denote the observed time. Let $(X_i^{\mathrm{T}}, Z_i^{\mathrm{T}})^{\mathrm{T}}$ be the $p \times 1$ covariate vector for subject i, where $X_i = (X_{i1}, \ldots, X_{ip_x})^{\mathrm{T}}$ is a $p_x \times 1$ vector of covariates, Z_i is a $p_z \times 1$ vector of covariates, and $p_x + p_z = p$.

For a variety of censoring mechanisms, statistical inference is based on the observed likelihood function $L = \prod_{i=1}^n L_i$ where

$$L_i = \{f(t_i|X_i, Z_i)\}^{\delta_i}\{S(t_i|X_i, Z_i)\}^{1-\delta_i}. \tag{3.7}$$

This formulation is derived by Lawless (2003, §2.2) under various censoring mechanisms, including the *independent censoring* for which all survival times and censoring times are mutually independent, given covariates. In this chapter, we focus the discussion on independent right censoring unless otherwise indicated. Under this censoring assumption, we examine the formulation (3.7) for two useful models.

Example 3.1. (*Proportional Hazards Model*)

Suppose that failure time T_i and covariates $\{X_i, Z_i\}$ are related by the Cox proportional hazards model. Namely, the conditional hazard function for T_i given $\{X_i, Z_i\}$ is modeled as

$$\lambda(t|X_i, Z_i) = \lambda_0(t)\exp(\beta_x^{\mathrm{T}} X_i + \beta_z^{\mathrm{T}} Z_i), \tag{3.8}$$

where $\lambda_0(t)$ is the baseline hazard function and $\beta = (\beta_x^{\mathrm{T}}, \beta_z^{\mathrm{T}})^{\mathrm{T}}$ is the vector of regression parameters to be estimated.

By (3.1), the logarithm of the observed likelihood (3.7) is

$$\ell = \sum_{i=1}^n \ell_i,$$

where

$$\ell_i = \delta_i \left\{\log \lambda_0(t_i) + \beta_x^{\mathrm{T}} X_i + \beta_z^{\mathrm{T}} Z_i\right\} - \exp(\beta_x^{\mathrm{T}} X_i + \beta_z^{\mathrm{T}} Z_i) \int_0^{t_i} \lambda_0(v)dv. \quad (3.9)$$

Example 3.2. (*Additive Hazards Model*)

Suppose that failure time T_i and covariates $\{X_i, Z_i\}$ are related by the additive hazards model, where the conditional hazard function of T_i, given $\{X_i, Z_i\}$, is modulated as

$$\lambda(t|X_i, Z_i) = \lambda_0(t) + \beta_x^{\mathrm{T}} X_i + \beta_z^{\mathrm{T}} Z_i \quad (3.10)$$

with $\lambda_0(t)$ being the baseline hazard function and $\beta = (\beta_x^{\mathrm{T}}, \beta_z^{\mathrm{T}})^{\mathrm{T}}$ the vector of unknown regression parameters.

Under this model, the logarithm of the observed likelihood function (3.7) is

$$\ell = \sum_{i=1}^{n} \left[\delta_i \log \left\{\lambda_0(t_i) + \beta_x^{\mathrm{T}} X_i + \beta_z^{\mathrm{T}} Z_i\right\} - \left\{(\beta_x^{\mathrm{T}} X_i + \beta_z^{\mathrm{T}} Z_i)t_i + \int_0^{t_i} \lambda_0(v)dv\right\}\right].$$

Inference about the model parameter β may be based on the log-likelihood function ℓ, following the same procedure as for the standard maximum likelihood method (Lawless 2003, §2.2.3). Large sample theory for maximum likelihood estimators may be applied as usual. This likelihood approach is straightforward to implement, but basically, requires modeling the baseline hazards function $\lambda_0(t)$.

3.1.6 Model-Dependent Inference Methods

The likelihood method based on the formulation (3.7) is applicable to a wide class of survival models, and it is not just restricted to proportional hazards and additive hazards models. Detailed implementation procedures were given by Lawless (2003, Ch. 6).

With specific model features available, special methods may be developed. We discuss two inference methods; one is applicable to the proportional hazards model while the other applies to the additive hazards model. These methods differ from the likelihood method described in §3.1.5 in that the baseline hazard function is left unattended to, thus viewed as *semiparametric regression methods*.

In addition to the notation in §3.1.5, for $i = 1, \ldots, n$, let

$$R_i(t) = I(t_i \geq t)$$

be the at risk indicator at time t for subject i, and

$$dN_i(t) = I\{T_i \in [t, t + \Delta t); \ \delta_i = 1\}$$

be the indicator variable for subject i who is alive and not censored before time t and has failure occurring right after time t, where Δt represents a infinitesimally small time. Write $\mathbb{T} = \{T_1, \ldots, T_n\}$, $\mathbb{C} = \{C_1, \ldots, C_n\}$, $\mathbb{X} = \{X_1, \ldots, X_n\}$, and $\mathbb{Z} = \{Z_1, \ldots, Z_n\}$.

Proportional Hazards Model

Treating the baseline hazard function $\lambda_0(t)$ in the proportional hazards model as a nuisance, Cox (1975) factorized the likelihood function as a product of a sequence of conditional probabilities for which some involve the regression parameters β alone. To conduct inference about parameter β in the absence of knowledge of the baseline hazard function $\lambda_0(t)$, Cox (1975) discarded those probabilities in the factorization that involve $\lambda_0(t)$ and used the product of the remaining pieces to conduct inference about β. This is the key idea of formulating the *partial likelihood* which has been extensively used in survival analysis (Kalbfleisch and Prentice 2002, §4.2).

Specifically, under model (3.8), the partial likelihood is given by

$$
\begin{aligned}
L_{\mathrm{P}}(\beta) &= \prod_{i=1}^{n} \left\{ \frac{\lambda(t_i|X_i, Z_i)}{\sum_{j=1}^{n} R_j(t_i)\lambda(t_i|X_j, Z_j)} \right\}^{\delta_i} \\
&= \prod_{i=1}^{n} \left\{ \frac{\exp(\beta_x^{\mathrm{T}} X_i + \beta_z^{\mathrm{T}} Z_i)}{\sum_{j=1}^{n} R_j(t_i)\exp(\beta_x^{\mathrm{T}} X_j + \beta_z^{\mathrm{T}} Z_j)} \right\}^{\delta_i}. \qquad (3.11)
\end{aligned}
$$

Although $L_{\mathrm{P}}(\beta)$ is not an authentic likelihood, it has properties similar to an ordinary likelihood. The score function, information matrix and likelihood ratio statistics based on $L_{\mathrm{P}}(\beta)$ behave as if they were obtained from a usual likelihood. Estimation of β may proceed by maximizing the log partial likelihood, and the resulting estimator is consistent and is, after a transformation, asymptotically normal under suitable conditions (Andersen et al. 1993).

Alternatively, define

$$
\begin{aligned}
S^{(0)}(t, \mathbb{X}, \mathbb{Z}; \beta) &= \frac{1}{n}\sum_{j=1}^{n} R_j(t)\exp(\beta_x^{\mathrm{T}} X_j + \beta_z^{\mathrm{T}} Z_j), \\
S^{(1)}(t, \mathbb{X}, \mathbb{Z}; \beta) &= \frac{1}{n}\sum_{j=1}^{n} R_j(t)\begin{pmatrix} X_j \\ Z_j \end{pmatrix}\exp(\beta_x^{\mathrm{T}} X_j + \beta_z^{\mathrm{T}} Z_j), \qquad (3.12)
\end{aligned}
$$

and

$$
S_{\mathrm{P}i}(t, \mathbb{X}, \mathbb{Z}; \beta) = \begin{pmatrix} X_i \\ Z_i \end{pmatrix} - \frac{S^{(1)}(t, \mathbb{X}, \mathbb{Z}; \beta)}{S^{(0)}(t, \mathbb{X}, \mathbb{Z}; \beta)}, \qquad (3.13)
$$

then the *partial score function* $U(\beta) = (\partial/\partial\beta)\log L_{\mathrm{P}}(\beta)$ is expressed as

$$
U(\beta) = \sum_{i=1}^{n} \delta_i S_{\mathrm{P}i}(t_i, \mathbb{X}, \mathbb{Z}; \beta). \qquad (3.14)
$$

Solving $U(\beta) = 0$ for β leads to an estimator, say $\widehat{\beta}$, of β. Under suitable conditions, $\sqrt{n}(\widehat{\beta} - \beta)$ has an asymptotic normal distribution with mean zero and a covariance matrix that is estimated by $nJ^{-1}(\widehat{\beta})$, where matrix $J(\beta) = -\partial^2 \log L_{\mathrm{P}}(\beta)/\partial\beta\partial\beta^{\mathrm{T}}$ is easily calculated to be

$$J(\beta) = \sum_{i=1}^{n} \delta_i \left\{ \frac{\sum_{j=1}^{n} R_j(t_i) \exp(\beta_x^{\mathrm{T}} X_j + \beta_z^{\mathrm{T}} Z_j)\{S_{\mathrm{P}j}(t_i, \mathbb{X}, \mathbb{Z}; \beta)\}^{\otimes 2}}{S^{(0)}(t_i, \mathbb{X}, \mathbb{Z}; \beta)} \right\},$$

and the operation $\otimes 2$ is defined as $a^{\otimes 2} = aa^{\mathrm{T}}$ for a column vector a. Detailed discussions on these expressions were given by Lawless (2003, §7.1).

The formulation of the partial likelihood is attractive because it allows us to leave the baseline hazard function $\lambda_0(t)$ unspecified. The partial likelihood is widely used to perform estimation of parameter β, especially when central interest lies in the covariate effects. Its implementation is available in standard statistical software packages, such as *coxph* and *survreg* in R and *PROC PHREG* in SAS.

Additive Hazards Model

In contrast to the proportional hazards model, the additive hazards model specifies the hazard function to be associated with covariates through the sum, rather than the product, of the baseline hazard function and the regression function of covariates. Analogous to the partial likelihood for the Cox proportional hazards model, estimation of the regression coefficients can be carried out with the baseline hazard function ignored. Lin and Ying (1994) proposed to use a *pseudo-score function* for inference about β.

Let $W_i = (X_i^{\mathrm{T}}, Z_i^{\mathrm{T}})^{\mathrm{T}}$ and

$$\overline{W}(t) = \frac{\sum_{j=1}^{n} R_j(t) \begin{pmatrix} X_j \\ Z_j \end{pmatrix}}{\sum_{j=1}^{n} R_j(t)}.$$

Under model (3.10), the pseudo-score function for parameter β is defined as

$$U_i(\beta) = \int_0^\infty \{W_i - \overline{W}(t)\}\{dN_i(t) - R_i(t)(\beta^{\mathrm{T}} W_i)dt\}. \tag{3.15}$$

Solving the estimating equation $\sum_{i=1}^{n} U_i(\beta) = 0$ for β gives the estimator, say $\widehat{\beta}$, of β, which is given by

$$\widehat{\beta} = \left[\sum_{i=1}^{n} \int_0^\infty \{W_i - \overline{W}(t)\}^{\otimes 2} R_i(t)dt\right]^{-1} \left[\sum_{i=1}^{n} \int_0^\infty \{W_i - \overline{W}(t)\}dN_i(t)\right].$$

Lin and Ying (1994) showed that under suitable conditions, $\sqrt{n}(\widehat{\beta} - \beta)$ asymptotically has a normal distribution with mean zero and a sandwich covariance matrix that is consistently estimated by $\widehat{\Gamma}\widehat{\Sigma}\widehat{\Gamma}^{-1}$, where

$$\widehat{\Gamma} = \frac{1}{n} \sum_{i=1}^{n} \int_0^\infty R_i(t)\{W_i - \overline{W}(t)\}^{\otimes 2} dt$$

and

$$\widehat{\Sigma} = \frac{1}{n}\sum_{i=1}^{n}\int_{0}^{\infty}\{W_i - \overline{W}(t)\}^{\otimes 2} dN_i(t).$$

3.2 Measurement Error Effects and Inference Framework

3.2.1 Induced Hazard Function

We discuss measurement error effects on changing the structures of survival models. Our discussion concentrates on two survival models: Cox proportional hazards and additive hazards models. This examination helps us understand the differences between the conditional distributions of survival times under the true and surrogate covariates, and also sheds light on developing valid inference approaches to accommodating measurement error effects.

Let X^* denote an observed version, or surrogate, of covariate X. We are interested in understanding how measurement error in X may affect the structure of the survival process of T. By the connections discussed in §3.1.1, we need only to investigate how replacing X with X^* may change the structure of the hazard function. In contrast to the conditional hazard function or its model, $\lambda(t|X, Z)$, of T given $\{X, Z\}$, we let $\lambda^*(t|X^*, Z)$ denote the conditional hazard function or its model, of T, given $\{X^*, Z\}$. We call $\lambda(t|X, Z)$ the *true* (conditional) hazard function and $\lambda^*(t|X^*, Z)$ the *induced* (conditional) hazard function.

Let $\lambda^{**}(t|X^*, X, Z)$ stand for the conditional hazard function or its model of T, given $\{X^*, X, Z\}$, defined by

$$\lambda^{**}(t|X^*, X, Z) = \lim_{\Delta t \to 0+} \frac{P(t \leq T < t + \Delta t | T \geq t, X^*, X, Z)}{\Delta t}.$$

Then the induced hazard function is given by

$$\lambda^*(t|X^*, Z) = E\{\lambda^{**}(t|X^*, X, Z)|T \geq t, X^*, Z)\}, \tag{3.16}$$

where the expectation is taken with respect to the conditional distribution, or its model, of X, given $\{T \geq t, X^*, Z\}$.

Consider the assumption

$$\lambda^{**}(t|X^*, X, Z) = \lambda(t|X, Z),$$

which suggests that given the true covariates $\{X, Z\}$, the observed covariate X^* has no predictive value for the hazard rate of survival time T. This assumption is related to the nondifferential measurement error mechanism to be discussed in §3.2.2 (see Problem 3.5). Under this assumption, the induced hazard function is identical to a conditional expectation of the true hazard function

$$\lambda^*(t|X^*, Z) = E\{\lambda(t|X, Z)|T \geq t, X^*, Z\}. \tag{3.17}$$

The expectation (3.17) is generally not equal to the true hazard function $\lambda(t|X, Z_i)$ with X replaced by X^*, which is attributed to its dependence on the distribution of survival time T through the conditioning requirement $T \geq t$ and the possible nonlinearity of $\lambda(t|X, Z)$. The function form $\lambda^*(t|X^*, Z)$ is usually more complex than the true hazard function $\lambda(t|X, Z)$ which often assumes an interpretable structure. For instance, under the proportional hazards model (3.8), the induced hazard function (3.17) is given by

$$\lambda^*(t|X^*, Z) = \lambda_0(t) \exp(\beta_z^{\mathrm{T}} Z) E\{\exp(\beta_x^{\mathrm{T}} X)|T \geq t, X^*, Z\}, \tag{3.18}$$

while under the additive hazards model (3.10), the induced hazard function is given by

$$\lambda^*(t|X^*, Z) = \lambda_0(t) + \beta_z^{\mathrm{T}} Z + E(\beta_x^{\mathrm{T}} X|T \geq t, X^*, Z). \tag{3.19}$$

None of these forms share the same structure as the original true hazard function $\lambda(t|X, Z)$ unless under some restrictive conditions, such as $\beta_x = 0$. The conditional expectations in (3.18) and (3.19) generally depend on the unknown baseline hazard function $\lambda_0(\cdot)$ due to the conditioning on $(T \geq t)$. Consequently, naively applying standard analysis procedures with X replaced by the observed version X^* would normally yield biased results because the structure of the hazard function is distorted. The degree of incurred biases is different from model to model. For instance, naive estimation of β based on the additive hazards model can be less biased than that for the proportional hazards model, because the former case misspecifies the conditional first moment $E(\beta_x^{\mathrm{T}} X|T \geq t, X^*, Z)$ to be $\beta_x^{\mathrm{T}} X^*$ while the latter case misuses $\exp(\beta_x^{\mathrm{T}} X^*)$ for the entire conditional moment generating function $E\{\exp(\beta_x^{\mathrm{T}} X)|T \geq t, X^*, Z\}$.

To visualize the differences in the structure between the induced and true hazard functions, we further examine a special situation where the failures are rare: the probability of survival beyond a time t, $P(T \geq t|X, Z)$, is close to 1 (Prentice 1982; Problem 3.5). Then the induced hazard function for the proportional and additive hazards models is approximated by

$$\lambda^*(t|X^*, Z) \approx \lambda_0(t) \exp(\beta_z^{\mathrm{T}} Z) E\{\exp(\beta_x^{\mathrm{T}} X)|X^*, Z\},$$

and

$$\lambda^*(t|X^*, Z) \approx \lambda_0(t) + \beta_z^{\mathrm{T}} Z + E(\beta_x^{\mathrm{T}} X|X^*, Z),$$

respectively.

To determine the induced hazard function, we need the conditional moment generating function of X, $M(\beta_x) = E\{\exp(\beta_x^{\mathrm{T}} X)|X^*, Z\}$, or the conditional expectation $E(\beta_x^{\mathrm{T}} X|X^*, Z)$, given the observed covariates $\{X^*, Z\}$. For example, if the measurement error process is characterized by a conditional normal distribution, $N(m(X^*, Z; \gamma), \Sigma^*)$, for X given $\{X^*, Z\}$, where $m(X^*, Z; \gamma)$ is a function of X^* and Z which may depend on parameter γ, and Σ^* is a nonnegative definite matrix, then the approximate induced hazard function for the proportional hazards model and the additive hazards model is given by

$$\lambda^*(t|X^*, Z) \approx \lambda_0^*(t) \exp\left\{\beta_x^{\mathrm{T}} m(X^*, Z; \gamma) + \beta_z^{\mathrm{T}} Z\right\} \tag{3.20}$$

and

$$\lambda^*(t|X^*, Z) \approx \lambda_0(t) + \beta_x^{\mathrm{T}} m(X^*, Z; \gamma) + \beta_z^{\mathrm{T}} Z, \tag{3.21}$$

respectively, where $\lambda_0^*(t) = \lambda_0(t)\exp(\beta_x^{\mathrm{T}}\Sigma^*\beta_x/2)$ is free of the covariates just as $\lambda_0(t)$ is.

We examine more specifically the structure of the induced hazard function under two measurement error models discussed in §2.6. First, we consider the Berkson error model (2.24) where the error term e is assumed to be normally distributed. By model (3.21), the induced hazard function for the additive hazards model is approximately identical to the true hazard function with X replaced by X^*. With the proportional hazards model, (3.20) indicates that the induced hazard function approximately has the same form as the true hazard function $\lambda(t|X, Z)$ with X replaced by X^*, but the baseline hazard function differs by a factor that depends on the degree of measurement error and the error-prone covariate effects β_x.

Next, we consider the classical additive error model (2.23) where $e \sim N(0, \Sigma_e)$ with covariance matrix Σ_e. Assume that conditional on Z, X has the distribution $N(\mu_x, \Sigma_x)$, where $\mu_x = \gamma_0 + \Gamma_z Z$, γ_0 is a column vector, Γ_z is a matrix of regression coefficients, and Σ_x is a nonnegative definite matrix. Define

$$\Omega = \Sigma_x(\Sigma_x + \Sigma_e)^{-1}$$

to be the *reliability matrix*. Then conditional on $\{X^*, Z\}$, X follows normal distribution $N(m(X^*, Z), (I_{p_x} - \Omega)\Sigma_x)$, where $m(X^*, Z) = (I_{p_x} - \Omega)\gamma_0 + \Omega X^* + (I_{p_x} - \Omega)\Gamma_z Z$ (see Problem 5.5(b) in Ch. 5).

By model (3.20), the approximate induced hazard function for the proportional hazards model is given by

$$\lambda^*(t|X^*, Z) \approx \lambda_0^{**}(t)\exp\left[\beta_x^{\mathrm{T}}\Omega X^* + \left\{\beta_x^{\mathrm{T}}(I_{p_x} - \Omega)\Gamma_z + \beta_z^{\mathrm{T}}\right\} Z\right] \tag{3.22}$$

with $\lambda_0^{**}(t) = \lambda_0(t)\exp\{\beta_x^{\mathrm{T}}(I_{p_x} - \Omega)(\Sigma_x\beta_x/2 + \gamma_0)\}$, whereas (3.21) yields the approximate induced hazard function for the additive hazards model:

$$\lambda^*(t|X^*, Z) \approx \lambda_0^{**}(t) + \beta_x^{\mathrm{T}}\Omega X^* + \left\{\beta_x^{\mathrm{T}}(I_{p_x} - \Omega)\Gamma_z + \beta_z^{\mathrm{T}}\right\} Z \tag{3.23}$$

with $\lambda_0^{**}(t) = \lambda_0(t) + \beta_x^{\mathrm{T}}(I_{p_x} - \Omega)\gamma_0$.

Comparing these approximate structures to the corresponding true hazard function reveals the impact of measurement error on changing the structure of the survival process. Examining the differences of the coefficients in (3.8) and (3.10), respectively, from those of (3.22) and (3.23) shows that measurement error in X would approximately attenuate estimation of β_x by the factor Ω and that measurement error effects on estimation of β_z may depend on the association between X and Z as well as covariate effect β_x. The induced baseline hazard function differs from the true baseline hazard function in general.

3.2.2 Discussion and Assumptions

The preceding discussion examines measurement error effects on the structure of the hazard function for the survival process alone. Special features, such as censoring, of survival data are not accommodated in the discussion. To understand measurement error effects in conjunction with censoring effects, one may directly examine the impact of measurement error on the estimation of the parameter governing the survival process. This can be, in principle, carried out using the strategies outlined in §1.4 to quantify asymptotic biases of estimation induced by the naive analysis with the difference between X^* and X ignored. Under special situations, discussion on this issue is available in the literature. For instance, under the proportional hazards model with a scalar error-prone covariate, Hughes (1993) and Küchenhoff, Bender and Langner (2007), respectively, investigated this problem for classical additive and Berkson error models. For multiple error-prone covariates under the proportional hazards model, Kong (1999) and Li and Ryan (2004) studied asymptotic biases under additive measurement error models. With the additive hazards model, Sun and Zhou (2008) discussed the asymptotic bias along the same line as Kong (1999).

In general, it is difficult to analytically quantify the nature and magnitude of asymptotic biases involved in the naive analysis which ignores measurement error. Asymptotic biases pertain to many factors, including the model forms for the survival and measurement error processes as well as the censoring mechanism and other features of survival data such as truncation. Other elements, including the dependence structure among covariates and the variability of covariates, may also affect asymptotic biases. Moreover, measurement error may have different impact on estimation of the same model parameters if different estimation procedures are employed (Yi and He 2006; Yi, Liu and Wu 2011).

It is sensible to conduct a case-by-case study in order to adequately accommodate measurement error effects. Although general strategies are outlined in §2.5, they are not directly applicable to deal with error-contaminated survival data due to their special features such as censoring or truncation. Usual mechanisms and assumptions imposed on either the measurement error process or survival analysis *alone* may become meaningless unless proper modifications are introduced. In principle, a valid inference method should be developed to reflect specific characteristics pertaining to mismeasurement and survival data processes as well as the observational scheme, which basically depends on the way we examine the data.

As an illustration, we consider right censored survival data with covariate X subject to measurement error. There are multiple ways of examining the joint distribution of $\{T, C, X^*, X, Z\}$ from which different model assumptions may arise. For example, one may consider any of the following factorizations:

$$h(t,c,x^*,x,z) = h(t,c,x^*|x,z)h(x,z); \tag{3.24}$$

$$h(t,c,x^*,x,z) = h(t,c|x^*,x,z)h(x^*,x,z); \tag{3.25}$$

$$h(t,c,x^*,x,z) = h(c|t,x^*,x,z)h(t,x^*,x,z); \tag{3.26}$$

among others.

These factorizations have different emphases on variables T, C and X^*. If we impose the conditional independence assumption

$$h(t,c,x^*|x,z) = h(t,c|x,z)h(x^*|x,z), \tag{3.27}$$

or equivalently,

$$h(t, c|x^*, x, z) = h(t, c|x, z), \tag{3.28}$$

then factorizations (3.24) and (3.25) reduce to the same expression:

$$h(t, c, x^*, x, z) = h(t, c|x, z)h(x^*, x, z). \tag{3.29}$$

This expression is advantageous in that the mismeasurement variable X^* is separated from the survival and censoring processes, thereby, measurement error models outlined in §2.6 may apply to describe $h(x^*, x, z)$ and modeling strategies in §3.1 may be directly employed to characterize $h(t, c|x, z)$ in conjunction with some simplistic assumptions. For example, T and C are often assumed to be conditionally independent, given $\{X, Z\}$:

$$h(t, c|x, z) = h(t|x, z)h(c|x, z). \tag{3.30}$$

This assumption allows us to not postulate the censoring time but to direct attention to describing $h(t|x, z)$ using the modeling strategies in §3.1. Many available inference methods in the literature are developed along these lines.

Conducting inferences based on factorization (3.26), on the other hand, may prompt different assumptions. For instance, when the distributions $h(c|t, x^*, x, z)$ and $h(t, x^*, x, z)$ are modeled parametrically, the associated model parameters are assumed to be distinct. If marginal analysis is conducted for the model parameter for $h(t, x^*, x, z)$, such as based on unbiased estimating functions, a specification of the model form of $h(c|t, x^*, x, z)$ may be needed. However, if the likelihood method is used for inference about the model parameter for $h(t, x^*, x, z)$, then modeling form of $h(c|t, x^*, x, z)$ can be left unattended to. In this case, the factorization

$$h(t, x^*, x, z) = h(t|x^*, x, z)h(x^*, x, z)$$

is usually employed and the assumption

$$h(t|x^*, x, z) = h(t|x, z) \tag{3.31}$$

is imposed so that models in §3.1 and §2.6 may be applied to portray the survival and measurement error processes.

In the following sections, we describe several methods to account for covariate measurement error effects under the framework based on (3.29), in combination with the independence censoring mechanism (3.30). Noting that the identities (3.27), (3.29) and (3.28) are all equivalent: assuming one identity yields the other two, we call a measurement error process satisfying any of these conditions *nondifferential*. This definition differs from that in §2.4, or the assumption (3.31). Identity (3.28) implies (3.31), but not vise versa. The nondifferential measurement error mechanism here says that the observed surrogate measurement X^* has no predictive value for either the survival or the censoring process if the true covariates $\{X, Z\}$ are controlled.

For the development of the rest of this chapter, we use the same notation or symbols defined in §3.1–§3.2 unless otherwise defined.

3.3 Approximate Methods for Measurement Error Correction

In §3.2.1, we demonstrate that ignoring measurement error in covariates may distort the structure of the hazard function and often produce biased inference results. In this section, we describe two methods that are frequently used in practice to *reduce* biases caused by measurement error in covariates.

3.3.1 Regression Calibration Method

The first approach is the *regression calibration* method, which is motivated by the similarity of the approximate structure of the induced hazard function (3.20) or (3.21) to the corresponding true hazard function. As opposed to the naive analysis by replacing X in the true hazard function with its observed surrogate X^* directly, the regression calibration method replaces unobserved X with its conditional expectation $E(X \mid X^*, Z)$.

Suppose the observed data consist of $\mathcal{O} = \{(t_i, \delta_i, X_i^*, Z_i) : i = 1, \ldots, n\}$ where the $(t_i, \delta_i, X_i^*, Z_i)$ are described in §3.1.5 and the measurements X_i^* are the surrogate versions of X_i. The regression calibration method comprises three steps:

- Step 1: Estimate $E(X_i|X_i^*, Z_i)$.
- Step 2: Run a standard survival analysis for the model $f(t_i|X_i, Z_i; \beta)$ with X_i replaced by the estimate of $E(X_i|X_i^*, Z_i)$ and obtain a point estimate of β. Let $\widehat{\beta}$ denote the resulting estimator of β.
- Step 3: Adjust the standard error associated with $\widehat{\beta}$ to account for the variability induced from estimation in Step 1.

Step 3 may be implemented using the bootstrap method and Step 2 is usually realized using existing statistical software packages, such as *coxph* or *survreg* in R, or *PROC PHREG* in SAS. At Step 1, estimation of $E(X_i|X_i^*, Z_i)$, the so-called *calibration function*, is determined by additional data that are used to characterize the measurement error process. With repeated surrogate measurements for X_i available, Xie, Wang and Prentice (2001) described a way to estimate the calibration function for the proportional hazards model. Under the classical additive error model, Carroll et al. (2006, §4.4) described methods of estimating the calibration function.

Here we examine a situation where an internal validation sample is available. Using the notation in §2.4, suppose that a validation subsample $\mathcal{D} = \{(t_i, \delta_i, X_i, X_i^*, Z_i) : i \in \mathcal{V}\}$ is available, in addition to the main study data $\{(t_i, \delta_i, X_i^*, Z_i) : i \in \mathcal{M}\}$, where $\mathcal{V}$ is a subset of $\mathcal{M}$. Let $\eta_i = I(i \in \mathcal{V})$ be the indicator variable whether or not subject i belongs to the validation subsample $\mathcal{V}$. To estimate the calibration function, we invoke standard regression analysis, such as linear regression, generalized linear regression or nonlinear regression, to the validation data $\mathcal{D}$.

For instance, we consider a regression model

$$X_i = m_x(X_i^*, Z_i; \gamma) + \epsilon_{xi} \quad \text{for } i \in \mathcal{V},$$

where error term ϵ_{xi} has mean zero and is independent of $\{X_i^*, Z_i, T_i, C_i\}$, γ is a vector of unknown parameters, and $m_x(\cdot)$ is a specified function. Let $\widehat{\gamma}$ denote the resultant estimate of γ obtained from using the validation data $\mathcal{D}$. The calibration function $E(X_i|X_i^*, Z_i)$ is then estimated by $m_x(X_i^*, Z_i; \widehat{\gamma})$.

For every subject $i \in \mathcal{M} = \{1, \ldots, n\}$ in the main study, define the *calibration measurement* for covariate X_i as

$$X_i^{**} = \eta_i X_i + (1 - \eta_i) m_x(X_i^*, Z_i; \widehat{\gamma}),$$

which is used in the standard survival analysis of Step 2. Calibration measurement X_i^{**} takes value X_i or $m_x(X_i^*, Z_i; \widehat{\gamma})$, depending on whether or not subject i is included in the validation subsample. Write $\mathbb{X}^{**} = \{X_1^{**}, \ldots, X_i^{**}\}$.

Example 3.3. Under the proportional hazards model (3.8), an estimating function for β is obtained from the partial score function by replacing X_i with X_i^{**}. Then solving

$$U^*(\beta) = \sum_{i=1}^{n} \delta_i \left\{ \begin{pmatrix} X_i^{**} \\ Z_i \end{pmatrix} - \frac{S^{(1)}(t_i, \mathbb{X}^{**}, \mathbb{Z}; \beta)}{S^{(0)}(t_i, \mathbb{X}^{**}, \mathbb{Z}; \beta)} \right\} = 0$$

for β results in an estimator, denoted $\widehat{\beta}$, of β, where $S^{(k)}(t, \mathbb{X}^{**}, \mathbb{Z}; \beta)$ is defined as (3.12) with $\mathbb{X}$ replaced by $\mathbb{X}^{**}$ for $k = 0, 1$.

Using the techniques of Andersen and Gill (1982), we can show that $\widehat{\beta}$ converges to β^* in probability as $n \to \infty$, where β^* is a root of $E\{U^*(\beta)\} = 0$, and the expectation is taken with respect to the model for the joint distribution of $\{\mathbb{T}, \mathbb{C}, \mathbb{X}, \mathbb{Z}, \mathbb{X}^*\}$ with $\mathbb{X}^* = \{X_1^*, \ldots, X_n^*\}$. As discussed in §2.5.2, the estimator $\widehat{\beta}$ is not exactly a consistent estimator of β and is just an approximately consistent estimator. From the numerical experience, it appears that β^* is often very close to β when $m_x(X_i^*, Z_i; \gamma)$ is reasonably estimated. A $\sqrt{n}$-consistent estimate of γ may be obtained using the validation data if the size n_{v} of the validation subsample satisfies $n_{\mathrm{v}}/n \to \rho$ as $n \to \infty$, where ρ is a constant greater than 0 (Wang et al. 1997).

Remark

The regression calibration algorithm is easy to implement by modifying existing software packages for survival data analysis. This procedure is attractive in that the distribution of the true covariates is left unspecified. Although the regression calibration method is initiated by Prentice (1982) for the proportional hazards model with error-prone covariates under the rare event assumption, as discussed in §3.2.1, this method has now been frequently employed for many parametric and semiparametric models with covariate measurement error. However, a major drawback makes this method less appealing, especially from the theoretical point of view. The regression calibration method cannot entirely correct for biases induced from measurement error; it can only produce *approximately* consistent estimators for general settings.

3.3.2 Simulation Extrapolation Method

The SIMEX method described in §2.5.3 may be used to reduce bias involved in the naive analysis which ignores measurement error in survival data. This method is used when the covariance matrix Σ_e in the error model (2.21) is known or estimated from a priori study or an additional data source.

In the presence of replicate surrogate measurements, the SIMEX method is applied with a modified simulation step. For $j = 1, \ldots, m_i$, let X_{ij}^* denote the repeated measurements for the true covariate X_i which are linked with X_i by the model

$$X_{ij}^* = X_i + e_{ij},$$

where the e_{ij} are independent of $\{X_i, Z_i, T_i, C_i\}$ and follow a normal distribution $N(0, \Sigma_e)$ with an unknown covariance matrix Σ_e, and m_i is a positive integer which may depend on i.

Instead of using (2.22) to generate $x_{ib}^*(c)$, we set, for given b and c,

$$x_{ib}^*(c) = \overline{x}_i^* + \sqrt{\frac{c}{m_i}} \cdot \sum_{j=1}^{m_i} c_{ij}(b) x_{ij}^*,$$

where $\overline{x}_i^* = m_i^{-1} \sum_{j=1}^{m_i} x_{ij}^*$ and the $c_i(b) = (c_{i1}(b), \ldots, c_{im_i}(b))^{\mathrm{T}}$ are normalized contrasts satisfying $\sum_{j=1}^{m_i} c_{ij}(b) = 0$ and $\sum_{j=1}^{m_i} c_{ij}^2(b) = 1$.

A simple way to generate such a contrast $c_i(b)$ is to use a normal variate generation. For each b and $i = 1, \ldots, n$, independently generate m_i normal random variables $d_{ij}(b)$ for $j = 1, \ldots, m_i$ from a standard normal distribution $N(0, 1)$, then setting

$$c_{ij}(b) = \frac{d_{ij}(b) - \overline{d}_i(b)}{\sqrt{\sum_{l=1}^{m_i} \{d_{il}(b) - \overline{d}_i(b)\}^2}}$$

results in the required contrasts $c_i(b)$ (Devanarayan and Stefanski 2002), where $\overline{d}_i(b) = m_i^{-1} \sum_{j=1}^{m_i} d_{ij}(b)$.

Like the regression calibration method, the second step of the SIMEX approach is often carried out using statistical software packages for survival analysis, such as *coxph* or *survreg* in R, or *PROC PHREG* in SAS. The extrapolation step is realized by usual regression analysis. The SIMEX method has been applied to analyze error-contaminated survival data under various models. A discussion on applications of this method is given in §3.9.

3.4 Methods Based on the Induced Hazard Function

The discussion in §3.2 shows that the induced hazard function $\lambda^*(t|X^*, Z)$ of T given the observed covariates $\{X^*, Z\}$ differs from the true hazard function $\lambda(t|X, Z)$ in structure or function form. The two functional methods described in §3.3, regression calibration and simulation extrapolation, are easy to implement but in many settings, they only partially correct for the bias induced from the naive analysis which disregards the difference between X^* and X. The performance of those approaches is fairly satisfactory when measurement error is not severe. If there is substantial measurement error involved, the performance may decay dramatically.

Alternatively, by capitalizing on the specific model features for survival data, we may develop valid inference methods to adjust for measurement error effects using the strategies sketched in §2.5. Here we describe the induced model strategy and defer other tactics to subsequent sections.

Our discussion is based on the methods developed by Zucker (2005) for the proportional hazards model (3.6), given by

$$S(t|X,Z) = \exp\{-\Lambda_0(t)g(X,Z;\beta)\},$$

where $\Lambda_0(\cdot)$ is an increasing, differentiable baseline cumulative hazard function whose form is unspecified, $g(X,Z;\beta)$ defines the covariate effects, and β is a vector of unknown parameters. Function $g(X,Z;\beta)$ is assumed to satisfy certain technical conditions such as $g(X,Z;0) = 1$ for all covariates so that $\beta = 0$ corresponds to no covariate effect. Often, $g(X,Z;\beta)$ is taken to be a function that is monotone in each component of $\{X,Z\}$ for all β. A classical choice is $g(X,Z;\beta) = \exp(\beta_x^{\mathrm{T}}X + \beta_z^{\mathrm{T}}Z)$ as in (3.8) with $\beta = (\beta_x^{\mathrm{T}}, \beta_z^{\mathrm{T}})^{\mathrm{T}}$.

To feature the measurement error model, we consider the conditional distribution of X given $\{X^*,Z\}$ and let $f(x|X^*,Z)$ denote the model for this conditional probability density or mass function with the parameter suppressed in the notation. To highlight estimation on β, we assume that $f(x|X^*,Z)$ and the associated parameter are known. In addition, the nondifferential measurement error mechanism is assumed.

3.4.1 Induced Likelihood Method

With the given model assumptions, the *induced* conditional survivor function of T given the observed covariates $\{X^*,Z\}$ is

$$\begin{aligned} S^*(t|X^*,Z) &= P(T > t|X^*,Z) \\ &= \int \exp\{-\Lambda_0(t)g(x,Z;\beta)\}f(x|X^*,Z)d\eta(x). \end{aligned}$$

Then applying identity (3.1) gives the induced hazard function

$$\lambda^*(t|X^*,Z) = \lambda_0(t)\exp\{\phi(X^*,Z;\beta,\Lambda_0(t))\},$$

where $\lambda_0(t) = (d/dt)\Lambda_0(t)$,

$$\begin{aligned} &\phi(X^*,Z;\beta,\Lambda_0(t)) \\ &= \log\left[\int \exp\{-\Lambda_0(t)g(x,Z;\beta)\}g(x,Z;\beta)f(x|X^*,Z)d\eta(x)\right] \\ &\quad - \log\left[\int \exp\{-\Lambda_0(t)g(x,Z;\beta)\}f(x|X^*,Z)d\eta(x)\right], \end{aligned} \tag{3.32}$$

and integration and differentiation are assumed to be exchangeable. This induced hazard function equals $\lambda_0(t)E\{g(X,Z;\beta)|T \geq t, X^*, Z\}$, as discussed in §3.2.1.

As a result, the model for the *induced* conditional probability density function of T given the observed covariates $\{X^*, Z\}$ is

$$f^*(t|X^*, Z) = \lambda^*(t|X^*, Z)S^*(t|X^*, Z),$$

which leads to the *induced* likelihood when used to the observed data $\mathcal{O}$ described in §3.3.1:

$$L^*(\beta) = \prod_{i=1}^{n} \{\lambda^*(t_i|X_i^*, Z_i)\}^{\delta_i} S^*(t_i|X_i^*, Z_i).$$

This likelihood, however, cannot be directly used for inference about β because of the involvement of the unknown baseline cumulative hazard function $\Lambda_0(t)$. To handle $\Lambda_0(t)$, one may employ a scheme outlined in §3.1.2. Alternatively, we may estimate $\Lambda_0(t)$ nonparametrically, following the description by Zucker (2005) where the Breslow cumulative hazard function estimator is used (Breslow 1974).

First, order all the observed survival times as s_k for $k = 1, \ldots, K$, where K is the number of distinct observed survival times. Let d_k represent the number of events at time s_k, and $\Delta\Lambda_0(s_k) = \Lambda_0(s_k) - \Lambda_0(s_{k-1})$ denote the difference, or the jump, of the baseline cumulative hazard function at adjacent observed times s_k and s_{k-1}, where $s_0 = 0$ and $\Lambda_0(s_0) = 0$. Then for a given value of β, we approximate $\Lambda_0(t)$ iteratively by a step function with jumps at the ordered observed event times s_k:

$$\widehat{\Lambda}_0(s_k) = \Delta\widehat{\Lambda}_0(s_k) + \widehat{\Lambda}_0(s_{k-1}),$$

where $\widehat{\Lambda}_0(s_0)$ is set as 0 and

$$\Delta\widehat{\Lambda}_0(s_k) = \frac{d_k}{\sum_{i=1}^{n} R_i(s_k) \exp\{\phi(X_i^*, Z_i; \beta, \widehat{\Lambda}_0(s_{k-1}))\}}$$

for $k = 1, \ldots, K$.

With continuous survival times T_i, all the d_k would be 1; in actual implementation, some d_k may be greater than 1 to allow for tied event times. Inference on β proceeds with the maximization of the induced likelihood $L^*(\beta)$ for which the $\Lambda_0(t)$ are replaced with their estimates $\widehat{\Lambda}_0(s_k)$ for $t \in (s_{k-1}, s_k]$.

3.4.2 Induced Partial Likelihood Method

Along the same line as for developing the partial likelihood (3.11) for the Cox proportional hazards model (Kalbfleisch and Prentice 2002, §4.2), we consider an analogue for the observed data $\mathcal{O}$ using the induced hazard function $\lambda^*(t|X^*, Z)$:

$$\begin{aligned} L_{\mathrm{P}}^*(\beta, \Lambda_0(\cdot)) &= \prod_{i=1}^{n} \left\{ \frac{\lambda^*(t_i|X_i^*, Z_i)}{\sum_{j=1}^{n} R_j(t_i)\lambda^*(t_i|X_j^*, Z_j)} \right\}^{\delta_i} \\ &= \prod_{i=1}^{n} \left[\frac{\exp\{\phi(X_i^*, Z_i; \beta, \Lambda_0(t_i))\}}{\sum_{j=1}^{n} R_j(t_i) \exp\{\phi(X_j^*, Z_j; \beta, \Lambda_0(t_i))\}} \right]^{\delta_i}, \end{aligned}$$

leading to the log *induced partial likelihood* function

$$\ell_{\mathrm{P}}^*(\beta, \Lambda_0(\cdot)) = \sum_{i=1}^{n} \ell_{\mathrm{P}i}^*(\beta, \Lambda_0(t_i)),$$

where

$$\begin{aligned}
&\ell_{\mathrm{P}i}^*(\beta, \Lambda_0(t_i)) \\
&= \delta_i \left(\phi(X_i^*, Z_i; \beta, \Lambda_0(t_i)) - \log \left[\sum_{j=1}^{n} R_j(t_i) \exp\{\phi(X_j^*, Z_j; \beta, \Lambda_0(t_i))\} \right] \right).
\end{aligned}$$

Unlike the standard partial likelihood (3.11) which is free of the baseline hazard function, $L_{\mathrm{P}}^*(\beta)$ depends on the cumulative baseline hazard function, in addition to the dependence on parameter β and the covariates. Therefore, estimation of parameter β based on $L_{\mathrm{P}}^*(\beta, \Lambda_0(\cdot))$ cannot be carried through unless $\Lambda_0(\cdot)$ is available. For a given value of β, let $\widehat{\Lambda}_0(t; \beta)$ be an estimate of $\Lambda_0(t)$ (e.g., the Breslow estimator in §3.4.1). Define $L_{\mathrm{P}}^*(\beta, \widehat{\Lambda}_0(\cdot; \beta))$ to be the function $L_{\mathrm{P}}^*(\beta, \Lambda_0(\cdot))$ with the estimate $\widehat{\Lambda}_0(t; \beta)$ in place of $\Lambda_0(t)$, which we call a *pseudo-partial likelihood*. Estimation of β is then based on this pseudo-partial likelihood.

Define

$$\psi(X_i^*, Z_i; \beta, c) = \frac{\partial}{\partial \beta}\phi(X_i^*, Z_i; \beta, c),\ \nu(X_i^*, Z_i; \beta, c) = \frac{\partial}{\partial c}\phi(X_i^*, Z_i; \beta, c),$$

$$Q(t; \beta) = \frac{\partial}{\partial \beta}\widehat{\Lambda}_0(t; \beta),\ \text{ and } \xi(X_i^*, Z_i; \beta, t) = \frac{\partial}{\partial \beta}\phi(X_i^*, Z_i; \beta, \widehat{\Lambda}_0(t; \beta)).$$

By the Chain Rule for derivatives, these functions are connected as follows:

$$\begin{aligned}
&\xi(X_i^*, Z_i; \beta, t) \\
&= \psi(X_i^*, Z_i; \beta, \widehat{\Lambda}_0(t; \beta)) + \nu(X_i^*, Z_i; \beta, \widehat{\Lambda}_0(t; \beta)) Q(t; \beta).
\end{aligned} \tag{3.33}$$

Let $U_i(\beta, \widehat{\Lambda}_0(t_i; \beta)) = (\partial/\partial\beta)\ell_{\mathrm{P}i}(\beta, \widehat{\Lambda}_0(t_i; \beta))$ be the *pseudo-partial score function* contributed from subject i, given by

$$\begin{aligned}
U_i(\beta, \widehat{\Lambda}_0(t_i; \beta)) = \delta_i \Bigg[&\xi(X_i^*, Z_i; \beta, t_i) \\
&- \frac{\sum_{j=1}^{n} R_j(t_i)\xi(X_j^*, Z_j; \beta, t_i) \exp\{\phi(X_j^*, Z_j; \beta, \widehat{\Lambda}_0(t_i; \beta))\}}{\sum_{j=1}^{n} R_j(t_i) \exp\{\phi(X_j^*, Z_j; \beta, \widehat{\Lambda}_0(t_i; \beta))\}} \Bigg],
\end{aligned}$$

where function $\xi(\cdot)$ is given by (3.33) and function $\phi(\cdot)$ is defined by (3.32).

Let

$$U(\beta, \widehat{\Lambda}_0(\cdot; \beta)) = \frac{1}{n} \sum_{i=1}^{n} U_i(\beta, \widehat{\Lambda}_0(t_i; \beta)),$$

then solving

$$U(\beta, \widehat{\Lambda}_0(\cdot; \beta)) = 0$$

for β leads to an estimate of β. Let $\widehat{\beta}$ denote the resultant estimator. Under regularity conditions of Zucker (2005), $\widehat{\beta}$ is a consistent estimator of β and $\sqrt{n}(\widehat{\beta} - \beta)$ is asymptotically normally distributed with mean 0. Inference about β is then conducted using this asymptotic result.

To see why the induced pseudo-partial likelihood method works, we sketch the lines of establishing this asymptotic result. As usual, we start with the identity $U(\widehat{\beta}, \widehat{\Lambda}_0(\cdot; \widehat{\beta})) = 0$ that leads to the estimator $\widehat{\beta}$. We examine how $U(\widehat{\beta}, \widehat{\Lambda}_0(\cdot; \widehat{\beta}))$ depends on the true values of β and $\Lambda_0(\cdot)$. Instead of looking at this dependence simultaneously on all the arguments, we examine it piece by piece with just one argument changing at a time. Specifically, we write

$$\begin{aligned} U(\widehat{\beta}, \widehat{\Lambda}_0(\cdot; \widehat{\beta})) = U(\beta, \Lambda_0(\cdot)) &+ \{U(\beta, \widehat{\Lambda}_0(\cdot; \beta)) - U(\beta, \Lambda_0(\cdot))\} \\ &+ \{U(\widehat{\beta}, \widehat{\Lambda}_0(\cdot; \widehat{\beta})) - U(\beta, \widehat{\Lambda}_0(\cdot; \beta))\}, \end{aligned} \tag{3.34}$$

which allows us to examine the difference induced by changing *one* argument with the others fixed. The first term is the function obtained by differentiating $\ell_{\text{p}}^*(\beta, \Lambda_0(\cdot))$ with respect to β; the second bracketed term indicates the variation induced from the estimation of the baseline cumulative hazard function $\Lambda_0(\cdot)$ for a given β; and the last bracketed term expresses the difference caused by estimator $\widehat{\beta}$ for a given estimate $\widehat{\Lambda}_0(\cdot; \cdot)$.

The asymptotic distribution of estimator $\widehat{\beta}$ is established by examining the limiting distribution of a scaled version of $U(\widehat{\beta}, \widehat{\Lambda}_0(\cdot; \widehat{\beta}))$, i.e., scaled by $\sqrt{n}$, which is done term by term for the expression (3.34). Applying the Taylor series expansion to the last bracketed term, scaled by $\sqrt{n}$, leads to its approximation $-\widehat{V} \cdot \sqrt{n}(\widehat{\beta} - \beta)$, where

$$\begin{aligned} \widehat{V} = \frac{1}{n} \sum_{i=1}^{n} \delta_i & \left[\frac{\sum_{j=1}^{n} R_j(t_i) \xi(X_j^*, Z_j; \beta, t_i)^{\otimes 2} \exp\{\phi(X_j^*, Z_j; \beta, \widehat{\Lambda}_0(t_i; \beta))\}}{\sum_{j=1}^{n} R_j(t_i) \exp\{\phi(X_j^*, Z_j; \beta, \widehat{\Lambda}_0(t_i; \beta))\}} \right. \\ & \left. \left\{ \frac{\sum_{j=1}^{n} R_j(t_i) \xi(X_j^*, Z_j; \beta, t_i) \exp\{\phi(X_j^*, Z_j; \beta, \widehat{\Lambda}_0(t_i; \beta))\}}{\sum_{j=1}^{n} R_j(t_i) \exp\{\phi(X_j^*, Z_j; \beta, \widehat{\Lambda}_0(t_i; \beta))\}} \right\}^{\otimes 2} \right] \Bigg|_{\beta = \widehat{\beta}}. \end{aligned}$$

Regarding the first and second bracketed terms, Zucker (2005) showed that they are asymptotically independent, and the scaled second bracketed term $\sqrt{n}\{U(\beta, \widehat{\Lambda}_0(\cdot; \beta)) - U(\beta, \Lambda_0(\cdot))\}$ is asymptotically normally distributed with mean 0 and a covariance matrix that is consistently estimated, say, by $\widehat{H}$. The scaled first term $\sqrt{n} U(\beta, \Lambda_0(\cdot))$ is shown, using the martingale arguments of Andersen and Gill (1982), to asymptotically follow a normal distribution with mean 0 and a covariance that is consistently estimated by $\widehat{V}$.

As a result, $\sqrt{n}(\widehat{\beta} - \beta)$ is asymptotically normally distributed with mean 0 and a covariance matrix that is consistently estimated by the matrix $\widehat{V}^{-1\text{T}} + \widehat{V}^{-1} \widehat{H} \widehat{V}^{-1\text{T}}$. Matrix $\widehat{V}^{-1}$ is similar to that arising from the classical Cox proportional hazards model and tends to be the dominant term (Zucker 2005). Extra variation pertaining to the estimation of $\Lambda_0(\cdot)$ is reflected in two places: the additional term $\widehat{V}^{-1}\widehat{H}\widehat{V}^{-1\mathrm{T}}$ and the involvement of the quantity $Q(\cdot;\beta)$ in $\widehat{V}^{-1}$.

Remark

Compared to the likelihood-based method in §3.4.1, the pseudo-partial likelihood approach seems likely to be less sensitive to the estimation of $\Lambda_0(\cdot)$. Some numerical experience suggests that the likelihood-based method tends to have convergence problems and yields estimates with higher variance than the pseudo-partial likelihood procedure does (Zucker 2005). In the aforementioned development, the distribution $f(x|X^*, Z)$ for the measurement error process is treated as known. This treatment is often not realistic, however. One must estimate $f(x|X^*, Z)$ using an additional source of data, such as a validation sample. It is necessary to modify the preceding development to account for the induced variability. With $f(x|X^*, Z)$ handled under the parametric framework, the principle outlined in §1.3.4 may be applied. Detailed discussion on this issue was given by Zucker (2005).

3.5 Likelihood-Based Methods

In contrast to the induced model strategy discussed in the previous section, we describe two strategies outlined in §2.5.2: the insertion correction and expectation correction methods. These methods root from using the true likelihood or the score function derived from the conditional distribution of T_i given $\{X_i, Z_i\}$. We illustrate the ideas by working with the proportion hazards model (3.8) for the observed data $\mathcal{O}$ described in §3.3.1.

3.5.1 Insertion Correction: Piecewise-Constant Method

In this subsection, we discuss the insertion correction strategy. Given the log-likelihood (3.9), we want to find a workable function, expressed in terms of the observed data $\mathcal{O}$ and the model parameters, so that it is connected with the true log-likelihood through (2.20). Since in (3.9), error-prone covariate X_i appears in polynomial, exponential or their product forms, we proceed with the use of the moment generating function of the measurement error model.

Suppose that the measurement error model assumes an additive form

$$X_i^* = X_i + e_i$$

for $i = 1, \ldots, n$, where conditional on $\{X_i, Z_i, T_i, C_i\}$, e_i has mean zero and the conditional moment generating function $M(v) = E\{\exp(v^{\mathrm{T}} e_i)|X_i, Z_i, T_i, C_i\}$. Under the nondifferential measurement error assumption in §3.2.2, we obtain that

$$E(e_i|X_i, Z_i) = 0 \text{ and } M(v) = E\{\exp(v^{\mathrm{T}} e_i)|X_i, Z_i\},$$

where the expectation is evaluated under the model for the distribution of e_i given $\{X_i, Z_i\}$.

For $i = 1, \ldots, n$, define

$$\ell_i^* = \delta_i\{\log \lambda_0(t_i) + \beta_x^{\mathrm{T}} X_i^* + \beta_z^{\mathrm{T}} Z_i\} \\ -\{M(\beta_x)\}^{-1} \exp(\beta_x^{\mathrm{T}} X_i^* + \beta_z^{\mathrm{T}} Z_i)\Lambda_0(t_i). \tag{3.35}$$

Then

$$\sum_{i=1}^{n} E\{\ell_i^* | X_i, Z_i, T_i, C_i\} = \ell,$$

where ℓ is the log-likelihood determined by (3.9), and the conditional expectation is taken with respect to the model for the conditional distribution of X_i^* given $\{X_i, Z_i, T_i, C_i\}$. Function ℓ_i^* is different from the naive log-likelihood obtained from (3.9) with X_i replaced by X_i^*. An additional term $\{M(\beta_x)\}^{-1}$is included in ℓ_i^* to reflect the adjustment of measurement error effects.

To use function ℓ_i^* for estimation of parameter β, we need to deal with the unknown baseline hazard function $\lambda_0(t)$. As discussed in §3.1.2, various schemes may be used to model $\lambda_0(t)$. Here we consider a weakly parametric scheme for modeling the baseline hazard function $\lambda_0(t)$, where $\lambda_0(t)$ is modeled by (3.2) and let $\rho = (\rho_1, \ldots, \rho_K)^{\mathrm{T}}$ denote the resulting parameter.

Let $\theta = (\rho^{\mathrm{T}}, \beta^{\mathrm{T}})^{\mathrm{T}}$ be the parameter associated with the survival model. We describe estimation procedures discussed by Augustin (2004) and Yi and Lawless (2007). To highlight the idea, we assume that the moment generating function $M(v)$ is known. For $i = 1, \ldots, n$, define $U_i^*(\theta) = \partial \ell_i^* / \partial \theta$. Solving

$$\sum_{i=1}^{n} U_i^*(\theta) = 0 \tag{3.36}$$

for θ leads to an estimate of parameter θ.

Let $\widehat{\theta}$ denote the resultant estimator of parameter θ. Under regularity conditions, $\sqrt{n}(\widehat{\theta} - \theta)$ has an asymptotic normal distribution with mean 0 and covariance matrix $\Gamma^{*-1}\Sigma^*\Gamma^{*-1\mathrm{T}}$, where $\Gamma^* = E\{\partial U_i^*(\theta)/\partial \theta^{\mathrm{T}}\}$, $\Sigma^* = E\{U_i^*(\theta)U_i^{*\mathrm{T}}(\theta)\}$, and the expectations are taken with respect to the model for the joint distribution of $\{T_i, C_i, X_i^*, X_i, Z_i\}$ which pertains to the response and measurement error models as well as the censoring process. As $n \to \infty$, Γ^* and Σ^* are consistently estimated by $\widehat{\Gamma}^* = n^{-1} \sum_{i=1}^{n} \{\partial U_i^*(\theta)/\partial \theta^{\mathrm{T}}\}|_{\theta=\widehat{\theta}}$, and $\widehat{\Sigma}^* = n^{-1} \sum_{i=1}^{n} \{U_i^*(\theta)U_i^{*\mathrm{T}}(\theta)\}|_{\theta=\widehat{\theta}}$, respectively.

The piecewise-constant modeling scheme offers flexibility to facilitate various types of baseline hazard functions. With an estimate $\widehat{\beta}$ for β available, an estimate of the baseline cumulative hazard function $\Lambda_0(t)$ is immediately derived as

$$\begin{aligned} \widehat{\Lambda}_0(t) &= \sum_{k=1}^{K} \widehat{\rho}_k u_k(t) \\ &= M(\widehat{\beta}_x) \sum_{k=1}^{K} \frac{\sum_{l=1}^{n} \delta_l I(t_l \in A_k)}{\sum_{l=1}^{n} \exp(\widehat{\beta}_x^{\mathrm{T}} X_l^* + \widehat{\beta}_z^{\mathrm{T}} Z_l) u_k(t_l)} \cdot u_k(t). \end{aligned}$$

A variance estimate for $\widehat{\Lambda}_0(t)$ at specified values of t may be obtained by applying the delta method to the estimated covariance matrix for $\widehat{\theta}$. Alternatively, the bootstrap algorithm may be employed to produce variance estimates.

Solving (3.36) gives, for fixed β_x and β_z, an estimator of ρ similar to that obtained from the profile likelihood:

$$\widehat{\rho}_k = M(\beta_x) \cdot \frac{\sum_{i=1}^n \delta_i I(t_i \in A_k)}{\sum_{i=1}^n \exp(\beta_x^{\mathrm{T}} X_i^* + \beta_z^{\mathrm{T}} Z_i) \cdot u_k(t_i)} \quad \text{for } k = 1, \ldots, K;$$

while $\widehat{\beta}$ can be solved from

$$\sum_{i=1}^n \widehat{U}_{i\beta_x}^*(\widehat{\rho}, \beta) = 0 \text{ and } \sum_{i=1}^n \widehat{U}_{i\beta_z}^*(\widehat{\rho}, \beta) = 0,$$

where $U_{i\beta_x}^*(\rho, \beta) = \partial \ell_i^* / \partial \beta_x$, $U_{i\beta_z}^*(\rho, \beta) = \partial \ell_i^* / \partial \beta_z$, and $\widehat{\rho} = (\widehat{\rho}_1, \ldots, \widehat{\rho}_K)^{\mathrm{T}}$.

The asymptotic distribution of $\sqrt{n}(\widehat{\theta} - \theta)$ described here does not take into account the cut point selection for modeling $\lambda_0(t)$ and treats them as fixed. Therefore, the inference method discussed here is regarded as a "conditional" analysis for given K and the a_k. Although it is expected that a larger K allows the ability to capture a more refined shape of the baseline hazard function, empirical evidence suggests that choosing K to be 4 to 6 would be adequate for many practical problems. A common strategy in selecting cut points a_k is to retain roughly equal numbers of observed failure times in each time interval $(a_{k-1}, a_k]$ (Lawless and Zhan 1998; He and Lawless 2003).

Let a_{K-1} be fixed at some large value beyond which failure times are essentially impossible. Using the same argument as in Lawless (2003, §7.4), we show that as $K \to \infty$ with the values $a_k - a_{k-1} \to 0$ for $k = 1, \ldots, K-1$, for the given data, $\widehat{U}_{\beta_x}^*(\widehat{\rho}, \beta)$ approaches

$$\begin{aligned} U_{\beta_x}^{**}(\beta) = \sum_{i=1}^n \delta_i \Bigg[X_i^* &- \frac{\sum_{l=1}^n R_l(t_i) X_l^* \exp(\beta_x^{\mathrm{T}} X_l^* + \beta_z^{\mathrm{T}} Z_l)}{\sum_{l=1}^n R_l(t_i) \exp(\beta_x^{\mathrm{T}} X_l^* + \beta_z^{\mathrm{T}} Z_l)} \\ &+ \{M(\beta_x)\}^{-1} \left\{ \frac{\partial M(\beta_x)}{\partial \beta_x} \right\} \Bigg], \end{aligned} \tag{3.37}$$

and $\widehat{U}_{\beta_z}^*(\beta, \widehat{\rho})$ approaches

$$U_{\beta_z}^{**}(\beta) = \sum_{i=1}^n \delta_i \left\{ Z_i - \frac{\sum_{l=1}^n R_l(t_i) Z_l \exp(\beta_x^{\mathrm{T}} X_l^* + \beta_z^{\mathrm{T}} Z_l)}{\sum_{l=1}^n R_l(t_i) \exp(\beta_x^{\mathrm{T}} X_l^* + \beta_z^{\mathrm{T}} Z_l)} \right\}, \tag{3.38}$$

where the constant factor accounting for the decreasing interval widths is omitted.

The limit form (3.38) is the same as the naive Cox partial score function for β_z, but the limit function (3.37) differs from the naive Cox partial score function for β_x

by the term $\{M(\beta_x)\}^{-1}\{\partial M(\beta_x)/\partial \beta_x\}$. Functions (3.37) and (3.38) were proposed heuristically by Nakamura (1992) to estimate β and justified by Kong and Gu (1999), where the measurement error process was modeled by (2.21).

We close this subsection with comments. In the case where the moment generating function $M(v)$ is unknown, one may use additional data sources, such as replicates or validation data, to estimate $M(v)$. The induced variation must then be taken into account; the procedures outlined in §1.3.4 may be applied for this purpose.

To illustrate this, we consider a situation where the moment generating function $M(v)$ has a known function form and involves an unknown vector of parameters, say α. In this case, function ℓ_i^* depends on not only θ but also α. Suppose for $i = 1, \ldots, n$, an unbiased estimating function of α, denoted by $\psi_i(\alpha)$, is available. Define $U_i^*(\alpha, \theta) = \partial \ell_i^* / \partial \theta$, then solving

$$\begin{pmatrix} \sum_{i=1}^n \psi_i(\alpha) \\ \sum_{i=1}^n U_i^*(\alpha, \theta) \end{pmatrix} = 0$$

for α and θ gives estimates for α and θ. Let $\widehat{\alpha}$ and $\widehat{\theta}$ denote the resulting estimators.

Define

$$Q_i^*(\alpha, \theta) = U_i^*(\alpha, \theta) - E\left\{\frac{\partial U_i^*(\alpha, \theta)}{\partial \alpha^{\mathrm{T}}}\right\}\left[E\left\{\frac{\partial \psi_i(\alpha)}{\partial \alpha^{\mathrm{T}}}\right\}\right]^{-1} \psi_i(\alpha),$$

and

$$\widetilde{\Sigma}^* = E\{Q_i^*(\alpha, \theta) Q_i^{*\mathrm{T}}(\alpha, \theta)\},$$

Applying (1.15) gives that $\sqrt{n}(\widehat{\theta} - \theta)$ has an asymptotic normal distribution with mean 0 and covariance matrix $\Gamma^{*-1}\widetilde{\Sigma}^*\Gamma^{*-1^{\mathrm{T}}}$, where $\Gamma^* = E\{\partial U_i^*(\alpha, \theta)/\partial \theta^{\mathrm{T}}\}$.

Finally, the inference scheme described here is likelihood-based and easy to be modified to handle other types of survival data. For instance, this approach is readily extended to deal with left truncation data when subjects are not followed up from the same entry points (Yi and Lawless 2007). Let v_i be the time for subject i to enter the study for $i = 1, \ldots, n$. Then the likelihood function contribution from subject i is

$$L_{\mathrm{LT}i} = \frac{\{f(t_i|X_i, Z_i)\}^{\delta_i}\{S(t_i|X_i, Z_i)\}^{1-\delta_i}}{S(v_i|X_i, Z_i)}.$$

Set

$$\ell_{\mathrm{LT}i}^*(\beta, \lambda_0) = \ell_i^*(\beta, \lambda_0) + \{M(\beta_x)\}^{-1}\Lambda_0(v_i)\exp(\beta_x^{\mathrm{T}} X_i^* + \beta_z^{\mathrm{T}} Z_i).$$

Then the conditional expectation $E\{\ell_{\mathrm{LT}i}^*(\beta, \lambda_0)|T_i, C_i, X_i, Z_i\}$ recovers the true log-likelihood function $\log L_{\mathrm{LT}i}$, where the conditional expectation is evaluated with respect to the model for the conditional distribution of X_i^* given $\{T_i, C_i, X_i, Z_i\}$. Inferential procedures are thus derived analogously to the foregoing development by using $\ell_{\mathrm{LT}i}^*(\beta, \lambda_0)$ for $i = 1, \ldots, n$.

3.5.2 Expectation Correction: Two-Stage Method

In contrast to the insertion correction strategy discussed in §3.5.1, we employ the expectation correction strategy, outlined in §2.5.2, to handle error-prone survival data where the nondifferential measurement error mechanism is assumed. We begin with a general description of the main idea and then elaborate on the details for the setup in §3.1.5 with the proportional hazards model (3.8).

Expectation Correction Strategy

For subject i, let L_i denote the likelihood function (3.7) and

$$S_{\theta i}(\theta; T_i, C_i, X_i, Z_i) = (\partial/\partial\theta) \log L_i$$

be the score function, where θ is the associated model parameter. The expectation correction strategy yields that the conditional expectation

$$U_i^*(\theta; T_i, C_i, X_i^*, Z_i) = E\{S_{\theta i}(\theta; T_i, C_i, X_i, Z_i)|T_i, C_i, X_i^*, Z_i\}$$

is unbiased and computable in the sense that it does not involve unobserved variables. The conditional expectation is taken with respect to the model $F(X_i|X_i^*, Z_i, T_i, C_i)$ for the conditional cumulative distribution of X_i, given $\{X_i^*, Z_i, T_i, C_i\}$, where the dependence on the model parameters is suppressed in the notation. Specifically,

$$dF(X_i|X_i^*, Z_i, T_i, C_i) = \frac{f(T_i, C_i|X_i, Z_i)f(X_i^*|X_i, Z_i)dF_{X|Z}(X_i|Z_i)}{\int f(T_i, C_i|x_i, Z_i)f(X_i^*|x_i, Z_i)dF_{X|Z}(x_i|Z_i)},$$

where $f(T_i, C_i|x, Z_i)$ is determined by $L_i = \exp(\ell_i)$, ℓ_i is given by (3.9), $f(X_i^*|X_i, Z_i)$ is the model for the conditional probability density or mass function of X_i^* given $\{X_i, Z_i\}$, and $F_{X|Z}(x_i|Z_i)$ is the model for the conditional cumulative distribution of X_i given Z_i.

Under regularity conditions, solving

$$\sum_{i=1}^{n} U_i^*(\theta; T_i, C_i, X_i^*, Z_i) = 0 \tag{3.39}$$

for θ yields a consistent estimator of θ which, after being subtracted θ and then re-scaled the difference by $\sqrt{n}$, has an asymptotic normal distribution.

This method requires modeling the full distribution form for all the three processes: the survival process, the measurement error process, and the covariate process of X_i given Z_i. The inference results are thus vulnerable to misspecification of any of the three models. In addition, this estimation procedure treats all the components of θ equally. However, in many applications, the parameters reflecting covariate effects associated with the survival model are of prime interest while the parameters associated with the baseline function are of secondary interest or even treated as a nuisance.

To alleviate the sensitivity of estimation to model misspecification, we use different ways to formulate estimating functions for different types of parameters. To highlight the idea, we assume that models $f(X_i^*|X_i, Z_i)$ and $F_{x|z}(X_i|Z_i)$ are known with the values of the associated parameters given, and concentrate on developing an estimation method for parameters of interest which is less sensitive to model misspecification than the method based on (3.39) is. Specifically, we divide the parameter vector θ into two subvectors, respectively, containing nuisance parameters and parameters of interest, and then develop a two-stage procedure with different ways directed to estimation of different types of parameters. In particular, we use a full set of model assumptions to estimate nuisance parameters and then use a robust approach to handle parameters of primary interest.

Two-Stage Estimation

To flesh out this idea explicitly, we look at the development of Li and Ryan (2006). The survival process is characterized by the Cox proportional hazards model (3.8), where the log baseline hazard function is posited by a piecewise-linear spline model

$$\log \lambda_0(t) = \rho_1 + \rho_2 t + \rho_3(t - a_1) + \ldots + \rho_K(t - a_{K-2})_+$$

with knots fixed at $0 = a_0 < a_1 < \ldots < a_{K-2}$ for a given K, where v_+ represents $\max(v, 0)$ and $\rho = (\rho_1, \ldots, \rho_K)^{\mathrm{T}}$ is the parameter.

Let $\theta = (\rho^{\mathrm{T}}, \beta^{\mathrm{T}})^{\mathrm{T}}$, where β is of prime interest. The observed likelihood function contributed from individual i is

$$L_i(T_i, C_i, X_i^*|Z_i; \rho, \beta) = \int f(T_i, C_i|x, Z_i) f(X_i^*|x, Z_i) dF_{x|z}(x|Z_i),$$

where the dependence of $f(T_i, C_i|x, Z_i)$ on θ is suppressed in the notation.

Define

$$U_\rho(\rho, \beta) = \sum_{i=1}^{n} \frac{\partial}{\partial \rho} \log L_i(T_i, C_i, X_i^*|Z_i; \rho, \beta) = 0$$

and

$$U_\beta(\rho, \beta) = \sum_{i=1}^{n} \frac{\partial}{\partial \beta} \log L_i(T_i, C_i, X_i^*|Z_i; \rho, \beta) = 0.$$

Joint estimation of ρ and β is carried out by simultaneously solving

$$U_\rho(\rho, \beta) = 0 \text{ and } U_\beta(\rho, \beta) = 0 \tag{3.40}$$

for ρ and β.

This method is straightforward to implement. However, estimation of β is at the risk of being seriously affected by incorrect modeling of the baseline hazard function. To achieve robustness, we wish to employ a function that is less sensitive to misspecification of the baseline hazard function. This motivates us to use the partial likelihood function for estimation of β.

Let

$$S_{\rm P}(\mathbb{T},\mathbb{C},\mathbb{X},\mathbb{Z};\beta) = \sum_{i=1}^{n} \int_0^{\tau} S_{{\rm P}i}(t,\mathbb{X},\mathbb{Z};\beta)dN_i(t),$$

where $S_{{\rm P}i}(t,\mathbb{X},\mathbb{Z};\beta)$ is given by (3.13); and τ is a constant satisfying $P(C_i > \tau) > 0$, which is often taken as the study duration. Define

$$U_{\rm P}^*(\theta;\mathbb{T},\mathbb{C},\mathbb{X}^*,\mathbb{Z}) = E_{\mathbb{X}|(\mathbb{T},\mathbb{C},\mathbb{X}^*,\mathbb{Z})}\{S_{\rm P}(\mathbb{T},\mathbb{C},\mathbb{X},\mathbb{Z};\beta)\},$$

where the expectation is taken with respect to the conditional distribution $F(\mathbb{X}|\mathbb{T},\mathbb{C},\mathbb{X}^*,\mathbb{Z})$, which equals $\prod_{i=1}^{n} F(X_i|X_i^*,Z_i,T_i,C_i)$ under the assumption that the $\{T_i,C_i,X_i,Z_i,X_i^*\}$ are independent. Then estimation of ρ and β is performed based on (3.40) with $U_\beta(\rho,\beta)$ replaced by $U_{\rm P}^*(\theta;\mathbb{T},\mathbb{C},\mathbb{X}^*,\mathbb{Z})$. That is, solving

$$\begin{pmatrix} U_\rho(\rho,\beta) \\ U_{\rm P}^*(\theta;\mathbb{T},\mathbb{C},\mathbb{X}^*,\mathbb{Z}) \end{pmatrix} = 0$$

for ρ and β gives an estimator $\widehat{\theta} = (\widehat{\rho}^{\rm T},\widehat{\beta}^{\rm T})^{\rm T}$ of θ.

If the baseline hazard function $\lambda_0(t)$ is correctly specified, then this set of estimating functions is unbiased, and consequently, yields a consistent estimator for θ, provided regularity conditions. When $\lambda_0(t)$ is misspecified, it is expected that the estimate of parameter β resulted from this scheme is much less affected than that directly obtained from solving (3.40). This estimation procedure requires evaluation of $U_{\rm P}^*(\theta;\mathbb{T},\mathbb{C},\mathbb{X}^*,\mathbb{Z})$, which typically involves intractable integrals. Li and Ryan (2006) discussed using a sampling importance resampling technique (McLachlan and Krishnan 1997, Ch. 6) to handle the integrals.

Under regularity conditions, $\sqrt{n}(\widehat{\theta}-\theta)$ has an asymptotic normal distribution with mean 0 and a sandwich covariance matrix. Direct estimation of this asymptotic covariance matrix is complicated. Li and Ryan (2006) suggested employing the bootstrap method to produce the standard errors for the estimator $\widehat{\theta}$.

3.6 Methods Based on Estimating Functions

In §3.5, we focus on correcting measurement error effects based on the likelihood function for the proportional hazards model. The likelihood-based methods are conceptually simple and the development of asymptotic properties is a straightforward application of standard estimating function theory. However, a major drawback of these methods involves modeling the baseline hazard function $\lambda_0(t)$, which is often of secondary or little interest for many applications. Model misspecification of $\lambda_0(t)$ places us at risk of producing biased inference results for parameter β. To adjust for measurement error effects, it is thereby desirable to directly introduce correction terms to the partial likelihood or unbiased estimating functions which are free of the baseline hazard function.

In this section, we explore inference methods for this purpose. Our discussion is directed to proportional hazards and additive hazards models under different measurement error scenarios.

3.6.1 Proportional Hazards Model

In this subsection, we consider the proportional hazards model (3.8) where the X_i are subject to measurement error. Three correction methods for measurement error effects are developed based on the true partial likelihood score function (3.14). These methods are described in conjunction with the availability of additional data sources for characterizing the measurement error process.

Extended Insertion Approach

The first strategy, called the *extended insertion method*, is similar in principal to the insertion correction strategy but different from that method in the way of specifying the conditioning variables. Rather than considering an expectation with respect to the measurement error model $f(x_i^*|T_i, C_i, X_i, Z_i)$ as in §3.5.1, we calculate an expectation with respect to the conditional distribution $f(x_i^*|\mathcal{H}_{t_i}^{\text{TC}}, \mathbb{X}, \mathbb{Z})$ of X_i^* given $\{\mathcal{H}_{t_i}^{\text{TC}}, \mathbb{X}, \mathbb{Z}\}$, where $\mathcal{H}_t^{\text{TC}}$ is the history of failures and censorings prior to t and the information of a failure occurring at t. We now elaborate on this method which modifies that of Buzas (1998).

Suppose that for any t, conditional on $\{\mathcal{H}_t^{\text{TC}}, \mathbb{X}, \mathbb{Z}\}$, the observed surrogate X_i^* is associated with the true covariate X_i by the model:

$$X_i^* = X_i + \Sigma_e^{1/2} e_i$$

for $i = 1, \ldots, n$, where the e_i have mean zero and an identity variance matrix, and are independent of each other and of the $\{X_i, T_i, C_i\}$. Assume that Σ_e is a nonnegative definite matrix which is known and that the moment generating function $M(\cdot)$ of e_i exists with a known form.

This measurement error model gives the conditional moment identities. For $j \neq i$ and a time point t,

$$\begin{aligned}
E\{X_j^*|\mathcal{H}_t^{\text{TC}}, \mathbb{X}, \mathbb{Z}\} &= X_j;\\
E\{\exp(\beta_x^{\text{T}} X_j^*)|\mathcal{H}_t^{\text{TC}}, \mathbb{X}, \mathbb{Z}\} &= M(\Sigma_e^{1/2}\beta_x)\exp(\beta_x^{\text{T}} X_j);\\
E\{X_i^* \exp(\beta_x^{\text{T}} X_j^*)|\mathcal{H}_t^{\text{TC}}, \mathbb{X}, \mathbb{Z}\} &= M(\Sigma_e^{1/2}\beta_x) X_i \exp(\beta_x^{\text{T}} X_j);\\
E\{X_j^* \exp(\beta_x^{\text{T}} X_j^*)|\mathcal{H}_t^{\text{TC}}, \mathbb{X}, \mathbb{Z}\} &= M(\Sigma_e^{1/2}\beta_x) X_j \exp(\beta_x^{\text{T}} X_j)\\
&\quad + \left\{\frac{\partial M(\Sigma_e^{1/2}\beta_x)}{\partial \beta_x}\right\} \exp(\beta_x^{\text{T}} X_j); \qquad (3.41)
\end{aligned}$$

where the conditional expectation is evaluated with respect to the model for the conditional distribution of $\mathbb{X}^*$ given $\{\mathcal{H}_t^{\text{TC}}, \mathbb{X}, \mathbb{Z}\}$.

Using these moment identities, we wish to construct an unbiased estimating function of β in terms of the observed variables. First, we examine the partial likelihood score function whose conditional expectation is zero (Kalbfleisch and Prentice 2002, §4.2):

$$E\left\{\delta_i S_{\text{P}i}(t_i, \mathbb{X}, \mathbb{Z}; \beta)|\mathcal{H}_{t_i}^{\text{TC}}, \mathbb{X}, \mathbb{Z}\right\} = 0, \qquad (3.42)$$

where $S_{\text{P}i}(t_i, \mathbb{X}, \mathbb{Z}; \beta)$ is given by (3.13).

As opposed to the quantities $S^{(k)}(t,\mathbb{X},\mathbb{Z};\beta)(k=0,1)$ defined by (3.12), we define

$$S_{i-}^{(0)}(t,\mathbb{X},\mathbb{Z};\beta)=\frac{1}{n}\sum_{j\neq i}R_j(t)\exp(\beta_x^{\mathrm{T}}X_j+\beta_z^{\mathrm{T}}Z_j)$$

and

$$S_{i-}^{(1)}(t,\mathbb{X},\mathbb{Z};\beta)=\frac{1}{n}\sum_{j\neq i}R_j(t)\begin{pmatrix}X_j\\ Z_j\end{pmatrix}\exp(\beta_x^{\mathrm{T}}X_j+\beta_z^{\mathrm{T}}Z_j)$$

for $i=1,\ldots,n$. Then $S_{\mathrm{P}i}(t,\mathbb{X},\mathbb{Z};\beta)$ is re-written as

$$S_{\mathrm{P}i}(t,\mathbb{X},\mathbb{Z};\beta)=\frac{\begin{pmatrix}X_i\\ Z_i\end{pmatrix}S_{i-}^{(0)}(t,\mathbb{X},\mathbb{Z};\beta)-S_{i-}^{(1)}(t,\mathbb{X},\mathbb{Z};\beta)}{S^{(0)}(t,\mathbb{X},\mathbb{Z};\beta)}. \tag{3.43}$$

Let $X_i^{**}=E(X_i|Z_i)$ and $\mathbb{X}^{**}=\{X_1^{**},\ldots,X_n^{**}\}$. Define

$$U_i^*(\beta;t_i,\mathbb{X}^*,\mathbb{Z})=\frac{\begin{pmatrix}X_i^*+D\\ Z_i\end{pmatrix}S_{i-}^{(0)}(t_i,\mathbb{X}^*,\mathbb{Z};\beta)-S_{i-}^{(1)}(t_i,\mathbb{X}^*,\mathbb{Z};\beta)}{S^{(0)}(t_i,\mathbb{X}^{**},\mathbb{Z};\beta)},$$

where $D=(\partial/\partial\beta_x)\{\log M(\Sigma_e^{1/2}\beta_x)\}$. We now show that estimating function

$$\sum_{i=1}^{n}\delta_i U_i^*(\beta;t_i,\mathbb{X}^*,\mathbb{Z})$$

is unbiased.

Noting that $S^{(0)}(t_i,\mathbb{X}^{**},\mathbb{Z};\beta)$ is a constant relative to the conditioning variables $\{\mathcal{H}_{t_i}^{\mathrm{TC}},\mathbb{X},\mathbb{Z}\}$, we obtain that

$$E\left\{\delta_i U_i^*(\beta;t_i,\mathbb{X}^*,\mathbb{Z})|\mathcal{H}_{t_i}^{\mathrm{TC}},\mathbb{X},\mathbb{Z}\right\}=$$
$$\frac{E\left[\delta_i\left\{\begin{pmatrix}X_i^*+D\\ Z_i\end{pmatrix}S_{i-}^{(0)}(t_i,\mathbb{X}^*,\mathbb{Z};\beta)-S_{i-}^{(1)}(t_i,\mathbb{X}^*,\mathbb{Z};\beta)\right\}\middle|\mathcal{H}_{t_i}^{\mathrm{TC}},\mathbb{X},\mathbb{Z}\right]}{S^{(0)}(t_i,\mathbb{X}^{**},\mathbb{Z};\beta)},$$

which equals, by (3.41) and (3.43),

$$\frac{M(\Sigma_e^{1/2}\beta_x)\delta_i S_{\mathrm{P}i}(t_i,\mathbb{X},\mathbb{Z};\beta)S^{(0)}(t_i,\mathbb{X},\mathbb{Z};\beta)}{S^{(0)}(t_i,\mathbb{X}^{**},\mathbb{Z};\beta)}.$$

Further evaluating the conditional expectation of this term, given $\{\mathcal{H}_{t_i}^{\mathrm{TC}},\mathbb{X},\mathbb{Z}\}$, gives

$$\frac{M(\Sigma_e^{1/2}\beta_x)E\{\delta_i S_{\mathrm{P}i}(t_i,\mathbb{X},\mathbb{Z};\beta)|\mathcal{H}_{t_i}^{\mathrm{TC}},\mathbb{X},\mathbb{Z}\}S^{(0)}(t_i,\mathbb{X},\mathbb{Z};\beta)}{S^{(0)}(t_i,\mathbb{X}^{**},\mathbb{Z};\beta)},$$

which equals zero by (3.42). Thus, we obtain that $\delta_i U_i^*(\beta;t_i,\mathbb{X}^*,\mathbb{Z})$ has zero expectation (see Problem 3.7).

To use $U_i^*(\beta; t_i, \mathbb{X}^*, \mathbb{Z})$, we need to calculate X_i^{**}. Noting that $E(X_i|Z_i)$ is identical to $E(X_i^*|Z_i)$, we then regress X_i^* on Z_i using the observed data to calculate X_i^{**}. Let α be the vector of parameters that are associated with the determination of $E(X_i^*|Z_i)$, and $\psi_i(\alpha; X_i^*, Z_i)$ be an associated unbiased estimating function of α contributed from subject i.

Define $\theta = (\alpha^{\mathrm{T}}, \beta^{\mathrm{T}})^{\mathrm{T}}$ and

$$\Psi_i(\theta) = \{\psi_i^{\mathrm{T}}(\alpha; X_i^*, Z_i), \delta_i U_i^{*\mathrm{T}}(\alpha, \beta; t_i, \mathbb{X}^*, \mathbb{Z})\}^{\mathrm{T}},$$

where the dependence of $U_i^*(t_i, \mathbb{X}^*, \mathbb{Z}; \beta)$ on α through $\mathbb{X}^{**}$ is now explicitly spelled out. Under suitable regularity conditions, solving

$$\sum_{i=1}^{n} \Psi_i(\theta) = 0$$

for θ yields a consistent estimator $\widehat{\theta}$, and $\sqrt{n}(\widehat{\theta} - \theta)$ has an asymptotic normal distribution with mean zero and a covariance matrix that may be consistently estimated by the sandwich formula $\widehat{\Gamma}^{-1}(\widehat{\theta})\widehat{\Sigma}(\widehat{\theta})\widehat{\Gamma}^{-1\mathrm{T}}(\widehat{\theta})$, where $\widehat{\Gamma}(\widehat{\theta}) = n^{-1}\sum_{i=1}^{n}(\partial/\partial\theta^{\mathrm{T}})\Psi_i(\theta)|_{\theta=\widehat{\theta}}$ and $\widehat{\Sigma}(\widehat{\theta}) = n^{-1}\sum_{i=1}^{n}\Psi_i(\widehat{\theta})\Psi_i^{\mathrm{T}}(\widehat{\theta})$.

The unbiasedness of $\delta_i U_i^*(\beta; t_i, \mathbb{X}^*, \mathbb{Z})$ basically comes from the zero expectation of its numerator. Any function of $\mathbb{Z}$ and β may replace its denominator $S^{(0)}(t_i, \mathbb{X}^{**}, \mathbb{Z}; \beta)$ to retain the unbiasedness. In this sense, the denominator is viewed as a weight function. Buzas (1998) discussed the feasibility of setting the weight function to be $S_i^{(0)}(t_i, \mathbb{X}^{**}, \mathbb{Z}; \beta)$.

We note that, as discussed in §3.5.1, the insertion correction method can be applied to the likelihood score function to produce an unbiased estimating function that is expressed in terms of the observed data, but this strategy cannot be *directly* applied to the partial likelihood score function to produce a workable unbiased estimating function. Stefanski (1989) and Nakamura (1990) discussed this issue. A main reason is due to the involvement of the fraction for which both the numerator and the denominator contain exponential functions of error-prone covariate X_i. However, by modifying the conditioning variables of the insertion correction method, the extended insertion method allows us to *separately* evaluate the conditional expectation for the numerator and the denominator which are involved in the fraction of the partial likelihood score. The difference in these two conditional expectation methods lies in the set of conditioning variables. In the insertion correction approach, the conditioning variables are only the subject-level covariates; whereas in the extended insertion method, the set of conditioning variables involves the entire sample information of the covariates and the history of survival and observation processes.

The extended insertion method assumes that the moment generating function $M(\cdot)$ for the measurement error model is known. This can be the case when conducting sensitivity analyses to evaluate the impact of different types of measurement error on the estimation of the response parameter, where one would specify a series of measurement error models with varying degrees of measurement error.

In the presence of additional data sources, such as a validation sample, $M(\cdot)$ may be estimated from using these additional data, where the principle to be discussed in §3.6.3 may be applied for this purpose.

3.6.2 Simulation Study

We conduct a simulation study to investigate the impact of ignoring measurement error on estimation and compare the performance of the methods which account for measurement error effects (Yi and Lawless 2007).

We set $n = 200$ and generate 1000 simulations for each parameter configuration. We consider a simple case where only a scalar covariate X_i is subject to error. The true covariate X_i is independently simulated from the standard normal distribution for $i = 1, \ldots, n$. Failure times are independently generated from the Cox proportional hazards model with the hazard function

$$\lambda(t_i|X_i) = \rho_1 \rho_2 t^{\rho_1 - 1} \exp(\beta X_i)$$

for $i = 1, \ldots, n$, where ρ_1 and ρ_2 are taken as 1.5 and 1.0, respectively; and parameter β is set as 0, 0.4, and 0.8 to represent unit, moderate, and high hazard ratios, respectively. A fixed censoring time C is generated for each subject so that about 70% of subjects are censored. For each generated X_i, its observed value X_i^* is generated from the normal distribution $N(X_i, \sigma_e^2)$ for $i = 1, \ldots, n$, where σ_e^2 is the variance.

First, we report on the performance of the naive method which disregards measurement error in X_i. Fig. 3.1 displays the average of the naive estimates for β against σ_e. When there is no covariate effect (i.e., $\beta = 0$), the naive method yields reasonable estimates regardless of the magnitude of measurement error. As expected, when $\beta \neq 0$, the naive method produces biased results. The resulting finite sample biases increase as measurement error becomes more severe as well as the covariate effect becomes more substantial.

Next, we compare the performance of the three methods which account for measurement error effects. Different configurations of σ_e are considered with $\sigma_e = 0.15, 0.25, 0.75$, featuring minor, moderate, and large measurement error, respectively. Method 1 is based on an unbiased partial likelihood score function discussed by Buzas (1998), Method 2 is the piecewise-constant approach discussed in §3.5.1, Method 3 is the same as Method 2 except for letting K approach ∞, where (3.37) and (3.38) are used in combination with a sandwich variance estimator for $\widehat{\beta}$, given by Nakamura (1992). For Method 2 we set $K = 5$. Cut points a_k are determined by the equations $\exp\{-\Lambda_0(a_k)\} = 0.8, 0.6, 0.4, 0.2$, respectively, for $k = 1, 2, 3, 4$.

We report on the results of the average of the estimates (EST), the empirical variance (EV), the average of the model-based variance estimates (MVE), and the coverage rate (CR) for 95% confidence intervals obtained by $\widehat{\beta} \pm 1.96 se(\widehat{\beta})$, where $se(\widehat{\beta})$ is the standard error of the estimate $\widehat{\beta}$. Table 3.1 presents the results for the case with $\beta = 0.4$. Estimates obtained from these three methods all appear to be consistent with small finite sample biases, though the magnitudes increase as the variance σ_e^2

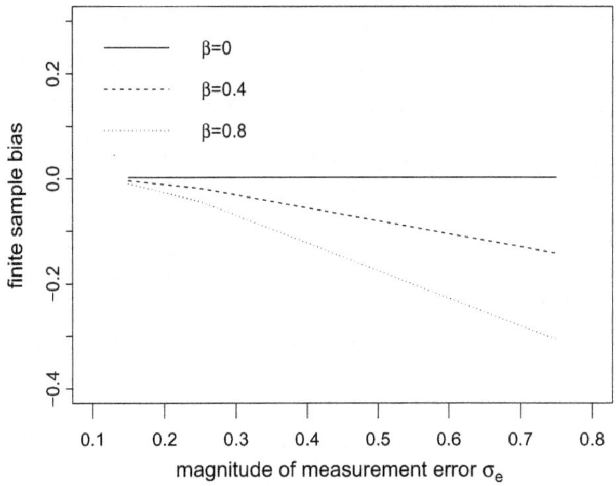

Fig. 3.1. *A Simulation Study of the Naive Method Which Ignores Measurement Error: Finite Sample Bias of the Naive Estimator for β Versus the Degree of Measurement Error σ_e*

increases. In spite of using only an approximately correct (piecewise constant) model for $\lambda_0(t)$, Method 2 appears to have slightly smaller biases than Methods 1 and 3. Model-based variance estimates obtained from all three methods agree well with the empirical variances, and Method 2 seems to yield smallest empirical variances. The three methods provide reasonable coverage rates that are close to the nominal level.

Table 3.1. *Simulation Results for Comparing the Performance of the Three Methods Accommodating Measurement Error Effects (Yi and Lawless 2007)*

σ_e	Method	EST	EV	MVE	CR (%)
0.15	1	0.407	0.018	0.018	94.0
	2	0.399	0.017	0.017	93.9
	3	0.406	0.018	0.018	94.0
0.25	1	0.407	0.019	0.019	94.2
	2	0.399	0.018	0.018	94.6
	3	0.406	0.019	0.018	94.2
0.75	1	0.420	0.034	0.033	93.9
	2	0.412	0.032	0.033	95.1
	3	0.421	0.035	0.034	94.2

3.6.3 Additive Hazards Model

In this section, we describe inference methods which account for measurement error effects under the additive hazards model (3.10), where covariate Z_i may be time-dependent and is now denoted as $Z_i(t)$. Specifically, we write the additive hazards model as

$$\lambda(t|X_i, Z_i(t)) = \lambda_0(t) + \beta_x^{\mathrm{T}} X_i + \beta_z^{\mathrm{T}} Z_i(t), \tag{3.44}$$

where $\lambda_0(t)$ is an unspecified baseline hazard function and $\beta = (\beta_x^{\mathrm{T}}, \beta_z^{\mathrm{T}})^{\mathrm{T}}$ is the vector of unknown regression parameters.

The discussion is directed to each of the three circumstances which are often encountered in practice: (1) parameters of the measurement error model are known from a priori studies or merely assumed to be given for conducting sensitivity analyses; (2) an internal validation sample is available; and (3) replicated measurements for X_i are collected.

In §3.6.1, we describe the extended insertion method for the Cox proportional hazards model with error-prone covariates. The principal idea there can also be applied to the additive hazards model with measurement error in covariates. Here we elaborate on the details.

Measurement Error Parameters Are Known

We consider the measurement error process for which there exist vectors of functions, denoted as $g_k(\cdot)$ for $k = 1, 2, 3$, such that for any i and $j \neq i$,

$$\begin{aligned} E\{g_1(X_i^*)|\mathcal{F}_\tau\} &= X_i; \\ E\{g_2(X_i^*; a)|\mathcal{F}_\tau\} &= (a^{\mathrm{T}} X_i) X_i; \\ E\{g_3(X_i^*, X_j^*; a)|\mathcal{F}_\tau\} &= (a^{\mathrm{T}} X_i) X_j; \end{aligned}$$

where $\mathcal{F}_\tau$ is the σ-field generated by the history of the failure, censoring, and the true covariates of all the subjects prior to the end of study time τ, and a is a vector of constants which is of the same dimension as X_i.

Let

$$\begin{aligned} \Psi_{1i}^*(t) &= \begin{pmatrix} g_1(X_i^*) \\ Z_i(t) \end{pmatrix}; \\ \Psi_{2i}^*(\beta_x; t) &= \begin{pmatrix} g_2(X_i^*; \beta_x) \\ \{\beta_x^{\mathrm{T}} g_1(X_i^*)\} Z_i(t) \end{pmatrix}; \\ \Psi_{3ij}^*(\beta_x; t) &= \begin{pmatrix} g_3(X_i^*, X_j^*; \beta_x) \\ \{\beta_x^{\mathrm{T}} g_1(X_i^*)\} Z_j(t) \end{pmatrix}. \end{aligned}$$

By the forms of X_i appearing in the pseudo-score function $U_i(\beta)$ given by (3.15), we construct an estimating function for β:

$$\begin{aligned} U_i^*(\beta) &= \int_0^\infty \left\{ \Psi_{1i}^*(t) - \frac{\sum_{j=1}^n R_j(t) \Psi_{1j}^*(t)}{\sum_{j=1}^n R_j(t)} \right\} \{dN_i(t) - R_i(t) \beta_z^{\mathrm{T}} Z_i(t) dt\} \\ &- \int_0^\infty \left\{ \Psi_{2i}^*(\beta_x; t) - \frac{\sum_{j \neq i} R_j(t) \Psi_{3ij}^*(\beta_x; t) + R_i(t) \Psi_{2i}^*(\beta_x; t)}{\sum_{j=1}^n R_j(t)} \right\} R_i(t) dt. \end{aligned}$$

Straightforward calculation shows that $E\{U_i^*(\beta)|\mathcal{F}_\tau\} = U_i(\beta)$, provided that integration and expectation are exchangeable. Because $E\{U_i(\beta)\} = 0$, $U_i^*(\beta)$ is then an unbiased estimating function. When the function form of $g_k(\cdot)$ is known for $k = 1, 2, 3$, solving

$$\sum_{i=1}^{n} U_i^*(\beta) = 0 \tag{3.45}$$

for β gives an estimate of β. Let $\widehat{\beta}$ denote the resulting estimator. Following the arguments of Kulich and Lin (2000), it can be shown that under regularity conditions, $\widehat{\beta}$ is a consistent estimator of β and $\sqrt{n}(\widehat{\beta} - \beta)$ has an asymptotically normal distribution with mean zero and a sandwich type covariance.

Construction of $U_i^*(\beta)$ basically hinges on identifying the correction functions $g_k(\cdot)(k = 1, 2, 3)$, which relegates to the form of the measurement error model. If the measurement error process satisfies the condition

$$E\{g(X_i^*, X_j^*)|\mathcal{F}_\tau\} = E\{g(X_i^*, X_j^*)|X_i, X_j\} \tag{3.46}$$

for any real-valued function $g(\cdot)$ and $i \neq j$, then finding functions $g_k(\cdot)(k = 1, 2, 3)$ is often straightforward. The condition (3.46) implies that given $\{X_i, X_j\}$, $\{X_i^*, X_j^*\}$ are independent of $N_i(t)$ and $R_i(t)$ for any t; it is pertinent to the nondifferential measurement error mechanism discussed in §3.2.2.

For example, assume that (3.46) holds. If the X_i are continuous covariates and linked with their surrogates by an additive error model

$$X_i^* = X_i + e_i \tag{3.47}$$

for $i = 1, \ldots, n$, where e_i is independent of $\{X_i, T_i, C_i\}$ and has mean zero and covariance matrix Σ_e. Then $g_1(\cdot)$, $g_2(\cdot)$ and $g_3(\cdot)$ are, respectively, taken as

$$\begin{aligned} g_1(X_i^*) &= X_i^*; \\ g_2(X_i^*; a) &= (a^{\mathrm{T}} X_i^*)X_i^* - \Sigma_e a; \\ g_3(X_i^*, X_j^*; a) &= (a^{\mathrm{T}} X_i^*)X_j^*. \end{aligned} \tag{3.48}$$

If X_i is, on the other hand, a scalar binary covariate with the (mis)classification probabilities $\pi_{00} = P(X_i^* = 0|X_i = 0)$ and $\pi_{11} = P(X_i^* = 1|X_i = 1)$, then functions $g_1(\cdot)$, $g_2(\cdot)$ and $g_3(\cdot)$ are set as

$$\begin{aligned} g_1(X_i^*) &= \frac{X_i^* - (1 - \pi_{00})}{\pi_{00} + \pi_{11} - 1}; \\ g_2(X_i^*; \beta_x) &= \beta_x g_1(X_i^*); \\ g_3(X_i^*, X_j^*; \beta_x) &= \beta_x g_1(X_i^*) g_1(X_j^*). \end{aligned} \tag{3.49}$$

Validation Sample Is Available

In the presence of an internal validation subsample considered in §3.3.1, estimating function $U_i^*(\beta)$ in (3.45) is refined to accommodate the true measurements of X_i from the validation sample.

Let

$$\Psi_{1i}^{**}(t) = \begin{pmatrix} \eta_i X_i + (1-\eta_i)\omega g_1(X_i^*) \\ Z_i(t) \end{pmatrix};$$

$$\Psi_{2i}^{**}(\beta_x;t) = \begin{pmatrix} \eta_i(\beta_x^{\mathrm{T}} X_i)X_i + (1-\eta_i)\omega g_2(X_i^*;\beta_x) \\ \eta_i(\beta_x^{\mathrm{T}} X_i)Z_i(t) + (1-\eta_i)\omega\{\beta_x^{\mathrm{T}} g_1(X_i^*)\}Z_i(t) \end{pmatrix};$$

$$\Psi_{3ij}^{**}(\beta_x;t) = \begin{pmatrix} \eta_i a_{ij}(\beta_x) + (1-\eta_i)\omega b_{ij}(\beta_x) \\ \eta_i(\beta_x^{\mathrm{T}} X_i)Z_j(t) + (1-\eta_i)\omega\{\beta_x^{\mathrm{T}} g_1(X_i^*)\}Z_j(t) \end{pmatrix};$$

where

$$a_{ij}(\beta_x) = (\beta_x^{\mathrm{T}} X_i)\{\eta_j X_j + (1-\eta_j)g_1(X_j^*)\};$$
$$b_{ij}(\beta_x) = \eta_j\{\beta_x^{\mathrm{T}} g_1(X_i^*)\}X_j + (1-\eta_j)g_3(X_i^*, X_j^*;\beta_x);$$

and ω is a weight specified to adjust for or downweigh the contribution from the subjects in the nonvalidation sample, taking a value between 0 and 1. Commonly, ω is set to be 1, reflecting equal contribution of the subjects from the validation subsample or the main study. If ω takes 0, then only the validation data are used for estimation.

Estimating function $U_i^*(\beta)$ in (3.45) is then modified to be

$$U_i^{**}(\beta) = \int_0^\infty \left\{ \Psi_{1i}^{**}(t) - \frac{\sum_{j=1}^n R_j(t)\Psi_{1j}^{**}(t)}{\sum_{j=1}^n R_j(t)} \right\} \{dN_i(t) - R_i(t)\beta_z^{\mathrm{T}} Z_i(t)dt\}$$
$$- \int_0^\infty \left\{ \Psi_{2i}^{**}(\beta_x;t) - \frac{\sum_{j\neq i} R_j(t)\Psi_{3ij}^{**}(\beta_x;t) + R_i(t)\Psi_{2i}^{**}(\beta_x;t)}{\sum_{j=1}^n R_j(t)} \right\} R_i(t)dt$$

so that $E\{U_i^{**}(\beta)|\mathcal{F}_\tau, \eta_i\} = U_i(\beta)$. Hence, $U_i^{**}(\beta)$ is an unbiased estimating function of β.

Furthermore, the validation subsample is used to characterize the measurement error information. Suppose we model the measurement error process parametrically and let α denote the vector of the associated parameters. Let $\psi_i(\alpha)$ be an unbiased estimating function of α contributed from subject i. Then estimation of α and β may proceed by using, respectively, the data from the validation subsample $\mathcal{V}$ and the main study sample $\mathcal{M}$ (i.e., $i \in \{1, \ldots, n\}$). Solving

$$\begin{pmatrix} \sum_{i\in\mathcal{V}} \psi_i(\alpha) \\ \sum_{i=1}^n U_i^{**}(\alpha,\beta) \end{pmatrix} = 0$$

for α and β gives estimates of α and β, where the dependence on α of $U_i^{**}(\beta)$ is explicitly spelled out. Asymptotic distributions of the resulting estimators may be established following the guideline of §1.3.4.

As examples of formulating $\psi_i(\alpha)$, we consider two scenarios where only a scalar covariate X_i is subject to measurement error or misclassification. First, suppose that X_i is continuous and that the measurement error model is given by (3.47) with the variance of e_i denoted as α. Then for subject $i \in \mathcal{V}$, estimating function $\psi_i(\alpha)$ is constructed as, by using the method of moments,

$$\psi_i(\alpha) = (X_i^* - X_i)^2 - \alpha.$$

Next, if X_i is a binary covariate with the (mis)classification probabilities $\pi_{00} = P(X_i^* = 0|X_i = 0)$ and $\pi_{11} = P(X_i^* = 1|X_i = 1)$, then π_{00} and π_{11} are naturally estimated by empirical frequencies

$$\widehat{\pi}_{00} = \frac{n_{00}}{n_{00} + n_{01}}; \ \widehat{\pi}_{11} = \frac{n_{11}}{n_{10} + n_{11}};$$

where $n_{jk} = \sum_{i=1}^{n} \eta_i I(X_i = j; X_i^* = k)$ is the counts in the validation sample $\mathcal{V}$ for $j, k = 0, 1$. Obviously, this is equivalent to solving the unbiased estimating equation:

$$\sum_{i \in \mathcal{V}} \psi_i(\alpha) = 0 \tag{3.50}$$

for α, where $\psi_i(\alpha) = \{(1 - X_i)(1 - X_i^*) - \pi_{00}(1 - X_i), X_i X_i^* - \pi_{11} X_i\}^{\mathrm{T}}$ and $\alpha = (\pi_{00}, \pi_{11})^{\mathrm{T}}$.

Replicates Are Available

Finally, we consider the case where the model parameter for the measurement error process is unknown and replicated surrogate measurements $\{X_{ik}^* : k = 1, \ldots, m_i\}$ are collected for X_i, where the number m_i of replicates may be subject-dependent. Different from the aforementioned extended insertion correction methods, we discuss another inference method to accommodating covariate measurement error.

Let $\mathcal{F}_t$ be the σ-field generated by the history of the failure, censoring and the true covariates of all the subjects prior to time t. Given $\mathcal{F}_t$ for any time t, we assume that the surrogates X_{ik}^* and the true covariate X_i are linked by an additive model:

$$X_{ik}^* = X_i + e_{ik} \tag{3.51}$$

for $k = 1, \ldots, m_i$, where the e_{ik} are independent of $\{X_i, T_i, C_i\}$ and have mean zero and covariance matrix Σ_e for $i = 1, \ldots, n$ and $k = 1, \ldots, m_i$. This assumption says that given $\mathcal{F}_t$ (which include the true covariates $\{X_i, Z_i(t)\}$ at any time t), T_i and C_i are independent of surrogate measurements $\{X_{ik}^* : k = 1, \ldots, m_i\}$.

With the replicates, Σ_e is empirically estimated by

$$\widehat{\Sigma}_e = \frac{\sum_{i=1}^{n} \sum_{k=1}^{m_i} (X_{ik}^* - \overline{X}_{i+}^*)^{\otimes 2}}{\sum_{i=1}^{n} (m_i - 1)},$$

where $\overline{X}_{i+}^* = m_i^{-1} \sum_{k=1}^{m_i} X_{ik}^*$.

Let $\Sigma = \text{diag}\{\Sigma_e, 0_{p_z \times p_z}\}$ be the block diagonal matrix and $\widehat{\Sigma} = \text{diag}\{\widehat{\Sigma}_e, 0_{p_z \times p_z}\}$. Because $E(\overline{X}_{i+}^*|\mathcal{F}_t) = X_i$ and $E(\overline{X}_{i+}^{*\otimes 2}|\mathcal{F}_t) = X_i^{\otimes 2} + m_i^{-1}\Sigma_e$, we obtain

$$E(\widehat{\Sigma}|\mathcal{F}_t) = \Sigma \text{ for any time } t. \tag{3.52}$$

To estimate β, one might be tempted to use the pseudo-score function (3.15) by substituting X_i with $\overline{X}_{i+}^*$. However, as shown in §3.2.1, this substitution does not ensure a consistent estimator of β because the resulting estimating function $U_{\text{NV}}(\beta)$ is not unbiased anymore, where $U_{\text{NV}}(\beta) = \sum_{i=1}^n U_{\text{NV}i}(\beta)$, and $U_{\text{NV}i}(\beta)$ is identical to the pseudo-scored function $U_i(\beta)$ of (3.15) except that X_i is replaced by $\overline{X}_{i+}^*$.

A remedy for this is to apply the subtraction correction strategy discussed in §2.5.2. We modify $U_{\text{NV}}(\beta)$ by subtracting its expectation $E\{U_{\text{NV}}(\beta)\}$ so that the resulting estimating function, $U_{\text{NV}}(\beta) - E\{U_{\text{NV}}(\beta)\}$, is unbiased. However, evaluation of the marginal expectation $E\{U_{\text{NV}}(\beta)\}$ is generally complicated due to the involvement of the joint distribution of the survival and censoring processes, thus making the modified estimating function $U_{\text{NV}}(\beta) - E\{U_{\text{NV}}(\beta)\}$ unappealing.

To get around this problem, we alternatively evaluate the conditional expectation of $U_{\text{NV}}(\beta)$, given $\mathcal{F}_\tau$. As indicated by Problem 3.9,

$$\begin{aligned} &E\{U_{\text{NV}}(\beta)|\mathcal{F}_\tau\} \\ &= U(\beta) - \int_0^\tau \left\{1 - \frac{1}{\sum_{j=1}^n R_j(t)}\right\} \sum_{i=1}^n \left\{\frac{R_i(t)\Sigma\beta}{m_i}\right\} dt, \end{aligned} \tag{3.53}$$

where $U(\beta) = \sum\limits_{i=1}^n U_i(\beta)$ and $U_i(\beta)$ is given by (3.15). This identity motivates us to consider the estimating function

$$U^*(\beta) = U_{\text{NV}}(\beta) + \int_0^\tau \left\{1 - \frac{1}{\sum_{j=1}^n R_j(t)}\right\} \sum_{i=1}^n \left\{\frac{R_i(t)\Sigma\beta}{m_i}\right\} dt$$

which satisfy $E\{U^*(\beta)\} = 0$ by (3.53) and the unbiasedness of $U(\beta)$. Thus, $U^*(\beta)$ is an unbiased estimating function.

To use $U^*(\beta)$ to estimate β, we need to replace Σ with its consistent estimate $\widehat{\Sigma}$; let $U^{**}(\beta)$ denote the resultant estimating function. One might expect that the substitution of $\widehat{\Sigma}$ for Σ would break down the unbiasedness of $U^*(\beta)$, but this is not the case with this method. Interchanging the conditional expectation and integration, we obtain that by (3.52),

$$\begin{aligned} E\{U^{**}(\beta)\} &= E\{U_{\text{NV}}(\beta)\} \\ &\quad + E\left(\int_0^\tau E\left[\left\{1 - \frac{1}{\sum_{j=1}^n R_j(t)}\right\} \sum_{i=1}^n \left\{\frac{R_i(t)\widehat{\Sigma}\beta}{m_i}\right\} \middle| \mathcal{F}_t\right] dt\right) \\ &= E\{U_{\text{NV}}(\beta)\} + E\left[\int_0^\tau \left\{1 - \frac{1}{\sum_{j=1}^n R_j(t)}\right\} \sum_{i=1}^n \left\{\frac{R_i(t)\Sigma\beta}{m_i}\right\} dt\right] \\ &= E\{U^*(\beta)\}, \end{aligned}$$

suggesting that $U^{**}(\beta)$ is still an unbiased estimating function.

Since $U^{**}(\beta)$ is unbiased, then under regularity conditions, solving

$$U^{**}(\beta) = 0$$

for β leads to a consistent estimator $\widehat{\beta}$ of β, given by

$$\begin{aligned}\widehat{\beta} = &\left[\sum_{i=1}^{n} \int_0^{\tau} R_i(t) \left\{W_i^*(t) - \overline{W}^*(t)\right\}^{\otimes 2} dt \right.\\ &\left. - \int_0^{\tau} \left\{1 - \frac{1}{\sum_{j=1}^{n} R_j(t)}\right\} \sum_{i=1}^{n} \left\{\frac{R_i(t)\widehat{\Sigma}}{m_i}\right\} dt \right]^{-1} \\ &\cdot \left[\sum_{i=1}^{n} \int_0^{\tau} \left\{W_i^*(t) - \overline{W}^*(t)\right\} dN_i(t)\right], \end{aligned} \tag{3.54}$$

where $W_i^*(t) = \{\overline{X}_{i+}^{*\mathrm{T}}, Z_i^{\mathrm{T}}(t)\}^{\mathrm{T}}$ and $\overline{W}^*(t) = \sum_{j=1}^{n} R_i(t) W_j^*(t) / \sum_{j=1}^{n} R_j(t)$.

The inverse matrix in (3.54) converges almost surely to a positive definite matrix under regularity conditions, thus when numerically calculating $\widehat{\beta}$, singularity does not occur in the asymptotic sense. Under certain regularity conditions, $\sqrt{n}(\widehat{\beta} - \beta)$ has the asymptotic normal distribution with mean zero and a sandwich-type covariance matrix. Details were provided by Yan and Yi (2016b).

3.6.4 An Example: Analysis of ACTG175 Data

To illustrate the method discussed in §3.6.3, we discuss the analysis results of Yan and Yi (2016b) for the data arising from the AIDS Clinical Trials Group (ACTG) 175 study (Hammer et al. 1996). The ACTG 175 study was a double-blind randomized clinical trial which evaluated the HIV treatment effects. It is of interest to understand how the survival time is associated with the treatment. Here the survival time T_i for subject i is defined to be the time to the occurrence of one of the events that CD4 counts decrease at least 50%, or disease progression to AIDS, or death, as considered by Hammer et al. (1996). Excluding the subjects who had missing values or unrecorded relevant information, we consider a subset of 2139 subjects in which about 75.6% of the outcome values are censored.

Let Z_i be the treatment assignment indicator for subject i, where $Z_i = 1$ if a subject received the treatment, and 0 otherwise. In the ACTG 175 study, the baseline measurements on CD4 were collected before randomization, ranging from 200 to 500 per cubic millimeter. Let X_i be a transformed version, log(CD4 counts + 1), of the true baseline CD4 counts which was not observed in the study. Forty-four subjects were measured once for the CD4 counts at the baseline, and 2095 subjects had two replicated baseline measurements of CD4 counts, denoted by X_{i1}^* and X_{i2}^* after the same transformation as for X_i.

The additive measurement error model (3.51) is specified to link the underlying transformed CD4 counts with the surrogate measurements. With the replicates, we estimate the variance of the measurement error model as $\widehat{\Sigma}_e = 0.035$.

The additive hazards model (3.44) is used to describe the dependence of T_i on covariates X_i and Z_i. For comparison, four methods are considered: the naive method (Naive) which uses the average of X_{i1}^* and X_{i2}^* (and the observed surrogate measurements for subjects who were measured once) to replace X_i in the standard analysis, the regression calibration method (RC), the method (SZS) by Sun, Zhang and Sun (2006), and the method (SUBTR) discussed in §3.6.3. Since the method by Sun, Zhang and Sun (2006) requires that every subject has replicates of surrogate measurements, for comparability we use two ways to look at the data: the subset of all the subjects with replicates (Subset) and the entire data set (Full). The analysis results are shown in Table 3.2.

The naive estimate of β_x is smaller than those obtained from the other methods, while the naive estimate of β_z is similar to those produced by the other methods. Although estimates of β_x and β_z differ from method to method, all the results suggest that both CD4 counts and treatment are statistically significant.

Table 3.2. *Analyses of the ACTG 175 Data Using Different Methods*

Data	Method	log(CD4 counts + 1)			Treatment		
		EST	MVE	95% CI	EST	MVE	95% CI
Subset	Naive	−4.67	2.15	(−5.58, −3.77)	−2.12	1.18	(−2.80, −1.45)
	SZS	−5.76	3.36	(−6.90, −4.63)	−2.16	1.19	(−2.84, −1.49)
	RC	−5.71	3.20	(−6.82, −4.60)	−2.14	1.18	(−2.81, −1.47)
	SUBTR	−5.78	3.40	(−6.93, −4.64)	−2.16	1.19	(−2.84, −1.49)
Full	Naive	−4.72	2.13	(−5.62, −3.81)	−2.15	1.16	(−2.81, −1.48)
	RC	−5.77	3.19	(−6.88, −4.67)	−2.16	1.16	(−2.83, −1.50)
	SUBTR	−5.85	3.41	(−7.00, −4.71)	−2.18	1.17	(−2.86, −1.51)

EST: estimates $\times 10^4$; MVE: model-based variance estimates $\times 10^9$; CI: confidence intervals $\times 10^4$

3.7 Misclassification of Discrete Covariates

The correction methods in the preceding sections are described for error-prone continuous covariates. These strategies are also applicable to discrete covariates which are subject to misclassification. In particular, the strategies discussed in §3.6 exemplify the fact that the estimating functions under the true model depend on X_i through polynomial or exponent forms. In this section, we develop correction methods for misclassified discrete covariates whose form can be arbitrary. For ease of exposition, we focus the discussion on a scalar discrete covariate X_i which is subject to misclassification. The development for multiple covariate X_i proceeds in the same manner though the notation would be more involved.

Suppose X_i is a discrete random variable with possible values $x_{(1)}, \ldots, x_{(r)}$, where r is a finite positive integer. Assume that X_i is not precisely observed; instead, X_i^* is the observed version of X_i so that $P(X_i^* = X_i) \leq 1$. Analogous to inferences with error-contaminated continuous covariates, a misclassification model is usually needed to supplement modeling of the response process in order to conduct valid inference about the response parameter. Similar to the structure of the classical additive and Berkson models for continuous covariates discussed in §2.6, the specification of misclassification probabilities may be done in two ways by using different conditioning variables. Given error-free covariate Z_i, one may characterize the dependence of X_i^* on X_i through the conditional distribution

$$P(X_i = x_{(k)} | X_i^* = x_{(l)}, Z_i),$$

or alternatively,

$$P(X_i^* = x_{(l)} | X_i = x_{(k)}, Z_i),$$

where $k, l = 1, \ldots, r$.

The former scheme was adopted by some authors (e.g., Zucker and Spiegelman 2004); here we use the latter modeling method. Let

$$\Pi_i = [\pi_{ikl}]_{r \times r}$$

be the $r \times r$ misclassification matrix, where $\pi_{ikl} = P(X_i^* = x_{(l)} | X_i = x_{(k)}, Z_i)$ for $i = 1, \ldots, n$ and $k, l = 1, \ldots, r$.

We discuss how to use the insertion correction strategy to correct for misclassification effects. Unlike the case where the insertion correction strategy cannot directly apply for some forms of continuous error-prone covariates, the insertion correction method works for any form of error-prone discrete covariates with a finite number of possible values. To see this, we begin with a universal device considered by Akazawa, Kinukawa and Nakamura (1998) and Zucker and Spiegelman (2008).

Suppose $g(X_i, Z_i)$ is a function of the true covariates. We wish to find a function, say $g^*(\cdot)$, which is expressed in terms of the observed covariates $\{X_i^*, Z_i\}$ and pertains to function $g(X_i, Z_i)$ via

$$E\{g^*(X_i^*, Z_i) | \mathcal{F}_\tau\} = g(X_i, Z_i).$$

If the measurement error process satisfies the condition

$$E\{\psi(X_i^*, Z_i) | \mathcal{F}_\tau\} = E\{\psi(X_i^*, Z_i) | X_i, Z_i\}, \tag{3.55}$$

for any function $\psi(\cdot)$, then it is sufficient to find a function $g^*(\cdot)$ to meet the following condition

$$E\{g^*(X_i^*, Z_i) | X_i, Z_i\} = g(X_i, Z_i). \tag{3.56}$$

Similar to the discussion for (3.46), condition (3.55) is ensured if misclassification is nondifferential.

Often, $g^*(\cdot)$ and $g(\cdot)$ assume different function forms due to the difference between X_i^* and X_i. In the case with continuous X_i, function $g^*(\cdot)$ may not exist if $g(\cdot)$ has a complex form (e.g., Stefanski 1989); when the existence of function $g^*(\cdot)$ is ensured, identification of its form is often done case by case, mainly based on examining the form of $g(\cdot)$ as well as the measurement error model. For the case with error-prone discrete covariates, however, things become much simpler. For any given function $g(\cdot)$, function $g^*(\cdot)$ always exists and is determined by

$$g^*(X_i^* = x_{(l)}, Z_i) = \sum_{k=1}^{r} \pi^{ilk} g(X_i = x_{(k)}, Z_i) \qquad (3.57)$$

for $l = 1, \ldots, r$, where π^{ilk} is the (l, k) element of the inverse matrix Π_i^{-1} whose existence is assumed. We express $X_i^* = x_{(l)}$ and $X_i = x_{(k)}$, respectively, for the arguments of $g^*(\cdot)$ and $g(\cdot)$ to stress individual values taken by the variables.

To illustrate the ideas, in the following development we focus on the proportional hazards model (3.8) although the procedure can also apply to other survival models.

3.7.1 Methods with Known Misclassification Probabilities

For this subsection, assume the misclassification matrix Π_i is known. Let $x_{(j)}$ denote the measured value of X_i^*. We describe two ways to apply the insertion correction strategy to handle estimation of parameter β for the proportional hazards model (3.8). Specifically, we examine how to introduce the error correction terms to the log-likelihood function (3.9) or the partial likelihood score function in (3.14).

Let $g_1(X_i, Z_i; \beta) = \beta_x^{\mathrm{T}} X_i + \beta_z^{\mathrm{T}} Z_i$ and $g_2(X_i, Z_i; \beta) = \exp(\beta_x^{\mathrm{T}} X_i + \beta_z^{\mathrm{T}} Z_i)$. By (3.57), the corresponding $g_1^*(\cdot)$ and $g_2^*(\cdot)$ are given by

$$g_1^*(X_i^* = x_{(j)}, Z_i; \beta) = \sum_{k=1}^{r} \pi^{ijk} (\beta_x^{\mathrm{T}} x_{(k)} + \beta_z^{\mathrm{T}} Z_i),$$

and

$$g_2^*(X_i^* = x_{(j)}, Z_i; \beta) = \sum_{k=1}^{r} \pi^{ijk} \exp(\beta_x^{\mathrm{T}} x_{(k)} + \beta_z^{\mathrm{T}} Z_i).$$

Then corresponding to the log-likelihood function (3.9), we take

$$\ell_i^* = \sum_{i=1}^{n} \delta_i \{\log \lambda_0(t_i) + g_1^*(X_i^* = x_{(j)}, Z_i; \beta)\} - g_2^*(X_i^* = x_{(j)}, Z_i; \beta) \int_0^{t_i} \lambda_0(v) dv.$$

Under the condition (3.55), we have

$$\begin{aligned} E(\ell_i^* | \mathcal{F}_\tau) &= E(\ell_i^* | X_i, Z_i) \\ &= \ell_i, \end{aligned}$$

suggesting that the conditional expectation of ℓ_i^*, $E(\ell_i^* | X_i, Z_i)$, recovers the log-likelihood (3.9).

Comparing this ℓ_i^* to function (3.35) for the case with continuous X_i, we see the difference in correcting effects induced from continuous measurement error and misclassification. Estimation β proceeds in the same manner as that in §3.5.1, and the asymptotic distribution of the resulting estimator is established accordingly. This approach basically requires attention to the baseline hazard function, which may be modeled parametrically or nonparametrically.

Alternatively, to leave the baseline function unattended to, one may work with the partial likelihood or partial likelihood score function to adjust for misclassification effects following the same procedure as in §3.6.1.

Let $g_0(X_i) = X_i$ and $g_3(X_i, Z_i; \beta) = X_i \exp(\beta_x^{\mathrm{T}} X_i + \beta_z^{\mathrm{T}} Z_i)$. Then (3.57) gives that

$$g_0^*(X_i^* = x_{(j)}) = \sum_{k=1}^{r} \pi^{ijk} x_{(k)},$$

and

$$g_3^*(X_i^* = x_{(j)}, Z_i; \beta) = \sum_{k=1}^{r} \pi^{ijk} x_{(k)} \exp(\beta_x^{\mathrm{T}} x_{(k)} + \beta_z^{\mathrm{T}} Z_i).$$

Let

$$S^{(0)*}(t, \mathbb{X}^*, \mathbb{Z}; \beta) = \frac{1}{n} \sum_{i=1}^{n} R_i(t) g_2^*(X_i^* = x_{(j)}, Z_i; \beta),$$

$$S^{(1)*}(t, \mathbb{X}^*, \mathbb{Z}; \beta) = \frac{1}{n} \sum_{i=1}^{n} R_i(t) \begin{pmatrix} g_3^*(X_i^* = x_{(j)}, Z_i; \beta) \\ Z_i g_2^*(X_i^* = x_{(j)}, Z_i; \beta) \end{pmatrix},$$

$$U_i^*(\beta; \mathbb{X}^*, \mathbb{Z}) = \int_0^{\tau} \left\{ \begin{pmatrix} g_0^*(X_i^* = x_{(j)}) \\ Z_i \end{pmatrix} - \frac{S^{(1)*}(t, \mathbb{X}^*, \mathbb{Z}; \beta)}{S^{(0)*}(t, \mathbb{X}^*, \mathbb{Z}; \beta)} \right\} dN_i(t),$$

and

$$U^*(\beta; \mathbb{X}^*, \mathbb{Z}) = \sum_{i=1}^{n} \delta_i U_i^*(\beta; \mathbb{X}^*, \mathbb{Z}). \tag{3.58}$$

Then solving

$$U^*(\beta; \mathbb{X}^*, \mathbb{Z}) = 0$$

for β gives an estimate of β. Let $\widehat{\beta}$ be the resulting estimator.

Requirement (3.57) indicates that for $k = 1, 2, 3$, individual expectation $E\{g_k^*(X_i^*, Z_i; \beta)|X_i, Z_i\}$ recovers the corresponding term $g_k(X_i, Z_i; \beta)$ in the partial score function $S_{\mathrm{P}i}(\mathbb{X}, \mathbb{Z}; \beta)$ defined by (3.13), in addition to $E\{g_0^*(X_i)|X_i, Z_i\} = g_0(X_i)$. Nevertheless, for the entire estimating function $U_i^*(\beta; \mathbb{X}^*, \mathbb{Z})$, the conditional expectation $E\{\delta_i U_i^*(\beta; \mathbb{X}^*, \mathbb{Z})|\mathbb{X}, \mathbb{Z}\}$ does not coincide to $\delta_i S_{\mathrm{P}i}(\mathbb{X}, \mathbb{Z}; \beta)$. On the other hand, following the same arguments as in Andersen and Gill (1982), $U^*(\beta; \mathbb{X}^*, \mathbb{Z})$ can be shown to be asymptotically unbiased. Under regularity conditions, $n^{1/2}(\widehat{\beta} - \beta)$ is asymptotically normally distributed with mean zero and a sandwich-type covariance (Zucker and Spiegelman 2008).

The preceding procedure works if the misclassification probabilities are known. When these probabilities are unknown, one needs to estimate them using additional data information, which introduces two extra issues. The first one is to develop an estimation method for handling the (mis)classification probabilities, and the second issue is to accommodate the induced variability into the asymptotic distribution of the estimator $\widehat{\beta}$. In the following two subsections, we discuss methods of estimating the misclassification probabilities. For ease of exposition, we focus the discussion on the case where X_i is a binary covariate subject to misclassification. Extensions to accommodating multiple discrete covariates proceed in a similar manner.

3.7.2 Method with a Validation Sample

Suppose an internal validation sample $\mathcal{V}$ is available as described in §3.3.1. Let $\pi_{i01} = P(X_i^* = 1|X_i = 0, Z_i)$ and $\pi_{i10} = P(X_i^* = 0|X_i = 1, Z_i)$ be the misclassification probabilities, which may depend on error-free covariate Z_i. Then the (mis)classification probability matrix is given by

$$\Pi_i = \begin{pmatrix} 1 - \pi_{i01} & \pi_{i01} \\ \pi_{i10} & 1 - \pi_{i10} \end{pmatrix},$$

yielding the inverse matrix

$$\Pi_i^{-1} = \begin{pmatrix} \pi^{i00} & \pi^{i01} \\ \pi^{i10} & \pi^{i11} \end{pmatrix},$$

where $\pi^{i00} = (1 - \pi_{i10})/(1 - \pi_{i01} - \pi_{i10})$, $\pi^{i11} = (1 - \pi_{i01})/(1 - \pi_{i01} - \pi_{i10})$, $\pi^{i01} = 1 - \pi^{i00}$, and $\pi^{i10} = 1 - \pi^{i11}$.

A regression model is often used to facilitate the dependence of misclassification probabilities on the covariates. For instance, consider logistic regression models

$$\text{logit}\, \pi_{i01} = \alpha_0^{\mathrm{T}} w_{i0}; \ \text{logit}\, \pi_{i10} = \alpha_1^{\mathrm{T}} w_{i1};$$

where α_k is the vector of regression parameters and w_{ik} is a subset of covariates $\{X_i = k, Z_i\}$ that reflects different misclassification mechanisms for $k = 0, 1$. In two extreme situations, w_{ik} is specified as the entire covariate vector $\{X_i = k, Z_i\}$ and constant 1, respectively; the latter scenario corresponds to homogeneous misclassification across all subjects, which was considered by Zucker and Spiegelman (2008). Let $\alpha = (\alpha_0^{\mathrm{T}}, \alpha_1^{\mathrm{T}})^{\mathrm{T}}$.

Estimation of α and β proceeds with a two-stage procedure. At the first stage, we apply the likelihood method to the validation sample to estimate α. For $i \in \mathcal{V}$, let

$$L_{\mathrm{v}i}(\alpha) = \left\{\pi_{i01}^{X_i^*}(1 - \pi_{i01})^{1-X_i^*}\right\}^{1-X_i} \cdot \left\{\pi_{i10}^{1-X_i^*}(1 - \pi_{i10})^{X_i^*}\right\}^{X_i}$$

be the likelihood contributed from subject i and $S_{\mathrm{v}i}(\alpha) = \partial \log L_{\mathrm{v}i}(\alpha)/\partial\alpha$ be the score function. Then solving

$$\sum_{i \in \mathcal{V}} S_{\mathrm{v}i}(\alpha) = 0$$

for α yields the maximum likelihood estimate $\widehat{\alpha}$ of α. This step is easily carried out using existing software such as SAS or R.

At the second stage, we estimate β by modifying the partial likelihood score function with misclassification effects accounted for. Let

$$g_0^{**}(X_i^* = x_{(j)}) = (1 - \eta_i)g_0^*(X_i^* = x_{(j)}) + \eta_i X_i,$$

$$S^{(0)**}(t; \alpha, \beta) = \frac{1}{n}\sum_{i=1}^{n} R_i(t)\{(1 - \eta_i)g_2^*(X_i^* = x_{(j)}, Z_i; \beta) + \eta_i \exp(\beta_x^{\mathrm{T}} X_i + \beta_z^{\mathrm{T}} Z_i)\},$$

and

$$S^{(1)**}(t; \alpha, \beta) = \frac{1}{n}\sum_{i=1}^{n} R_i(t)\left\{(1 - \eta_i)\begin{pmatrix} g_3^*(X_i^* = x_{(j)}, Z_i; \beta) \\ Z_i g_2^*(X_i^* = x_{(j)}, Z_i; \beta) \end{pmatrix}\right.$$
$$\left. + \eta_i \begin{pmatrix} X_i \exp(\beta_x^{\mathrm{T}} X_i + \beta_z^{\mathrm{T}} Z_i) \\ Z_i \exp(\beta_x^{\mathrm{T}} X_i + \beta_z^{\mathrm{T}} Z_i) \end{pmatrix}\right\}.$$

Define

$$U_i^{**}(\alpha, \beta) = \int_0^{\tau} \left\{ \begin{pmatrix} g_0^{**}(X_i^* = x_{(j)}) \\ Z_i \end{pmatrix} - \frac{S^{(1)**}(t; \alpha, \beta)}{S^{(0)**}(t; \alpha, \beta)} \right\} dN_i(t).$$

Then estimation of β is obtained by solving

$$\sum_{i=1}^{n} \delta_i U_i^{**}(\widehat{\alpha}, \beta) = 0$$

for β, where $U_i^{**}(\widehat{\alpha}, \beta)$ is $U_i^{**}(\alpha, \beta)$ with α replaced by $\widehat{\alpha}$. Let $\widehat{\beta}$ be the resultant estimator of β.

Because the score function $S_{\mathrm{v}i}(\alpha)$ is free of β, this two-stage estimation algorithm is equivalent to the joint estimation procedure by solving

$$\begin{pmatrix} \sum_{i=1}^{n} \eta_i S_{\mathrm{v}i}(\alpha) \\ \sum_{i=1}^{n} \delta_i U_i^{**}(\alpha, \beta) \end{pmatrix} = 0$$

for α and β. If the size n_{v} of the validation sample and sample size n of the main study are of the same order, i.e., n_{v}/n approaches a nonzero constant when $n \to \infty$, the asymptotic distribution of $\widehat{\beta}$ can be established following the same lines for the result (1.15).

3.7.3 Method with Replicates

We discuss an estimation method in the presence of replicated measurements for the misclassified binary covariate. Suppose binary X_i is measured m_i times with replicate measurements X_{ij}^* that are not necessarily identical to X_i, where $j = 1, \ldots, m_i$. We assume that the (mis)classification probabilities are homogeneous among all subjects, which is often feasible when a risk factor is assessed repeatedly using the same device.

Let $\pi_{ilk,1-k} = P(X_{il}^* = 1 - k | X_i = k)$ be the misclassification probabilities for $k = 0, 1$ and $l = 1, \ldots, m_i$. Conditional on X_i, the X_{il}^* are assumed to be independent and identically distributed so that $\pi_{ilk,1-k} = \pi_{k,1-k}$ for all $l = 1, \ldots, m_i$ and $i = 1, \ldots, n$, where $\pi_{k,1-k}$ is a constant between 0 and 1 for $k = 0, 1$.

Consider the total $X_{i+}^* = \sum_{l=1}^{m_i} X_{il}^*$. Then conditional on $X_i = k$, the total X_{i+}^* follows a binomial distribution $\text{BIN}(m_i, p_k)$, where p_k equals $1 - \pi_{10}$ if $k = 1$ and π_{01} if $k = 0$. Let $\widetilde{\pi} = P(X_i = 1)$ be the marginal probability of X_i. Then the marginal probability of the total X_{i+}^* is

$$\begin{aligned} P(X_{i+}^* = x_i^*) &= \sum_{k=0,1} P(X_{i+}^* = x_i^* | X_i = k) P(X_i = k) \\ &= \widetilde{\pi} \binom{m_i}{x_i^*} (1 - \pi_{10})^{x_i^*} \pi_{10}^{m_i - x_i^*} + (1 - \widetilde{\pi}) \binom{m_i}{x_i^*} \pi_{01}^{x_i^*} (1 - \pi_{01})^{m_i - x_i^*}, \end{aligned}$$

where $x_i^* = 0, \ldots, m_i$.

Let $\alpha = (\widetilde{\pi}, \pi_{01}, \pi_{10})^{\mathrm{T}}$ be the associated parameter, and $L_{\mathrm{T}i} = P(X_{i+}^* = x_i^*)$ be the likelihood function contributed from subject i, and $S_{\mathrm{T}i}(\alpha) = \partial \log L_{\mathrm{T}i} / \partial \alpha^{\mathrm{T}}$ be the score function. Solving

$$\sum_{i=1}^{n} S_{\mathrm{T}i}(\alpha) = 0$$

for α gives the maximum likelihood estimate $\widehat{\alpha}$ of α. Then estimation of β is obtained by solving

$$\widehat{U}^*(\beta; \mathbb{X}^*, \mathbb{Z}) = 0$$

for β, where $\widehat{U}^*(\beta; \mathbb{X}^*, \mathbb{Z})$ is determined by (3.58) with the (mis)classification probabilities replaced by the corresponding estimates.

The discussion here is addressed to a binary covariate X_i. Extensions to accommodating more general settings are possible by using a similar idea. For instance, if X_i assumes r values with $r \geq 3$, then the preceding argument applies with the conditional binomial distribution replaced by a conditional multinomial distribution. The independence assumption for the replicates X_{il}^* may also be relaxed to allow some dependence structures by following the discussions of Torrance-Rynard and Walter (1997) and Zucker and Spiegelman (2008).

3.8 Multivariate Survival Data with Covariate Measurement Error

Relative to extensive attention on univariate error-prone survival data, research on multivariate or clustered survival data with covariate measurement error is limited. In this section, we briefly describe issues concerning covariate measurement error for multivariate or clustered survival data, focusing on three modeling and inference frameworks.

Suppose the sample includes n units each experiencing m types of failure. For $i = 1, \ldots, n$ and $j = 1, \ldots, m$, let T_{ij} be the jth failure time of unit i and C_{ij} be the corresponding censoring time. Denote $t_{ij} = \min(T_{ij}, C_{ij})$ and $\delta_{ij} = I(T_{ij} \leq C_{ij})$. Let $R_{ij}(t) = I(t_{ij} \geq t)$ be the indicator that the jth failure for unit i remains at risk at time t, and $\{X_{ij}, Z_{ij}\}$ be the covariates corresponding to the jth failure for unit i. Covariate X_{ij} is time-independent but Z_{ij} may be time-independent or time-varying. Sometimes we write $Z_{ij}(t)$ to emphasize that the Z_{ij} are time-dependent. Suppose that X_{ij} is measured with error, and Z_{ij} is accurately measured. Let X_{ij}^* be the surrogate measurement of X_{ij}.

Write $t_i = (t_{i1}, \ldots, t_{im})^{\mathrm{T}}$, $\delta_i = (\delta_{i1}, \ldots, \delta_{im})^{\mathrm{T}}$, $T_i = (T_{i1}, \ldots, T_{im})^{\mathrm{T}}$, $C_i = (C_{i1}, \ldots, C_{im})^{\mathrm{T}}$, $X_i = (X_{i1}^{\mathrm{T}}, \ldots, X_{im}^{\mathrm{T}})^{\mathrm{T}}$, $X_i^* = (X_{i1}^{*\mathrm{T}}, \ldots, X_{im}^{*\mathrm{T}})^{\mathrm{T}}$, $Z_i = (Z_{i1}^{\mathrm{T}}, \ldots, Z_{im}^{\mathrm{T}})^{\mathrm{T}}$, and $Z_i(t) = (Z_{i1}^{\mathrm{T}}(t), \ldots, Z_{im}^{\mathrm{T}}(t))^{\mathrm{T}}$ for any time t. Within each unit i, the T_{ij} may be correlated for $j = 1, \ldots, m$; but the $\{T_i, C_i, X_i, Z_i(t) : t \geq 0\}$ are independent for $i = 1, \ldots, n$. For each i, conditional on the true covariates, T_i, C_i and X_i^* are assumed to be independent.

3.8.1 Marginal Approach

Here we discuss a marginal modeling approach and consider the case where error-free covariate $Z_i(t)$ is time-dependent. For $i = 1, \ldots, n$ and $j = 1, \ldots, m$, the failure time T_{ij} follows a marginal model with the hazard function determined by

$$\lambda_{ij}(t|X_{ij}, Z_{ij}(t)) = \lambda_{0j}(t) \exp\{\beta_x^{\mathrm{T}} X_{ij} + \beta_z^{\mathrm{T}} Z_{ij}(t)\}, \tag{3.59}$$

where $\lambda_{0j}(t)$ is the baseline hazard function for the jth type of failure and β_x and β_z are the regression coefficients. Write $\beta = (\beta_x^{\mathrm{T}}, \beta_z^{\mathrm{T}})^{\mathrm{T}}$.

If X_{ij} were precisely measured, estimation of parameter β may be realized using the marginal partial likelihood by ignoring possible association of the failure times within the same unit (Wei, Lin and Weissfeld 1989; Cai and Prentice 1995). Let

$$S_{ij}^{(0)}(t_{ij}; \beta) = \frac{1}{n} \sum_{k=1}^{n} R_{kj}(t_{ij}) \exp\{\beta_x^{\mathrm{T}} X_{kj} + \beta_z^{\mathrm{T}} Z_{kj}(t_{ij})\},$$

and

$$S_{ij}^{(1)}(t_{ij}; \beta) = \frac{1}{n} \sum_{k=1}^{n} R_{kj}(t_{ij}) \begin{pmatrix} X_{kj} \\ Z_{kj}(t_{ij}) \end{pmatrix} \exp\{\beta_x^{\mathrm{T}} X_{kj} + \beta_z^{\mathrm{T}} Z_{kj}(t_{ij})\}.$$

Define

$$U(\beta) = \sum_{i=1}^{n} \sum_{j=1}^{m} \delta_{ij} \left\{ \begin{pmatrix} X_{ij} \\ Z_{ij}(t_{ij}) \end{pmatrix} - \frac{S_{ij}^{(1)}(t_{ij}; \beta)}{S_{ij}^{(0)}(t_{ij}; \beta)} \right\}$$

to be the *pseudo-partial likelihood score* function. In the instance where for any unit i, all the failure times T_{ij} are independent for $j = 1, \ldots, m$, function $U(\beta)$ is identical to the usual partial likelihood score function. Under regularity conditions of Wei, Lin and Weissfeld (1989), solving

$$U(\beta) = 0 \tag{3.60}$$

for β leads to a consistent estimator of β.

When X_{ij} is subject to measurement error, directly replacing X_{ij} with its surrogate measurement X^*_{ij} in (3.60) usually results in a biased estimator of β. Depending on the form of measurement error models or the availability of data sources, various bias correction methods may be developed along the same lines as discussed in §3.3, §3.6.1 or §3.7. For example, Greene and Cai (2004) explored the simulation-extrapolation method for the case where measurement error model is given by $X^*_{ij} = X_{ij} + e_{ij}$; the e_{ij} are independent of each other and of $\{X_i, T_i, C_i, Z_i(t) : t \geq 0\}$, and the e_{ij} follow a normal distribution $N(0, \Sigma_e)$ with a known covariance matrix Σ_e.

These marginal methods are easy modifications of their univariate counterparts, and their implementation is fairly straightforward. These approaches are useful when our primary interest lies in inference about the marginal model parameter β. The association strength among the T_{ij} is typically ignored in these methods. In the next two subsections, we discuss methods which accommodate the association among the T_{ij}.

3.8.2 Dependence Parameter Estimation of Copula Models

We consider a modeling framework which explicitly facilitates the clustering effects among the failure times T_{ij} via copula models (Nelsen 2006). This modeling allows us to explicitly express the marginal survivor functions as well as the association parameter. We consider the case with $m = 2$. Let $S_j(\cdot)$ be the model for the marginal survivor function of T_{ij}, and $C(\cdot, \cdot; \phi)$ be a copula function indexed by parameter ϕ which may be a scalar or a vector. Then the model for the joint survivor function of (T_{i1}, T_{i2}) is given by

$$S(t_1, t_2) = C(S_1(t_1), S_2(t_2); \phi). \tag{3.61}$$

As a result, the model for the joint probability density function of (T_{i1}, T_{i2}) is

$$f(t_1, t_2) = c(S_1(t_1), S_2(t_2); \phi) f_1(t_1) f_2(t_2),$$

where $c(\cdot; \phi)$ is the density function corresponding to the distribution $C(\cdot; \phi)$, and $f_j(\cdot)$ is the model for the marginal density function of T_{ij} for $j = 1, 2$.

Assume that given covariates $\{X_{ij}, Z_{ij}\}$ for the jth type of failure, covariates $\{X_{ik}, Z_{ik}\}$ with $k \neq j$ have no predictive value for the failure time T_{ij}, i.e., $h_j(t|X_i, Z_i) = h_j(t|X_{ij}, Z_{ij})$, where $h_j(t|\cdot)$ is the conditional probability density function of T_{ij} given the covariates indicated by the arguments. To facilitate the covariate information, we postulate the marginal survivor functions of the T_{ij} using the regression strategies discussed in §3.1, and let β denote the associated parameter vector of the marginal models $S_j(\cdot)$ for $j = 1, 2$. Let $\theta = (\beta^{\mathrm{T}}, \phi^{\mathrm{T}})^{\mathrm{T}}$ denote the parameter for the joint survival model.

If X_{ij} were precisely measured, inference on θ is carried out using the likelihood method. The likelihood function of θ contributed from unit i is

$$L_i(\theta) = \{f(t_{i1}, t_{i2})\}^{\delta_{i1}\delta_{i2}} \left\{ -\frac{\partial S(t_{i1}, t_{i2})}{\partial t_{i1}} \right\}^{\delta_{i1}(1-\delta_{i2})} \left\{ -\frac{\partial S(t_{i1}, t_{i2})}{\partial t_{i2}} \right\}^{(1-\delta_{i1})\delta_{i2}}$$
$$\cdot \{S(t_{i1}, t_{i2})\}^{(1-\delta_{i1})(1-\delta_{i2})},$$

where the dependence on the parameter θ is suppressed in the symbols of the right-hand side.

Define

$$U_{\beta i}(\theta) = \frac{\partial \log L_i(\theta)}{\partial \beta} \text{ and } U_{\phi i}(\theta) = \frac{\partial \log L_i(\theta)}{\partial \phi}. \tag{3.62}$$

Under regularity conditions, solving

$$\begin{pmatrix} \sum_{i=1}^{n} U_{\beta i}(\theta) \\ \sum_{i=1}^{n} U_{\phi i}(\theta) \end{pmatrix} = 0$$

for θ gives a consistent estimator of θ.

The likelihood method is straightforward in principle. However, it can be computationally demanding. Alternatively, a two-stage estimation algorithm is used with β and ϕ being separately estimated at each step (Hougaard 1986; Shih and Louis 1995). At the first stage, we ignore the dependence structure among the T_{ij} and merely use the marginal models to estimate β; at the second stage, we estimate parameter ϕ using the joint model with β replaced by the estimate obtained from the first stage.

Specifically, let

$$L_{ij}^*(\beta) = \left\{ \frac{-\partial S_j(t_{ij})}{\partial t_{ij}} \right\}^{\delta_{ij}} \{S_j(t_{ij})\}^{1-\delta_{ij}}$$

be the marginal likelihood pertinent to T_{ij} for $j = 1, 2$. Define

$$L_i^*(\beta) = L_{i1}^*(\beta) L_{i2}^*(\beta)$$

to be the pseudo-likelihood contributed from unit i for which T_{i1} and T_{i2} are pretended to be independent. Let $U_{\beta i}^*(\beta) = \partial \log L_i^*(\beta) / \partial \beta$. At the first stage, solving

$$\sum_{i=1}^{n} U_{\beta i}^*(\beta) - 0 \tag{3.63}$$

for β gives an estimate, say $\widehat{\beta}$, of β. At the second stage, we solve

$$\sum_{i=1}^{n} U_{\phi i}(\widehat{\beta}, \phi) = 0 \tag{3.64}$$

for ϕ to obtain an estimate of ϕ, where $U_{\phi i}(\widehat{\beta}, \phi)$ is determined by (3.62) with β replaced by $\widehat{\beta}$.

Glidden (2000) applied this approach to the Clayton–Oakes model and showed that the two-stage estimator is consistent and has the asymptotic normality property under regularity conditions. Andersen (2005) generalized the discussion to copula models where marginal survivor functions are modeled parametrically or semiparametrically.

In the presence of measurement error in X_{ij}, naively applying existing approaches with X_{ij} replaced by X_{ij}^* may lead to seriously biased results. It is necessary to take into account the measurement error effects when developing estimation procedures for θ. Relative to the univariate case, adjusting for the impact of covariate measurement error on analysis of multivariate error-prone survival data is more complex. Although copula model (3.61) separates the marginal structures from the association parameter, correction for measurement error effects cannot necessarily be done separately, even when a two-stage estimation procedure is performed to separately estimate the marginal model parameter β and the dependence parameter ϕ.

To see this, we consider the setting discussed by Gorfine, Hsu and Prentice (2003) with replicated surrogate measurements X_{ijk}^* taken for X_{ij}, where $k = 1, \ldots, K$, and K is an integer no smaller than 2. Suppose marginal models $S_j(\cdot)$ for failure times T_{ij} are specified as (3.59) with $\lambda_{0j}(\cdot) = \lambda_0(\cdot)$ for $j = 1, 2$ and the joint survivor model is given by the Clayton–Oakes model

$$S(t_1, t_2) = \{S_1(t_1)^{-\phi} + S_2(t_2)^{-\phi} - 1\}^{-1/\phi},$$

where ϕ is the dependence parameter which is positive (Clayton 1978; Cox and Oakes 1984, Ch. 10; He 2014).

The dependence parameter ϕ is interpreted as the ratio of the conditional hazard functions evaluated under different conditions:

$$\phi = \frac{\lambda_{\mathrm{T}_{i1}|\mathrm{T}_{i2}}(t|T_{i2} = t_2)}{\lambda_{\mathrm{T}_{i1}|\mathrm{T}_{i2}}(t|T_{i2} \geq t_2)} - 1 = \frac{\lambda_{\mathrm{T}_{i2}|\mathrm{T}_{i1}}(t|T_{i1} = t_1)}{\lambda_{\mathrm{T}_{i2}|\mathrm{T}_{i1}}(t|T_{i1} \geq t_1)} - 1,$$

where $\lambda_{\mathrm{T}_{ij}|\mathrm{T}_{ik}}(\cdot|\cdot)$ represents the model for the hazard function of the conditional distribution of T_{ij}, given T_{ik}; $j \neq k$ and $j, k = 1, 2$.

If we use the two-stage procedure to estimate β and ϕ, it is possible to produce a consistent estimator for the marginal model parameter β by modifying estimating function $U_{\beta i}^*(\beta)$ in (3.63) using the schemes developed in the previous sections for univariate error-contaminated data. For instance, one may introduce correction terms of measurement error effects individually to each of the marginal score functions of T_{i1} and T_{i2}. The resulting estimating function of β at the first stage can still be unbiased or asymptotically unbiased, hence yielding a consistent estimator of β under regularity conditions. However, the measurement error correction terms at the first stage may not fully accommodate measurement error effects on using the score function $U_{\phi i}(\beta, \phi)$ in (3.64) for estimation of the dependence parameter ϕ, thus the estimator of ϕ obtained at the second stage is not necessarily consistent. The induced bias in estimating ϕ may be examined using the strategy outlined in §1.4. To reduce the induced bias in estimating ϕ at the second stage, Gorfine, Hsu and Prentice (2003) proposed to use the second-order Taylor series expansion of the score function $U_{\phi i}(\beta, \phi)$. For details, see Gorfine, Hsu and Prentice (2003).

3.8.3 EM Algorithm with Frailty Measurement Error Model

Another useful tool for modeling multivariate failure times is frailty models. Association among failure times within units is facilitated by frailties (or random effects).

Here we describe a frailty measurement error model to illustrate how error-prone multivariate survival data may be analyzed.

Conditional on the unit-specific frailty u_i and the covariates, the failure times T_{ij} are assumed to be independent and have the conditional proportional hazards functions modeled as

$$\lambda_{ij}(t|u_i, X_{ij}, Z_{ij}) = \lambda_0(t)\exp(u_i^{\mathrm{T}} B_{ij} + \beta_x^{\mathrm{T}} X_{ij} + \beta_z^{\mathrm{T}} Z_{ij}), \tag{3.65}$$

where $\lambda_0(t)$ is the (conditional) baseline hazard function that is common for all the units, β_x and β_z are fixed effects associated with covariates $\{X_{ij}, Z_{ij}\}$, and the B_{ij} are covariates associated with the frailty and measured without error. The frailties u_i are assumed to be independent of each other and of the covariates and censoring times; and the distribution of u_i is modeled by $f(u_i;\phi)$ with the associated parameter ϕ. Common choices of $f(u_i;\phi)$ include log-Gamma and multivariate normal distributions (e.g., Clayton and Cuzick 1985).

Let $\Lambda_0(t) = \int_0^t \lambda_0(v)dv$ be the cumulative baseline hazard function. Under model (3.65), the likelihood contributed from the ith unit is

$$\begin{aligned} L_i(t_i, \delta_i|X_i, Z_i) = \int \prod_{j=1}^{m} \Big[& \{\lambda_0(t_{ij})\exp(u_i^{\mathrm{T}} B_{ij} + \beta_x^{\mathrm{T}} X_{ij} + \beta_z^{\mathrm{T}} Z_{ij})\}^{\delta_{ij}} \\ & \cdot \exp\{-\Lambda_0(t_{ij})\exp(u_i^{\mathrm{T}} B_{ij} + \beta_x^{\mathrm{T}} X_{ij} + \beta_z^{\mathrm{T}} Z_{ij})\} \Big] \\ & \cdot f(u_i;\phi)d\eta(u_i). \end{aligned} \tag{3.66}$$

Inference on the model parameter cannot be directly based on (3.66) because the covariates X_{ij} are not observed. Instead, it must be conducted based on the observed surrogate measurements X_{ij}^*, along with the observed failure times or censoring times, and the observed covariates $\{Z_{ij}, B_{ij}\}$. Under the nondifferential measurement error mechanism, the likelihood based on the observed data is given by

$$L_i(t_i, \delta_i|X_i^*, Z_i) = \int L_i(t_i, \delta_i|x_i, Z_i) f(x_i|X_i^*, Z_i)d\eta(x_i), \tag{3.67}$$

or

$$L_i(t_i, \delta_i, X_i^*|Z_i) = \int L_i(t_i, \delta_i|x_i, Z_i) f(X_i^*|x_i, Z_i) f(x_i|Z_i)d\eta(x_i), \tag{3.68}$$

depending on the form of the measurement error model, where $L_i(t_i, \delta_i|X_i, Z_i)$ is determined by (3.66), and $f(\cdot|\cdot)$ represents the model for the conditional probability density or mass function of the corresponding variables.

If conditional model $f(x_i|X_i^*, Z_i)$ is given, then inferences may be conducted using (3.67). In contrast, if conditional model $f(x_i^*|X_i, Z_i)$ is specified, then inferences are based on (3.68) which further requires specification of the conditional distribution of X_i, given Z_i. In either case, it is necessary to have knowledge of the conditional distribution of X_i given $\{X_i^*, Z_i\}$ or of X_i given Z_i.

Given that the models are all posited, each with a full distributional form specified, inferences are then carried out by maximizing the observed likelihood

$$L_o = \prod_{i=1}^{n} L_i(t_i, \delta_i | X_i^*, Z_i)$$

with respect to the model parameter, where $L_i(t_i, \delta_i | X_i^*, Z_i)$ is determined by (3.67) or (3.68).

Alternatively, estimation of the model parameter may proceed by using the EM algorithm. To see this, we discuss a case where X_{ij} and Z_{ij} are scalar for ease of exposition, and the classical additive error model is assumed. X_{ij}^* and X_{ij} are linked by

$$X_{ij}^* = X_{ij} + e_{ij},$$

where the e_{ij} are independent of $\{T_i, C_i, Z_i\}$ and follow the distribution $N(0, \sigma_e^2)$ with an unknown variance σ_e^2.

For the unit-level covariate vector X_i we consider a linear regression model:

$$X_i = \mu_x 1_m + \mu_z Z_i + \epsilon_{xi}$$

where the ϵ_{xi} are independent of $\{T_i, C_i, Z_i\}$ as well as the e_{ij} and follow distribution $N(0, \sigma_x^2 I_m)$, and μ_x, μ_z and σ_x^2 are scalar parameters.

In (3.65), we assume that u_i follows a normal distribution $N(0, \Sigma_u)$ where covariance matrix Σ_u contains a vector of parameters ϕ. Let $\theta = (\beta_x, \beta_z, \mu_x, \mu_z, \sigma_x^2, \sigma_e^2, \phi^{\mathrm{T}})^{\mathrm{T}}$. With the preceding distributional assumptions, the log-likelihood for the complete data is, omitting an additive constant,

$$\ell_c(\theta) = \sum_{i=1}^{n} \ell_{ci}(\theta; t_i, \delta_i, X_i^*, Z_i, X_i, u_i),$$

where

$$\begin{aligned}
&\ell_{ci}(\theta; t_i, \delta_i, X_i^*, Z_i, X_i, u_i) \\
&= \sum_{j=1}^{m} \left[\delta_{ij} \left\{\log \lambda_0(t_{ij}) + u_i^{\mathrm{T}} B_{ij} + \beta_x X_{ij} + \beta_z Z_{ij}\right\} - \Lambda_{ij}(t_{ij})\right] \\
&\quad -\frac{m}{2} \log(\sigma_e^2) - \frac{1}{2\sigma_e^2}(X_i^* - X_i)^{\mathrm{T}}(X_i^* - X_i) \\
&\quad -\frac{m}{2} \log(\sigma_x^2) - \frac{1}{2\sigma_x^2}(X_i - \mu_x 1_m - \mu_x Z_i)^{\mathrm{T}}(X_i - \mu_x 1_m - \mu_x Z_i) \\
&\quad -\frac{1}{2} \log|\Sigma_u| - u_i^{\mathrm{T}} \Sigma_u^{-1} u_i
\end{aligned} \tag{3.69}$$

and $\Lambda_{ij}(t) = \Lambda_0(t) \exp(u_i^{\mathrm{T}} B_{ij} + \beta_x X_{ij} + \beta_z Z_{ij})$.

In implementing the E-step at iteration $(k+1)$, the terms involving unobserved X_i and u_i are replaced with their conditional expectations taken with respect to the model, $f(X_i, u_i | t_i, \delta_i, X_i^*, Z_i; \theta^{(k)})$, for the conditional distribution of $\{X_i, u_i\}$ given the observable variables $\{t_i, \delta_i, X_i^*, Z_i\}$, where $\theta^{(k)}$ is the estimate of θ obtained at the kth iteration. This evaluation typically involves integrals that have no analytical forms. An option is to use Monte Carlo simulations to approximate the expectations by generating variables from the conditional distribution

$$f(X_i, u_i | t_i, \delta_i, X_i^*, Z_i; \theta^{(k)}) = \frac{\exp \ell_{ci}(\theta^{(k)}; t_i, \delta_i, X_i^*, Z_i, X_i, u_i)}{\int \exp \ell_{ci}(\theta^{(k)}; t_i, \delta_i, X_i^*, Z_i, X_i, u_i) d\eta(X_i) d\eta(u_i)},$$

where $\ell_{ci}(\theta^{(k)}; t_i, \delta_i, X_i^*, Z_i, X_i, u_i)$ is determined by (3.69) with θ replaced by $\theta^{(k)}$.

The M-step updates θ by maximizing the resultant expectation

$$\sum_{i=1}^{n} E\{\ell_{ci}(\theta; t_i, \delta_i, X_i^*, Z_i, X_i, u_i) | t_i, \delta_i, X_i^*, Z_i; \theta^{(k)}\}$$

with respect to θ, which may be realized by using, for instance, the algorithm of Liu and Rubin (1994).

Let $\widehat{\theta}$ be the resulting estimator of θ. The associated variance estimate of $\widehat{\theta}$ may be calculated using the formula of Louis (1982), which partitions the complete data information into two parts: the information associated with the observed data and the information associated with the missing data. Alternatively, one may employ the approximate formula discussed by Liu and Wu (2007). Let $S_{ci} = \partial \ell_{ci}(\theta; t_i, \delta_i, X_i^*, Z_i, X_i, u_i)/\partial\theta$, then an approximation of the covariance matrix of $\widehat{\theta}$ is given by

$$\left[\sum_{i-1}^{n} E(S_{ci} | t_i, \delta_i, X_i^*, Z_i; \widehat{\theta}) \{E(S_{ci} | t_i, \delta_i, X_i^*, Z_i; \widehat{\theta})\}^{\mathrm{T}}\right]^{-1},$$

where the expectation is evaluated with respect to $f(X_i, u_i | t_i, \delta_i, X_i^*, Z_i; \widehat{\theta})$, the model for the conditional distribution of $\{X_i, u_i\}$ given $\{t_i, \delta_i, X_i^*, Z_i\}$, with θ replaced by $\widehat{\theta}$. The expectation may again be handled with the Monte Carlo method.

To implement the Monte Carlo EM (MCEM) algorithm, one needs to deal with the baseline hazards function $\lambda_0(t)$. This baseline hazards function may be modeled parametrically, semiparametrically or nonparametrically. Different modeling schemes may induce varying difficulties in implementation and establishment of asymptotic properties. If $\lambda_0(t)$ is modeled parametrically or weakly parametrically as discussed in §3.5.1, then the preceding discussion carries through with parameter θ modified to include the associated parameter of modeling $\lambda_0(t)$. However, if $\lambda_0(t)$ is treated nonparametrically, as discussed by Li and Lin (2000), developing asymptotic results can be challenging.

Finally, we note that the method described here requires modeling the distribution of the error-prone covariate X_i. To relax this assumption, Li and Lin (2003a) explored the SIMEX method. The results are robust to potential misspecification of the distribution of X_i. This method, however, can only partially correct for measurement error effects on inferential procedures, which is the price paid for achieving the robustness.

3.9 Bibliographic Notes and Discussion

Since Prentice (1982) proposed the regression calibration approach for the proportional hazards model with covariate measurement error, there has been increasing interest in accommodating measurement error effects into inferential procedures when analyzing error-prone survival data. Many authors investigated the impact of ignoring measurement error on inferential procedures, and a large number of methods have been developed to correct for measurement error effects. For instance, see Hughes (1993), Pepe, Self and Prentice (1989), Gong, Whittemore and Grosser (1990), Wang et al. (1997), Augustin and Schwarz (2002), Gorfine, Hsu and Prentice (2004), Wang (2008), Küchenhoff, Bender and Langner (2007), Zucker and Spiegelman (2004, 2008), Cheng and Crainiceanu (2009), Zhang, He and Li (2014), and Yan (2014), among many others.

Although the regression calibration method can only partially remove the bias induced from covariate measurement error, generality and easy implementation make this strategy popular. In the literature, extensions of this method are available. With a single covariate subject to measurement error, Thurston et al. (2005) compared the asymptotic relative efficiency of several regression calibration methods for studies with internal validation data. Kipnis et al. (2012) investigated the performance of the regression calibration method for settings with more surrogates than mismeasured variables. Xie, Wang and Prentice (2001) proposed the *risk set regression calibration* approach for time-invariant covariates subject to measurement error. Liao et al. (2011) extended the risk set regression calibration approach to settings with time-varying covariates subject to measurement error. Shaw and Prentice (2012) developed the risk set calibration approach under a general measurement error model considered by Prentice et al. (2002).

The SIMEX method is another useful approach which has been widely used in practice. In survival analysis with error-prone covariates, a number of authors explored the use of this approach for various survival models. For instance, He, Yi and Xiong (2007) and Yi and He (2012) explored the SIMEX method for analysis of error-prone survival data under AFT models and proportional odds models, respectively. An R package of implementing the SIMEX method for AFT models was developed by He, Xiong and Yi (2012). The use of the SIMEX approach appears in other contexts as well. For example, Kim and Gleser (2000) discussed using the SIMEX method for estimation of the area under the *receiver operating characteristic* (ROC) curve in the presence of measurement error in variables. Delaigle and Hall (2008) explored using the SIMEX method for selecting smoothing parameters when applying nonparametric methods to errors-in-variables regression. Other applications of the SIMEX procedure have been reported by Lin and Carroll (1999), Staudenmayer and Ruppert (2004) and Luo, Stefanski and Boos (2006), among others.

Regarding the expectation correction strategies, there are a number of different versions. Huang and Wang (2000), Hu and Lin (2002, 2004), Augustin (2004), and Song and Huang (2005) extended the "corrected" score methods, initially discussed by Nakamura (1990, 1992), to settings with various types of measurement error models. Under the additive hazards model, Kulich and Lin (2000), Sun, Zhang and Sun

(2006), and Sun and Zhou (2008) developed inference algorithms using the expectation correction strategy. Yan and Yi (2015) proposed a corrected profile likelihood approach for the Cox model with error-contaminated covariates, and their approach unifies several existing methods under the same framework. Ma and Yin (2008) developed corrected score based approaches for cure rate models with mismeasured covariates. Other work related to the expectation correction scheme can be found in Zhou and Pepe (1995), Zhou and Wang (2000), Wang and Pepe (2000), and Li and Ryan (2006), among many others.

In terms of the likelihood-based methods which typically require distributional specification for the true covariates X_i, many authors, including Hu, Tsiatis and Davidian (1998), Dupuy (2005), and Wen (2010), explored inferential procedures for the proportional hazards model. He, Xiong and Yi (2011) considered the proportional odds model for error-prone survival data, and compared the performance of the likelihood method and the regression calibration approach. Sun, Song and Mu (2012) extended the induced partial likelihood method by Zucker (2005) from the proportional hazards model to the additive hazards model. Cheng and Wang (2001) developed inference procedures under linear transformation models (Dabrowska and Doksum 1988) using the generalized estimating equation approach. Wang and Song (2013) investigated an approximate induced hazard estimator and proposed an expected estimating equation estimator via the EM algorithm.

Relative to extensive attention on univariate survival data with covariate measurement error, research on multivariate or clustered survival data with covariate measurement error is limited. Li and Lin (2000) proposed a structural approach to correct the bias induced by covariate measurement error. They subsequently developed a functional approach using the SIMEX algorithm (Li and Lin 2003a). Greene and Cai (2004) considered a marginal model setup and explored the SIMEX method for inferences. Hu and Lin (2004) analyzed multivariate survival data with measurement error under shared frailty models. Gorfine, Hsu and Prentice (2003) proposed a bias reduction technique for error-prone bivariate survival data under copula models. Under accelerated lifetime regression models with mismeasured covariates, Choi, Yi and Matthews (2006) developed a functional method, and Yi and He (2006) proposed structural marginal methods. Kim, Li and Spiegelman (2016) proposed a semiparametric copula approach for consistent estimation of the effect of an error-prone covariate.

The discussion on measurement error is directed to the case where only covariates are subject to mismeasurement and the survival times are precisely measured. For some practical problems, measurement of survival times may also be subject to error. In this instance, it is necessary to investigate such error effects and develop valid inference methods accordingly. Research on this topic, however, is rather scarce, although some authors investigated this problem (e.g., Meier, Richardson and Hughes 2003).

3.10 Supplementary Problems

3.1.

(a) In §3.1.3, we describe that proportional hazards and proportional odds models are defined using the structure of (3.5). Now we look at an alternative structure that accommodates both types of models. Show that both proportional hazards and proportional odds models can be written as

$$\psi\{S(t|X,Z)\} = \psi\{S_0(t)\} + \phi(X,Z;\beta)$$

for some monotone function $\psi(\cdot)$ and function $\phi(\cdot)$, where β is the associated parameter. Clearly define the meaning of functions $S(t|X,Z)$ and $S_0(t)$. Identify function forms of $\psi(\cdot)$ and $\phi(\cdot)$ for proportional hazards and proportional odds models.

(b) Show that the only models for the distribution of T given $\{X,Z\}$ that fall in both the proportional hazards family (3.6) and the accelerated failure time family (3.4) must follow a Weibull distribution.

(c) Show that the survivor function of the log-logistic regression model for the distribution of T given $\{X,Z\}$ may be written in the form

$$S(t|X,Z) = [1 + \{t/\psi(X,Z)\}^{\alpha}]^{-1} \qquad (3.70)$$

for some function $\psi(\cdot)$ and parameter α. Show that this is both a proportional odds (PO) model and an accelerated failure time (AFT) model. Show that any regression model that is in both the PO and AFT families must be of the form (3.70).

(Lawless 2003, Ch. 6)

3.2. Suppose that a censored random sample consists of data $\{(y_i, \delta_i, X_i, Z_i) : i = 1, \ldots, n\}$, where for $i = 1, \ldots, n$, $y_i = \log t_i$, $t_i = \min(T_i, C_i)$, T_i is the lifetime, C_i is the censoring time, and $\{X_i, Z_i\}$ are covariates. Assume that the survivor function of T_i given $\{X_i, Z_i\}$ is postulated by a location-scale model discussed in §3.1.3:

$$S(y|X_i,Z_i) = S_0\left(\frac{y - m(X_i,Z_i;\beta)}{\sigma}\right) \quad \text{for } -\infty < y < \infty,$$

where β and σ are unknown parameters, $m(\cdot)$ is a function, and $S_0(\cdot)$ is a survivor function of a given form, such as the one for a standard normal, extreme value or logistic distribution. Assume that

$$m(X_i,Z_i;\beta) = \beta_0 + \beta_x^{\mathrm{T}} X_i + \beta_z^{\mathrm{T}} Z_i,$$

where $\beta = (\beta_0, \beta_x^{\mathrm{T}}, \beta_z^{\mathrm{T}})^{\mathrm{T}}$ is the vector of regression parameters. Let $\theta = (\beta^{\mathrm{T}}, \sigma)^{\mathrm{T}}$.

(a) Let $f_0(t)$ be the probability density function corresponding to the survivor function $S_0(t)$. Show that if $\log f_0(t)$ is concave, i.e.,

$$\frac{d^2}{dt^2}\log f_0(t) < 0 \text{ for all } t,$$

then $\log S_0(t)$ is also concave.

(b) Identify assumptions for the censoring mechanism so that the following likelihood formulation can be used for inference about θ:

$$L(\theta) = \prod_{i=1}^{n} \left\{ \frac{1}{\sigma} f_0\left(\frac{y_i - m(X_i, Z_i; \beta)}{\sigma} \right) \right\}^{\delta_i} \left\{ S_0\left(\frac{y_i - m(X_i, Z_i; \beta)}{\sigma} \right) \right\}^{1-\delta_i}.$$

(c) Show that the MLE does not necessarily exist for all location-scale models.

(d) Discuss conditions for which the MLE exists for location-scale models. Using the result in (b), show that if $S_0(t)$ takes the form of the standard extreme value, normal or logistic distribution, and that if the MLE exists, then the MLE is unique.

(e) When the MLE exists, determine the asymptotic distribution of the maximum likelihood estimator $\widehat{\theta}$.

(f) Perform a statistical test for the null hypothesis $H_o : \beta_x = 0$.

(Lawless 2003, Ch. 6)

3.3. For the data in Problem 3.2, assume that the hazard function of survival times is modeled as

$$\lambda(t|X_i, Z_i) = \lambda_0(t; \rho) \exp(\beta_x^{\mathrm{T}} X_i + \beta_z^{\mathrm{T}} Z_i),$$

where $\lambda_0(t; \rho)$ is the baseline hazard function that is indexed by a parameter vector ρ, and $\beta = (\beta_x^{\mathrm{T}}, \beta_z^{\mathrm{T}})^{\mathrm{T}}$. Let $\theta = (\beta^{\mathrm{T}}, \rho^{\mathrm{T}})^{\mathrm{T}}$.

(a) Find the likelihood function of θ and specify the associated assumptions.

(b) Assume that $\lambda_0(t; \rho)$ is specified as $\lambda_0(t; \rho) = \rho_1 \rho_2 (\rho_1 t)^{\rho_2 - 1}$, where ρ_1 and ρ_2 are positive parameters and $\rho = (\rho_1, \rho_2)^{\mathrm{T}}$. Find the asymptotic distribution of the maximum likelihood estimator $\widehat{\theta}$.

(c) Assume that $\lambda_0(t; \rho)$ is specified by the piecewise-constant method described in §3.1.2. Find the asymptotic distribution of the maximum likelihood estimator $\widehat{\theta}$.

(d) Let K be the number of the cut points of modeling $\lambda_0(t; \rho)$ in (c). Find the likelihood score function for β when $K \to \infty$. Compare this function with the partial score function for β.

(Lawless 2003, §6.5, §7.4)

3.4. Verify (3.16) in §3.2.1.

3.5. Suppose T is the failure time of an individual and X is the vector of associated covariates which are subject to measurement error. Let X^* be the observed measurement of X.

(a) Let $h(\cdot|\cdot)$, $\lambda(\cdot|\cdot)$ and $S(\cdot|\cdot)$ denote the conditional probability density function, hazard function and survivor function for the corresponding variables, respectively. Show that

$$\begin{aligned} h(t|X, X^*) &= h(t|X) \\ \text{if and only if } \lambda(t|X, X^*) &= \lambda(t|X) \\ \text{if and only if } S(t|X, X^*) &= S(t|X). \end{aligned}$$

(b) Suppose $g(\cdot)$ is a real-valued function.

(i) Show that $E\{g(X) \mid X^*, T \geq t\} = E\{g(X) \mid X^*\}$ if

$$P(T \geq t \mid X, X^*) = E_{X|X^*}\{P(T \geq t \mid X, X^*)\}.$$

(ii) Show that $E\{g(X) \mid X^*, T \geq t\} = E\{g(X) \mid X^*\}$ if

$$P(T \geq t \mid X, X^*) = P(T \geq t \mid X^*).$$

(iii) Show that $E\{g(X) \mid X^*, T \geq t\} \approx E\{g(X) \mid X^*\}$ if

$$P(T \geq t \mid X, X^*) \approx 1.$$

3.6. Verify (3.22) and (3.23) in §3.2.1.

3.7.

(a) Verify (3.41).

(b) Suppose that U, V and W are random variables and that $g(u, v, w)$ is a real-valued function. Show that

$$E_{(U,V)|W}\{g(U, V, W)\} = E_{V|W}\left[E_{U|(V,W)}\{g(U, V, W)\}\right].$$

(c) Show in detail that $\delta_i U_i^*(\beta; t_i, \mathbb{X}^*, \mathbb{Z})$ in §3.6.1 has zero expectation.

3.8.

(a) Show that $E\{U_i^*(\beta)|\mathcal{F}_\tau\} = U_i(\beta)$, where $U_i^*(\beta)$ and $U_i(\beta)$ are defined by (3.45) and (3.15), respectively.

(b) Verify the validity of (3.48).

(c) Verify the validity of (3.49).

(d) Show the equivalence in (3.50).

3.9.

(a) Verify (3.52) in §3.6.3.

(b) Prove the identity (3.53) in §3.6.3.

3.10. Verify that in §3.7, (3.57) satisfies (3.56).

3.11. Suppose the observed data consist of $\{(t_i, \delta_i, X_i^*, Z_i) : i = 1, \ldots, n\}$, as described in §3.3.1, where the measurements X_i^* are the surrogate versions of X_i. Consider the semiparametric linear transformation model for survival times T_i:

$$g(T_i) = -\beta_0 - \beta_x^{\mathrm{T}} X_i - \beta_z^{\mathrm{T}} Z_i + \epsilon_i, \tag{3.71}$$

where $\beta = (\beta_0, \beta_x^{\mathrm{T}}, \beta_z^{\mathrm{T}})^{\mathrm{T}}$ is the vector of regression parameters of interest, $g(\cdot)$ is an unspecified strictly increasing function, and ϵ_i has a given distribution function $F(\cdot)$.

Assume that the measurement error mechanism is nondifferential and the measurement error model is given by

$$X_i^* = X_i + e_i, \tag{3.72}$$

where e_i is independent of $\{T_i, C_i, X_i, Z_i\}$ and follows a normal distribution with mean 0 and covariance matrix Σ_e.

(a) Analogous to the development in §3.6, construct an unbiased estimating function which is expressed in terms of the observed data to perform estimation of parameter β.
(b) Work out the asymptotic distribution of the resultant estimators under suitable regularity conditions.

3.12. Suppose the observed data consist of $\{(t_i, \delta_i, X_i^*, Z_i) : i = 1, \ldots, n\}$, as described in §3.3.1, where X_i^* is the surrogate version of X_i. Assume that T_i and the true covariates $\{X_i, Z_i\}$ are related by the proportional hazards model (3.8).

Assume that measurement error is nondifferential and the measurement error model is given by a Berkson model

$$X_i = X_i^* + e_i, \tag{3.73}$$

where e_i is independent of $\{X_i^*, Z_i, T_i, C_i\}$ and follows distribution $N(0, \Sigma_e)$ with covariance matrix Σ_e.

(a) What might be the effects of ignoring measurement error in covariate X_i on estimation of β?
(b) To conduct estimation of β, can you construct a likelihood function expressed in terms of the observed data? What conditions do you need?
(c) What is the asymptotic distribution of the resultant estimator for β?
(d) How many possible ways can you think of to perform inference about β? Elaborate on them.
(e) How would you handle the baseline hazard function $\lambda_0(t)$?

3.13. Suppose the observed data consist of $\{(t_i, \delta_i, X_i^*, Z_i) : i = 1, \ldots, n\}$, as described in §3.3.1, where X_i^* is the surrogate version of X_i. Response variable $Y_i = \log T_i$ is characterized by the model

$$Y_i = \beta_0 + \beta_x^{\mathrm{T}} X_i + \beta_z^{\mathrm{T}} Z_i + \alpha \epsilon_i,$$

where $\beta = (\beta_0, \beta_x^{\mathrm{T}}, \beta_z^{\mathrm{T}})^{\mathrm{T}}$ is the vector of regression parameters, α is a scale parameter, and ϵ_i is independent of $\{X_i, Z_i, T_i, C_i\}$ and has a standard normal distribution $N(0, 1)$.
Assume that the measurement error model is given by (3.72).

(a) Analogously to the estimating function approaches discussed in §3.6, develop unbiased estimating functions that are expressed by the observed data to perform estimation of parameter β. What assumptions do you need to make?
(b) Develop asymptotic distributions of the resultant estimators under suitable regularity conditions.
(c) If the measurement error model is, instead, given by (3.73), repeat the discussion in (a) and (b).

4

Recurrent Event Data with Measurement Error

Recurrent event data arise commonly in public health and medical studies. While analysis of such data has similarities to that of survival data for many settings, recurrent event data have their own special features. Compared to the extensive attention given to survival data with covariate measurement error, there are relatively limited discussions on analysis of error-prone recurrent event data. In this chapter, we discuss several models and methods to shed light on this topic.

The layout of this chapter is similar to the previous chapter. The framework and modeling strategies are first set up for the error-free context, and analysis methods then follow to address measurement error problems. The chapter is closed with bibliographic notes and supplementary exercises.

4.1 Analysis Framework for Recurrent Events

A *recurrent event process* is a process which repeatedly generates events over time; data arising from such a process are called *recurrent event data*. Examples include repeated seizures of epileptic patients, successive tumors in cancer patients, and multiple births in women's lifetimes, etc.

Interests in analyzing such data vary from problem to problem. Sometimes we are interested in understanding individual event processes themselves, while other times we may focus on determining the relationship between risk factors (or covariates) and event occurrence. A broad variety of models and methods have been developed to address different scientific questions. The analysis of recurrent event data has been covered by a number of monographs, such as Cox and Lewis (1966), Hougaard (2000), Kalbfleisch and Prentice (2002), Martinussen and Scheike (2006), and Sun (2006). A comprehensive discussion of this topic was given by Cook and Lawless (2007).

Following Cook and Lawless (2007), here we briefly outline some standard modeling strategies for recurrent event data in the absence of measurement error.

G. Y. Yi, *Statistical Analysis with Measurement Error or Misclassification*,
Springer Series in Statistics, DOI 10.1007/978-1-4939-6640-0_4

4.1.1 Notation and Framework

Recurrent events may occur in either *continuous time* or *discrete time*. For events occurring in continuous time, a mathematically convenient assumption is commonly adopted: more than one events cannot occur simultaneously. Methods for handling processes that do not satisfy this assumption were discussed by Cook and Lawless (2007). In this chapter, we mainly concentrate on continuous time models, while discrete time models are considered occasionally.

Modeling of recurrent events may be approached from multiple perspectives, but the strategies basically pertain to two fundamental approaches: modeling *event counts* or modeling *waiting times* between successive events. While the choice of a particular modeling scheme is often driven by the objective of analysis, a clear framework may be immediately evident from the nature of the event process itself, such as the scale of the event frequency. When individuals frequently experience events, modeling of event counts is usually useful, whereas modeling gap times between successive events may be preferred if the event occurs infrequently.

For $i = 1, \ldots, n$, suppose individual i experiences an event process starting at time origin $t = 0$. For $j = 1, 2, \ldots$, let T_{ij} denote the time of the jth event for individual i, and the difference $W_{ij} = T_{ij} - T_{i,j-1}$ be defined as the *waiting time*, also called *gap time* or *elapsed time*, between events $(j - 1)$ and j for individual i, where $T_{i0} = 0$.

Alternatively, we let $N_i(t)$ denote the number of events experienced by subject i over time interval $[0, t]$, leading to a *counting process* $\{N_i(t) : t \geq 0\}$ which records the cumulative number of events generated by the process for subject i. Often, counting processes are defined to be right-continuous, i.e., $N_i(t^+) = N_i(t)$ for $t \geq 0$, where t^+ denotes a time that is infinitesimally bigger than t. This is illustrated in Fig. 4.1. The number of events occurring over an interval, say $(s, t]$, is then given by $N_i(s, t) = N_i(t) - N_i(s)$, where $0 \leq s < t$.

For convenience we often assume that $T_{i1} > 0$ or $N_i(0) = 0$. The event times, the frequencies and the waiting times are linked by the identities

$$N_i(t) = \sum_{j=1}^{\infty} I(T_{ij} \leq t)$$

and

$$T_{in_i} = W_{i1} + \ldots + W_{in_i},$$

where n_i is the number of events experienced by subject i. Moreover, the probability connection

$$P\{N_i(t) \geq n_i\} = P(T_{in_i} \leq t)$$

suggests the equivalence between modeling event counts and modeling event times.

Define $dN_i(t) = N_i(t) - N_i(t^-)$, where t^- denotes a time that is infinitesimally smaller than t. Sometimes, we write

$$\Delta N_i(t) = N_i\{(t + \Delta t)^-\} - N_i(t^-)$$

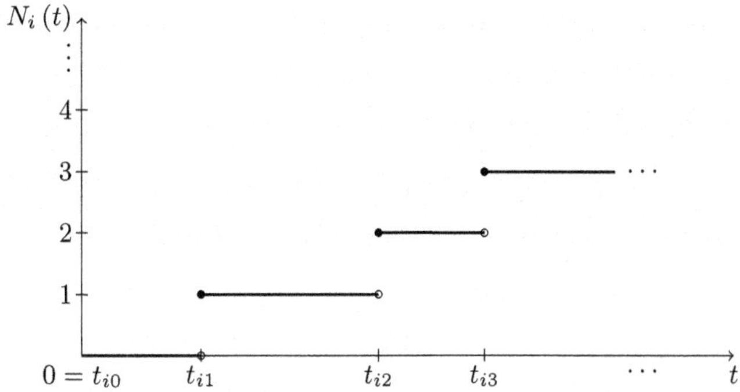

Fig. 4.1. *Illustration of a Counting Process*

for the number of events experienced by subject i over the time interval $[t, t + \Delta t)$, where Δt represents a positive (often small) time increment. Let $\mathcal{H}_{it}^{\mathrm{N}} = \{N_i(v) : 0 \le v < t\}$ denote the history of the event process until (but not including) time t for subject i.

There are multiple objectives for analyzing recurrent event data. Sometimes our interest centers around special characteristics of the process, such as expected event counts; sometimes it is compelling to delineate the distribution of the entire event process. Analyses of recurrent events may be distinguished by the nature of the modeling assumption - whether or not the modeling assumption can fully or partially determine the event process. Two important concepts, *intensity function* and *mean function*, are frequently used to describe recurrent event processes. The intensity function completely determines an event process, whereas the mean function facilitates only marginal features of a process.

Intensity Function

Conditional on the process history, the event intensity function gives the instantaneous probability of an event occurring at a time point. For each subject i with history $\mathcal{H}_{it}^{\mathrm{N}}$, the (conditional) *intensity function* is defined as

$$\lambda(t|\mathcal{H}_{it}^{\mathrm{N}}) = \lim_{\Delta t \to 0+} \frac{P\{\Delta N_i(t) = 1|\mathcal{H}_{it}^{\mathrm{N}}\}}{\Delta t} \quad \text{for } t > 0.$$

Conventionally, an intensity function is assumed to be bounded and continuous except for a finite number of points over a finite time interval. With the intensity function available, statistical inference may be carried out using the likelihood method. The following results describe how the intensity function is related to probability calculations.

Theorem 4.1. *Suppose subject i experiences recurrent events over a given time interval $[0, \tau_i]$. Let $0 < t_{i1} < \ldots < t_{in_i}$ denote the observed event times. Assume that the intensity function $\lambda(t|\mathcal{H}_{it}^{\mathrm{N}})$ is integrable. Then the following results hold.*

(a) *The probability density function for the outcome that n_i events occur over time interval* $[0, \tau_i]$ *is*

$$\left\{\prod_{j=1}^{n_i} \lambda(t_{ij}|\mathcal{H}^{\mathrm{N}}_{it_{ij}})\right\} \exp\left\{-\int_0^{\tau_i} \lambda(v|\mathcal{H}^{\mathrm{N}}_{iv})dv\right\}.$$

(b) *For the waiting times, we have the conditional probability*

$$P\left(W_{ij} > w \,\middle|\, T_{i,j-1} = t_{i,j-1}, \mathcal{H}^{\mathrm{N}}_{it_{i,j-1}}\right) = \exp\left\{-\int_{t_{i,j-1}}^{t_{i,j-1}+w} \lambda(v|\mathcal{H}^{\mathrm{N}}_{iv})dv\right\},$$

where w is a given positive values, $t_{i0} = 0$, and $j = 1, 2, \ldots$.

Mean Function

In principle, the intensity function completely determines the characteristics of an event process. Knowledge of the intensity function allows us to readily work out the probabilities or conditional probabilities for an event process or inter-event times, as described in Theorem 4.1. Some features, such as mean and variance functions, of the event process, however, may not be straightforward enough to be derived from the intensity function of the process. Directly modeling those features would be sufficient and more transparent when our objective centers around the marginal analysis.

In contrast to using the likelihood for inferences when intensity functions are modeled, unbiased estimating functions are commonly used to perform inferences when mean functions are postulated. A notable advantage for using marginal features over fully modeling the processes is the minimal model assumption, which allows the inference results to be more robust to model misspecification. The marginal method, however, requires the observation process and the event process to be independent.

Suppose there is a random sample of n individuals who are each under observation from time $t = 0$ to a stopping or censoring time. For $i = 1, \ldots, n$, let τ_i denote the stopping time for subject i, and $R_i(t) = I(t \le \tau_i)$ be the at risk indicator showing whether or not subject i is observed at time t. By convention, $R_i(t)$ is assumed to be left-continuous with $R_i(t^-) = R_i(t)$ for any time t. We define

$$\mu(t) = E\{N_i(t)\}$$

to be the *mean function* at time t and

$$\mu'(t) = \frac{d\mu(t)}{dt}$$

to be the *rate function* at time t. The mean function gives the expected cumulative number of events at time t, while the rate function indicates the marginal instantaneous probability of an event at time t.

For subject i, assume that the observation process $\{R_i(t) : t \ge 0\}$ and the event process $\{N_i(t) : t \ge 0\}$ are independent, i.e., for any $t \ge 0$ and a nonnegative integer k,

$$P\{N_i(t) = k|R_i(t) = 1\} = P\{N_i(t) = k\}.$$

Given a time t, then we have that for $v \in [0, t]$,

$$E[R_i(v)\{dN_i(v) - d\mu(v)\}] = 0$$

for $i = 1, \ldots, n$. Hence with the entire sample information included, an unbiased estimating equation for $d\mu(v)$ is set as

$$\sum_{i=1}^{n} R_i(v)\{dN_i(v) - d\mu(v)\} = 0,$$

which gives the estimator

$$d\widehat{\mu}(v) = \frac{dN_+(v)}{R_+(v)},$$

where $dN_+(v) = \sum_{i=1}^{n} R_i(v)dN_i(v)$ is the total number of the observed events, and $R_+(v) = \sum_{i=1}^{n} R_i(v)$ is the total number of subjects at risk at time v.

Provided that $E\{dN_i(v)|R_1(v), \ldots, R_n(v)\} = E\{dN_i(v)|R_i(v)\}$ for each i, the estimator is unbiased with

$$E\{d\widehat{\mu}(v)\} = d\mu(v). \tag{4.1}$$

Assume that $R_+(v) > 0$ for $0 \le v \le t$. Then by the identity $\mu(t) = \int_0^t d\mu(v)$, we obtain an estimator for $\mu(t)$ as

$$\widehat{\mu}(t) = \int_0^t d\widehat{\mu}(v) = \int_0^t \frac{dN_+(v)}{R_+(v)} = \sum_{k:t_{(k)} \le t} \frac{dN_+(t_{(k)})}{R_+(t_{(k)})},$$

where $t_{(k)}$ represents the kth distinct event time across all the individuals in the sample. The variance of $\widehat{\mu}(t)$ is given by

$$\begin{aligned} \text{var}[\sqrt{n}\{\widehat{\mu}(t) - \mu(t)\}] &= n \cdot \text{var}\left\{\int_0^t \frac{dN_+(v)}{R_+(v)}\right\} \\ &= n \sum_{i=1}^{n} \int_0^t \int_0^t \frac{R_i(v_1)R_i(v_2)}{R_+(v_1)R_+(v_2)} \text{cov}\{dN_i(v_1), dN_i(v_2)\}. \end{aligned}$$

For all $v \in [0, t]$, if $R_+(v)/n \to g(v)$ for some function $g(\cdot) > 0$ as $n \to \infty$, then the variance $\text{var}[\sqrt{n}\{\widehat{\mu}(t) - \mu(t)\}]$ may be estimated by the sample counterpart

$$n \sum_{i=1}^{n} \int_0^t \int_0^t \frac{R_i(v_1)R_i(v_2)}{R_+(v_1)R_+(v_2)} \{dN_i(v_1) - d\widehat{\mu}(v_1)\}\{dN_i(v_2)) - d\widehat{\mu}(v_2)\}.$$

4.1.2 Poisson Process and Renewal Process

Recurrent event data may be described through two standard processes: *Poisson* and *renewal* processes. The Poisson process focuses on modeling the *event frequency* over a given sequence of time intervals, whereas the renewal process emphasizes describing the *elapsed time* between events. Both processes require certain types of independence assumptions. For the Poisson process, we assume that events occur randomly in such a way that the event counts over nonoverlapping time intervals are independent. The renewal process, on the other hand, requires the elapsed times between successive events to be independent. These two processes are relatively easy to handle mathematically, and they can be defined in different but equivalent ways. They are, of course, not tenable for many applications due to the restrictive independence assumptions. Various extensions have been developed to enhance the flexibility and generality. For more details, see Cook and Lawless (2007). Here we confine our attention to these two processes only.

Poisson processes can be described by requiring the intensity function to be independent of the process history:

$$\lambda(t|\mathcal{H}_{it}^{\mathrm{N}}) = \rho(t),$$

where $\rho(t)$ is a function of time t alone. For this process the mean function is written as

$$\mu(t) = \int_0^t \rho(v)dv,$$

or equivalently,

$$\rho(t) = \frac{d\mu(t)}{dt}$$

is the marginal rate function.

The Poisson process is the only process for which the mean rate function $\rho(t)$ equals the conditional intensity function $\lambda\{t|\mathcal{H}_{it}^{\mathrm{N}}\}$. The following properties for the Poisson process may be derived by definition and Theorem 4.1. They are useful for conducting statistical inference.

Theorem 4.2. *Suppose $\{N_i(t) : t \geq 0\}$ is a Poisson process with the mean function $\mu(t)$. Then*

(a) mean and variance functions are identical, i.e.,

$$E\{N_i(t)\} = \mathrm{var}\{N_i(t)\};$$

(b) $N_i(s,t)$ has a Poisson distribution with mean

$$\mu(s,t) = \mu(t) - \mu(s) \ \ \text{for } 0 \leq s < t;$$

(c) if $(s_1, t_1]$ and $(s_2, t_2]$ are nonoverlapping intervals, then $N_i(s_1, t_1)$ and $N_i(s_2, t_2)$ are independent random variables;

(d) the conditional probability for the waiting times is given by

$$P(W_{ij} > w|T_{i,j-1} = t_{i,j-1}) = \exp[-\{\mu(t_{i,j-1} + w) - \mu(t_{i,j-1})\}]$$

for $j = 1, 2, \ldots$, where w is a given positive value.

The results imply that for a Poisson process, event counts over nonoverlapping intervals are independent, but the gap times between successive events are not necessarily independent. Therefore, a Poisson process is generally not a renewal process. However, in a special situation with the rate function $\rho(t)$ being a constant, say ρ, the gap times are independent, and also identically distributed with the survivor function $P(W_{ij} > w) = \exp(-\rho w)$ for $w > 0$. A Poisson process with a constant rate function $\rho(t) = \rho$ is called a *homogeneous Poisson process.*

As opposed to a Poisson process whose gap times are generally not independent, a renewal process is defined to be the one for which the gap times W_{ij} are independent and identically distributed. Renewal processes can also be contrasted with Poisson processes from another perspective based on the characteristic of the intensity function. The intensity function of a Poisson process is independent of the process history, but the intensity function of a renewal process depends on the process history via the most recent time. That is,

$$\lambda(t|\mathcal{H}_{it}^{\mathrm{N}}) = g(t - T_{iN_i(t-)})$$

for some function $g(\cdot)$ and $t > 0$.

This says that the intensity function $\lambda(t|\mathcal{H}_{it}^{\mathrm{N}})$ for a renewal process is a function of the elapsed time since the most recent event before t. Function $g(\cdot)$ is the *hazard function* for the variables W_{ij}. That is, if $f(\cdot)$ and $S(\cdot)$ are the probability density and survivor functions for W_{ij}, respectively, then

$$g(w) = \lim_{\Delta w \to 0+} \frac{P(W_{ij} < w + \Delta w | W_{ij} > w)}{\Delta w} = \frac{f(w)}{S(w)}.$$

Finally, a homogeneous Poisson process links Poisson and renewal processes because it possesses the features from both types of processes. Such a process, however, may be too restrictive for application. A quick extension is to relax the constant rate function required by a homogeneous Poisson process. For instance, using the piecewise-constant approach discussed in §3.1.2, we define a model to be *the Poisson model with piecewise-constant rates* if its intensity function is given by

$$\lambda(t|\mathcal{H}_{it}^{\mathrm{N}}) = \rho_k \tag{4.2}$$

for $t \in (a_{k-1}, a_k]$, where $0 = a_0 < a_1 < \ldots < a_{K-1} < a_K = \infty$ is a pre-specified sequence of constants for a given K.

4.1.3 Covariates and Extensions

In application, event processes are often analyzed in conjunction with covariates that are fixed or time-varying. It is customary to use X_i or Z_i to denote fixed covariates, and $X_i(t)$ or $Z_i(t)$ for time-varying covariates for $i = 1, \ldots, n$. Time-varying covariates may be distinguished to be *external* or *internal*, as in Cook and Lawless (2007, §2.5). Fixed covariates are regarded as external. Methods developed for external covariates are usually more tractable than those for internal covariates. In this chapter, we consider fixed or external covariates only.

Let $\mathcal{H}_{it}^{\text{XZ}} = \{(X_i(v), Z_i(v)) : 0 \le v \le t\}$ denote the history of the covariate process up to and including time t for subject i. It is often assumed that

$$P[\Delta N_i(t) = 1|\mathcal{H}_{it}^{\text{N}}, \{\mathcal{H}_{iv}^{\text{XZ}} : v \ge 0\}] = P\{\Delta N_i(t) = 1|\mathcal{H}_{it}^{\text{N}}, \mathcal{H}_{it}^{\text{XZ}}\},$$

which says that given the history of events and covariates, the number of events experienced by subject i over time interval $[t, t + \Delta t)$ is independent of covariate values after time t.

The definition of intensity and mean functions, $\lambda(t|\mathcal{H}_{it}^{\text{N}})$ and $\mu(t)$ in §4.1.1, is now modified as

$$\lambda(t|\mathcal{H}_{it}^{\text{N}}, \mathcal{H}_{it}^{\text{XZ}}) = \lim_{\Delta t \to 0+} \frac{P\{\Delta N_i(t) = 1|\mathcal{H}_{it}^{\text{N}}, \mathcal{H}_{it}^{\text{XZ}}\}}{\Delta t}$$

and

$$\mu(t|\mathcal{H}_{it}^{\text{XZ}}) = E\{N_i(t)|\mathcal{H}_{it}^{\text{XZ}}\},$$

where the covariate history is included as conditioning variables.

To facilitate the dependence on covariates, regression models are employed to postulate the (conditional) intensity function $\lambda(t|\mathcal{H}_{it}^{\text{N}}, \mathcal{H}_{it}^{\text{XZ}})$ or the (conditional) mean function $\mu(t|\mathcal{H}_{it}^{\text{XZ}})$. For example, multiplicative models may be, respectively, used to describe the intensity and mean functions for a process:

$$\lambda(t|\mathcal{H}_{it}^{\text{N}}, \mathcal{H}_{it}^{\text{XZ}}) = \lambda_0(t|\mathcal{H}_{it}^{\text{N}})g(\mathcal{H}_{it}^{\text{XZ}}; \beta)$$

and

$$\mu(t|\mathcal{H}_{it}^{\text{XZ}}) = \mu_0(t)g(\mathcal{H}_{it}^{\text{XZ}}; \beta),$$

where $\lambda_0(t|\mathcal{H}_{it}^{\text{N}})$ is the baseline intensity function that may depend on the event history, $\mu_0(t)$ represents the baseline mean function, $g(\mathcal{H}_{it}^{\text{XZ}}; \beta)$ is a nonnegative function that contains information of covariates, and β is the vector of regression coefficients which are often of prime interest. For more detailed modeling schemes, see Cook and Lawless (2007).

Gap Times and Covariates

Because gap times are positive values just like survival times, models used for survival analysis may be employed to describe various types of relationship between gap times and covariates. Two useful regression models are the *proportional hazards model* and the *accelerated failure time model*. For example, with fixed covariates, the hazard function of the elapsed times W_{ij} is marginally modeled as

$$\lambda(w|X_i, Z_i) = \lambda_0(w)\exp(\beta_x^{\text{T}} X_i + \beta_z^{\text{T}} Z_i)$$

for the *proportional hazards model* and

$$\lambda(w|X_i, Z_i) = \lambda_0\{w\exp(\beta_x^{\text{T}} X_i + \beta_z^{\text{T}} Z_i)\}\exp(\beta_x^{\text{T}} X_i + \beta_z^{\text{T}} Z_i)$$

for the *accelerated failure time model*, where $\lambda_0(\cdot)$ is the baseline hazard function that is positive-valued and β_x and β_z are parameters.

In application, gap times are usually dependent, even after associated covariates are being controlled. Several strategies are useful to feature dependence structures of gap times. One way is to form models by conditioning on the history of gap times, together with the covariates. Hence the dependence among gap times is accommodated by the conditional structure. For instance, one may specify the conditional distribution of W_{ij}, given prior gap times $W_{i1}, \ldots, W_{i,j-1}$ and the covariates, to be of a given form, such as a log-normal distribution for $j = 2, 3, \ldots$.

An alternative strategy of facilitating associations among gap times is to introduce random effects at the subject-level, say u_i, for $i = 1, \ldots, n$. Conditional on random effects u_i and the covariates, the gap times $\{W_{ij} : j = 1, 2, \ldots\}$ are assumed to be independent with a conditional hazard function, say, given by

$$\lambda(w|u_i, X_i, Z_i) = u_i \lambda_0(w) \exp(\beta_x^{\mathrm{T}} X_i + \beta_z^{\mathrm{T}} Z_i),$$

where $\lambda_0(\cdot)$ is the baseline hazard function that is positive-valued and β_x and β_z are parameters. Because random effects are not observed, the u_i are usually assumed to be independent and identically distributed with a given distribution. Inferences are then based on the observed likelihood obtained by integrating out the u_i from the model for the joint conditional distribution of W_{ij} and u_i for each i, given $\{X_i, Z_i\}$.

A third approach to describing correlated gap times is to invoke multivariate survival models, such as *copula models*, for a specified set of gap times. Discussion of this method was provided by Cook and Lawless (2007, Ch. 4).

Poisson Processes with Covariates

A useful model for describing Poisson processes with associated covariates is the *multiplicative model*, given by

$$\lambda(t|\mathcal{H}_{it}^{\mathrm{N}}, \mathcal{H}_{it}^{\mathrm{XZ}}) = \lambda_0(t) \exp\{\beta^{\mathrm{T}} V_i(t)\},$$

where $V_i(t)$ is a covariate vector that is based on the covariate history $\mathcal{H}_{it}^{\mathrm{XZ}}$ and $\lambda_0(t)$ is the baseline intensity function that is free of the event history. A simple form of $V_i(t)$ is taken as $V_i(t) = \{X_i^{\mathrm{T}}(t), Z_i^{\mathrm{T}}(t)\}^{\mathrm{T}}$.

In practice, recurrent events often exhibit heterogeneity among subjects. A common treatment on this feature is to introduce random effects into the model (e.g., Lawless 1987; Therneau and Grambsch 2000). In particular, *mixed Poisson processes* are a convenient framework for handling nonhomogeneous processes.

For illustrations, we consider the case with fixed covariates. Conditional on a nonnegative random effect u_i and the covariates, $\{N_i(t) : t \geq 0\}$ is assumed to follow a nonhomogeneous Poisson process with the intensity function modeled as

$$\lambda(t|u_i, X_i, Z_i) = u_i \lambda_0(t) \exp(\beta_x^{\mathrm{T}} X_i + \beta_z^{\mathrm{T}} Z_i), \tag{4.3}$$

where β_x and β_z are parameters, $\lambda_0(t)$ is the baseline intensity function, and the u_i are assumed to be independent of $\{X_i, Z_i\}$ and identically distributed. Since $\lambda_0(t)$ may include an arbitrary scale parameter, without loss of generality, the mean of u_i is assumed to be 1.

The random effect u_i, also called *"frailty"*, is introduced to facilitate the subject-specific heterogeneity that is not explained by the covariates. Inclusion of this frailty, however, breaks down the identity between the mean and variance for the Poisson process (Cook and Lawless 2007, §2.2.3).

To see this, we write $\mu_i(t) = \int_0^t \lambda_0(v)\exp(\beta_x^{\mathrm{T}} X_i + \beta_z^{\mathrm{T}} Z_i)dv$, then the conditional mean and variance of $N_i(t)$, given $\{u_i, X_i, Z_i\}$, are

$$E\{N_i(t)|u_i, X_i, Z_i\} = \mathrm{var}\{N_i(t)|u_i, X_i, Z_i\} = u_i\mu_i(t).$$

Since the marginal mean and variance of $N_i(t)$ are related to the conditional mean and variance via

$$E\{N_i(t)|X_i, Z_i\} = E[E\{N_i(t)|u_i, X_i, Z_i\}] \tag{4.4}$$

and

$$\mathrm{var}\{N_i(t)|X_i, Z_i\} = E[\mathrm{var}\{N_i(t)|u_i, X_i, Z_i\}] + \mathrm{var}[E\{N_i(t)|u_i, X_i, Z_i\}], \tag{4.5}$$

therefore,

$$E\{N_i(t)|X_i, Z_i\} = \mu_i(t)$$

and

$$\mathrm{var}\{N_i(t)|X_i, Z_i\} = \mu_i(t) + \phi\mu_i(t),$$

suggesting that the mean and variance of $N_i(t)$ are not equal unless $\phi = 0$, where ϕ represents the variance of u_i.

In some settings, count data exhibit patterns that may be better explained by two distinct subpopulations in which one includes individuals with no events. A special mixed Poisson model, called the *zero-inflated Poisson model*, may be used. This model is defined as follows.

Let u_i be a binary latent (unobserved) random variable with

$$P(u_i = 1) = \widetilde{\pi} \text{ and } P(u_i = 0) = 1 - \widetilde{\pi}$$

for $i = 1, \ldots, n$, where $\widetilde{\pi}$ is between 0 and 1. Then conditional on $u_i = 1$, $\{N_i(t) : t \geq 0\}$ is assumed to be a Poisson process with mean function $\mu_i(t)$; and conditional on $u_i = 0$, $N_i(t)$ is zero for any time t, i.e.,

$$P\{N_i(\infty) = 0|u_i = 0\} = 1.$$

Consequently, the model for the marginal distribution of $N_i(t)$ is a mixed Poisson process which accommodates an excessive number of zeros, and the mean and variance of $N_i(t)$ are

$$\begin{aligned} E\{N_i(t)\} &= \mu_i(t)\widetilde{\pi}; \\ \mathrm{var}\{N_i(t)\} &= \mu_i(t)\widetilde{\pi} + \mu_i^2(t)\widetilde{\pi}(1 - \widetilde{\pi}). \end{aligned} \tag{4.6}$$

Interval Count Data

In many studies, exact event times are not observed; subjects are only examined periodically and interval count data are thereby collected. Suppose that subject i is observed over a sequence of time intervals $B_{ij} = (b_{i,j-1}, b_{ij}]$ for $j = 1, \ldots, K_i$, with $N_{ij} = N_i(b_{ij}) - N_i(b_{i,j-1})$ events being observed in interval j, where $b_{i0} = 0$, $b_{iK_i} = \tau_i$, and K_i is a positive integer. The sequence of intervals $B_{ij} = (b_{i,j-1}, b_{ij}]$ may be pre-specified or random but has to satisfy certain conditions as discussed in the sequel.

In principle, modeling and inference typically depend on the relationship between the observation times b_{ij} and the event processes. For $j = 1, \ldots, K_i$, let $\mathcal{H}_{ij}^{b\text{N}} = \{b_{i1}, N_{i1}; \ldots; b_{i,j-1}, N_{i,j-1}\}$ be the history of both recurrent events and observation times up to (but not including) the jth assessment. Then the joint distribution of the observations times and event counts for subject i is given by

$$L_i = \prod_{j=1}^{K_i} P(b_{ij}, N_{ij} | \mathcal{H}_{ij}^{b\text{N}}),$$

which is factorized as

$$L_i = \prod_{j=1}^{K_i} P(N_{ij} | b_{ij}, \mathcal{H}_{ij}^{b\text{N}}) P(b_{ij} | \mathcal{H}_{ij}^{b\text{N}}), \tag{4.7}$$

where $P(\cdot|\cdot)$ is the conditional probability function for the corresponding variables.

When the inspection times are independent of the event process, inference may be performed by ignoring the terms $P(b_{ij} | \mathcal{H}_{ij}^{b\text{N}})$ in (4.7). This reflects scenarios where subjects are scheduled to be examined at pre-specified assessment times. It is often useful to assume that

$$P(N_{ij} | b_{ij}, \mathcal{H}_{ij}^{b\text{N}}) = P(N_{ij} | N_{i1}, \ldots, N_{i,j-1}),$$

which says that given the event history, the occurrence of the next event is independent of the inspection times. This assumption allows us to conduct inferences based only on

$$\prod_{i=1}^{n} \prod_{j=1}^{K_i} P(N_{ij} | N_{i1}, \ldots, N_{i,j-1}). \tag{4.8}$$

For settings where inspection times depend on the observed events, the conditional probabilities $P(b_{ij} | \mathcal{H}_{ij}^{b\text{N}})$ may be omitted if they do not contain the parameter associated with the conditional probabilities $P(N_{ij} | b_{ij}, \mathcal{H}_{ij}^{b\text{N}})$. Detailed discussion on dependent observation times was provided by Gruger, Kay and Schumacher (1991), Lawless and Zhan (1998), Sun and Wei (2000), Wang, Qin and Chiang (2001), Zeng and Cai (2010), Chen, Yi and Cook (2010a, 2011), and others.

In analysis, modeling the event process is frequently the emphasis, whereas the observation process is left unmodeled with certain assumptions imposed. Following the same ideas outlined in the previous subsections, modeling strategies on count data may be applied to analyze interval count data. Technical details for various settings were presented by Cook and Lawless (2007, Ch. 7).

We close this section with an example for which count data are generated from a mixed Poisson process, and the observation process satisfies the conditions outlined by Lawless and Zhan (1998) so that inference about the regression parameters is merely based on the conditional distribution $P(N_{ij}|N_{i1},\ldots,N_{i,j-1})$ for the counting process, as shown in (4.8).

Conditional on a nonnegative random effect u_i and the covariates, $\{N_i(t) : t \geq 0\}$ is assumed to follow a nonhomogeneous Poisson process with the intensity function modeled as

$$\lambda(t|u_i, X_i, Z_i) = u_i \lambda_0(t) \exp(\beta_x^{\mathrm{T}} X_i + \beta_z^{\mathrm{T}} Z_i), \tag{4.9}$$

where β_x and β_z are parameters, $\lambda_0(t)$ is the baseline intensity function, and the u_i are independent of $\{X_i, Z_i\}$ and identically distributed with a probability density or mass function modeled by $f(u;\phi)$ with parameter ϕ. As explained previously, it is a convention to assume $E(u_i) = 1$.

Consequently, the count data N_{ij} follow Poisson distributions with

$$N_{ij} \sim \text{Poisson}(u_i \mu_{ij}),$$

where $\mu_{ij} = \mu_{0ij} \exp(\beta_x^{\mathrm{T}} X_i + \beta_z^{\mathrm{T}} Z_i)$ and $\mu_{0ij} = \int_{b_{i,j-1}}^{b_{ij}} \lambda_0(v) d\eta(v)$. Thus, the likelihood contributed from subject i is

$$L_i = \int_0^\infty \prod_{j=1}^{K_i} \exp(-u_i \mu_{ij})(u_i \mu_{ij})^{N_{ij}} f(u_i;\phi) d\eta(u_i). \tag{4.10}$$

As a result, inferences proceed with the likelihood method by maximizing the likelihood $\prod_{i=1}^n L_i$ with respect to the model parameters.

In a special but useful case, the distribution of u_i is modeled by a gamma distribution, Gamma(ϕ, ϕ^{-1}), with scale parameter ϕ^{-1} and shape parameter ϕ so that the mean of u_i is 1. With this distributional assumption, L_i in (4.10) is simplified as

$$L_i \propto \left[\prod_{j=1}^{K_i} \left\{ \mu_{0ij} \exp(\beta_x^{\mathrm{T}} X_i + \beta_z^{\mathrm{T}} Z_i) \right\}^{N_{ij}} \right] \cdot \frac{\Gamma(N_{i+} + \phi^{-1}) \phi^{N_{i+}}}{\Gamma(\phi^{-1})\{1 + \phi \mu_{0i+} \exp(\beta_x^{\mathrm{T}} X_i + \beta_z^{\mathrm{T}} Z_i)\}^{N_{i+} + \phi^{-1}}}, \tag{4.11}$$

where $N_{i+} = \sum_{j=1}^{K_i} N_{ij}$, $\mu_{0i+} = \sum_{j=1}^{K_i} \mu_{0ij}$, and $\Gamma(\cdot)$ is the Gamma function defined as $\Gamma(a) = \int_0^\infty v^{a-1} \exp(-v) dv$ for $a > 0$ (Lawless and Zhan 1998).

4.2 Measurement Error Effects on Poisson Process

We discuss how covariate measurement error may affect the structure of the process and point estimation. In addition to the notation defined in §4.1, let X_i^* be a surrogate measurement of X_i. In subsequent development we consider the case where covariates X_i and Z_i are fixed and the nondifferential measurement error mechanism is assumed:

$$P\{N_i(t)|X_i, X_i^*, Z_i\} = P\{N_i(t)|X_i, Z_i\} \text{ for } t \geq 0.$$

Overdispersion Effect

Conditional on the true covariates, $\{N_i(t) : t \geq 0\}$ is assumed to follow a Poisson process with the mean function

$$\mu_i(t) = E\{N_i(t)|X_i, Z_i\}$$

for $t \geq 0$. A unique property for the Poisson process is the equality of mean and variance:

$$E\{N_i(t)|X_i, Z_i\} = \text{var}\{N_i(t)|X_i, Z_i\}$$

for any time t. This property, however, does not necessarily hold if X_i is replaced with its surrogate X_i^*. In fact, the conditional variance of $N_i(t)$, given the observed covariate measurements $\{X_i^*, Z_i\}$, is

$$\begin{aligned}
&\text{var}\{N_i(t)|X_i^*, Z_i\} \\
&= E_{X_i|(X_i^*,Z_i)}[\text{var}\{N_i(t)|X_i, X_i^*, Z_i\}] + \text{var}_{X_i|(X_i^*,Z_i)}[E\{N_i(t)|X_i, X_i^*, Z_i\}] \\
&= E_{X_i|(X_i^*,Z_i)}[\text{var}\{N_i(t)|X_i, Z_i\}] + \text{var}_{X_i|(X_i^*,Z_i)}[E\{N_i(t)|X_i, Z_i\}] \\
&= E_{X_i|(X_i^*,Z_i)}[E\{N_i(t)|X_i, Z_i\}] + \text{var}_{X_i|(X_i^*,Z_i)}[E\{N_i(t)|X_i, Z_i\}],
\end{aligned}$$

where the second step comes from the nondifferential error assumption and the third step is due to the equality between mean and variance for the Poisson process. Here we use both $\text{var}_{U|V}\{g(U, V)\}$ and $\text{var}\{g(U, V)|V\}$ to refer to the conditional variance of $g(U, V)$ taken with respect to the model for the conditional distribution of U, given V, where $g(U, V)$ is a function of any random variables U and V.

Since

$$E_{X_i|(X_i^*,Z_i)}[E\{N_i(t)|X_i, Z_i\}] = E\{N_i(t)|X_i^*, Z_i\}, \tag{4.12}$$

we obtain

$$\text{var}\{N_i(t)|X_i^*, Z_i\} = E\{N_i(t)|X_i^*, Z_i\} + \text{var}_{X_i|(X_i^*,Z_i)}[E\{N_i(t)|X_i, Z_i\},$$

suggesting that

$$\text{var}\{N_i(t)|X_i^*, Z_i\} \geq E\{N_i(t)|X_i^*, Z_i\}.$$

Therefore, over-dispersion may exist in the relationship between the response and the observed covariates $\{X_i^*, Z_i\}$ even if the process linking the response and the true covariates $\{X_i, Z_i\}$ is a Poisson process. The degree of over-dispersion is determined by the quantity $\text{var}_{X_i|(X_i^*,Z_i)}[E\{N_i(t)|X_i, Z_i\}]$, which depends on the event process as well as the measurement error process.

To further see this, consider an example with a log-linear model for the (conditional) mean function $\mu(t|X_i, Z_i)$, or denoted as $\mu_i(t)$ for simplicity,

$$\mu_i(t) = \mu_0(t)\exp(\beta_x^{\mathrm{T}} X_i + \beta_z^{\mathrm{T}} Z_i), \tag{4.13}$$

where $\mu_0(t)$ is the baseline mean function that possibly depends on time and β_x and β_z are regression coefficients.

Assume that the surrogate X_i^* is linked with X_i through a Berkson error model

$$X_i = X_i^* + e_i \tag{4.14}$$

for $i = 1, \ldots, n$, where e_i is independent of $\{X_i^*, Z_i, N_i(t) : t \geq 0\}$ and has a distribution $N(0, \Sigma_e)$ with covariance matrix Σ_e. Then the variance and mean for the observed process, $\text{var}\{N_i(t)|X_i^*, Z_i\}$ and $E\{N_i(t)|X_i^*, Z_i\}$, differ by the amount

$$\begin{aligned} &\text{var}_{X_i|(X_i^*,Z_i)}[E\{N_i(t)|X_i, Z_i\}] \\ &= \mu_0(t)\exp(2\beta_x^{\mathrm{T}} X_i^* + \beta_z^{\mathrm{T}} Z_i)\exp(\beta_x^{\mathrm{T}} \Sigma_e \beta_x)\{\exp(\beta_x^{\mathrm{T}} \Sigma_e \beta_x) - 1\}, \end{aligned}$$

thus, leading to

$$\begin{aligned} \text{var}\{N_i(t)|X_i^*, Z_i\} = &\ E\{N_i(t)|X_i^*, Z_i\} \\ &\cdot \exp(\beta_x^{\mathrm{T}} X_i^* + \beta_x^{\mathrm{T}} \Sigma_e \beta_x/2)\{\exp(\beta_x^{\mathrm{T}} \Sigma_e \beta_x) - 1\}. \end{aligned} \tag{4.15}$$

Expression (4.15) shows that the degree of over-dispersion, contained in the relationship between the event process and the observed covariate measurements $\{X_i^*, Z_i\}$, depends on the degree of measurement error, the magnitude of the covariate effect β_x associated with X_i as well as measurement X_i^* itself.

Effect on Point Estimate

To illustrate the possible impact of measurement error on point estimation, we consider an event process $\{N_i(t) : t \geq 0\}$ with the mean function specified by model (4.13).

Suppose we ignore measurement error in X_i and replace it with X_i^* in the data analysis. That is, we take the same model structure as (4.13) for the conditional process of $N_i(t)$ given $\{X_i^*, Z_i\}$:

$$E\{N_i(t)|X_i^*, Z_i\} = \mu_0^*(t)\exp(\beta_x^{*\mathrm{T}} X_i^* + \beta_z^{*\mathrm{T}} Z_i), \tag{4.16}$$

where $\mu_0^*(t)$ represents the baseline mean function and β_x^* and β_z^* represent the covariate effects for which the naive analysis aims to estimate. These quantities potentially differ from $\{\mu_0(t), \beta_x, \beta_z\}$ in the true model (4.13) due to the difference between X_i^* and X_i.

On the other hand, $E\{N_i(t)|X_i^*, Z_i\}$ pertains to the true model (4.13) via the conditional expectation (4.12), so

$$E\{N_i(t)|X_i^*, Z_i\} = \mu_0(t)\exp(\beta_z^{\mathrm{T}} Z_i) E_{X_i|(X_i^*, Z_i)}\{\exp(\beta_x^{\mathrm{T}} X_i)\}. \tag{4.17}$$

Equating (4.16) and (4.17) gives

$$\begin{aligned}&\mu_0^*(t)\exp(\beta_z^{*\mathrm{T}} Z_i + \beta_x^{*\mathrm{T}} X_i^*)\\&= \mu_0(t)\exp(\beta_z^{\mathrm{T}} Z_i) E_{X_i|(X_i^*, Z_i)}\{\exp(\beta_x^{\mathrm{T}} X_i)\}.\end{aligned} \tag{4.18}$$

Identity (4.18) quantifies the relationship between $\{\mu_0^*(t), \beta_x^*, \beta_z^*\}$ and $\{\mu_0(t), \beta_x, \beta_z\}$, which is determined by the conditional moment generating function of X_i given $\{X_i^*, Z_i\}$. We look at two examples to further examine (4.18).

Example 4.3. If the surrogate X_i^* is linked with X_i through the Berkson model (4.14), then the conditional moment generating function of X_i given $\{X_i^*, Z_i\}$ is

$$E_{X_i|(X_i^*, Z_i)}\{\exp(\beta_x^{\mathrm{T}} X_i)\} = \exp(\beta_x^{\mathrm{T}} X_i^* + \beta_x^{\mathrm{T}} \Sigma_e \beta_x / 2).$$

Consequently, (4.18) gives that

$$\beta_x^* = \beta_x, \ \beta_z^* = \beta_z$$

and

$$\mu_0^*(t) = \mu_0(t)\exp(\beta_x^{\mathrm{T}} \Sigma_e \beta_x / 2).$$

Therefore, under the Berkson model (4.14), the naive analysis with the difference between X_i^* and X_i ignored still yields consistent estimates for the covariate effects β_x and β_z, but the estimate of the baseline function is inflated by the factor $\exp(\beta_x^{\mathrm{T}} \Sigma_e \beta_x / 2)$.

Example 4.4. Suppose that X_i is a binary variable, and let

$$\pi_{01}^* = P(X_i = 1|X_i^* = 0, Z_i) \text{ and } \pi_{10}^* = P(X_i = 0|X_i^* = 1, Z_i)$$

be the (mis)classification probabilities. Then the conditional moment generating of X_i given $\{X_i^*, Z_i\}$ is

$$E_{X_i|(X_i^*, Z_i)}\{\exp(\beta_x X_i)\} = P(X_i = 0|X_i^*, Z_i) + \exp(\beta_x) P(X_i = 1|X_i^*, Z_i).$$

Therefore, corresponding to $X_i^* = 0$ and $X_i^* = 1$, applying identity (4.18) leads to

$$\mu_0^*(t)\exp(\beta_z^{*\mathrm{T}} Z_i) = \mu_0(t)\exp(\beta_z^{\mathrm{T}} Z_i)\{(1 - \pi_{01}^*) + \pi_{01}^* \exp(\beta_x)\}$$

and

$$\mu_0^*(t)\exp(\beta_x^* + \beta_z^{*\mathrm{T}} Z_i) = \mu_0(t)\exp(\beta_z^{\mathrm{T}} Z_i)\{\pi_{10}^* + (1 - \pi_{10}^*)\exp(\beta_x)\}.$$

As a result, we obtain

$$\beta_x^* = \log\left\{\frac{\pi_{10}^* + (1 - \pi_{10}^*)\exp(\beta_x)}{(1 - \pi_{01}^*) + \pi_{01}^* \exp(\beta_x)}\right\}, \ \beta_z^* = \beta_z,$$

and

$$\mu_0^*(t) = \mu_0(t)\{(1 - \pi_{01}^*) + \pi_{01}^* \exp(\beta_x)\}.$$

These examples illustrate that covariate measurement error may or may not affect point estimates for the response model parameters; this basically depends on the relationship between the surrogate measurement X_i^* and the true covariates $\{X_i, Z_i\}$. Estimation of the baseline mean function $\mu_0(t)$ is affected in general if measurement error is ignored. Furthermore, comparison between (4.17) and (4.13) shows that the mean structure for the process linking $N_i(t)$ with the true covariates $\{X_i, Z_i\}$ differs from that for the process linking $N_i(t)$ with the observed covariate measurements $\{X_i^*, Z_i\}$, because the conditional expectation $E_{X_i|(X_i^*, Z_i)}\{\exp(\beta_x^{\mathrm{T}} X_i)\}$ is generally not equal to $\exp(\beta_x^{\mathrm{T}} X_i^*)$.

In subsequent sections, we describe inference methods to account for measurement error effects for different circumstances.

4.3 Directly Correcting Naive Estimators When Assessment Times are Discrete

Consider settings where n subjects are observed at discrete observation time points: $1, \ldots, K$. For $i = 1, \ldots, n$ and $k = 1, \ldots, K$, let N_{ik} be the number of events for subject i observed at time point k, and R_{ik} be the indicator that subject i is at risk prior to time point k. Let X_{ik} and Z_{ik} be vectors of covariates for subject i at time point k. Define $N_i = (N_{i1}, \ldots, N_{iK})^{\mathrm{T}}$, $R_i = (R_{i1}, \ldots, R_{iK})^{\mathrm{T}}$, $X_i = (X_{i1}^{\mathrm{T}}, \ldots, X_{iK}^{\mathrm{T}})^{\mathrm{T}}$, and $Z_i = (Z_{i1}^{\mathrm{T}}, \ldots, Z_{iK}^{\mathrm{T}})^{\mathrm{T}}$.

Suppose the counting process $\{N_{ik} : k = 1, \ldots, K\}$ follows a random effects model with the conditional multiplicative mean structure

$$E(N_{ik}|R_i, X_i, Z_i, u_i) = R_{ik} u_{ik} \lambda_k \exp(\beta_x^{\mathrm{T}} X_{ik} + \beta_z^{\mathrm{T}} Z_{ik}) \tag{4.19}$$

for $k = 1, \ldots, K$, where u_{ik} represents a positive random effect, $u_i = (u_{i1}, \ldots, u_{iK})^{\mathrm{T}}$, $\beta = (\beta_x^{\mathrm{T}}, \beta_z^{\mathrm{T}})^{\mathrm{T}}$ is the vector of regression coefficients, and λ_k represents the discrete baseline intensity at time point k. Moreover, given u_i and $\{R_i, X_i, Z_i\}$, the N_{ik} are assumed to be conditionally independent.

Conditional mean model (4.19) and its analogue in the continuous time scale are commonly used in practice. There are two roles of random effects in the model. Those random effects not only facilitate the dependence among the event counts N_{ik}, but also feature additional heterogeneity among subjects that is not explained by the covariates.

Model (4.19) involves a tacit assumption

$$E(N_{ik}|R_i, X_i, Z_i, u_i) = E(N_{ik}|R_{ik}, X_{ik}, Z_{ik}, u_{ik}),$$

which says that, given the information of the covariates, random effects and the at risk indicator at time k, the mean count of N_{ik} is not affected by $\{R_{ik'}, X_{ik'}, Z_{ik'}, u_{ik'}\}$ for $k' \neq k$.

A conventional assumption

$$E(u_{ik}|R_i, X_i, Z_i) = 1$$

is often made for $i = 1, \ldots, n$ and $k = 1, \ldots, K$. Without this assumption, random effects would be arbitrary, which would lead to unrestricted conditional mean responses. Combining this assumption with model (4.19) gives the convenient marginal log-linear model

$$E(N_{ik}|R_i, X_i, Z_i) = R_{ik}\lambda_k \exp(\beta_x^{\mathrm{T}} X_{ik} + \beta_z^{\mathrm{T}} Z_{ik}). \tag{4.20}$$

Suppose covariate X_{ik} is error-contaminated and is measured with surrogate measurement X_{ik}^*. Let $X_i^* = (X_{i1}^{*\mathrm{T}}, \ldots, X_{iK}^{*\mathrm{T}})^{\mathrm{T}}$. For the measurement error process, we assume that for $i = 1, \ldots, n$ and $k = 1, \ldots, K$,

$$E(N_{ik}|R_i, X_i, Z_i, X_i^*, u_i) = E(N_{ik}|R_i, X_i, Z_i, u_i)$$

and

$$E(u_i|R_i, X_i, Z_i, X_i^*) = E(u_i|R_i, X_i, Z_i).$$

To estimate parameter β, it is ideal to base estimation on the true model that generates the data. But in reality, this model is unknown. One has to adopt a *working* model that is thought to well approximate the true data generation process. However, specifying a sensible working model is difficult due to the lack of knowledge of the true distribution for generating the data. Convenience and tractability may then drive us to choose a particular working model.

In the problem we consider here, we might blindly choose a working model by imposing convenient assumptions on the data. Specifically, we consider a working model by ignoring the existence of random effects and naively assuming that conditional on $\{R_i, X_i, Z_i\}$, the N_{ik} are independent, and further imposing Poisson distributions as the marginal distributions for the N_{ik}. Moreover, we ignore the differences between X_i^* and X_i when specifying the working model.

This working model is simple to implement and can yield a quick estimation of β by using the likelihood method, but the results are expected to incur considerable biases. To obtain valid estimation results, proper care is required to adjust for the estimator derived from this working model, as elaborated next.

The working model assumes that given $\{R_i, X_i, Z_i\}$, the N_{ik} are independent and $N_{ik} \sim \text{Poisson}(\mu_{ik}^*)$ with the marginal mean

$$\mu_{ik}^* = R_{ik}\lambda_k^* \exp(\beta_x^{*\mathrm{T}} X_{ik}^* + \beta_z^{*\mathrm{T}} Z_{ik})$$

for $k = 1, \ldots, K$, where the asterisks indicate that the symbols potentially differ from their counterparts in the true model (4.20).

Let $\theta^* = (\lambda^{*\mathrm{T}}, \beta^{*\mathrm{T}})^{\mathrm{T}}$ with $\beta^* = (\beta_x^{*\mathrm{T}}, \beta_z^{*\mathrm{T}})^{\mathrm{T}}$ and $\lambda^* = (\lambda_1^*, \ldots, \lambda_K^*)^{\mathrm{T}}$. Then the likelihood resulted from the working model for subject i is

$$L_i^*(\theta^*) = \prod_{k=1}^{K} \left\{ \frac{\mu_{ik}^{*N_{ik}} \exp(-\mu_{ik}^*)}{N_{ik}!} \right\}^{R_{ik}},$$

yielding the working score functions

$$\frac{\partial \ell_i^*}{\partial \lambda_k^*} = R_{ik}\left\{\frac{N_{ik}}{\lambda_k^*} - \exp(\beta_x^{*\mathrm{T}} X_{ik}^* + \beta_z^{*\mathrm{T}} Z_{ik})\right\} \text{ for } k = 1, \ldots, K$$

and

$$\frac{\partial \ell_i^*}{\partial \beta^*} = \sum_{k=1}^{K}\left[R_{ik}\left\{N_{ik}\begin{pmatrix} X_{ik}^* \\ Z_{ik}\end{pmatrix} - \lambda_k^*\begin{pmatrix} X_{ik}^* \\ Z_{ik}\end{pmatrix}\exp(\beta_x^{*\mathrm{T}} X_{ik}^* + \beta_z^{*\mathrm{T}} Z_{ik})\right\}\right],$$

where $\ell_i^* = \log L_i^*(\theta^*)$.

Solving $\sum_{i=1}^{n} \partial \ell_i^*/\partial \theta^* = 0$ for θ^* leads to a naive estimate of θ. Let $\widehat{\theta}^* = (\widehat{\lambda}^{*\mathrm{T}}, \widehat{\beta}^{*\mathrm{T}})^{\mathrm{T}}$ denote the resultant estimator of θ. The naive estimator $\widehat{\theta}^*$ potentially incurs biases in estimating θ. To see how to remove such biases, we invoke the theory in §1.4 by evaluating the expectation of the working score functions under the true model.

Let E_{J} represent the expectation taken with respect to the model for the joint distribution of $\{R_i, u_i, N_i, X_i, Z_i, X_i^*\}$. Then set

$$E_{\mathrm{J}}\left(\frac{\partial \ell_i^*}{\partial \lambda_k^*}\right) = 0 \text{ for } k = 1, \ldots, K$$

and

$$E_{\mathrm{J}}\left(\frac{\partial \ell_i^*}{\partial \beta^*}\right) = 0.$$

These identities are simplified as

$$\lambda_k E\{R_{ik}\exp(\beta_x^{\mathrm{T}} X_{ik} + \beta_z^{\mathrm{T}} Z_{ik})\} = \lambda_k^* E\{R_{ik}\exp(\beta_x^{*\mathrm{T}} X_{ik}^* + \beta_z^{*\mathrm{T}} Z_{ik})\}$$

and

$$\begin{aligned}
&\sum_{k=1}^{K}\lambda_k E\left\{R_{ik}\begin{pmatrix} X_{ik}^* \\ Z_{ik}\end{pmatrix}\exp(\beta_x^{\mathrm{T}} X_{ik} + \beta_z^{\mathrm{T}} Z_{ik})\right\} \\
&= \sum_{k=1}^{K}\lambda_k^* E\left\{R_{ik}\begin{pmatrix} X_{ik}^* \\ Z_{ik}\end{pmatrix}\exp(\beta_x^{*\mathrm{T}} X_{ik}^* + \beta_z^{*\mathrm{T}} Z_{ik})\right\},
\end{aligned} \tag{4.21}$$

where the expectations are evaluated with respect to the model for the joint distribution of $\{R_i, X_i, Z_i, X_i^*\}$.

These identities link the naive estimator with the estimator derived from the true model. For general situations, it is difficult to obtain analytical connections between the naive estimator $\widehat{\theta}^*$ and the estimator obtained from the true model. But under special circumstances, closed-form results are possible, suggested as follows.

Theorem 4.5. *In addition to the preceding assumptions, we assume the following conditions:*

(a) the follow-up process R_i is independent of $\{X_i, Z_i, X_i^*\}$ and $E(R_{ik})$ is a common positive constant for $k = 1, \ldots, K$;

(b) the true covariates and their surrogate measurements are time-independent with

$$X_{ik} = X_{i0};\ X_{ik}^* = X_{i0}^*;\ Z_{ik} = Z_{i0}$$

for all $k = 1, \ldots, K$, *where* X_{i0}, Z_{i0} *and* X_{i0}^* *represent the baseline measurements;*

(c) the baseline covariate X_{i0} *follows a conditional normal distribution*

$$X_{i0}|(X_{i0}^*, Z_{i0}) \sim N(C_0 + C_x^{\mathrm{T}} X_{i0}^* + C_z^{\mathrm{T}} Z_{i0}, \Sigma_e),$$

where C_0 *is a vector,* C_x *and* C_z *are matrices, and* Σ_e *is a positive definite matrix.*

Then we have

$$\begin{aligned}
\lambda_k^* &= \lambda_k \exp(C_0^{\mathrm{T}} \beta_x + \beta_x^{\mathrm{T}} \Sigma_e \beta_x / 2) \ \textit{for}\ k = 1, \ldots, K; \\
\beta_x^* &= C_x \beta_x; \\
\beta_z^* &= \beta_z + C_z \beta_x.
\end{aligned}$$

An immediate result is that $\beta_z = \beta_z^*$ if Z_i is independent of X_i (hence, $C_z = 0$), which is practically useful. For example, if Z_i is a treatment assignment variable in a randomized trial and is, by design, independent of covariate X_i and the follow-up process, then the treatment effect can still be consistently estimated by the naive estimator which is derived from neglecting measurement error and random effects. Regarding error-prone covariates, we note that $\beta_x = \beta_x^*$ if X_i and X_i^* follow a Berkson error model for which $C_0 = 0$, $C_z = 0$, and C_x is the identity matrix. It is interesting to compare this result with the conclusion in §4.2. Although the mean structure of the true model is not preserved by the model linking the outcome to the observed covariate measurements $\{X_i^*, Z_i\}$, the point estimates produced by the naive analysis are sometimes still identical to those obtained from using the true model.

Finally, using the relationship established in Theorem 4.5, we adjust for the native estimator $\widehat{\theta}^*$ to obtain a consistent estimator $\widehat{\theta} = (\widehat{\lambda}_1, \ldots, \widehat{\lambda}_K, \widehat{\beta}_x^{\mathrm{T}}, \widehat{\beta}_z^{\mathrm{T}})^{\mathrm{T}}$, given by

$$\begin{aligned}
\widehat{\lambda}_k &= \widehat{\lambda}_k^* \exp(-C_0^{\mathrm{T}} C_x^{-1} \widehat{\beta}_x^* - \widehat{\beta}_x^{*\mathrm{T}} C_x^{\mathrm{T}-1} \Sigma_e C_x^{-1} \widehat{\beta}_x^* / 2) \ \text{ for } k = 1, \ldots, K; \\
\widehat{\beta}_x &= C_x^{-1} \widehat{\beta}_x^*; \\
\widehat{\beta}_z &= \widehat{\beta}_z^* - C_z C_x^{-1} \widehat{\beta}_x^*;
\end{aligned}$$

where C_x is assumed to be invertible.

This is an example of using the *naive estimator correction strategy*, outlined in §2.5.3, to correct for covariate measurement error effects on point estimation. This approach is easy to implement, but it does not provide us with variance estimates for the adjusted estimators. To complete inferential procedures, one may employ the bootstrap method to calculate associated standard errors for estimators $\widehat{\lambda}_k$ ($k = 1, \ldots, K$), $\widehat{\beta}_x$ and $\widehat{\beta}_z$. The details were given by Jiang, Turnbull and Clark (1999).

4.4 Counting Processes with Observed Event Times

In contrast to discrete counting processes in the previous section, we discuss counting processes which may be continuous or discrete. Assume that the follow-up process is independent of the event process, given the covariate process (Cook and Lawless 2007, §2.6). Using the notation in §4.1, for $t > 0$, we consider a multiplicative model

$$E[dN_i(t)|\{R_i(v): 0 \le v \le t\}, \mathcal{H}_{it}^{\mathrm{N}}, \mathcal{H}_{it}^{\mathrm{XZ}}] = R_i(t)\lambda\{t|X_i(t), Z_i(t)\}d\eta(t)$$

with

$$\lambda\{t|X_i(t), Z_i(t)\} = \lambda_0(t|\mathcal{H}_{it}^{\mathrm{N}})\exp\{\beta_x^{\mathrm{T}}X_i(t) + \beta_z^{\mathrm{T}}Z_i(t)\}, \tag{4.22}$$

where $\lambda\{t|X_i(t), Z_i(t)\}$ is the intensity function for subject i, $\beta = (\beta_x^{\mathrm{T}}, \beta_z^{\mathrm{T}})^{\mathrm{T}}$ is the regression parameter that is of interest, $\lambda_0(t|\mathcal{H}_{it}^{\mathrm{N}})$ is the baseline intensity function which may depend on the event history (e.g., the renewal process discussed in Cook and Lawless (2007, §2.3, §5.4)), and $d\eta(t)$ is the measure featuring a continuous or a discrete time process. This multiplication model allows us to separate the covariate effects from the event history.

We consider settings where the event times for each subject are observed. Let N_i be the number of events experienced by subject i, and $0 < t_{i1} < \ldots < t_{iN_i} \le \tau_i$ be the observed event times for subject i, where τ_i is the length of the study period for subject i.

It is straightforward to express the likelihood function contributed from subject i as

$$L_i = \left[\prod_{j=1}^{N_i} \lambda\{t_{ij}|X_i(t_{ij}), Z_i(t_{ij})\}\right] \cdot \exp\left[-\int_0^\infty R_i(v)\lambda\{v|X_i(v), Z_i(v)\}d\eta(v)\right]. \tag{4.23}$$

Assume that the baseline intensity function $\lambda_0(t|\mathcal{H}_{it}^{\mathrm{N}})$ in (4.22) is postulated as a parametric model $\lambda_0(t;\rho)$, where ρ is the associated parameter vector.

Time-Independent Covariates

First, we consider the case where the true covariates and their surrogate measurements are time-independent; they are, respectively, denoted as $\{X_i, Z_i\}$ and X_i^*, where X_i^* is an observed measurement for X_i. With covariates being time-independent, the log-likelihood, resulted from (4.23), is given by

$$\ell_i = \sum_{j=1}^{N_i}\{\log\lambda_0(t_{ij};\rho) + \beta_x^{\mathrm{T}}X_i + \beta_z^{\mathrm{T}}Z_i\} - \exp(\beta_x^{\mathrm{T}}X_i + \beta_z^{\mathrm{T}}Z_i)\int_0^\infty R_i(v)\lambda_0(v;\rho)d\eta(v),$$

which resembles the log-likelihood (3.9) for the proportional hazards model.

To incorporate measurement error effects into inferential procedures, we consider the insertion correction strategy discussed in §2.5.2 and §3.5.1. In light of the form of ℓ_i, which depends on X_i through linear or exponent terms, we need only to find functions $g_k(X_i^*; \beta_x)$ for $k = 1, 2$ such that

$$\begin{aligned} E\{g_1(X_i^*; \beta_x)|X_i, Z_i, N_i\} &= \beta_x^{\mathrm{T}} X_i; \\ E\{g_2(X_i^*; \beta_x)|X_i, Z_i, N_i\} &= \exp(\beta_x^{\mathrm{T}} X_i); \end{aligned} \tag{4.24}$$

where the expectations are taken with respect to the model for the conditional distribution of X_i^* given $\{X_i, Z_i, N_i\}$.

Define

$$\begin{aligned} \ell_i^* = & \sum_{j=1}^{N_i} \{\log \lambda_0(t_{ij}; \rho) + g_1(X_i^*; \beta_x) + \beta_z^{\mathrm{T}} Z_i\} \\ & - g_2(X_i^*; \beta_x) \exp(\beta_z^{\mathrm{T}} Z_i) \int_0^\infty R_i(v) \lambda_0(v; \rho) d\eta(v), \end{aligned}$$

then it is immediate that $E(\ell_i^*|X_i, Z_i, N_i) = \ell_i$.

Let $\theta = (\rho^{\mathrm{T}}, \beta^{\mathrm{T}})^{\mathrm{T}}$. Estimation of parameter θ is performed by solving

$$\sum_{i=1}^{n} \frac{\partial \ell_i^*}{\partial \theta} = 0$$

for θ. Let $\widehat{\theta}$ denote the resulting estimator of θ. The asymptotic normality of $\widehat{\theta}$ is readily established by applying the standard theory of estimating functions, provided regularity conditions.

This estimation method relies on the availability of functions $g_1(\cdot)$ and $g_2(\cdot)$. As discussed in Chapter 3, determination of functions $g_1(\cdot)$ and $g_2(\cdot)$ calls for knowledge of the mismeasurement process. In addition, functions $g_1(\cdot)$ and $g_2(\cdot)$ may involve parameters associated with the model of the mismeasurement process. Estimation of such parameters normally requires additional data sources, such as a validation sample or replicates. The induced variability in estimation of such parameters needs to be accounted for in establishing the asymptotic distribution of the estimator $\widehat{\theta}$. This may be done using the procedures outlined in §1.3.4.

To illustrate the choice of function $g_k(\cdot)$ for $k = 1, 2$, we consider a simple case where X_i is a scalar binary variable. Let $\pi_{01} = P(X_i^* = 1|X_i = 0, Z_i)$ and $\pi_{10} = P(X_i^* = 0|X_i = 1, Z_i)$ be the (mis)classification probabilities. By the result in Problem 2.10, we take

$$g_1(X_i^*; \beta_x) = \frac{\beta_x(\pi_{01} - X_i^*)}{\pi_{01} + \pi_{10} - 1}$$

and

$$g_2(X_i^*; \beta_x) = \frac{X_i^*\{1 - \exp(\beta_x)\} + \pi_{01}\exp(\beta_x) - (1 - \pi_{10})}{\pi_{01} + \pi_{10} - 1}$$

so that (4.24) is satisfied.

Time-Varying Covariates

When error-prone covariates are time varying, correcting measurement error effects is usually difficult, and certain assumptions are often imposed to ease development. To see this, we consider a special case with time-varying covariates.

Let $X_i(t)$ denote the vector of error-prone covariates and $Z_i(t)$ be the vector of precisely measured covariates. Suppose that $X_i(t)$ takes constant values between two consecutive observation times, i.e., for $j = 1, \ldots, N_i$,

$$X_i(t) = X_i(t_{i,j-1}) \text{ for } t \in [t_{i,j-1}, t_{ij}), \tag{4.25}$$

where $t_{i0} = 0$. Suppose $X_i(t)$ is only assessed at time points t_{ij} for $j = 1, \ldots, N_i$ and $X_i^*(t_{ij})$ is the corresponding surrogate measurement.

The log-likelihood, resulted from (4.23), becomes

$$\begin{aligned} \ell_i = & \sum_{j=1}^{N_i} \{\log \lambda_0(t_{ij}; \rho) + \beta_x^{\mathrm{T}} X_i(t_{ij}) + \beta_z^{\mathrm{T}} Z_i(t_{ij})\} \\ & - \sum_{j=1}^{N_i} \exp\{\beta_x^{\mathrm{T}} X_i(t_{i,j-1})\} \int_{t_{i,j-1}}^{t_{ij}} R_i(v)\lambda_0(v;\rho)\exp\{\beta_z^{\mathrm{T}} Z_i(v)\} d\eta(v). \end{aligned}$$

Applying the same strategy as for the case with time-independent covariates, we define

$$\begin{aligned} \ell_i^* = & \sum_{j=1}^{N_i} \left[\log \lambda_0(t_{ij}; \rho) + g_1\{X_i^*(t_{ij}); \beta_x\} + \beta_z^{\mathrm{T}} Z_i(t_{ij})\right] \\ & - \sum_{j=1}^{N_i} g_2\{X_i^*(t_{i,j-1}); \beta_x\} \int_{t_{i,j-1}}^{t_{ij}} R_i(v)\lambda_0(v;\rho)\exp\{\beta_z^{\mathrm{T}} Z_i(v)\} d\eta(v), \end{aligned}$$

where functions $g_1\{X_i^*(t); \beta_x\}$ and $g_2\{X_i^*(t); \beta_x\}$ satisfy

$$E[g_1\{X_i^*(t); \beta_x\} | X_i(t), Z_i(t), N_i] = \beta_x^{\mathrm{T}} X_i(t)$$

and

$$E[g_2\{X_i^*(t); \beta_x\} | X_i(t), Z_i(t), N_i] = \exp\{\beta_x^{\mathrm{T}} X_i(t)\}. \tag{4.26}$$

The expectations here are evaluated with respect to the model for the conditional distribution of $X_i^*(t)$ given $\{X_i(t), Z_i(t), N_i\}$ for time point t.

It is easily seen that $E\{\ell_i^* | X_i(t), Z_i(t), N_i\} = \ell_i$. Then by the insertion correction scheme discussed in §2.5.2, estimation of θ proceeds by solving

$$\sum_{i=1}^{n} \frac{\partial \ell_i^*}{\partial \theta} = 0$$

for θ.

As an example of choosing functions $g_k(\cdot)(k = 1, 2)$, we consider an additive measurement error model. Given time t, we model $X_i^*(t)$ as

$$X_i^*(t) = X_i(t) + e_i(t),$$

where $e_i(t)$ is independent of $\{X_i(t), Z_i(t), N_i\}$ and has mean zero and the moment generating function $M(\cdot)$. Then setting

$$g_1\{X_i^*(t); \beta_x\} = \beta_x^{\mathrm{T}} X_i^*(t)$$

and

$$g_2\{X_i^*(t); \beta_x\} = M^{-1}(\beta_x) \exp\{\beta_x^{\mathrm{T}} X_i^*(t)\}$$

makes (4.26) be satisfied.

If $X_i(t)$ varies with time in a more complex dynamic form than (4.25), the preceding procedure based on moments correction usually breaks down. In this case, a possible strategy for correcting measurement error effects is to employ the likelihood method for the *joint modeling* analysis, which is to be discussed in §5.6.

4.5 Poisson Models for Interval Counts

The insertion correction scheme discussed in the previous section can be modified to handle error-contaminated interval count data. Using the notation in §4.1.3, we assume that the sequence of time intervals $\{B_{ij} : B_{ij} = (b_{i,j-1}, b_{ij}]; j = 1, \ldots, K_i\}$ satisfies the conditions outlined by Lawless and Zhan (1998). Consider the setting where covariates are time-independent. Assume that the counting process $\{N_i(t) : t \geq 0\}$ is a Poisson process with the intensity function modeled as

$$\lambda(t|X_i, Z_i) = \lambda_0(t) \exp(\beta_x^{\mathrm{T}} X_i + \beta_z^{\mathrm{T}} Z_i), \tag{4.27}$$

where $\lambda_0(t)$ is the baseline intensity function, $\beta = (\beta_x^{\mathrm{T}}, \beta_z^{\mathrm{T}})^{\mathrm{T}}$ is the vector of regression coefficients, X_i is the vector of error-prone covariates, and Z_i is the vector of precisely observed covariates.

By Theorem 4.2, the counts N_{ij} over time intervals B_{ij} are independent and follow Poisson distributions:

$$N_{ij} \sim \text{Poisson}(\mu_{ij}),$$

where $\mu_{ij} = \mu_{0ij} \exp(\beta_x^{\mathrm{T}} X_i + \beta_z^{\mathrm{T}} Z_i)$ and $\mu_{0ij} = \int_{b_{i,j-1}}^{b_{ij}} \lambda_0(v) d\eta(v)$. Therefore, the likelihood contributed from subject i is given by, with the factor $(\prod_{j=1}^{K_i} N_{ij}!)^{-1}$ omitted,

$$L_i = \prod_{j=1}^{K_i} \exp(-\mu_{ij}) \mu_{ij}^{N_{ij}},$$

giving the log-likelihood function contributed from subject i

$$\ell_i = \sum_{j=1}^{K_i} N_{ij} \log(\mu_{0ij}) + N_{i+}(\beta_x^{\mathrm{T}} X_i + \beta_z^{\mathrm{T}} Z_i) - \mu_{0i+} \exp(\beta_x^{\mathrm{T}} X_i + \beta_z^{\mathrm{T}} Z_i),$$

where $N_{i+} = \sum_{j=1}^{K_i} N_{ij}$ and $\mu_{0i+} = \sum_{j=1}^{K_i} \mu_{0ij}$.

Suppose X_i is not directly observed and its surrogate measurement X_i^* is available. Noting that X_i appears in linear or exponent form in ℓ_i, we use the same strategy as in §4.4 and define

$$\ell_i^* = \sum_{j=1}^{K_i} N_{ij} \log(\mu_{0ij}) + N_{i+}\{g_1(X_i^*; \beta_x) + \beta_z^{\mathrm{T}} Z_i\} - \mu_{0i+} g_2(X_i^*; \beta_x) \exp(\beta_z^{\mathrm{T}} Z_i),$$

where $g_1(\cdot)$ and $g_2(\cdot)$ are determined by (4.24) with conditioning variable N_i replaced by $\{N_{i1}, \ldots, N_{iK_i}\}$. That is,

$$\begin{aligned} E[g_1(X_i^*; \beta_x) | X_i, Z_i, \{N_{i1}, \ldots, N_{iK_i}\}] &= \beta_x^{\mathrm{T}} X_i; \\ E[g_2(X_i^*; \beta_x) | X_i, Z_i, \{N_{i1}, \ldots, N_{iK_i}\}] &= \exp(\beta_x^{\mathrm{T}} X_i). \end{aligned} \tag{4.28}$$

It is easily seen that

$$E(\ell_i^* | X_i, Z_i, N_{i1}, \ldots, N_{iK_i}) = \ell_i, \tag{4.29}$$

where the expectation is taken with respect to the model for the conditional distribution of X_i^*, given $\{X_i, Z_i, N_{i1}, \ldots, N_{iK_i}\}$.

As ℓ_i^* is computable and satisfies (4.29), then by the arguments in §2.5.2, working with ℓ_i^* produces a consistent estimator of β if suitable regularity conditions are satisfied. But since the baseline mean function μ_{0ij} is unknown, we cannot directly use the function ℓ_i^* to estimate parameter β. To circumvent this, we need to deal with the baseline mean function μ_{0ij}, or equivalently, the baseline intensity function $\lambda_0(t)$.

To avoid strong parametric assumptions about the baseline intensity function $\lambda_0(t)$, we use the flexible piecewise-constant approach, as discussed in §4.1.2. Let the baseline intensity function be modeled as

$$\lambda_0(t) = \rho_k \tag{4.30}$$

for $t \in A_k = (a_{k-1}, a_k]$, where $0 = a_0 < a_1 < \ldots < a_{K-1} < a_K = \infty$ is a pre-specified sequence of constants for a given K and $\rho = (\rho_1, \ldots, \rho_K)^{\mathrm{T}}$ is the parameter. Then, as demonstrated in Fig. 4.2, the baseline mean function is given by

$$\mu_{0ij} = \sum_{k=1}^{K} \rho_k u_k(i, j), \tag{4.31}$$

where $u_k(i, j) = \max\{0, \min(a_k, b_{ij}) - \max(a_{k-1}, b_{i,j-1})\}$ is the length of the intersection of interval B_{ij} with interval A_k.

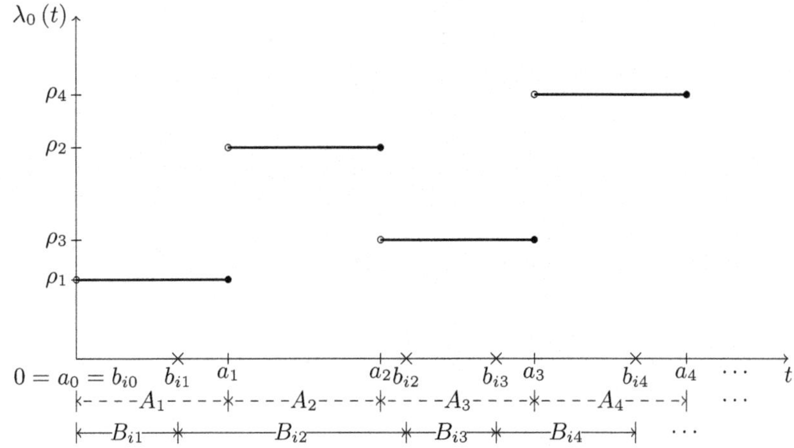

Fig. 4.2. *Piecewise-Constant Model for the Baseline Intensity Function and Observation Times for Interval Count Data*

As a result, the partial derivatives of ℓ_i^* are given by

$$\frac{\partial \ell_i^*}{\partial \beta_x} = N_{i+}\frac{\partial g_1(X_i^*;\beta_x)}{\partial \beta_x} - \mu_{0i+}\frac{\partial g_2(X_i^*;\beta_x)}{\partial \beta_x}\exp(\beta_z^{\mathrm{T}} Z_i);$$
$$\frac{\partial \ell_i^*}{\partial \beta_z} = N_{i+}Z_i - \mu_{0i+}g_2(X_i^*;\beta_x)Z_i\exp(\beta_z^{\mathrm{T}} Z_i);$$
$$\frac{\partial \ell_i^*}{\partial \rho_k} = \sum_{j=1}^{K_i}\frac{N_{ij}}{\mu_{0ij}}u_k(i,j) - u_k(i,+)g_2(X_i^*;\beta_x)\exp(\beta_z^{\mathrm{T}} Z_i)$$

for $k = 1, \ldots, K$; where $u_k(i,+) = \sum_{j=1}^{K_i} u_k(i,j)$.

Write $\partial \ell_i^*/\partial \rho = (\partial \ell_i^*/\partial \rho_1, \ldots, \partial \ell_i^*/\partial \rho_K)^{\mathrm{T}}$, then solving

$$\sum_{i=1}^{n}\frac{\partial \ell_i^*}{\partial \beta_x} = 0;\ \sum_{i=1}^{n}\frac{\partial \ell_i^*}{\partial \beta_z} = 0;\ \sum_{i=1}^{n}\frac{\partial \ell_i^*}{\partial \rho} = 0 \tag{4.32}$$

for β and ρ gives their estimates. Let $\widehat{\beta}$ and $\widehat{\rho}$ denote the resultant estimators of β and ρ, respectively.

Assuming that the differentiation and expectation operations can change the order, then the property (4.29) implies that the functions in (4.32) are unbiased estimating functions. Applying the standard theory of estimating functions outlined in §1.3.2, we can readily establish the asymptotic normality for estimator $(\widehat{\beta}^{\mathrm{T}}, \widehat{\rho}^{\mathrm{T}})^{\mathrm{T}}$.

4.6 Marginal Methods for Interval Count Data with Measurement Error

The method discussed in §4.5 is likelihood-based and assumes the underlying process of generating interval counts is a Poisson process. Likelihood-based inference is generally useful for handling error-contaminated interval count data because of its efficiency and well-established asymptotic properties. However, this approach may suffer from sensitivity to model misspecification. In this section, we discuss a marginal inference procedure which requires modeling mean functions only and leaves the underlying distribution unspecified.

Suppose that the observation scheme is the same as that of §4.5. Using the same notation as in §4.5, we assume that the conditional mean, $\mu_{ij} = E(N_{ij}|X_i, Z_i)$, of N_{ij} given $\{X_i, Z_i\}$, is given by

$$\mu_{ij} = \mu_{0ij} \exp(\beta_x^{\mathrm{T}} X_i + \beta_z^{\mathrm{T}} Z_i), \tag{4.33}$$

where μ_{0ij} is modeled as (4.31).

Let $\widetilde{N}_i = (N_{i1}, \ldots, N_{iK_i})^{\mathrm{T}}$. Assume that the conditional covariance matrix $V_i = \mathrm{var}(\widetilde{N}_i|X_i, Z_i)$ for the interval count vector $\widetilde{N}_i$ is given by

$$V_i = C_i + \phi \mu_i \mu_i^{\mathrm{T}}, \tag{4.34}$$

where $C_i = \mathrm{diag}\{\mu_{i1}, \ldots, \mu_{iK_i}\}$, $\mu_i = (\mu_{i1}, \ldots, \mu_{iK_i})^{\mathrm{T}}$, and ϕ is a dispersion parameter.

Models (4.33) and (4.34) provide a class of useful models for interval count data. For instance, interval count data generated from a mixed Poisson process, say the one modeled by (4.9), have the mean structure (4.33) and covariance matrix (4.34), which is easily seen using (4.4) and (4.5). Interval count data generated from the Poisson process modeled by (4.27) are accommodated by (4.33) and (4.34) as well where dispersion parameter $\phi = 0$.

Let $\theta = (\rho^{\mathrm{T}}, \beta^{\mathrm{T}})^{\mathrm{T}}$. Given the mean and covariance structures of $\widetilde{N}_i$, estimation of θ is naturally performed using the GEE method, as formulated in (1.9),

$$U_1 = \sum_{i=1}^{n} D_i V_i^{-1}(\widetilde{N}_i - \mu_i) = 0,$$

where $D_i = \partial \mu_i^{\mathrm{T}} / \partial \theta$. More specifically, this formulation gives three sets of estimating functions (Lawless and Zhan 1998):

$$U_1 = \begin{pmatrix} \sum_{i=1}^n U_{1\rho i} \\ \sum_{i=1}^n U_{1xi} \\ \sum_{i=1}^n U_{1zi} \end{pmatrix} \tag{4.35}$$

with

$$\begin{aligned} U_{1\rho i} &= \exp(\beta_x^{\mathrm{T}} X_i + \beta_z^{\mathrm{T}} Z_i) \\ &\quad \cdot \left\{ \sum_{j=1}^{K_i} \frac{N_{ij} - \mu_{ij}}{\mu_{ij}} u(i, j) - \frac{\phi(N_{i+} - \mu_{i+})}{1 + \phi \mu_{i+}} u(i, +) \right\}; \end{aligned}$$

$$U_{1xi} = \frac{N_{i+} - \mu_{i+}}{1 + \phi\mu_{i+}} X_i;$$
$$U_{1zi} = \frac{N_{i+} - \mu_{i+}}{1 + \phi\mu_{i+}} Z_i;$$

where $u(i,j) = \{u_1(i,j), \ldots, u_K(i,j)\}^{\mathrm{T}}, u(i,+) = \sum_{j=1}^{K_i} u(i,j)$, and $\mu_{i+} = \sum_{j=1}^{K_i} \mu_{ij}$.

Interestingly, estimating function (4.35) coincides with the score function derived from the likelihood function (4.11) in §4.1.3. However, the validity of (4.35) does not require the recurrent event process to be a mixed Poisson process from which likelihood (4.11) is derived. The unbiasedness of estimating function (4.35) requires only the correct specification of (4.33).

When the X_i are subject to measurement error with surrogate measurements X_i^* available, estimation based on estimating function U_1 with X_i replaced by X_i^* commonly incurs bias. One strategy to correct for the induced bias is to employ the insertion correction method, as described in §2.5.2. In particular, we consider a weight version of U_1.

For $i = 1, \ldots, n$, let $U_{1i} = (U_{1\rho i}^{\mathrm{T}}, U_{1xi}^{\mathrm{T}}, U_{1zi}^{\mathrm{T}})^{\mathrm{T}}$. Define

$$U_{1\mathrm{w}i} = w_{1i}(\phi, \theta; X_i, Z_i) U_{1i},$$

where $w_{1i}(\phi, \theta; X_i, Z_i)$ is the weight taken as $1 + \phi\mu_{i+}$. Let $g_1(\cdot)$ and $g_2(\cdot)$ be the functions satisfying (4.28), and $g_3(\cdot)$ be a function satisfying

$$E\{g_3(X_i^*; \beta_x) | X_i, Z_i, \widetilde{N}_i\} = X_i \exp(\beta_x^{\mathrm{T}} X_i).$$

Define

$$U_{1\rho i}^* = \sum_{j=1}^{K_i} \frac{N_{ij}}{\mu_{0ij}} u(i,j) + g_2(X_i^*; \beta_x) \exp(\beta_z^{\mathrm{T}} Z_i) \cdot \left\{ \phi\mu_{0i+} \sum_{j=1}^{K_i} \frac{N_{ij}}{\mu_{0ij}} u(i,j) - (1 + \phi N_{i+}) u(i,+) \right\};$$

$$U_{1xi}^* = N_{i+} g_1(X_i^*; 1) - \mu_{0i+} g_3(X_i^*; \beta_x) \exp(\beta_z^{\mathrm{T}} Z_i);$$
$$U_{1zi}^* = N_{i+} Z_i - g_2(X_i^*; \beta_x) Z_i \exp(\beta_z^{\mathrm{T}} Z_i).$$

Let $U_{1i}^* = (U_{1\rho i}^{*\mathrm{T}}, U_{1xi}^{*\mathrm{T}}, U_{1zi}^{*\mathrm{T}})^{\mathrm{T}}$. It is readily verified that

$$E(U_{1i}^* | X_i, Z_i, \widetilde{N}_i) = U_{1\mathrm{w}i}. \tag{4.36}$$

If ϕ is known, then solving

$$\sum_{i=1}^{n} U_{1i}^* = 0 \tag{4.37}$$

for θ yields an estimate for θ.

When ϕ is unknown, it must be estimated. Here we invoke the method of moments to estimate ϕ. Let $\sigma_{i+}^2 = \text{var}(N_{i+})$, then by (4.34), $\sigma_{i+}^2 = \mu_{i+} + \phi\mu_{i+}^2$. Define

$$U_{2i} = w_{2i}(\phi, \theta; X_i, Z_i)\{(N_{i+} - \mu_{i+})^2 - \sigma_{i+}^2\},$$

where $w_{2i}(\phi, \theta; X_i, Z_i)$ is a weight free of N_{ij}. Particular choices of weight function $w_{2i}(\phi, \theta; X_i, Z_i)$ are $1, 1/\sigma_{i+}^2$, and μ_{i+}^2/σ_{i+}^4, as considered by Lawless and Zhan (1998). Let

$$U_2 = \sum_{i=1}^{n} U_{2i}, \tag{4.38}$$

then U_2 is unbiased and used for estimation of ϕ.

Since (4.38) is expressed in terms of the unobserved covariates X_i, we need to find a function U_{2i}^* that is workable. In the same manner as the preceding discussion, we use the moment generating function for the measurement error to construct U_{2i}^* such that it is expressed as a function of ϕ and the observed data. As long as

$$E(U_{2i}^*|X_i, Z_i, \widetilde{N}_i) = U_{2i}, \tag{4.39}$$

working with $\sum_{i=1}^{n} U_{2i}^*$ leads to a consistent estimator for ϕ under regularity conditions.

As an example, we take $w_{2i}(\phi, \theta; X_i, Z_i)$ as 1. Then setting

$$\begin{aligned} U_{2i}^* &= N_{i+}^2 - (2N_{i+} + 1)\mu_{0i+} g_2(X_i^*; \beta_x) \exp(\beta_z^{\mathrm{T}} Z_i) \\ &\quad + (1 - \phi)\mu_{0i+}^2 g_2(X_i^*; 2\beta_x) \exp(2\beta_z^{\mathrm{T}} Z_i) \end{aligned}$$

makes (4.39) be met. Then pairing

$$\sum_{i=1}^{n} U_{2i}^* = 0 \tag{4.40}$$

with (4.37) and solving them for the parameters gives estimates of ϕ and θ. Let $\widehat{\phi}$ and $\widehat{\theta}$ be the resulting estimators of ϕ and θ, respectively. Identities (4.36) and (4.39) ensure that $\widehat{\phi}$ and $\widehat{\theta}$ are consistent estimators, provided suitable regularity conditions.

To complete estimation steps, we need to work out the expressions for functions $g_1(\cdot)$, $g_2(\cdot)$ and $g_3(\cdot)$, which generally depend on the measurement error process. We illustrate this by considering a scenario where replicate measurements for the X_i are available.

Example 4.6. For $i = 1, \ldots, n$, let $X_{il}^* = (X_{i1l}^*, \ldots, X_{ip_xl}^*)^{\mathrm{T}}$ be m_i independent surrogate measurements of X_i, where $l = 1, \ldots, m_i$ and p_x is the dimension of X_i. Suppose that X_{il}^* and X_i are linked by the model

$$X_{il}^* = X_i + e_{il} \tag{4.41}$$

for $l = 1, \ldots, m_i$, where the e_{il} have mean zero and are independent of each other and of $\{X_i, Z_i\}$ and the event process.

Let $\bar{e}_{i+} = m_i^{-1} \sum_{l=1}^{m_i} e_{il}$, and $M_i(v) = E\{\exp(v^{\mathrm{T}}\bar{e}_{i+})\}$ be the moment generating function for $\bar{e}_{i+}$. For $j = 1, \ldots, p_x$, let $\overline{X}^*_{ij+} = m_i^{-1} \sum_{l=1}^{m_i} X^*_{ijl}$, and write $X_i^* = (\overline{X}^*_{i1+}, \ldots, \overline{X}^*_{ip_x+})^{\mathrm{T}}$. Then functions $g_1(\cdot)$, $g_2(\cdot)$ and $g_3(\cdot)$ are given as

$$
\begin{aligned}
g_1(X_i^*; \beta_x) &= \beta_x^{\mathrm{T}} X_i^*;\\
g_2(X_i^*; \beta_x) &= \exp(\beta_x^{\mathrm{T}} X_i^*)\{M_i(\beta_x)\}^{-1};\\
g_3(X_i^*; \beta_x) &= X_i^* \exp(\beta_x^{\mathrm{T}} X_i^*)\{M_i(\beta_x)\}^{-1}\\
&\quad - \exp(\beta_x^{\mathrm{T}} X_i^*)\{M_i(\beta_x)\}^{-2} \left\{\frac{\partial M_i(\beta_x)}{\partial \beta_x}\right\}.
\end{aligned}
$$

If the error terms e_{il} in model (4.41) follow a normal distribution $N(0, \Sigma_e)$, where Σ_e is the covariance matrix with unknown (j,k) element α_{jk}, then

$$
M_i(\beta_x) = \exp\left(\frac{1}{2m_i}\beta_x^{\mathrm{T}} \Sigma_e \beta_x\right),
$$

and the parameters α_{jk} are estimated empirically from the replicates:

$$
\widehat{\alpha}_{jk} = \frac{1}{n}\sum_{i=1}^{n}\left\{\frac{1}{m_i - 1}\sum_{l=1}^{m_i}(X^*_{ijl} - \overline{X}^*_{ij+})(X^*_{ikl} - \overline{X}^*_{ik+})\right\}, \tag{4.42}
$$

where $j, k = 1, \ldots, p_x$.

When developing asymptotic properties for estimators $\widehat{\theta}$ and $\widehat{\phi}$, variability induced in estimating measurement error model parameters should be taken into account. Suppose α is the vector of parameters associated with the measurement error model and $\psi_i(\alpha)$ is a set of unbiased estimating functions of α contributed from subject i. For instance, in Example 4.6, α represents $(\alpha_{jk} : 1 \le j \le k \le p_x)^{\mathrm{T}}$, and $\psi_i(\alpha)$ is taken as $\{\psi_{ijk}(\alpha) : 1 \le j \le k \le p_x\}^{\mathrm{T}}$ where

$$
\psi_{ijk}(\alpha) = \alpha_{jk} - \frac{1}{m_i - 1}\sum_{l=1}^{m_i}(X^*_{ijl} - \overline{X}^*_{ij+})(X^*_{ikl} - \overline{X}^*_{ik+})
$$

for $1 \le j \le k \le p_x$.

Let $\zeta = (\phi, \theta^{\mathrm{T}})^{\mathrm{T}}$ and $\widehat{\zeta} = (\widehat{\phi}, \widehat{\theta}^{\mathrm{T}})^{\mathrm{T}}$. Define $U_i^*(\alpha, \zeta) = (U_{1i}^{*\mathrm{T}}(\alpha, \zeta), U_{2i}^{*\mathrm{T}}(\alpha, \zeta))^{\mathrm{T}}$ and

$$
Q_i^*(\alpha, \zeta) = U_i^*(\alpha, \zeta) - E\left(\frac{\partial U_i^*(\alpha, \zeta)}{\partial \alpha^{\mathrm{T}}}\right)\left\{E\left(\frac{\partial \psi_i(\alpha)}{\partial \alpha^{\mathrm{T}}}\right)\right\}^{-1}\psi_i(\alpha),
$$

where the dependence on α is explicitly spelled out in the notation. Applying the strategy outlined in §1.3.4 yields that, under regularity conditions, $\sqrt{n}(\widehat{\zeta} - \zeta)$ has an asymptotic multivariate normal distribution with mean 0 and covariance matrix $\Gamma^{-1}(\alpha, \zeta)\Sigma(\alpha, \zeta)\Gamma^{-1\mathrm{T}}(\alpha, \zeta)$, where $\Gamma(\alpha, \zeta) = E(\partial U_i^*(\alpha, \zeta)/\partial \zeta^{\mathrm{T}})$, $\Sigma(\alpha, \zeta) = E\{Q_i^*(\alpha, \zeta)Q_i^{*\mathrm{T}}(\alpha, \zeta)\}$, and the expectation is taken with respect to the model for the joint distribution of $\{\widetilde{N}_i, X_i^*, Z_i\}$.

4.7 An Example: rhDNase Data

In this section, we illustrate some of the preceding methods with the rhDNase data described in §2.7.2. We are interested in evaluating whether the treatment has the desired effect on reducing the incidence of exacerbations and how error-prone covariate FEV is associated with exacerbations. In the first analysis, we cast the data as coming from an event process whose event times are observed, i.e., we use the framework discussed in §4.4, where column B j in Table 2.2 records the event times for the jth exacerbation. Fig. 4.3 displays histograms of the number of exacerbations for the treatment and placebo groups. The "corrected" likelihood formulation in §4.4 is employed to conduct inference.

Next, we treat the data as interval count data where columns B j and E j in Table 2.2 represent the cut points b_{ij} for interval count data as defined in §4.1.3. We consider two model assumptions. First, we assume that the underlying process for the interval count data is a Poisson process, as in §4.5; estimating equations (4.32) are used for estimation. Second, we relax the Poisson distribution assumption and incorporate possible heterogeneity among subjects by introducing random effects, as modeled by (4.9); estimating equations (4.37) and (4.40) in §4.6 are used for estimation.

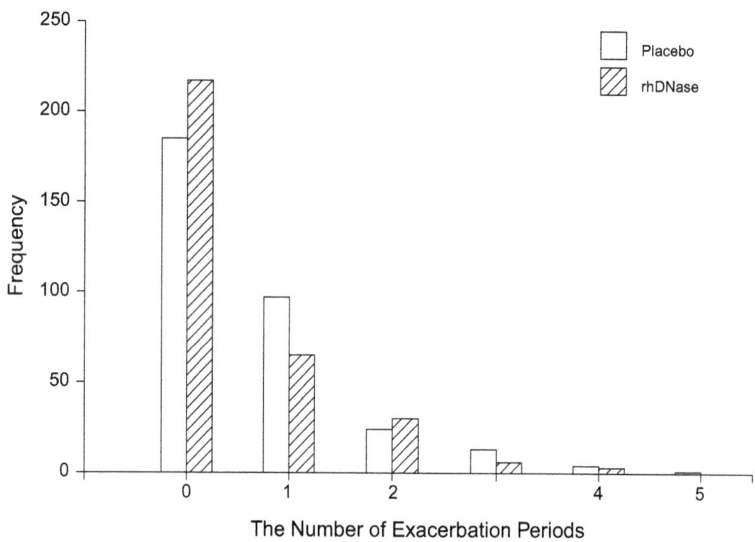

Fig. 4.3. *Back-to-Back Histogram of the Number of Exacerbations for the Treatment and Placebo Groups*

In all these analyses, we model the baseline intensity function with the piecewise-constant approach as described by (4.30). Specifically, we cut the study period into six pieces, yielding the subintervals (in days): (0, 28], (28, 56], (56, 84], (84, 112], (112, 140], and $(140, \infty)$.

The measurement error for covariate FEV is specified by model (4.41) with $e_{il} \sim N(0, \sigma_e^2)$ for $l = 1, 2$, where parameter σ_e is estimated from the repeated measurements FEV1 and FEV2 according to (4.42).

Table 4.1 reports the analysis results presented by Yi and Lawless (2012). Under different modeling strategies, all the analyses lead to very similar results regarding both point estimates and standard errors. Both the error-prone covariate FEV and the error-free covariate TRT are statistically significant, having anticipated effects on reducing the incidence of exacerbations. There is evidence that ϕ is statistically significant, suggesting the existence of heterogeneity among subjects.

Table 4.1. *Analyses of the rhDNase Data with Various Methods*

Method	Parameter	EST	SE	95% CI	p-value
Method of §4.4	FEV (β_x)	−0.017	0.003	(−0.022, −0.011)	<0.001
	TRT (β_z)	−0.274	0.121	(−0.511, −0.036)	0.024
Method of §4.5	FEV (β_x)	−0.016	0.004	(−0.024, −0.009)	<0.001
	TRT (β_z)	−0.266	0.126	(−0.514, −0.019)	0.035
Method of §4.6	FEV (β_x)	−0.016	0.003	(−0.022, −0.011)	<0.001
	TRT (β_z)	−0.266	0.120	(−0.501, −0.031)	0.026
	ϕ	0.401	0.130	(0.145, 0.656)	0.002

4.8 Bibliographic Notes and Discussion

Research concerning error-contaminated recurrent event data has been limited. Discussion of recurrent event data with covariate measurement error mostly focuses on count data. Little research has been directed to analysis of waiting times with error-prone covariates, although techniques of handling survival data with covariate measurement error can shed light on or even be directly applied.

Turnbull, Jiang and Clark (1997) considered the mixed Poisson process for count data subject to measurement error. They proposed a method of correcting measurement error effects by directly adjusting for the naive estimator obtained from ignoring measurement error. Jiang, Turnbull and Clark (1999) explored inference methods for events occurring in discrete time where covariates are subject to measurement error. Their approaches are developed under semiparametric Poisson and mixed Poisson models, which are summarized in §4.3.

Yi and Lawless (2012) explored methods which account for measurement error in covariates under a class of models, including general counting processes with multiplicative intensity functions and mixed Poisson models. They discussed likelihood-based inference and robust inference based on estimating equations and considered both continuous and interval-count data. Those methods are summarized in this chapter.

Other relevant work is available but limited. For instance, Veierød and Laake (2001) and Guo and Li (2002) investigated misclassification and covariate measurement error effects on Poisson regression. Zeger and Edelstein (1989) discussed a likelihood method for handling the Poisson regression model with covariate measurement error. Fung and Krewski (1999) empirically studied two adjustment methods, SIMEX and regression calibration algorithms, for Poisson regression with replicates of surrogate measurements for X_i. Assuming the availability of a validation subsample, Kim (2007) considered a mean model for the event count data and discussed a correction method using kernel estimates for the case with categorical surrogate measurements. Numerical studies were provided to assess the performance of this method whereas asymptotic properties for the resultant estimator were not explored.

4.9 Supplementary Problems

4.1. Prove the identity (4.1) and discuss associated conditions.

4.2. Prove Theorems 4.1 and 4.2.

(Cook and Lawless 2007, Ch. 2)

4.3. Suppose there is a random sample of n subjects who are observed over time intervals $[0, \tau_i]$ for $i = 1, \ldots, n$. Conditional on a nonnegative random effect u_i, $\{N_i(t) : t \geq 0\}$ is assumed to follow a nonhomogeneous Poisson process with mean function

$$\mu_i(t) = u_i \mu(t),$$

where $\mu(t)$ is a nonnegative function.

(a) Suppose that the u_i follow a Gamma distribution with the probability density function

$$f(u) = \frac{1}{\phi^{\phi^{-1}} \Gamma(\phi^{-1})} u^{\phi^{-1}-1} \exp(-u/\phi) \quad \text{for } u > 0, \tag{4.43}$$

where ϕ is a positive parameter. Show that the marginal distribution of $N_i(t)$ is a negative binomial distribution.

(b) Show that the marginal distribution of $N_i(t)$ becomes a Poisson distribution as $\phi \to 0$.

(c) Develop a procedure for testing the hypothesis $H_o : \phi = 0$.

(Cook and Lawless 2007, §2.2, §3.7)

4.4. (Test for *homogeneity* or *trend* for Poisson models) Suppose there is a random sample of n subjects who are observed over time intervals $[0, \tau_i]$ for $i = 1, \ldots, n$.

(a) Suppose that $\{N_i(t) : t \geq 0\}$ is characterized as the Poisson model with piecewise-constant rates, given by (4.2). We are interested in testing the null hypothesis

$$H_o : \rho_k = \rho \text{ for } k = 1, \ldots, K,$$

which corresponds to a homogeneous Poisson model. Here ρ is a given positive constant. Derive a test procedure for testing H_o.

(b) Suppose that $\{N_i(t) : t \geq 0\}$ is a Poisson process with a rate function

$$\lambda(t) = \exp(\rho_0 + \rho_1 t),$$

where ρ_0 and ρ_1 are parameters. Derive a test procedure for testing the null hypothesis $H_o : \rho_1 = 0$.

(Cook and Lawless 2007, Ch. 3)

4.5. (Test for *trend* or *homogeneity* for Poisson models in the presence of measurement error) Suppose there is a random sample of n subjects who are observed over time intervals $[0, \tau_i]$ for $i = 1, \ldots, n$ and subject i is observed at event times $0 < t_{i1} < \ldots < t_{in_i}$ for $i = 1, \ldots, n$. Let $N_i(t)$ be the number of events experienced by subject i over interval $[0, t]$, and $\{X_i, Z_i\}$ be the associated covariates. Suppose that conditional on $\{X_i, Z_i\}$, $\{N_i(t) : t \geq 0\}$ follows a Poisson process with intensity function

$$\lambda(t|X_i, Z_i) = \lambda_0(t) \exp(\beta_x^{\mathrm{T}} X_i + \beta_z^{\mathrm{T}} Z_i),$$

where $\lambda_0(t)$ is the baseline intensity function and β_x and β_z are regression coefficients.

(a) Suppose that for subject $i = 1, \ldots, n$, the observed data consist of $\{(N_i(t), X_i, Z_i) : t = t_{i1}, \ldots, t_{n_i}; i = 1, \ldots, n\}$. Using these observed data, derive a test procedure for the following hypothesis.

(i) Consider that $\lambda_0(t)$ is modeled as piecewise-constant rates, defined as (4.30). We are interested in testing the null hypothesis

$$H_o : \rho_k = \rho \text{ for } k = 1, \ldots, K,$$

where ρ is a given positive constant.

(ii) Consider that $\lambda_0(t)$ is modeled as

$$\lambda_0(t) = \exp(\rho_0 + \rho_1 t),$$

where ρ_0 and ρ_1 are parameters. We are interested in testing the null hypothesis $H_o : \rho_1 = 0$.

(b) Assume that the X_i are measured with error, and let X_i^* be the actual measurement of X_i. Based on the observed data $\{(N_i(t), X_i^*, Z_i) : t = t_{i1}, \ldots, t_{n_i}; i = 1, \ldots, n\}$, derive a test procedure for each null hypothesis in (a). What additional assumptions are needed in the development?

(c) Compare the test procedures between (a) and (b).

4.6. Let $\mu_i(t) = E\{N_i(t)|X_i, Z_i\}$ be the conditional mean function of the event process $\{N_i(t) : t \geq 0\}$, given covariates $\{X_i, Z_i\}$. Suppose that the mean function $\mu_i(t)$ is specified as a log-linear model:

$$\mu_i(t) = \mu_0(t) \exp(\beta_x^{\mathrm{T}} X_i + \beta_z^{\mathrm{T}} Z_i),$$

where $\mu_0(t)$ is the baseline mean function and β_x and β_z are parameters.

Suppose that X_i is subject to measurement error and X_i^* is the observed version of X_i. For the following situations, discuss the bias induced from the naive analysis where the difference between X_i and X_i^* is ignored.

(a) Assume that X_i is a binary covariate and the (mis)classification probabilities are

$$\pi_{01} = P(X_i^* = 1|X_i = 0, Z_i) \text{ and } \pi_{10} = P(X_i^* = 0|X_i = 1, Z_i).$$

(b) Assume that X_i is a scalar categorical covariate with K levels where $K \geq 3$ and that the (mis)classification probabilities are

$$\pi_{jk} = P(X_i^* = k|X_i = j, Z_i) \quad \text{for } j, k = 1, \ldots, K.$$

(c) Assume that X_i is a scalar categorical covariate with K levels where $K \geq 3$ and that the (mis)classification probabilities are

$$\pi_{jk}^* = P(X_i = k|X_i^* = j, Z_i) \quad \text{for } j, k = 1, \ldots, K.$$

(d) Generalize the discussion in (a)-(c) to the case where X_i is a vector of multiple binary or categorical variables.

(e) Discuss misclassification effects on the variance of the naive estimators in (a)–(d).

4.7. Suppose $(X_1, Z_1, N_1), \ldots, (X_n, Z_n, N_n)$ are independently and identically distributed. Let $\mu_i = E(N_i|X_i, Z_i)$ be the conditional mean of N_i given covariates X_i and Z_i. Consider a Poisson regression model with

$$N_i|(X_i, Z_i) \sim \text{Poisson}(\mu_i)$$

where the mean is modeled as

$$\log \mu_i = \beta_x^{\mathrm{T}} X_i + \beta_z^{\mathrm{T}} Z_i \tag{4.44}$$

with the vector of regression parameters $\beta = (\beta_x^{\mathrm{T}}, \beta_z^{\mathrm{T}})^{\mathrm{T}}$.

Suppose that X_i is subject to measurement error with a surrogate variable X_i^*. The measurement error is given as

$$X_i^* = X_i + e_i, \tag{4.45}$$

where e_i is independent of $\{X_i, Z_i, N_i\}$.

(a) Let $\ell_i(\beta; X_i, Z_i, N_i)$ be the log-likelihood function for β under model (4.44) contributed by subject i. Assume the error terms e_i in (4.45) follow a normal distribution $N(0, \Sigma_e)$ with covariance matrix Σ_e.

(i) Find a function $\ell_i^*(\beta; X_i^*, Z_i, N_i)$ of β and the observed data $\{X_i^*, Z_i, N_i\}$ such that

$$E\{\ell_i^*(\beta; X_i^*, Z_i, N_i)|X_i, Z_i, N_i\} = \ell_i(\beta; X_i, Z_i, N_i).$$

(ii) Let $\widehat{\beta}$ be the estimator of β obtained by maximizing

$$\sum_{i=1}^{n} \ell_i^*(\beta; X_i^*, Z_i, N_i)$$

with respect to β. Find the asymptotic distribution of the estimator $\widehat{\beta}$. What assumptions are needed?

(b) Assume that $e_i \sim Gamma(\kappa, \tau)$ with the probability density function

$$f(e) = \frac{1}{\Gamma(\kappa)\tau^\kappa} e^{\kappa-1} \exp\{-e/\tau\} \text{ for } e > 0,$$

and $X_i \sim Gamma(\delta, \tau)$ with the probability density function

$$f(x) = \frac{1}{\Gamma(\delta)\tau^\delta} x^{\delta-1} \exp\{-x/\tau\} \text{ for } x > 0,$$

where κ, δ and τ are positive parameters. Can you develop an estimation procedure for β using the likelihood method? What assumptions are needed?

(c) Suppose the measurement error model is not given by (4.45), but instead, is characterized by

$$X_i = X_i^* + e_i,$$

where e_i is independent of $\{X_i^*, Z_i, N_i\}$. Can the discussion in (a) and (b) be repeated?

4.8.

(a) Verify the identity (4.15).
(b) Verify the identities in (4.21).
(c) Prove Theorem 4.5.

4.9. Consider the model setup in §4.3. As opposed to the working model in §4.3, we consider another working model which is less naive in a sense that heterogeneity among subjects is not ignored. Specifically, we assume that conditional on random effects u_i and $\{R_i, X_i, X_i^*, Z_i\}$, the N_{ik} are independent and follow a Poisson distribution with mean $\mu_{uik}^* = E(N_{ik}|R_i, X_i^*, Z_i, u_i)$ which is modeled as

$$\mu_{uik}^* = R_{ik} u_i \lambda_k^* \exp(\beta_x^{*\mathrm{T}} X_{ik} + \beta_z^{*\mathrm{T}} Z_{ik}). \tag{4.46}$$

Here, adding an asterisk to each parameter indicates that the symbols may be possibly different from their counterparts in the true model (4.20). Furthermore, we assume that the u_i follow a Gamma distribution with the probability density function (4.43).

(a) Find the likelihood function obtained from this working model.
(b) Discuss the relationship between the estimators derived from the working model (4.46) and the true model (4.19).
(c) In contrast to the development in §4.3, can you use the *naive estimator correction strategy* to construct a consistent estimator of β by adjusting for the working estimator obtained from the working likelihood function in (a)?

4.10. In contrast to the interval count data which follow model (4.27) in §4.5, we consider the situation where interval count data are generated from an underlying nonhomogeneous Poisson process. Conditional on a nonnegative random effect u_i and the covariates, $\{N_i(t) : t \geq 0\}$ is assumed to follow a nonhomogeneous Poisson process with intensity function

$$\lambda_i(t|u_i, X_i, Z_i) = u_i \lambda_0(t) \exp(\beta_x^{\mathrm{T}} X_i + \beta_z^{\mathrm{T}} Z_i),$$

where the u_i are assumed to follow a Gamma distribution with the probability density function (4.43), $\lambda_0(t)$ is the baseline intensity function, and $\beta = (\beta_x^{\mathrm{T}}, \beta_z^{\mathrm{T}})^{\mathrm{T}}$ is the vector of regression parameters.

Suppose that X_i is subject to measurement error with repeatedly measured surrogate measurements X_{ij}^* for $j = 1, \ldots, m_i$, where m_i is a positive integer greater than 1. Assume that the X_{ij}^* are linked with the X_i by the model

$$X_{ij}^* = X_i + e_{ij},$$

where the e_{ij} are independent of each other and of $\{X_i, Z_i, N_i(t) : t \geq 0\}$ and $e_{ij} \sim N(0, \Sigma_e)$ with covariance matrix Σ_e.

(a) Develop the SIMEX procedure for conducting estimation of β.
(b) Develop an inferential procedure for β using the regression calibration method.
(c) Develop the EM algorithm for conducting estimation of β.
(d) Compare these inference procedures.
(e) Is it possible to develop an estimation procedure for β using the insertion correction method or the expectation correction method described in §2.5.2?
(f) Develop a test procedure for testing the null hypothesis

$$H_0 : \beta_x = 0.$$

4.11. Verify (4.36).

4.12.

(a) Verify that U_2 in (4.38) is an unbiased estimating function.
(b) Verify that U_2^* in (4.40) is an unbiased estimating function.

4.13. Consider the setup in §4.6.

(a) If the weight $w_{2i}(\phi, \theta, X_i, Z_i)$ in the estimating function (4.38) is set as one of the following forms, can you develop an estimating function for parameter ϕ ?
  (i) $w_{2i}(\phi, \theta, X_i, Z_i) = 1/\sigma_{i+}^2$;
  (ii) $w_{2i}(\phi, \theta, X_i, Z_i) = \mu_{i+}^2/\sigma_{i+}^4$.

(b) Relative to the estimating function in (4.40), discuss the asymptotic efficiency of each estimating function in (a).

(c) Pairing each estimating function in (a) with estimating function (4.37) for β, develop inference procedures for parameters β and ϕ. Compare the efficiency of the resultant estimators of β.

4.14. As in §4.1.1, for $i = 1, \ldots, n$ and $j = 2, 3, \ldots$, let $W_{ij} = T_{ij} - T_{i,j-1}$ be defined as the gap time between events $(j-1)$ and j for subject i. For subject i, let Z_i be a vector of precisely measured covariates, and X_i be a vector of error-prone covariates with an observed surrogate measurement X_i^*.

Let $Y_{ij} = \log W_{ij}$. Conditional on random effects u_i and covariates $\{X_i, Z_i\}$, the Y_{ij} are independent and follow the model

$$Y_{ij} = \beta_0 + \beta_x^{\mathrm{T}} X_i + \beta_z^{\mathrm{T}} Z_i + u_i + \epsilon_{ij}, \tag{4.47}$$

where $\beta = (\beta_0, \beta_x^{\mathrm{T}}, \beta_z^{\mathrm{T}})^{\mathrm{T}}$ is the parameter vector of interest; u_i has mean zero and variance σ_u^2; the ϵ_{ij} are independent of each other and of $\{X_i, Z_i, u_i\}$ and are identically distributed with mean 0 and variance σ^2.

Assume the nondifferential measurement error mechanism. Suppose the measurement error model is given by

$$X_i^* = X_i + e_i, \tag{4.48}$$

where the e_i are independent of $\{X_i, Z_i, u_i, \epsilon_{ij} : j = 2, 3, \ldots\}$ and have mean zero and covariance matrix Σ_e.

(a) Compute $E(Y_{ij}|X_i, Z_i)$, $\mathrm{var}(Y_{ij}|X_i, Z_i)$ and $\mathrm{cov}(Y_{ij}, Y_{i,j-k}|X_i, Z_i)$ for $k = 1, \ldots, j-1$; $j = 2, \ldots, n_i$, where n_i is the number of events experienced by subject i.

(b) Assume that ϵ_{ij}, u_i and e_i all follow normal distributions and that the conditional distribution of X_i, given Z_i, is a normal distribution with mean μ_x and covariance matrix Σ_x. Conduct likelihood inference about parameter β.

(c) Without the distributional assumptions in (b), can you construct unbiased estimating functions for estimation of parameter β?

4.15. In Problem 4.14, suppose measurement error model (4.48) is not true, but X_i is a scalar binary variable with a surrogate measurement X_i^*. Let

$$\pi_{01} = P(X_i^* = 1|X_i = 0, Z_i) \text{ and } \pi_{10} = P(X_i^* = 0|X_i = 1, Z_i)$$

be the (mis)classification probabilities.

(a) Can you construct unbiased estimating functions for estimation of parameter β?

(b) McGilchrist and Aisbett (1991) and Cook and Lawless (2007, p. 157) discussed the recurrent event data, given in Table 4.2. The data consist of the recurrence times to infection at point of insertion of the catheter for kidney patients using a portable dialysis equipment. For each patient the first two gap times to infection are given; either of them may be censored (1=infection occurs; 0=censored) because catheters were sometimes removed for reasons other than infection. Precisely measured covariates Z include age (in year) and sex (1=male; 2=female); and misclassification-prone covariate X is the type of kidney disease, coded as 0 if GN or AN and 1 otherwise. Assuming a sequence of plausible values of the misclassification probabilities, conduct sensitivity analyses of the data using the method developed in (a).

4.16. In Problem 4.14, suppose the response model is not (4.47), but is given as follows. Conditional on $\{X_i, Z_i\}$,

$$Y_{i1} = \beta_0 + \beta_x^{\mathrm{T}} X_i + \beta_z^{\mathrm{T}} Z_i + \epsilon_{i1};$$

and for $j = 2, \ldots, n_i$, conditional on $\{\mathcal{H}_{ij}^{\mathrm{Y}}, X_i, Z_i\}$,

$$Y_{ij} = \beta_0 + \beta_x^{\mathrm{T}} X_i + \beta_z^{\mathrm{T}} Z_i + \beta_y Y_{i,j-1} + \epsilon_{ij};$$

where $\mathcal{H}_{ij}^{\mathrm{Y}} = \{Y_{i1}, \ldots, Y_{i,j-1}\}$ for $j = 2, \ldots, n_i$, $\beta = (\beta_0, \beta_x^{\mathrm{T}}, \beta_z^{\mathrm{T}}, \beta_y)^{\mathrm{T}}$ is the parameter vector of interest, and the ϵ_{ij} are independent and identically distributed with mean 0 and variance σ^2 for $j = 1, \ldots, n_i$.

Assume that the nondifferential measurement error mechanism holds, and that the measurement error model is specified as (4.48).

(a) Can you compute $E(Y_{ij}|X_i, Z_i)$, $\text{var}(Y_{ij}|X_i, Z_i)$ and $\text{cov}(Y_{ij}, Y_{i,j-k}| X_i, Z_i)$ for $k = 1, \ldots, j-1$ and $j = 2, \ldots, n_i$?

(b) Assume that ϵ_{ij} follows a normal distribution $N(0, \sigma^2)$ with variance σ^2, e_i has a normal distribution $N(0, \Sigma_e)$ with covariance matrix Σ_e, and the conditional distribution of X_i given Z_i is a normal distribution with mean μ_x and covariance matrix Σ_x. Conduct likelihood inference on parameter β.

(c) Without distributional assumptions in (b), can you construct an unbiased estimating function for estimation of parameter β?

(d) Can the development in (b) or (c) be extended to the case with time-dependent covariates $X_i(t)$? Discuss potential issues.
(e) Use the developed methods to analyze the rhDNase data described in §2.7.2.

4.17. Consider the zero-inflated Poisson model defined in §4.1.3 (on page 160).
(a) Verify (4.6).
(b) Suppose that X_i is subject to measurement error, and let X_i^* be its observed measurement. Assume that the nondifferential measurement error mechanism holds. Suppose that the measurement error model assumes the same form as (4.48), where e_i is independent of $\{X_i, Z_i, u_i, N_i(t) : t \geq 0\}$ and follows a normal distribution with mean zero and covariance matrix Σ_e.
(i) Develop an EM algorithm for estimation of parameters β_x, β_z and $\widetilde{\pi}$.
(ii) Can you develop an estimation procedure using the estimating equations approach?
(iii) Repeat the development in (i) and (ii) for the case where X_i is a binary covariate.

4.18. For $i = 1, \ldots, n$, suppose individual i experiences two event processes $\{N_{i1}(t) : t \geq 0\}$ and $\{N_{i2}(t) : t \geq 0\}$. Let $0 \leq t_{ij1} < t_{ij2} < \ldots < t_{ijn_{ij}}$ denote the event times for process $N_{ij}(t)$ where $j = 1, 2$. Let X_i and Z_i be the covariates for subject i where $i = 1, \ldots, n$.

Suppose that conditional on a nonnegative random effect u_i, processes $\{N_{i1}(t) : t \geq 0\}$ and $\{N_{i2}(t) : t \geq 0\}$ are independent and, respectively, follow nonhomogeneous Poisson processes with the mean functions

$$\mu_{i1}(t) = u_i \mu_{01}(t) \exp(\beta_{x1}^{\mathrm{T}} X_i + \beta_{z1}^{\mathrm{T}} Z_i)$$

and

$$\mu_{i2}(t) = u_i \mu_{02}(t) \exp(\beta_{x2}^{\mathrm{T}} X_i + \beta_{z2}^{\mathrm{T}} Z_i),$$

where for $j = 1, 2$, $\beta_j = (\beta_{xj}^{\mathrm{T}}, \beta_{zj}^{\mathrm{T}})^{\mathrm{T}}$ is the vector of coefficients, and $\mu_{0j}(t)$ is the baseline mean function which is modeled with the piecewise-constant approach. Suppose that u_i follows a Gamma distribution with the probability density function (4.43).

Suppose that X_i is subject to measurement error with a surrogate variable X_i^*. Assume that the nondifferential measurement error mechanism holds. Suppose that the measurement error model assumes the same form as (4.48), where e_i is independent of $\{X_i, Z_i, u_i, N_{i1}(t), N_{i2}(t) : t \geq 0\}$ and follows a normal distribution with mean zero and covariance matrix Σ_e. Assume that Σ_e is known.

(a) Find the likelihood function of $\beta = (\beta_1^{\mathrm{T}}, \beta_2^{\mathrm{T}})^{\mathrm{T}}$, using the measurements of $\{X_i, Z_i\}$ and $\{N_{ij}(t) : j = 1, 2;\ t = t_{ij1}, \ldots, t_{ijn_{ij}}\}$.
(b) Can you use the likelihood function in (a) to develop a "corrected" likelihood for β based on the measurements of $\{X_i^*, Z_i\}$ and $\{N_{ij}(t) : j = 1, 2; t = t_{ij1}, \ldots, t_{ijn_{ij}}\}$?

(c) Applying the induced likelihood method outlined in §2.5.1, derive the likelihood function based on the observed measurements of $\{X_i^*, Z_i\}$ and $\{N_{ij}(t) : j = 1, 2;\ t = t_{ij1}, \ldots, t_{ijn_{ij}}\}$. What assumptions do you need?
(d) Can you develop a robust estimation method for β?
(e) Can you proceed with (a)–(d) by treating the baseline functions nonparametrically?
(f) Repeat the foregoing discussion for the case where Σ_e is unknown and a validation sample is available.

Table 4.2. *Infection Data of Kidney Patients*

Patient number	Gap times	Event types	Age	Sex	Disease type
1	8, 16	1, 1	28	1	1
2	23, 13	1, 0	48	2	0
3	22, 28	1, 1	32	1	1
4	447, 318	1, 1	31–32	2	1
5	30, 12	1, 1	10	1	1
6	24, 245	1, 1	16–17	2	1
7	7, 9	1, 1	51	1	0
8	511, 30	1, 1	55–56	2	0
9	53, 196	1, 1	69	2	0
10	15, 154	1, 1	51–52	1	0
11	7, 333	1, 1	44	2	0
12	141, 8	1, 0	34	2	1
13	96, 38	1, 1	35	2	0
14	149, 70	0, 0	42	2	0
15	536, 25	1, 0	17	2	1
16	17, 4	1, 0	60	1	0
17	185, 177	1, 1	60	2	1
18	292, 114	1, 1	43–44	2	1
19	22, 159	0, 0	53	2	0
20	15, 108	1, 0	44	2	1
21	152, 562	1, 1	46–47	1	1
22	402, 24	1, 0	30	2	1
23	13, 66	1, 1	62–63	2	0
24	39, 46	1, 0	42–43	2	0
25	12, 40	1, 1	43	1	0
26	113, 201	0, 1	57 58	2	0
27	132, 156	1, 1	10	2	0
28	34, 30	1, 1	52	2	0
29	2, 25	1, 1	53	1	0
30	130, 26	1, 1	54	2	0
31	27, 58	1, 1	56	2	0
32	5, 43	0, 1	50–51	2	0
33	152, 30	1, 1	57	2	1
34	190, 5	1, 0	44–45	2	0
35	119, 8	1, 1	22	2	1
36	54, 16	0, 0	42	2	1
37	6, 78	0, 1	52	2	1
38	63, 8	1, 0	60	1	1

5

Longitudinal Data with Covariate Measurement Error

Longitudinal studies are routinely conducted in various fields, including epidemiology, health research, and clinical trials. A variety of modeling and inference approaches are available for longitudinal data analysis. The validity of these methods relies on an important requirement that variables are precisely measured. This assumption is, however, often violated in practice.

This chapter highlights methods for handling longitudinal data with covariate measurement error. We begin this chapter with a brief review of the modeling framework and analysis schemes which are used in the error-free context for longitudinal data analysis. Illustrations of measurement error effects are then presented to stress the necessity and importance of accommodating measurement error in the analysis. Inference methods dealing with error-prone longitudinal data are described in subsequent sections. Bibliographic notes and discussion, together with supplementary problems, conclude this chapter.

5.1 Error-Free Inference Frameworks

Longitudinal studies are useful for examining the change of time-dependent response variables and their relationships with relevant covariates. They are often designed to collect measurements for subjects in the study repeatedly over a time period. Two features make longitudinal data analysis different from the analysis of univariate independent data. As each individual in the study contributes a set of repeated measurements on the outcome variable (together with possibly repeated covariate measurements), addressing the association among response components may become necessary. On the other hand, observation times may be associated with the response process, thus may come into play when formulating models and estimation procedures.

Suppose subject i is assessed at time points $0 \leq t_{i1} < \ldots < t_{im_i}$ for $i = 1, \ldots, n$. Let $Y_i(t_{ij})$ be the response measurement for subject i at time t_{ij},

G. Y. Yi, *Statistical Analysis with Measurement Error or Misclassification*, Springer Series in Statistics, DOI 10.1007/978-1-4939-6640-0_5

and $X_i(t_{ij})$ and $Z_i(t_{ij})$ be the associated covariates. Let $A_i = (t_{i1}, \ldots, t_{im_i})^{\mathrm{T}}$, $Y_i = \{Y_i(t_{i1}), \ldots, Y_i(t_{im_i})\}^{\mathrm{T}}$, $X_i = \{X_i^{\mathrm{T}}(t_{i1}), \ldots, X_i^{\mathrm{T}}(t_{im_i})\}^{\mathrm{T}}$, and $Z_i = \{Z_i^{\mathrm{T}}(t_{i1}), \ldots, Z_i^{\mathrm{T}}(t_{im_i})\}^{\mathrm{T}}$.

Covariates may be time-dependent or time-independent. If covariates, say $X_i(t_{ij})$, are time-independent, we write $X_i(t_{ij}) = X_i$. The number m_i of observation times may be the same or different across subjects. Both equally spaced and irregularly occurring observation times are allowed. If time gaps are not an issue, we often use simplified notation, such as $Y_{ij} = Y_i(t_{ij})$, $X_{ij} = X_i(t_{ij})$, and $Z_{ij} = Z_i(t_{ij})$, to indicate the longitudinal response and covariates; otherwise, explicit dependence on time point, i.e., $Y_i(t_{ij})$, $X_i(t_{ij})$, and $Z_i(t_{ij})$, is preferred.

We now briefly outline some modeling frameworks in regard to the treatment of the observation process and defer elaboration on accounting for the association of response components to the following subsections.

In principle, valid inferences should originate from the consideration of all the relevant variables involved. Let $h(y_i, x_i, z_i, a_i)$ be the joint distribution of $\{Y_i, X_i, Z_i, A_i\}$ that governs the data collection and observation processes. One may view $h(y_i, x_i, z_i, a_i)$ by separating the observation process from the response and covariate processes using the factorization

$$h(y_i, x_i, z_i, a_i) = h(a_i | y_i, x_i, z_i) h(y_i, x_i, z_i),$$

where $h(y_i, x_i, z_i)$ stands for the joint distribution for the data generation process of $\{Y_i, X_i, Z_i\}$, and $h(a_i | y_i, x_i, z_i)$ represents the conditional distribution for the observation process given the data.

This decomposition enables the joint distribution $h(y_i, x_i, z_i)$ to be explicitly spelled out, and allows us to make assumptions about the observation process to simplify modeling and inference procedures. In many settings, the observation process is assumed to be *noninformative* in the sense that it is independent of the response and covariate processes without carrying information about $h(y_i, x_i, z_i)$. Under this inspection scheme, inference procedures is developed by modeling the response and covariate processes while ignoring the observation process.

Specifically, inference on $h(y_i, x_i, z_i)$ can be carried out based on the factorization

$$f(y_i, x_i, z_i; \beta, \alpha) = f(y_i | x_i, z_i; \beta) f(x_i, z_i; \alpha), \tag{5.1}$$

where $f(y_i, x_i, z_i; \beta, \alpha)$ represents the model for $h(y_i, x_i, z_i)$ which is formulated through the conditional model $f(y_i | x_i, z_i; \beta)$ for Y_i given $\{X_i, Z_i\}$, and the marginal model $f(x_i, z_i; \alpha)$ for $\{X_i, Z_i\}$. Conventionally, the models for the response and covariate processes are assumed to be governed by distinct parameters, say, β and α. As a result, if interest centers on β, conditional analysis based on model $f(y_i | x_i, z_i; \beta)$ alone is performed.

The noninformative observational process assumption is reasonable in many applications. For example, in observational studies, observation times of individual measurements are often not determined by the outcome of patients' measurements. In many longitudinal studies, assessment times are pre-specified for all subjects in the study, thus, they are independent of the response and covariate processes.

In other circumstances, assessment times may be related to the measurements of the variables. To examine the joint stochastic process $h(y_i, x_i, z_i, a_i)$, alternative perspectives of (5.1) are required and modeling of the inspection times is often needed. For example, if Z_i is a vector of time-invariant covariates which determines the observation process, one may consider the factorization

$$h(y_i, x_i, z_i, a_i) = h(y_i, x_i | z_i, a_i) h(a_i | z_i) h(z_i), \tag{5.2}$$

where $h(y_i, x_i | z_i, a_i)$ represents the conditional distribution of $\{Y_i, X_i\}$ given $\{Z_i, A_i\}$, $h(a_i | z_i)$ is the conditional distribution of A_i given Z_i, and $h(z_i)$ is the marginal distribution of Z_i. Based on (5.2), modeling of the response and covariate processes may be introduced together with modeling of the inspection process.

Formulations (5.1) and (5.2) provide two examples of frameworks for handling longitudinal data. In this chapter, our development is embedded in the framework (5.1) where the observation process is not modeled and the conditional model $f(y_i | x_i, z_i; \beta)$ is employed to describe the conditional distribution of Y_i given $\{X_i, Z_i\}$.

When introducing conditional model $f(y_i | x_i, z_i; \beta)$, one needs to deal with the association among the components of Y_i. While a multivariate distribution may be directly specified as $f(y_i | x_i, z_i; \beta)$ (e.g., a multivariate normal distribution may be employed for continuous random vector Y_i), three modeling strategies are commonly used in the literature, leading to the three class of models, called *marginal models*, *random effects models*, and *transition models*, respectively. The first two types of models are discussed in this section, whereas transition models are deferred to Chapter 6. Comprehensive discussions on modeling and analysis of longitudinal data can be found in Davidian and Giltinan (1995), Diggle et al. (2002), Skrondal and Rabe-Hesketh (2004), Molenberghs and Verbeke (2005), Fitzmaurice et al. (2009), and the references therein.

5.1.1 Estimating Functions Based on Mean Structure

Marginal models are useful when we are interested in inference on quantities at the population-level, such as population mean or variance. For $i = 1, \ldots, n$ and $j = 1, \ldots, m_i$, let $\mu_{ij} = \mathrm{E}(Y_{ij} | X_{ij}, Z_{ij})$ and $v_{ij} = \mathrm{var}(Y_{ij} | X_{ij}, Z_{ij})$ be the conditional expectation and variance of Y_{ij}, respectively, given the subject-time-specific covariates X_{ij} and Z_{ij}.

We model the influence of the covariates on the marginal response mean using a regression model

$$g(\mu_{ij}) = \beta_0 + \beta_x^{\mathrm{T}} X_{ij} + \beta_z^{\mathrm{T}} Z_{ij}, \tag{5.3}$$

where $\beta = (\beta_0, \beta_x^{\mathrm{T}}, \beta_z^{\mathrm{T}})^{\mathrm{T}}$ is the vector of regression parameters which is of prime interest, and $g(\cdot)$ is a specified monotone function.

Frequently, the conditional variance v_{ij} is assumed to be a function of μ_{ij} with $v_{ij} = k(\mu_{ij}; \phi)$, where $k(\cdot)$ is a specified function and ϕ is the dispersion or scale parameter that is known or to be estimated. For instance, with binary data, ϕ is taken as 1 and $v_{ij} = \mu_{ij}(1 - \mu_{ij})$.

Model (5.3) is called a *marginal mean* or *population-average* model. The regression parameter β is interpreted as the changes in the transformed mean response of the study population as the covariates change by a unit vector.

With the only assumptions on mean and variance structures, the GEE method is the most natural to be used to perform estimation of β, as outlined in §1.3.2. For $i = 1, \ldots, n$, let $\mu_i = (\mu_{i1}, \ldots, \mu_{im_i})^{\mathrm{T}}$, and $D_i = \partial \mu_i^{\mathrm{T}}/\partial \beta$ be the matrix of the derivatives of the mean vector μ_i with respect to β. Let V_i be the conditional covariance matrix of Y_i, given $\{X_i, Z_i\}$.

Define

$$U_i(\beta) = D_i V_i^{-1}(Y_i - \mu_i). \tag{5.4}$$

Then solve

$$\sum_{i=1}^{n} U_i(\beta) = 0 \tag{5.5}$$

for β. Let $\widehat{\beta}$ denote the resulting estimator. By the unbiasedness of $U_i(\beta)$, estimator $\widehat{\beta}$ is a consistent estimator of β and $\sqrt{n}(\widehat{\beta}-\beta)$ is asymptotically normally distributed with mean 0 and covariance matrix

$$\left\{E\left(\frac{\partial U_i(\beta)}{\partial \beta^{\mathrm{T}}}\right)\right\}^{-1} E\{U_i(\beta)U_i^{\mathrm{T}}(\beta)\} \left\{E\left(\frac{\partial U_i(\beta)}{\partial \beta^{\mathrm{T}}}\right)\right\}^{-1\mathrm{T}},$$

provided regularity conditions. In implementation of solving (5.5), covariance matrix V_i is often decomposed as $V_i = B_i^{1/2} C_i B_i^{1/2}$, where C_i is the correlation matrix of Y_i given $\{X_i, Z_i\}$, and $B_i = \mathrm{diag}\{v_{ij} : j = 1, \ldots, m_i\}$ for which

$$\mathrm{var}(Y_{ij}|X_i, Z_i) = \mathrm{var}(Y_{ij}|X_{ij}, Z_{ij}) \tag{5.6}$$

is implicitly assumed. In application, correlation matrix C_i is often replaced with a working matrix.

Although there is no universal agreement on choosing a suitable working matrix for C_i, common choices are roughly classified into several categories by their temporal features. For example, setting C_i as an identity matrix leads to the *independence* working matrix; specifying all the diagonal elements to be 1 and off-diagonal elements to be a common constant for C_i results in the *exchangeable* working matrix. In both matrices, the association among repeated response components is regarded as time-invariant. To feature time-dependent association among response components, an *autoregressive* working matrix may be used for C_i, where for instance, the (j, k) element of C_i is set as $\rho^{|j-k|}$, and ρ is a parameter. Sometimes, an *unstructured* working matrix is adopted for C_i where the elements of C_i are treated as distinct parameters. Cautious notes on the specification of the working matrix were provided by Crowder (1995). Statistical software packages, such as *PROC GENMOD* in SAS and *gee* in R, are available for the implementation of the GEE method.

It is important to note that the validity of the GEE method is ensured by the two conditions: (1) the correct specification of the mean structure (5.3), and (2) the "independence" assumption that

$$\mathrm{E}(Y_{ij}|X_i, Z_i) = \mathrm{E}(Y_{ij}|X_{ij}, Z_{ij})$$

if the working matrix for C_i is not diagonal.

Condition (2) may be viewed as the price paid for not fully specifying the distribution of the response vector when performing inference about the model parameter. This assumption implies that at a time point, the dependence of the response mean on the subject-level covariates $\{X_i, Z_i\}$ is completely reflected by the subject-time-specific covariates $\{X_{ij}, Z_{ij}\}$, which is effectively the same as that given $\{X_{ij}, Z_{ij}\}$, the mean of Y_{ij} is independent of $\{X_{ik}, Z_{ik}\}$ for $j \neq k$. This assumption was discussed by Pepe and Anderson (1994), Pepe and Couper (1997), and Lai and Small (2007) (e.g., see Problem 5.1).

When the feasibility of condition (2) is in doubt, two strategies may help. One scheme is to use the working independence matrix to replace V_i in (5.4), which always ensures consistent estimation as stated in Problem 5.1 (although this does not guarantee ideal efficiency). Alternatively, one may directly model $E(Y_{ij}|X_i, Z_i)$ and $\mathrm{var}(Y_{ij}|X_i, Z_i)$, rather than $E(Y_{ij}|X_{ij}, Z_{ij})$ and $\mathrm{var}(Y_{ij}|X_{ij}, Z_{ij})$. That is, we redefine μ_{ij} to be $E(Y_{ij}|X_i, Z_i)$ and v_{ij} to be $\mathrm{var}(Y_{ij}|X_i, Z_i)$, then we modify model (5.3) by extending *subject-time-specific* covariates to the *subject-specific* covariates over the entire observation course. Formulation (5.4) then carries through.

The GEE approach is attractive because modeling the full distribution of the response vector Y_i is not needed; only the first two moments of the response vector are required to be modeled. When Y_i follows a multivariate normal distribution, $U_i(\beta)$ formulated by (5.4) is identical to the score function derived from the likelihood formulation, hence we have the identities

$$E\{U_i(\beta)\} = 0 \tag{5.7}$$

and

$$E\{U_i(\beta)U_i^{\mathrm{T}}(\beta)\} = E\left\{-\frac{\partial U_i(\beta)}{\partial \beta^{\mathrm{T}}}\right\}, \tag{5.8}$$

which are analogous to (1.4) and (1.5) in §1.3.1.

For general cases, estimating function $U_i(\beta)$ formulated by (5.4) still satisfies these two identities if V_i is the true covariance matrix of Y_i given $\{X_i, Z_i\}$. When V_i is misspecified or replaced by a working matrix, say V_i^*, then the resulting estimating function, say $U_i^*(\beta)$, does not satisfy the second identity (5.8), and efficiency loss may incur for estimation of the mean parameter. To improve the efficiency in this instance, Qu, Lindsay and Li (2000) proposed a method based on *quadratic inference functions*; their method does not involve direct estimation of the correlation parameter and retains certain optimality even if the working correlation structure is misspecified.

When V_i is replaced by a working matrix V_i^* in the formulation of (5.4) (regardless of the assumption (5.6)), as long as Conditions (1) and (2) for the GEE method are satisfied, the first identity (5.7) still holds for $U_i^*(\beta)$ with $E\{U_i^*(\beta)\} = 0$. This implies that under regularity conditions, the consistency of the resulting estimator is retained regardless of the validity of (5.8); this property has been widely used in application.

Although primary interest frequently lies in making inference about the parameters in regression models for marginal means, sometimes we are interested in inference about association parameters as well. In this instance, second-order GEEs are usually constructed for estimation of association parameters. Many authors exploited using two sets of GEEs for inference about the mean and association parameters; see Prentice (1988), Liang, Zeger and Qaqish (1992), Yi and Cook (2002), Hardin and Hilbe (2012), and the references therein. A brief account of this method is covered in §8.7.1.

5.1.2 Generalized Linear Mixed Models

In contrast to the average change at the *population*-level described by (5.3) for each time point, one may be interested in specific features at the *subject*-level. Heterogeneity among subjects is a concern. This feature is commonly described by means of introducing random effects into usually specified population-level models, such as *generalized linear models* (GLMs) (McCullagh and Nelder 1989) or nonlinear regression models (Wu 2009). Consequently, this, respectively, leads to *generalized linear mixed models* (GLMMs) and *nonlinear mixed models*, the two useful classes of *random effects models*. We discuss GLMMs in this subsection and defer nonlinear mixed models to the next subsection.

GLMMs are formulated via a two-stage modeling procedure. At Stage 1, assume that conditional on random effects u_i as well as covariates $\{X_i, Z_i\}$, the Y_{ij} are independent and modeled by a distribution of the exponential family with the probability density or mass function

$$f(y_{ij}|u_i, x_i, z_i; \xi_{ij}, \phi) = \exp\left\{\frac{y_{ij}\xi_{ij} - b(\xi_{ij})}{a(\phi)} + c(y_{ij}; \phi)\right\}, \tag{5.9}$$

where $a(\cdot)$, $b(\cdot)$, and $c(\cdot)$ are known functions and ϕ is the dispersion parameter.

It is noted that

$$E(Y_{ij}|u_i, X_i, Z_i) = b'(\xi_{ij}) \text{ and } \mathrm{var}(Y_{ij}|u_i, X_i, Z_i) = a(\phi)b''(\xi_{ij}),$$

where $b'(\cdot)$ and $b''(\cdot)$ represent the first and second derivatives of $b(\cdot)$, respectively. Parameter ξ_{ij}, sometimes called the *canonical* or *natural* parameter, is further modeled to facilitate within-subject variability via covariates, as described at the next stage.

At Stage 2, postulate the conditional mean $\mu_{uij} = E(Y_{ij}|u_i, X_i, Z_i)$ by

$$g(\mu_{uij}) = \beta_0 + \beta_x^{\mathrm{T}} X_{ij} + \beta_z^{\mathrm{T}} Z_{ij} + u_i^{\mathrm{T}} F_{ij}, \tag{5.10}$$

where $g(\cdot)$ is a link function and $\beta = (\beta_0, \beta_x^{\mathrm{T}}, \beta_z^{\mathrm{T}})^{\mathrm{T}}$ is the vector of regression parameters. Quantity F_{ij} takes a certain form to reflect the study design or is a covariate vector that may be part of $\{X_i, Z_i\}$. Random effects u_i are assumed to be independent of $\{X_i, Z_i\}$ and their distributions are modeled as $f(u_i; \gamma)$ with γ denoting the associated parameters. Often, a multivariate normal distribution $N(0, D(\gamma))$ is assumed for random effects u_i, where $D(\gamma)$ is the covariance matrix with a vector γ of parameters; the elements of γ are sometimes called *variance components*.

As opposed to the name of *random effects* for u_i, components of β are called *fixed effects* or *fixed covariate effects*. This β has a different interpretation from β in the marginal mean model (5.3). Parameter β in the conditional model (5.10) describes the transformed mean response change for an *individual* as covariates change by a unit vector, while β in the marginal mean model (5.3) represents the average change of the transformed *population* mean as covariates change by a unit vector. These two changes are generally different, as mathematically suggested by the inequality

$$E(Y_{ij}|u_i, X_i, Z_i) \neq E(Y_{ij}|X_i, Z_i).$$

Let $\theta = (\beta^{\mathrm{T}}, \gamma^{\mathrm{T}})^{\mathrm{T}}$. Inference on parameter θ proceeds based on the marginal likelihood with random effects integrated out. The marginal likelihood contributed from subject i is

$$L_i = \int \prod_{j=1}^{m_i} f(y_{ij}|u_i, x_i, z_i) f(u_i) d\eta(u_i), \tag{5.11}$$

where $f(u_i)$ is the model for the probability density or mass function of u_i, $f(y_{ij}|u_i, x_i, z_i)$ is determined by (5.9) in conjunction with (5.10), and the model parameter is supposed in the notation.

In special situations, such as when both the conditional distribution of the response components and the marginal distribution of random effects are normal, the marginal likelihood (5.11) may have a closed form. The maximum likelihood method is then directly implemented. In situations where the integrals in (5.11) have no analytical expressions, numerical algorithms, such as the Monte Carlo method, Gaussian quadratures, or Laplace approximations, are routinely used to handle the integrals in (5.11). For details, see Jiang (2007), Wu (2009), Halimi (2009), and Stroup (2012).

We conclude this subsection with comments on the role of random effects u_i. In postulating model (5.10), the assumption that

$$E(Y_{ij}|u_i, X_i, Z_i) = E(Y_{ij}|u_i, X_{ij}, Z_{ij})$$

is implicitly made.

In the formulation of (5.11), the conditional independence of the Y_{ij} given u_i and $\{X_i, Z_i\}$ allows us to simply use the product

$$\prod_{j=1}^{m_i} f(y_{ij}|u_i, x_i, z_i)$$

to compute the conditional probability density or mass function $f(y_i|u_i, x_i, z_i)$ for the entire response vector Y_i, given u_i and $\{X_i, Z_i\}$. This assumption implies that the association among repeated response components Y_{ij} is fully responsible by subject-level random effects u_i when covariates $\{X_i, Z_i\}$ are controlled.

Other ways of using random effects to characterize the response and covariate processes and their association are also possible. For instance, one may introduce random effects, say v_i, to facilitate the dependence among the $\{Y_{ij}, X_{ij}, Z_{ij}\}$. Conditional on random effects v_i, the $\{Y_{ij}, X_{ij}, Z_{ij}\}$ are assumed to be independent for $j = 1, \ldots, m_i$. Then the marginal likelihood contributed from subject i is written as

$$L_i = \int \prod_{j=1}^{m_i} f(y_{ij}, x_{ij}, z_{ij} | v_i) f(v_i) d\eta(v_i),$$

where $f(v_i)$ is the model for the probability density or mass function of v_i, and $f(y_{ij}, x_{ij}, z_{ij}|v_i)$ is the model for the conditional distribution of $\{Y_{ij}, X_{ij}, Z_{ij}\}$ given v_i. Quantity $f(y_{ij}, x_{ij}, z_{ij}|v_i)$ is further factorized as

$$f(y_{ij}, x_{ij}, z_{ij}|v_i) = f(y_{ij}|x_{ij}, z_{ij}, v_i) f(x_{ij}, z_{ij}|v_i)$$

so that available models may be used for $f(y_{ij}|x_{ij}, z_{ij}, v_i)$ and $f(x_{ij}, z_{ij}|v_i)$.

5.1.3 Nonlinear Mixed Models

When the objective aims at making inference about individuals rather than the target population, GLMMs offer a useful modeling framework in which the regression parameters typically appear in a linear form in the transformed response mean model. With more liberal specification of function forms, *nonlinear mixed models* provide a flexible venue to accommodate more complex nonlinearity relationships. Aligning with the formulation of GLMMs, nonlinear mixed models are developed through two stages, featuring *intra-individual* variability and *inter-individual* variability, respectively.

At Stage 1, an *intra-individual* model, often formed as a nonlinear regression model, is used to characterize the mean and covariance structure of the response over time for each individual. Let ξ_i represent individual-specific regression parameters for $i = 1, \ldots, n$. Given ξ_i, the response components Y_{ij} assume the model

$$Y_{ij} = g(X_{ij}, Z_{ij}; \xi_i) + \sigma k\{g(X_{ij}, Z_{ij}; \xi_i); \theta\}\epsilon_{ij}, \tag{5.12}$$

where error terms ϵ_{ij} are independent of $\{X_{ij}, Z_{ij}\}$ and have mean 0 and variance 1. Functions $g(\cdot)$ and $k(\cdot)$ are smooth functions which are user-specified to feature different types of data. Although functions $g(\cdot)$ and $k(\cdot)$ are common for all individual responses, differences among individual longitudinal trajectories are facilitated by different regression parameters ξ_i and the covariates at the subject-time-specific level. Constant parameters σ and θ, called *intra-individual variance parameters*, are assumed to reflect the belief that the pattern of within-individual variation is comparable across individuals (Wang and Davidian 1996).

Model (5.12) implies that the intra-individual mean and variance are

$$E(Y_{ij}|\xi_i, X_{ij}, Z_{ij}) = g(X_{ij}, Z_{ij}; \xi_i)$$

and

$$\text{var}(Y_{ij}|\xi_i, X_{ij}, Z_{ij}) = \sigma^2 k^2\{g(X_{ij}, Z_{ij}; \xi_i); \theta\}$$

for $j = 1, \ldots, m_i$. Common models for the intra-individual variance include $k(g;\theta) = 1$ and the power model $k(g;\theta) = g^\theta$.

Let

$$G(X_i, Z_i; \xi_i) = \{g(X_{i1}, Z_{i1}; \xi_i), \ldots, g(X_{im_i}, Z_{im_i}; \xi_i)\}^{\mathrm{T}},$$

$$K\{X_i, Z_i; \xi_i; \theta\} = \mathrm{diag}(k\{g(X_{i1}, Z_{i1}; \xi_i); \theta\}, \ldots, k\{g(X_{im_i}, Z_{im_i}; \xi_i); \theta\}),$$

and $\epsilon_i = (\epsilon_{i1}, \ldots, \epsilon_{im_i})^{\mathrm{T}}$. Model (5.12) is then expressed in the vector form

$$Y_i = G(X_i, Z_i; \xi_i) + \sigma K\{X_i, Z_i; \xi_i; \theta\}\epsilon_i, \tag{5.13}$$

Random vectors ϵ_i are frequently assumed to have a multivariate normal distribution $N(0, V_i)$ with covariance matrix V_i. Although the dimension of V_i is $m_i \times m_i$, which is subject-dependent, covariance matrices V_i are often assumed to contain common parameters for $i = 1, \ldots, n$. Unlike the first stage of formulating GLMMs which imposes conditional independence on response components Y_{ij}, here covariance matrix V_i does not have to be diagonal; the ϵ_{ij} in (5.12) are not necessarily assumed to be independent of each other (Fitzmaurice et al. 2009, Ch. 2).

At Stage 2, an *inter-individual model* is postulated to describe individual-specific regression parameters ξ_i via

$$\xi_i = d(X_i, Z_i, u_i; \beta), \tag{5.14}$$

where $d(\cdot)$ is a specified vector-valued function, β is the parameter representing fixed effects, and the u_i represent random effects which are assumed to be independent of the ϵ_i, X_i and Z_i. Often, the u_i are assumed to follow a multivariate normal distribution with mean 0 and covariance matrix Σ_u, although other ramifications of this choice are available (e.g., Fitzmaurice et al. 2009, Ch. 6).

In addition to inference about parameters σ and θ, it is of principal interest to carry out inference about β and Σ_u. Inference on Σ_u addresses random inter-individual variation, while parameter β facilitates variation in ξ_i explained by the covariates. Interpretation of β is *subject-specific*, just like that of the fixed effects in GLMMs. Subject-specific parameters ξ_i are allowed to be either linear or nonlinear functions of fixed effects β as well as the covariates. The marginal mean response does not have a closed-form expression in general.

Inference about the model parameters is based on the marginal distribution for the response vector Y_i:

$$f(y_i|x_i, z_i) = \int f(y_i|x_i, z_i, u_i) f(u_i) d\eta(u_i),$$

where $i = 1, \ldots, n$; $f(y_i|x_i, z_i, u_i)$ is the model for the conditional distribution of Y_i, given $\{X_i, Z_i, u_i\}$, determined by models (5.13) and (5.14); and $f(u_i)$ is the model for the distribution of random effects u_i. The dependence on the parameters is suppressed in the notation.

Although inference about the model parameters is often of central interest, predications or estimates of random effects may be needed, especially when there is interest in predication of subject-specific evolutions. Inference for the random effects is usually based on their posterior distribution

$$f(u_i|y_i, x_i, z_i) = \frac{f(y_i|x_i, z_i, u_i)f(u_i)}{\int f(y_i|x_i, z_i, u_i)f(u_i)d\eta(u_i)},$$

where the mean of the posterior distribution of u_i is used as estimates for u_i. Such estimates are called *empirical Bayes estimates* of random effects u_i.

5.2 Measurement Error Effects

Measurement error has multiple effects on statistical inference. It may alter the estimates of the response model parameters, distort the association structure among response components, change the dependence nature between response and covariate variables, and more generally, vary the distributional form of the response vector. Broadly speaking, the impact of measurement error varies with a number of factors, including the model form for the response and measurement error processes, and it depends on the nature of an inference method as well. In this section, we investigate these issues under different situations to unveil the complex nature of measurement error effects.

5.2.1 Marginal Analysis Based on GEE with Independence Working Matrix

We examine the marginal setup given in §5.1.1 with the assessment times taken as common. That is, the sample includes n individuals who are scheduled to have m visits. At visit j, measurements on the variables $\{Y_{ij}, X_{ij}, Z_{ij}\}$ are collected, where Y_{ij} is the response variable, Z_{ij} is the vector of precisely observed covariates, and X_{ij} is the vector of covariates which are not exactly measured but their surrogates X_{ij}^* are gathered. Let $Y_i = (Y_{i1}, \ldots, Y_{im})^{\mathrm{T}}$, $X_i = (X_{i1}^{\mathrm{T}}, \ldots, X_{im}^{\mathrm{T}})^{\mathrm{T}}$, $Z_i = (Z_{i1}^{\mathrm{T}}, \ldots, Z_{im}^{\mathrm{T}})^{\mathrm{T}}$, and $X_i^* = (X_{i1}^{*\mathrm{T}}, \ldots, X_{im}^{*\mathrm{T}})^{\mathrm{T}}$.

Consider regression model (5.3) which postulates the population mean at each time point as a function of subject-time-specific covariates.

As discussed in §5.1.1, in the absence of measurement error, it is conventional to assume that $E(Y_{ij}|X_i, Z_i) = E(Y_{ij}|X_{ij}, Z_{ij})$, which is ensured if Y_{ij} is independent of $\{X_{ik}, Z_{ik}\}$ for $j \neq k$, given $\{X_{ij}, Z_{ij}\}$; such covariates are called *Type I covariates* by Lai and Small (2007). However, in the presence of measurement error, the property of Type I covariates may be lost for the observed covariates, as illustrated in the following example.

Example 5.1. Suppose that the response model is given by

$$Y_{ij} = \beta X_{ij} + \epsilon_{ij}$$

for $j = 1, \ldots, m$, where $\epsilon_i = (\epsilon_{i1}, \ldots, \epsilon_{im})^{\mathrm{T}}$ follows a normal distribution $N(0, \Sigma)$ with a diagonal covariance matrix Σ and ϵ_i is independent of X_i. Then the Type I assumption holds for the regression mean of Y_{ij} on X_i:

$$E(Y_{ij}|X_i) = E(Y_{ij}|X_{ij}) \text{ for } j = 1, \ldots, m.$$

Suppose further that $X_i \sim N(0, I_m)$ and that

$$X_i^* = X_i + e_i,$$

where $e_i \sim N(0, \Sigma_e)$ with covariance matrix Σ_e and e_i is independent of X_i and ϵ_i.

Then, as long as Σ_e is not diagonal and $\beta \neq 0$, the Type I covariates property fails for the observed data (see Problem 5.2), i.e.,

$$E(Y_{ij}|X_i^*) \neq E(Y_{ij}|X_{ij}^*).$$

This example demonstrates that the Type I independence structure of the response on the true covariates can be destroyed when the true covariates are replaced with their surrogate measurements.

Next, we examine measurement error effects on estimation of the response parameters. When X_i is subject to measurement error and unobservable, naively applying estimating equation (5.5) with X_i replaced by surrogates X_i^* often leads to biased estimates. To quantify asymptotic biases of the naive method, one may apply the arguments discussed in §1.4.

Let $U_i^*(\beta^*)$ be the surrogate version of estimating function $U_i(\beta)$ in (5.4) with X_i replaced by X_i^* and β replaced by β^*, where symbol β^* is used to show regression coefficients are possibly different from the original parameter β in model (5.3) when using the replacement X_i^* for X_i.

Solving

$$\sum_{i=1}^{n} U_i^*(\beta^*) = 0$$

for β^* gives a naive estimator, denoted by $\widehat{\beta}^*$, of the model parameter β. Estimator $\widehat{\beta}^*$ is not necessarily a consistent estimator of β. Instead, $\widehat{\beta}^*$ converges in probability to a limit which is the solution to

$$E\{U_i^*(\beta^*)\} = 0, \tag{5.15}$$

where the expectation, typically depending on β, is taken under the response model together with the measurement error model.

The relationship between β^* and β, portrayed by (5.15), is generally not expressed in an analytically closed-form. Under special situations, however, working with (5.15) can shed light on the measurement error effects on estimation.

As discussed in §5.1.1, to ensure the validity of the GEE method, the Type I covariates assumption is required if the working matrix for V_i is not an independence working matrix. The Type I covariates assumption, as illustrated by Example 5.1, may break down for the model linking Y_i and $\{X_i^*, Z_i\}$. To narrow down the discussion on measurement error effects on estimation, we then consider a simple estimation scenario where the Type I covariates assumption is not needed, and we estimate the response parameters using estimating equation (5.5) with covariance matrix V_i replaced by the independence working matrix $\text{diag}\{v_{ij} : j = 1, \ldots, m\}$. The details are given in the following example.

Example 5.2. Suppose that the response model is given by model (5.3) with $g(\cdot)$ set as an identity function and that X_{ij} and Z_{ij} are scalar:

$$Y_{ij} = \beta_0 + \beta_x X_{ij} + \beta_z Z_{ij} + \epsilon_{ij} \tag{5.16}$$

for $j = 1, \ldots, m$, where the ϵ_{ij} are independent of each other and of $\{X_{ij}, Z_{ij}\}$ and have mean 0 and a constant variance σ^2.

Under this model and using the independence working matrix to replace V_i, estimating function (5.4) becomes

$$\left(\frac{\partial \mu_i^{\mathrm{T}}}{\partial \beta}\right) B_i^{-1}(Y_i - \mu_i),$$

where $B_i = \mathrm{diag}\{\sigma^2, \ldots, \sigma^2\}$ is an $m \times m$ matrix, $\mu_i = (\mu_{i1}, \ldots, \mu_{im})^{\mathrm{T}}$, and $\mu_{ij} = \beta_0 + \beta_x X_{ij} + \beta_z Z_{ij}$ for $j = 1, \ldots, m$.

Since B_i is a diagonal matrix with diagonal elements being a common constant, then solving equation (5.15) is equivalent to solving

$$\sum_{j=1}^{m} E\left\{\left(\frac{\partial \mu_{ij}^*}{\partial \beta^*}\right)(Y_{ij} - \mu_{ij}^*)\right\} = 0, \tag{5.17}$$

where the expectation is taken with respect to the model $f(y_{ij}, x_{ij}, z_{ij}, x_{ij}^*)$ for the joint distribution of $\{Y_{ij}, X_{ij}, Z_{ij}, X_{ij}^*\}$, and μ_{ij}^* is the surrogate version of μ_{ij} with X_{ij} replaced by X_{ij}^* and β replaced by β^*.

Assume that the measurement error model is given by

$$X_{ij}^* = X_{ij} + e_{ij} \tag{5.18}$$

for $j = 1, \ldots, m$, where the e_{ij} are independent of each other and of $\{X_{ij}, Z_{ij}, \epsilon_{ij}\}$ and have mean 0 and a common variance σ_e^2.

By the given modeling format, we evaluate the expectation in (5.17) by a sequence of expectations with respect to the conditional models $f(x_{ij}^*|y_{ij}, x_{ij}, z_{ij})$ and $f(y_{ij}|x_{ij}, z_{ij})$ together with the marginal model $f(x_{ij}, z_{ij})$. As a result, (5.17) gives

$$(\beta_x - \beta_x^*)\sum_{j=1}^{m} E(X_{ij}) + (\beta_z - \beta_z^*)\sum_{j=1}^{m} E(Z_{ij}) + (\beta_0 - \beta_0^*) = 0;$$

$$(\beta_x - \beta_x^*)\sum_{j=1}^{m} E(X_{ij}^2) + (\beta_z - \beta_z^*)\sum_{j=1}^{m} E(X_{ij}Z_{ij}) + (\beta_0 - \beta_0^*)\sum_{j=1}^{m} E(X_{ij}) - m\beta_x^*\sigma_e^2 = 0;$$

$$(\beta_x - \beta_x^*)\sum_{j=1}^{m} E(X_{ij}Z_{ij}) + (\beta_z - \beta_z^*)\sum_{j=1}^{m} E(Z_{ij}^2) + (\beta_0 - \beta_0^*)\sum_{j=1}^{m} E(Z_{ij}) = 0;$$

where the expectations are evaluated under the marginal model $f(x_{ij}, z_{ij})$ for the distribution of covariates $\{X_{ij}, Z_{ij}\}$.

For ease of notation, let $\mu_{xz} = \sum_{j=1}^{m} E(X_{ij}Z_{ij})$, $\mu_{xk} = \sum_{j=1}^{m} E(X_{ij}^k)$, and $\mu_{zk} = \sum_{j=1}^{m} E(Z_{ij}^k)$ for $k = 1, 2$. Define

$$\begin{aligned}
\Delta_0 &= \mu_{x2}\mu_{z2} - \mu_{xz}^2 - \mu_{x2}\mu_{z1}^2 - \mu_{x1}^2\mu_{z2} + 2\mu_{xz}\mu_{x1}\mu_{z2};\\
R_x &= 1 + m\sigma_e^2(\mu_{z2} - \mu_{z1}^2)/\Delta_0;\\
R_z &= m\sigma_e^2(\mu_{xz} - \mu_{x1}\mu_{z1})/\Delta_0;\\
R_0 &= m\sigma_e^2(\mu_{x1}\mu_{z2} - \mu_{xz}\mu_{z1})/\Delta_0;
\end{aligned}$$

then solving the preceding equations yields

$$\beta_x^* = R_x^{-1}\beta_x,\ \beta_z^* = \beta_z + R_z R_x^{-1}\beta_x,\ \text{and}\ \beta_0^* = \beta_0 + R_0 R_x^{-1}\beta_x. \tag{5.19}$$

Identities in (5.19) quantify the difference between β^* and β and demonstrate that asymptotic biases incurred in the naive estimator $\widehat{\beta}^*$ depend on the magnitude σ_e^2 of measurement error and the mean and variance of X_{ij} and Z_{ij} as well as the correlation between X_{ij} and Z_{ij}. The number of longitudinal assessments also affects the asymptotic biases. In a special situation where X_i and Z_i are uncorrelated and both X_{ij} and Z_{ij} have zero mean, we have

$$\begin{aligned}
\beta_x^* &= \left\{\frac{\sum_{j=1}^m \operatorname{var}(X_{ij})}{\sum_{j=1}^m \operatorname{var}(X_{ij}) + m\sigma_e^2}\right\}\beta_x;\\
\beta_z^* &= \beta_z;\\
\beta_0^* &= \beta_0.
\end{aligned}$$

When the relationship between the surrogate measurement X_{ij}^* and the true covariate X_{ij} is modeled differently, asymptotic biases induced in the naive estimation may be different (see Problem 5.4).

5.2.2 Mixed Effects Models

Bias analysis is complex when the response process is characterized via a multiple stage of modeling. For instance, if the response process is determined by a random effects model, then measurement error effects induced by replacing X_i with X_i^* may not be as transparent as those in the marginal analysis discussed in §5.2.1.

To understand how measurement error may alter structures of mixed effects models, we consider the response model which is formulated by a two-stage modeling procedure outlined in §5.1.2. Conditional on random effects u_i and covariates $\{X_i, Z_i\}$, the Y_{ij} are assumed to be independent. This conditional independence allows us to use the product of the $f(y_{ij}|x_i, z_i, u_i)$ to express the conditional model for Y_i given $\{u_i, X_i, Z_i\}$, thus leading to the conditional model (5.11) for Y_i given $\{X_i, Z_i\}$.

In §5.2.1, we examine measurement error effects on point estimation when a marginal method is employed. Here we are concerned about the impact of ignoring the difference between X_i^* and X_i on changing the model structures. Let $f(y_{ij}|x_i, z_i)$ be the model for the conditional distribution of Y_{ij} given $\{X_i, Z_i\}$, where the dependence on parameters is suppressed in the notation. We are interested in the following questions which are pertinent to the *marginal* and *association* features of the response components:

- Does replacing X_i with X_i^* alter the *mean structure* of $f(y_{ij}|x_i, z_i)$? That is, do $E(Y_{ij}|X_i^*, Z_i)$ and $E(Y_{ij}|X_i, Z_i)$ have the same structure?
- Does replacing X_i with X_i^* change the *variance structure* of $f(y_{ij}|x_i, z_i)$? That is, do $\mathrm{var}(Y_{ij}|X_i^*, Z_i)$ and $\mathrm{var}(Y_{ij}|X_i, Z_i)$ have the same structure?
- Given random effects u_i, does replacing X_i with X_i^* change the *conditional independence* among the Y_{ij}? That is, conditioning on the observed covariates $\{X_i^*, Z_i\}$ and random effects u_i, are the Y_{ij} still independent?
- More generally, can the conditional distribution of Y_i given $\{X_i^*, Z_i\}$ be modeled through the same *two-stage procedure* as that of Y_i given $\{X_i, Z_i\}$ with certain random effects introduced?

To answer these questions, we consider a linear mixed model where X_{ij}, Z_{ij} and random effects u_i all are scalar. Conditional on random effects u_i and covariates $\{X_i, Z_i\}$, the Y_{ij} are independent and modeled as

$$Y_{ij} = \beta_0 + \beta_x X_{ij} + \beta_z Z_{ij} + u_i F_{ij} + \epsilon_{ij}, \tag{5.20}$$

where the ϵ_{ij} are independent of each other and of the $\{X_{ij}, Z_j, u_i\}$ and normally distributed with mean 0 and variance σ^2; the u_i are random effects with mean 0 and variance σ_u^2 and are independent of the $\{X_{ij}, Z_{ij}, \epsilon_{ij}\}$; and F_{ij} is an error-free scalar which features different types of random effects.

This model implicitly assumes that $f(y_{ij}|x_i, z_i, u_i) = f(y_{ij}|x_{ij}, z_{ij}, u_i)$, where $f(y_{ij}|x_{ij}, z_{ij}, u_i)$ represents the model for the conditional distribution of Y_{ij} given $\{X_{ij}, Z_{ij}, u_i\}$. Equivalently, model (5.20) is written in the vector form

$$Y_i = B_0 + B_x X_i + B_z Z_i + u_i F_i + \epsilon_i, \tag{5.21}$$

where $B_0 = \beta_0 1_{m_i}$, $B_x = \beta_x I_{m_i}$, $B_z = \beta_z I_{m_i}$, $F_i = (F_{i1}, \ldots, F_{im_i})^{\mathrm{T}}$, and $\epsilon_i = (\epsilon_{i1}, \ldots, \epsilon_{im_i})^{\mathrm{T}}$. Conditional independence of the Y_{ij}, given $\{X_i, Z_i, u_i\}$, is reflected by the diagonal form of the covariance matrix $\mathrm{var}(\epsilon_i) = \sigma^2 I_{m_i}$.

By model (5.21), we obtain the conditional mean and variance of Y_i, given $\{X_i, Z_i\}$:

$$E(Y_i|X_i, Z_i) = \beta_0 1_{m_i} + \beta_x X_i + \beta_z Z_i \tag{5.22}$$

and

$$\mathrm{var}(Y_i|X_i, Z_i) = \sigma_u^2 F_i F_i^{\mathrm{T}} + \sigma^2 I_{m_i}. \tag{5.23}$$

Assume that the measurement error process is featured by an additive model

$$X_i^* = X_i + e_i,$$

where e_i has mean 0 and covariance matrix Σ_{ei} and is independent of random variables in model (5.20). Assume that X_i has covariance matrix Σ_{xi}.

Quantities Σ_{ei} and Σ_{xi} depend on i through the dimension m_i while unknown parameters in those quantities are assumed free of i. Let

$$\Omega_i = \Sigma_{xi}\{\Sigma_{xi} + \Sigma_{ei}\}^{-1},$$

where the inverse matrix is assumed to exist. Matrix Ω_i is sometimes called the *reliability matrix*.

If we further impose a normality assumption for e_i, X_i and u_i, then by the result in Problem 5.5 (c)(iii), the conditional model of Y_i, given the observed covariates $\{X_i^*, Z_i\}$ and random effects u_i, is

$$Y_i = B_0^* + B_x^* X_i^* + B_z^* Z_i + u_i F_i + \epsilon_i^*, \tag{5.24}$$

where $\{B_0^*, B_x^*, B_z^*\}$ and $\{\beta_0, \beta_x, \beta_z\}$ are connected by

$$\begin{aligned} B_0^* &= \beta_0 1_{m_i} + \beta_x (I_{m_i} - \Omega_i)\mu_{xi}; \\ B_x^* &= \beta_x \Omega_i; \\ B_z^* &= \beta_z I_{m_i}; \end{aligned} \tag{5.25}$$

and ϵ_i^* has mean zero and covariance matrix

$$\text{var}(\epsilon_i^*) = \sigma^2 I_{m_i} + \beta_x^2 (I_{m_i} - \Omega_i)\Sigma_{xi}. \tag{5.26}$$

To compare the mean structure between models $f(y_i|x_i^*, z_i)$ and $f(y_i|x_i, z_i)$, we use the property

$$E(Y_i|X_i^*, Z_i) = E\{E(Y_i|X_i^*, Z_i, u_i)\}$$

and the assumption $E(u_i) = 0$, and then obtain that

$$E(Y_i|X_i^*, Z_i) = B_0^* + B_x^* X_i^* + B_z^* Z_i. \tag{5.27}$$

Comparing (5.27) to (5.22) and (5.25) shows that the changes in the conditional mean structure of Y_i, given $\{X_i^*, Z_i\}$, are reflected by the intercept B_0^* and coefficient B_x^* of the X_i^* but not by the coefficient of Z_i. The coefficients in model (5.21) are common for all the components of X_i, but the coefficients in model (5.24) vary with the components of X_i^*, which is affected by reliability matrix Ω_i.

Regarding the comparison of the variance structure between models $f(y_i|x_i^*, z_i)$ and $f(y_i|x_i, z_i)$, we apply the fact

$$\text{var}(Y_i|X_i^*, Z_i) = E\{\text{var}(Y_i|X_i^*, Z_i, u_i)\} + \text{var}\{E(Y_i|X_i^*, Z_i, u_i)\},$$

in combination with (5.24) and (5.26), and then comparing to (5.23) shows that $\text{var}(Y_i|X_i^*, Z_i)$ and $\text{var}(Y_i|X_i, Z_i)$ have different structures.

Comparing the covariance matrices of the error terms in (5.21) and (5.24) uncovers that the conditional independence property would disappear when X_i is replaced by its surrogate X_i^*, because the off-diagonal elements of $\text{var}(\epsilon_i^*)$ in (5.26) are not necessarily zero. The precise effect of the measurement error on the between- and within-subject variance structures is, however, not entirely clear by this comparison, because the same random effects u_i for the formulation of $f(y_i|x_i, z_i)$ are used as an intermediate step to examine model $f(y_i|x_i^*, z_i)$. In general, we are interested in whether or not there exist some random effects, say $\widetilde{u}_i$, which can, along with the observed covariates $\{X_i^*, Z_i\}$, completely capture the association among response components Y_{ij}.

To answer this question we further assume that X_i is modeled as

$$X_i = \vartheta_0 1_{m_i} + \vartheta_z Z_i + \epsilon_{xi},$$

where ϑ_0 and ϑ_z are scalar parameters, the ϵ_{xi} are independent of each other and of $\{Z_i, u_i, \epsilon_i, e_i\}$, and $\epsilon_{xi} \sim N(0, \Sigma_{xi})$ with covariance matrix Σ_{xi} which is identical to that of X_i.

By the normality assumption for both ϵ_{xi} and e_i, we obtain that

$$E(X_i|X_i^*, Z_i) = (I_{m_i} - \Omega_i)(\vartheta_0 1_{m_i} + \vartheta_z Z_i) + \Omega_i X_i^*.$$

Define

$$u_i^* = X_i - E(X_i|X_i^*, Z_i),$$

then

$$X_i = (I_{m_i} - \Omega_i) 1_{m_i} \vartheta_0 + (I_{m_i} - \Omega_i)\vartheta_z Z_i + \Omega_i X_i^* + u_i^*. \tag{5.28}$$

Furthermore, it can be shown that

$$\begin{aligned} u_i^* &= (I_{m_i} - \Omega_i)\epsilon_{xi} - \Omega_i e_i, \\ u_i^* &\sim N(0, (I_{m_i} - \Omega_i)\Sigma_{xi}), \end{aligned}$$

and u_i^* is independent of $\{X_i^*, Z_i\}$ and u_i (see Problem 5.7). Expression (5.28) indicates that for each j, the jth component of X_i can be written as

$$X_{ij} = \alpha_{0j} + \vartheta_z \alpha_{zj}^{\mathrm{T}} Z_i + \alpha_{x^*j}^{\mathrm{T}} X_i^* + C_{ij}^{\mathrm{T}} u_i^*, \tag{5.29}$$

where α_{0j} is the jth element of $(I_{m_i} - \Omega_i)1_{m_i}\vartheta_0$, α_{zj}^{T} is the jth row of $(I_{m_i} - \Omega_i)$, $\alpha_{x^*j}^{\mathrm{T}}$ is the jth row of Ω_i, and C_{ij}^{T} is the jth row of the identity matrix I_{m_i}.

Substituting (5.29) into (5.20) yields the conditional model of Y_{ij} given $\{X_i^*, Z_i, u_i, u_i^*\}$,

$$\begin{aligned} Y_{ij} = {} & (\beta_0 + \alpha_{0j}\beta_x) + \beta_x \alpha_{x^*j}^{\mathrm{T}} X_i^* + (\beta_z Z_{ij} + \beta_x \vartheta_z \alpha_{zj}^{\mathrm{T}} Z_i) \\ & + (u_i F_{ij} + \beta_x C_{ij}^{\mathrm{T}} u_i^*) + \epsilon_{ij}. \end{aligned} \tag{5.30}$$

As noted earlier, (5.24) shows that the conditional independence of the Y_{ij} breaks down if merely conditioning on the initial random effects u_i along with the observed covariates $\{X_i^*, Z_i\}$, because the covariance matrix of ϵ_i^* is not diagonal. This phenomenon is actually explained by the structure of (5.30). Expression (5.30) reveals that when replacing X_i with X_i^*, association among the Y_{ij} is not fully captured by the random effects u_i, the quantities which suffice for describing the association among the Y_{ij} when conditioned on $\{X_i, Z_i\}$; the residual u_i^* facilitates the association between X_i and X_i^*, thus containing the dependence structure of repeated response components Y_{ij} via covariates X_i. It is seen that if taking

$$\widetilde{u}_i = (u_i, u_i^{*\mathrm{T}})^{\mathrm{T}}$$

as new random effects, then the conditional independence of the Y_{ij} can be preserved, if conditioned on $\widetilde{u}_i$ and $\{X_i^*, Z_i\}$.

Moreover, comparison of (5.30) to (5.20) shows that ignoring the difference between X_i and X_i^* would result in misspecification of both the fixed-effects and random-effects structures. Model (5.20) shows that the conditional expectation $E(Y_{ij}|X_i, Z_i, u_i)$ merely depends on subject-time-specific covariates, while model (5.30) suggests that the expectation of Y_{ij}, conditional on $\{X_i^*, Z_i\}$ and random effects $\widetilde{u}_i$, does depend not only on subject-time-specific covariates X_{ij}^* and Z_{ij}, but also on subject-specific observations X_i^* and Z_i. If X_i and Z_i are independent (hence $\vartheta_z = 0$), then the naive analysis with X_i^* replacing X_i does not change the point estimates of the fixed effects for the Z_{ij} covariates. Random effects $\widetilde{u}_i$ in model (5.30) are determined by

$$\widetilde{u}_i \sim N\left(\begin{pmatrix} 0 \\ 0_{m_i} \end{pmatrix}, \begin{pmatrix} \sigma_u^2 & 0_{m_i}^{\mathrm{T}} \\ 0_{m_i} & (I_{m_i} - \Omega_i)\Sigma_{xi} \end{pmatrix}\right),$$

where variance components differ from variance component σ_u^2 for model (5.20). In addition, the cluster size m_i also plays a role in the change of the model structures when X_i is replaced with X_i^*.

5.3 Estimating Function Methods

Marginal analysis based on unbiased estimating functions is often conducted when inference interest lies in the population-average. The choice of a marginal analysis over a likelihood method may also be driven by the concerns of robustness to misspecification of a full distributional model and computational simplicity. Marginal analysis under measurement error models commonly comprises two basic steps. At the first step, an estimating function (frequently, unbiased) is built under the model linking the responses and the true covariates. At the second step, proper adjustments based on the measurement error model are introduced to modify the estimating function to be workable and valid.

While the first step is usually realized using standard marginal modeling schemes for error-free contexts, the second step embraces variability of different strategies of incorporating measurement error effects, which typically depends on the form of a measurement error model. In this section, we discuss two approaches concerning the second step, which are elaborations on the *expectation correction strategy* and the *insertion correction method* outlined in §2.5.2.

Suppose at the first step, the response model is given by the marginal model (5.3), and we construct an unbiased estimating function $U_i(\beta; Y_i, X_i, Z_i)$ using (5.4) where the dependence on $\{Y_i, X_i, Z_i\}$ is explicitly spelled out. The *expectation correction strategy* is to evaluate

$$E\{U_i(\beta; Y_i, X_i, Z_i)|Y_i, X_i^*, Z_i\}, \tag{5.31}$$

while the *insertion correction method* is to find a function, say $U_i^*(\beta; Y_i, X_i^*, Z_i)$, which is expressed in terms of the observed covariates $\{X_i^*, Z_i\}$ as well as response variable Y_i and parameter β, so that

$$E\{U_i^*(\beta; Y_i, X_i^*, Z_i)|Y_i, X_i, Z_i\} = U_i(\beta; Y_i, X_i, Z_i). \tag{5.32}$$

Then estimation of the response parameter β proceeds with solving

$$\sum_{i=1}^{n} U_i^*(\beta; Y_i, X_i^*, Z_i) = 0$$

for β, where $U_i^*(\beta; Y_i, X_i^*, Z_i)$ is either set as (5.31) or is determined by (5.32).

This procedure generally requires the knowledge of model $f(x_i|y_i, x_i^*, z_i)$ (or $f(x_i^*|y_i, x_i, z_i)$) for the distribution of the *entire* covariate vector X_i (or X_i^*), given other random variables. This information is, however, often not available when conducting a marginal analysis.

To get around this problem, we consider an alternative way to construct estimating functions. Instead of finding an unbiased estimating function at the *subject-specific* level jointly for $\{Y_i, X_i, Z_i\}$, we construct an estimating function, say $U_{ij}(\beta; y_{ij}, x_{ij}, z_{ij})$, at the *subject-time-specific* level for each time point j and each subject i. For example, with the marginal mean $\mu_{ij} = E(Y_{ij}|X_{ij}, Z_{ij})$ and variance $v_{ij} = \text{var}(Y_{ij}|X_{ij}, Z_{ij})$ given, it is natural to work with the estimating function of β:

$$U_{ij}(\beta; Y_{ij}, X_{ij}, Z_{ij}) = \left(\frac{\partial \mu_{ij}}{\partial \beta}\right) v_{ij}^{-1}(Y_{ij} - \mu_{ij}) \tag{5.33}$$

for $j = 1, \ldots, m_i$ and $i = 1, \ldots, n$. Then we use the expectation correction strategy or the insertion correction method to identify an estimating function $U_{ij}^*(\beta; y_{ij}, x_{ij}^*, z_{ij})$ at the subject-time-specific level for each time point j and each subject i. These methods normally require the knowledge of model $f(x_{ij}|y_{ij}, x_{ij}^*, z_{ij})$ (or $f(x_{ij}^*|y_{ij}, x_{ij}, z_{ij})$) for the distribution of X_{ij} (or X_{ij}^*), given other random variables at time j.

Consequently, estimation of β is based on the sequence of these functions $U_{ij}^*(\beta; y_{ij}, x_{ij}^*, z_{ij})$. The generalized method of moments, described in §1.3.3, is employed to combine those estimating functions to enhance efficiency. Let

$$U_i^*(\beta) = (U_{ij}^{*\text{T}}(\beta; Y_{ij}, X_{ij}^*, Z_{ij}), \ldots, U_{im_i}^{*\text{T}}(\beta; Y_{im_i}, X_{im_i}^*, Z_{im_i}))^{\text{T}},$$

and

$$U^*(\beta) = \frac{1}{n}\sum_{i=1}^{n} U_i^*(\beta).$$

Then a GMM estimator of β is obtained by minimizing $U^{*\text{T}}(\beta) W U^*(\beta)$, where W is a weight matrix. The asymptotically optimal weight matrix W is given by the inverse matrix of the covariance matrix of $U_i^*(\beta)$.

Alternatively, let $\Gamma = E\{(\partial/\partial\beta^{\text{T}})U_i^*(\beta)\}$, $\Sigma = E\{U_i^*(\beta)U_i^{\text{T}*}(\beta)\}$ and

$$U_i^{**}(\beta) = \Gamma^{\text{T}}\Sigma^{-1}U_i^*(\beta).$$

Under regular situations, the GMM estimator solves the estimating equation

$$\sum_{i=1}^{n} U_i^{**}(\beta) = 0 \tag{5.34}$$

for β.

It is noted that the form of $U_i^{**}(\beta)$ is also justified by Theorem 1.8. For the implementation of (5.34), Γ and Σ are usually replaced by their consistent estimates, given by $\widehat{\Gamma} = n^{-1}\sum_{i=1}^n (\partial/\partial\beta^{\mathrm{T}})U_i^*(\beta)$ and $\widehat{\Sigma} = n^{-1}\sum_{i=1}^n U_i^*(\beta)U_i^{*\mathrm{T}}(\beta)$, respectively. Set $\widehat{U}_i^{**}(\beta) = \widehat{\Gamma}^{\mathrm{T}}\widehat{\Sigma}^{-1}U_i^*(\beta)$. Then solving $\sum_{i=1}^n \widehat{U}_i^{**}(\beta) = 0$ for β leads to an estimator of β.

When applying the preceding strategies, unknown parameter, say α, associated with the measurement error model, is normally involved. To complete estimation of the response model parameter β that is of primary interest, we need to estimate parameter α using additional available data sources, such as validation data or replicates; the principles discussed in Chapter 3 may be applied for this purpose.

Depending on the nature of the modeling setup, one strategy might be easier to implement than the other. Generally speaking, the expectation correction strategy is implemented if there is a conditional distributional assumption on X_{ij} given $\{Y_{ij}, X_{ij}^*, Z_{ij}\}$. The insertion correction method, on the other hand, has the appeal in that the distribution of X_{ij} is often not modeled. This approach, however, does not necessarily suggest an easy scheme to construct $U_i^*(\beta)$, and in some situations, an analytical form for such an estimating function does not even exist.

In the following subsections, we elaborate on the construction of estimating function $U_{ij}^*(\beta; Y_{ij}, X_{ij}^*, Z_{ij})$ using the expectation correction or the insertion correction strategy.

5.3.1 Expected Estimating Equations

For each time point j and estimating function $U_{ij}(\beta; Y_{ij}, X_{ij}, Z_{ij})$, define

$$U_{ij}^* = E\{U_{ij}(\beta; Y_{ij}, X_{ij}, Z_{ij})|Y_{ij}, X_{ij}^*, Z_{ij}\}.$$

Evaluation of U_{ij}^* only requires model $f(x_{ij}|y_{ij}, x_{ij}^*, z_{ij})$ for the conditional distribution of X_{ij}, given $\{Y_{ij}, X_{ij}^*, Z_{ij}\}$. This considerably weakens the model assumptions, as opposed to calculating the conditional expectation in (5.31) which generally needs model $f(x_i|y_i, x_i^*, z_i)$ for the distribution of X_i, given $\{Y_i, X_i^*, Z_i\}$.

Under suitable conditions, the GMM estimator of β obtained by setting the weight matrix W to be Σ^{-1} is equivalent to solving (5.34). In a special case where W is set to be the unit matrix, the GMM estimator of β may be obtained by solving a modified version of (5.34) with $E(\partial U_{ij}^*/\partial\beta^{\mathrm{T}})$ dropped:

$$\sum_{i=1}^{n}\sum_{j=1}^{m_i} E\{U_{ij}(\beta; Y_{ij}, X_{ij}, Z_{ij})|Y_{ij}, X_{ij}^*, Z_{ij}\} = 0; \tag{5.35}$$

equation (5.35) was discussed by Wang and Pepe (2000).

Under the nondifferential measurement error mechanism, the kth element of $U_{ij}^*(\beta; Y_{ij}, X_{ij}, Z_{ij})$ is given by

$$\begin{aligned} &E\{U_{ijk}(\beta; Y_{ij}, X_{ij}, Z_{ij})|Y_{ij}, X_{ij}^*, Z_{ij}\} \\ &= \frac{\int U_{ijk}(\beta; Y_{ij}, x_{ij}, Z_{ij}) f(Y_{ij}|x_{ij}, Z_{ij}) f(x_{ij}, X_{ij}^*|Z_{ij}) d\eta(x_{ij})}{\int f(Y_{ij}|x_{ij}, Z_{ij}) f(x_{ij}, X_{ij}^*|Z_{ij}) d\eta(x_{ij})}, \end{aligned} \tag{5.36}$$

where $U_{ijk}(\beta; Y_{ij}, x_{ij}, Z_{ij})$ is the kth element of $U_{ij}(\beta; Y_{ij}, x_{ij}, Z_{ij})$ and $k = 1, \ldots, p$ with p being the dimension of β.

Depending on the form of the measurement error model, the model $f(x_{ij}, x_{ij}^*|z_{ij})$ in (5.36) for the joint distribution of $\{X_{ij}, X_{ij}^*\}$, given Z_{ij}, is further factorized as

$$f(x_{ij}, x_{ij}^*|z_{ij}) = f(x_{ij}|x_{ij}^*, z_{ij}) f(x_{ij}^*|z_{ij}) \tag{5.37}$$

or

$$f(x_{ij}, x_{ij}^*|z_{ij}) = f(x_{ij}^*|x_{ij}, z_{ij}) f(x_{ij}|z_{ij}). \tag{5.38}$$

Evaluation of (5.36) requires knowledge of the conditional distribution of the response component Y_{ij}, given the true covariates $\{X_{ij}, Z_{ij}\}$, and the measurement error process at each time point j. In special situations, this requirement may be relaxed to weaker conditions that are merely pertinent to the marginal structures of the response and measurement error processes, as illustrated by the following example.

Example 5.3. Suppose Y_{ij} is a binary variable and X_{ij} is scalar. Assume that each response component is marginally modeled by a logistic regression model

$$\text{logit}\, \mu_{ij} = \beta_0 + \beta_x X_{ij} + \beta_z^{\mathrm{T}} Z_{ij},$$

where $\mu_{ij} = E(Y_{ij}|X_{ij}, Z_{ij})$ and $\beta = (\beta_0, \beta_x, \beta_z^{\mathrm{T}})^{\mathrm{T}}$ is the vector of regression coefficients.

Consequently, the conditional variance $v_{ij} = \text{var}(Y_{ij}|X_{ij}, Z_{ij})$ equals $\mu_{ij}(1 - \mu_{ij})$, and the conditional model of Y_{ij}, given $\{X_{ij}, Z_{ij}\}$, is given by $f(y_{ij}|x_{ij}, z_{ij}) = \mu_{ij}^{y_{ij}}(1 - \mu_{ij})^{(1-y_{ij})}$. For each time point j, unbiased estimating function (5.33) becomes

$$U_{ij}(\beta; Y_{ij}, X_{ij}, Z_{ij}) = \begin{pmatrix} 1 \\ X_{ij} \\ Z_{ij} \end{pmatrix} (Y_{ij} - \mu_{ij}). \tag{5.39}$$

We consider two scenarios of measurement error in covariate X_{ij}. First, we examine the case where X_{ij} is continuous and the measurement error model is given by

$$X_{ij} = X_{ij}^* + e_{ij}$$

for $j = 1, \ldots, m_i$, where the e_{ij} are independent of each other and of $\{X_{ij}^*, Z_{ij}, Y_{ij}\}$ and $e_{ij} \sim N(0, \sigma_e^2)$ with variance σ_e^2. In this instance, using (5.36) in combination with (5.37), we may determine $U_{ij}^*(\beta; Y_{ij}, X_{ij}^*, Z_{ij})$.

Next, we consider the case where X_{ij} is a binary covariate with the misclassification probabilities

$$\pi_{01} = P(X_{ij}^* = 1|X_{ij} = 0, Z_{ij});\ \ \pi_{10} = P(X_{ij}^* = 0|X_{ij} = 1, Z_{ij});$$

and the marginal probability $\widetilde{\pi} = P(X_{ij} = 1|Z_{ij})$. In this case, using (5.36) in combination with (5.38) yields the construction of $U_{ij}^*(\beta; Y_{ij}, X_{ij}^*, Z_{ij})$.

5.3.2 Corrected Estimating Functions

The expectation correction approach discussed in §5.3.1 generally calls for distributional assumptions for the X_{ij}, which may be difficult to specify in application. Alternatively, we proceed with a correction approach which is functional-oriented in terms of its way of treating the X_{ij}. The idea is to construct an estimating function, say $U_{ij}^*(\beta; Y_{ij}, X_{ij}^*, Z_{ij})$, using the observed surrogate measurements X_{ij}^* together with other observed variables, such that

$$E\{U_{ij}^*(\beta; Y_{ij}, X_{ij}^*, Z_{ij})|Y_{ij}, X_{ij}, Z_{ij}\} = U_{ij}(\beta; Y_{ij}, X_{ij}, Z_{ij}). \tag{5.40}$$

The unbiasedness of $U_{ij}(\beta; Y_{ij}, X_{ij}, Z_{ij})$ under the initial model setup ensures unbiasedness of workable estimating function $U_{ij}^*(\beta; Y_{ij}, X_{ij}^*, Z_{ij})$.

This strategy is often used when the nondifferential measurement error mechanism is adopted and the conditional model $f(x_{ij}^*|x_{ij}, z_{ij})$ of X_{ij}^*, given $\{X_{ij}, Z_{ij}\}$, is specified to characterize the measurement error process. For instance, suppose that surrogate X_{ij}^* is given by

$$X_{ij}^* = X_{ij} + e_{ij} \tag{5.41}$$

for $j = 1, \ldots, m_i$, where the error terms e_{ij} have mean 0 and covariance matrix Σ_e and are independent of each other and of the $\{X_{ij}, Z_{ij}, Y_{ij}\}$.

If e_{ij} has a moment generating function $M(v) = E\{\exp(v^{\mathrm{T}} e_{ij})\}$ where v is a vector of real numbers, then the moment identities may be used to construct estimating function $U_{ij}^*(\beta; Y_{ij}, X_{ij}^*, Z_{ij})$ so that (5.40) is satisfied. In particular, for regression models where X_{ij} appears in an exponential or polynomial form, the following identities are useful:

$$E(X_{ij}^* X_{ij}^{*\mathrm{T}} - \Sigma_e|X_{ij}, Z_{ij}) = X_{ij} X_{ij}^{\mathrm{T}},$$

$$E[\{M(v)\}^{-1} \exp(v^{\mathrm{T}} X_{ij}^*)|X_{ij}, Z_{ij}] = \exp(v^{\mathrm{T}} X_{ij}),$$

and

$$E\left(\{M(v)\}^{-1}\left[X_{ij}^* - \{M(v)\}^{-1}\left\{\frac{dM(v)}{dv}\right\}\right]\exp(v^{\mathrm{T}} X_{ij}^*)\middle| X_{ij}, Z_{ij}\right)$$
$$= X_{ij}\exp(v^{\mathrm{T}} X_{ij}),$$

where $M(v)$ is assumed differentiable over a certain region. We illustrate this approach with the following examples where the measurement error model is given by (5.41).

Example 5.4. (*Linear Regression Models*)

Suppose a continuous response component Y_{ij} is modeled by the linear regression model

$$Y_{ij} = \mu_{ij} + \epsilon_{ij}$$

with

$$\mu_{ij} = \beta_0 + \beta_x^{\mathrm{T}} X_{ij} + \beta_z^{\mathrm{T}} Z_{ij}, \tag{5.42}$$

where ϵ_{ij} is a random error with mean 0 and variance σ^2 and $\beta = (\beta_0, \beta_x^{\mathrm{T}}, \beta_z^{\mathrm{T}})^{\mathrm{T}}$ is the vector of regression parameters.

For each time point j, taking (5.33) as an estimating function for β gives

$$U_{ij} = \frac{1}{\sigma^2}\begin{pmatrix} 1 \\ X_{ij} \\ Z_{ij} \end{pmatrix}(Y_{ij} - \mu_{ij}).$$

Let

$$\begin{aligned}
U^*_{ij\beta_0} &= (\sigma^2)^{-1}(Y_{ij} - \beta_0 - \beta_x^{\mathrm{T}} X^*_{ij} - \beta_z^{\mathrm{T}} Z_{ij}); \\
U^*_{ij\beta_x} &= (\sigma^2)^{-1}\left\{X^*_{ij} Y_{ij} - X^*_{ij}\beta_0 - (X^*_{ij} X^{*\mathrm{T}}_{ij} - \Sigma_e)\beta_x - X^*_{ij}\beta_z^{\mathrm{T}} Z_{ij}\right\}; \\
U^*_{ij\beta_z} &= (\sigma^2)^{-1} Z_{ij}(Y_{ij} - \beta_0 - \beta_x^{\mathrm{T}} X^*_{ij} - \beta_z^{\mathrm{T}} Z_{ij});
\end{aligned}$$

then $U^*_{ij} = (U^*_{ij\beta_0}, U^{*\mathrm{T}}_{ij\beta_x}, U^{*\mathrm{T}}_{ij\beta_z})^{\mathrm{T}}$ satisfies (5.40) and, thus, is an unbiased estimating function for β.

In constructing U^*_{ij} for linear regression models, we employ only the model for the conditional mean and variance of X^*_{ij} given $\{X_{ij}, Z_{ij}\}$; no model assumption for the full distribution of X^*_{ij} given $\{X_{ij}, Z_{ij}\}$ is needed. In addition, this marginal method does not require specific distributional assumption for the error term ϵ_{ij} in the response model (5.42).

Example 5.5. (*Log-Linear Models*)

Suppose the response component Y_{ij} records counts with the mean given by a log-linear model

$$\log \mu_{ij} = \beta_0 + \beta_x^{\mathrm{T}} X_{ij} + \beta_z^{\mathrm{T}} Z_{ij}$$

and variance $\mathrm{var}(Y_{ij}|X_{ij}, Z_{ij}) = \mu_{ij}$, where $\beta = (\beta_0, \beta_x^{\mathrm{T}}, \beta_z^{\mathrm{T}})^{\mathrm{T}}$ is the parameter vector. This framework accommodates Poisson distributions as a special case.

For each time point j, setting (5.33) as an estimating function gives

$$U_{ij} = \begin{pmatrix} 1 \\ X_{ij} \\ Z_{ij} \end{pmatrix}(Y_{ij} - \mu_{ij}).$$

Let

$$U^*_{ij\beta_0} = Y_{ij} - \{M(\beta_x)\}^{-1}\exp(\beta_0 + \beta_x^{\mathrm{T}} X^*_{ij} + \beta_z^{\mathrm{T}} Z_{ij});$$

$$
\begin{aligned}
U^*_{ij\beta_x} &= Y_{ij}X^*_{ij} - \{M(\beta_x)\}^{-1}\exp(\beta_0 + \beta_x^{\mathrm{T}}X_{ij} + \beta_z^{\mathrm{T}}Z_{ij}) \\
&\quad \cdot \left[X^*_{ij} - \frac{dM(\beta_x)}{d\beta_x}\cdot\{M(\beta_x)\}^{-1}\right]; \\
U^*_{ij\beta_z} &= Y_{ij}Z_{ij} - \{M(-\beta_x)\}^{-1}\exp(\beta_0 + \beta_x^{\mathrm{T}}X_{ij} + \beta_z^{\mathrm{T}}Z_{ij});
\end{aligned}
$$

then $U^*_{ij} = (U^*_{ij\beta_0}, U^{*\mathrm{T}}_{ij\beta_x}, U^{*\mathrm{T}}_{ij\beta_z})^{\mathrm{T}}$ satisfies (5.40) and, thus, is an unbiased estimating function for β.

5.4 Likelihood-Based Inference

In longitudinal data analysis, models are often built for the response $Y_i(t)$ and covariate measurements $\{X_i(t), Z_i(t)\}$ that are measured at the same time points. In application, however, some covariates, say $X_i(t)$, may be measured at times different from the response (e.g., Lin, Scharfstein and Rosenheck 2004). To reflect this difference, for subject i let $0 \le t_{i1} < \ldots < t_{im_i}$ be the observation times for response $Y_i(t)$ and covariates $Z_i(t)$, and $0 \le t^*_{i1} < \ldots < t^*_{in_i}$ be the observation times for covariates $X_i(t)$, where time points $\{t_{i1}, \ldots, t_{im_i}\}$ can be identical or different from time points $\{t^*_{i1}, \ldots, t^*_{in_i}\}$. In situations where some observation times for the covariates differ from those for the response variable and m_i and n_i are reasonably comparable, we may cast the problem as a covariate measurement error problem.

For a given observation time t_{ij} for the response variable (and covariates $Z_i(t)$ as well), let t^*_{ik} be the nearest assessment time point for covariates $X_i(t)$, then take the observed measurement $X_i(t^*_{ik})$ as a surrogate version for covariate $X_i(t_{ij})$ whose measurement is unavailable. We set $X^*_i(t_{ij}) = X_i(t^*_{ik})$, and admit that $X^*_i(t_{ij})$ may not be exactly identical to $X_i(t_{ij})$ and is just a surrogate measurement of $X_i(t_{ij})$. Using the notation consistent with that in §5.2 and §5.3, we write $Y_{ij} = Y_i(t_{ij}), X_{ij} = X_i(t_{ij})$, and $X^*_{ij} = X^*_i(t_{ij})$ for $j = 1, \ldots, m_i$. We assume $n_i \le m_i$ so that every observed covariate measurement $X_i(t^*_{ik})$ can potentially serve as a surrogate covariate measurement for (at least) one observed response measurement. When $n_i > m_i$, some observed covariate measurements $X_i(t^*_{ik})$ cannot be matched with any of the observed response measurements. In this case, the problem may be embedded into the setting where the response variable is subject to missingness and covariates are error-contaminated. This topic is to be discussed in §5.5.

We describe inference procedures using likelihood-based methods where the response model is postulated by a nonlinear mixed model following the modeling steps for (5.12) and (5.14). For ease of exposition, we consider the following model where X_{ij} is a scalar covariate.

For $j = 1, \ldots, m_i$,

$$Y_{ij} = g(X_{ij}, Z_{ij}; \xi_i) + \sigma\epsilon_{ij} \tag{5.43}$$

and

$$\xi_i = d(B_i, u_i; \beta), \tag{5.44}$$

where ξ_i is a vector (say, of dimension r) which describes the subject-specific trajectory for subject i, the ϵ_{ij} are independent of each other and of the $\{X_{ij}, Z_{ij}\}$ as well as of the ξ_i, $\epsilon_{ij} \sim N(0, 1)$, $g(\cdot)$ is a nonlinear function, σ is a scale parameter, $d(\cdot)$ is an r-dimensional function which characterizes the relationship of ξ_i and the subject-level covariates B_i based on a vector of regression parameters β, the u_i are random effects whose distribution is modeled as $N(0, \Sigma_u)$ with covariance matrix Σ_u, and the u_i are independent of each other and of the $\{X_{ij}, Z_{ij}, \epsilon_{ij}\}$ (Fitzmaurice et al. 2009, Ch. 5).

Assume that the measurement error mechanism is nondifferential. Suppose that X_{ij}^* is modeled as a function of X_{ij} with an additive form

$$X_{ij}^* = X_{ij} + e_{ij}, \tag{5.45}$$

where the e_{ij} are independent of each other and of $\{X_{ij}, Z_{ij}, \epsilon_{ij}, u_i\}$, and $e_{ij} \sim N(0, \sigma_e^2)$ with variance σ_e^2.

Furthermore, we employ a polynomial random effects model to portray the covariate process. Conditional on Z_{ij} and random effects v_i, X_{ij} is given as

$$X_{ij} = \vartheta^{\mathrm{T}} T_{ij} + v_i^{\mathrm{T}} S_{ij}, \tag{5.46}$$

where T_{ij} and S_{ij} include error-free covariate Z_{ij} or its subset and possibly other quantities such as functions of time t_{ik}^*. Here ϑ is the regression parameter, the v_i are random effects whose distribution is modeled by normal distribution $N(0, \Sigma_v)$ with covariance matrix Σ_v, and the v_i are assumed to be independent of each other and of the $\{Z_{ij}, \epsilon_{ij}, u_i\}$.

Let θ denote the parameter associated with the response model, which includes $\{\beta^{\mathrm{T}}, \sigma^2\}$ and those in Σ_u; and let α denote the parameter related to the measurement error and covariate processes, which includes ϑ, σ_e^2 and those in Σ_v.

5.4.1 Observed Likelihood

Combining the response models (5.43) and (5.44) with the covariate model (5.46), we set

$$L_1(y_i | u_i, v_i, Z_i; \theta, \alpha) = \prod_{j=1}^{m_i} \frac{1}{\sqrt{2\pi\sigma^2}} \exp\left[-\frac{\{y_{ij} - g(X_{ij}, Z_{ij}; \xi_i)\}^2}{2\sigma^2} \right]$$

with ξ_i replaced by (5.44) and X_{ij} replaced by (5.46), which gives a model for the conditional distribution of response vector Y_i, given random effects u_i and v_i as well as precisely observed covariates Z_i.

Write

$$L_2(u_i; \Sigma_u) = \frac{1}{\sqrt{2\pi}|\Sigma_u|^{1/2}} \exp\left(-\frac{1}{2} u_i^{\mathrm{T}} \Sigma_u^{-1} u_i \right).$$

Plugging (5.46) into (5.45) gives

$$X_{ij}^* = \vartheta^{\mathrm{T}} T_{ij} + v_i^{\mathrm{T}} S_{ij} + e_{ij}, \tag{5.47}$$

we then define

$$L_3(X_i^*|v_i, Z_i; \vartheta, \sigma_e^2) = \prod_{j=1}^{m_i} \frac{1}{\sqrt{2\pi}\sigma_e} \exp\left\{-\frac{(X_{ij}^* - \vartheta^{\mathrm{T}} T_{ij} - v_i^{\mathrm{T}} S_{ij})^2}{2\sigma_e^2}\right\}.$$

Let

$$L_4(v_i; \Sigma_v) = \frac{1}{\sqrt{2\pi}|\Sigma_v|^{1/2}} \exp\left(-\frac{1}{2} v_i^{\mathrm{T}} \Sigma_v^{-1} v_i\right).$$

Then the likelihood of the observed data contributed from subject i is given by

$$L(y_i, X_i^*|Z_i; \theta, \alpha) = \int\int L_1(y_i|u_i, v_i, Z_i; \theta, \alpha) L_2(u_i; \Sigma_u) \cdot L_3(X_i^*|v_i, Z_i; \vartheta, \sigma_e^2) L_4(v_i; \Sigma_v) du_i dv_i.$$

Inference about θ and α is, in principle, carried out by maximizing the observed likelihood for the sample data

$$L(\theta, \alpha) = \prod_{i=1}^{n} L(y_i, X_i^*|Z_i; \theta, \alpha) \tag{5.48}$$

with respect to θ and α. The integrals involved in (5.48) usually do not have closed forms, partially due to nonlinearity in the response model. Maximization of $L(\theta, \alpha)$ often has to rely on numerical methods, such as the Monte Carlo simulation approach or the Gibbs sampling method.

5.4.2 Three-Stage Estimation Method

Due to the high dimensionality and nonlinearity in the integrals, directly maximizing likelihood (5.48) with respect to all the model parameters θ and α can be computationally intensive. To circumvent this difficulty, multiple stage estimation methods may be employed to simplify computation. Here we outline a three-stage algorithm for parameter estimation by approximating the observed likelihood (5.48).

We use a matrix representation to describe this procedure. Let $Y_i = (Y_{i1}, \ldots, Y_{im_i})^{\mathrm{T}}$, $\mathbb{Y} = (Y_1^{\mathrm{T}}, \ldots, Y_n^{\mathrm{T}})^{\mathrm{T}}$, $\epsilon_i = (\epsilon_{i1}, \ldots, \epsilon_{im_i})^{\mathrm{T}}$, $\epsilon = (\epsilon_1^{\mathrm{T}}, \ldots, \epsilon_n^{\mathrm{T}})^{\mathrm{T}}$, $e_i = (e_{i1}, \ldots, e_{im_i})^{\mathrm{T}}$, and $e = (e_1^{\mathrm{T}}, \ldots, e_n^{\mathrm{T}})^{\mathrm{T}}$. Similar symbols are defined for Z_i, X_i, X_i^*, T_i, S_i, $\mathbb{Z}$, $\mathbb{X}$, $\mathbb{X}^*$, $\mathbb{B}$, $\mathbb{T}$, and $\mathbb{S}$.

Let $\xi = (\xi_1^{\mathrm{T}}, \ldots, \xi_n^{\mathrm{T}})^{\mathrm{T}}$ and $u = (u_1^{\mathrm{T}}, \ldots, u_n^{\mathrm{T}})^{\mathrm{T}}$. Define

$$G_i(X_i, Z_i; \xi_i) = \{g(X_{i1}, Z_{i1}; \xi_i), \ldots, g(X_{im_i}, Z_{im_i}; \xi_i)\}^{\mathrm{T}};$$
$$G(\mathbb{X}, \mathbb{Z}; \xi) = \{G_1^{\mathrm{T}}(X_1, Z_1; \xi_1), \ldots, G_n^{\mathrm{T}}(X_n, Z_n; \xi_n)\}^{\mathrm{T}};$$
$$d(\mathbb{B}, u; \beta) = \{d_1^{\mathrm{T}}(B_1, u_1; \beta), \ldots, d_n^{\mathrm{T}}(B_n, u_n; \beta)\}^{\mathrm{T}}.$$

Then models (5.43), (5.44), (5.45), and (5.46) are written as

$$\mathbb{Y} = G(\mathbb{X}, \mathbb{Z}; \xi) + \sigma\epsilon; \tag{5.49}$$

$$\xi = d(\mathbb{B}, u; \beta); \tag{5.50}$$

$$\mathbb{X}^* = \mathbb{X} + e; \tag{5.51}$$

$$\mathbb{X} = \mathbb{V} + \mathbb{W}, \tag{5.52}$$

respectively, where

$$\begin{aligned}
\epsilon &\sim N(0, \text{diag}(I_{m_i} : i = 1, \dots, n)); \\
u &\sim N(0, [\text{diag}(\Sigma_u)]_n); \\
e &\sim N(0, \text{diag}(\sigma_e^2 I_{m_i} : i = 1, \dots, n)); \\
\mathbb{V} &= (V_1^{\mathrm{T}}, \dots, V_n^{\mathrm{T}})^{\mathrm{T}} \text{ with } V_i = (\vartheta^{\mathrm{T}} T_{i1}, \dots, \vartheta^{\mathrm{T}} T_{im_i})^{\mathrm{T}}; \\
\mathbb{W} &= (W_1^{\mathrm{T}}, \dots, W_n^{\mathrm{T}})^{\mathrm{T}} \text{ with } W_i = (v_i^{\mathrm{T}} S_{i1}, \dots, v_i^{\mathrm{T}} S_{im_i})^{\mathrm{T}};
\end{aligned}$$

and $[\text{diag}\{\Sigma_u\}]_n$ is the diagonal block matrix with n identical block matrix Σ_u.

Using a presentation slightly different from the observed likelihood (5.48), we consider the following observed likelihood, expressed in terms of the entire data set,

$$\begin{aligned}
&L(\mathbb{Y}|\mathbb{X}^*, \mathbb{Z}; \theta, \alpha) \\
&= \int\int L_1(\mathbb{Y}|u, \mathbb{X}, \mathbb{Z}; \theta) L_2(u; \theta) L_3(\mathbb{X}|\mathbb{X}^*, \mathbb{Z}; \alpha) d\mathbb{X} du,
\end{aligned} \tag{5.53}$$

where $L_1(\mathbb{Y}|u, \mathbb{X}, \mathbb{Z}; \theta)$ is determined by (5.49) and (5.50); $L_2(u; \theta)$ is determined by the model $N(0, [\text{diag}(\Sigma_u)]_n)$ for u; and $L_3(\mathbb{X}|\mathbb{X}^*, \mathbb{Z}; \alpha)$ characterizes the conditional model of $\mathbb{X}$, given $\{\mathbb{X}^*, \mathbb{Z}\}$, which can be worked out using the conditional model (5.51) of $\mathbb{X}^*$, given $\{\mathbb{X}, \mathbb{Z}\}$, and the conditional model (5.52) of $\mathbb{X}$, given $\mathbb{Z}$.

To estimate the model parameter using (5.53), Li et al. (2004) proposed an estimation procedure based on multiple steps of approximations to (5.53). The procedure consists of three steps. The first step estimates α in $L_3(\mathbb{X}|\mathbb{X}^*, \mathbb{Z}; \alpha)$. A regular algorithm is utilized to fit the linear mixed model (5.47) to obtain the maximum likelihood estimator $\widehat{\alpha}$ for parameter α. Conditional mean $E(\mathbb{X}|\mathbb{X}^*, \mathbb{Z}; \alpha)$ is then evaluated with α replaced by $\widehat{\alpha}$, and let $E(\mathbb{X}|\mathbb{X}^*, \mathbb{Z}; \widehat{\alpha})$ denote the resulting value. The second step handles the inner integral of (5.53); this integral is approximated using the Solomon–Cox approximation (Solomon and Cox 1992), where the integrand is taken as a function of $\mathbb{X}$ and a quadratic expansion of the integrand about the conditional mean $E(\mathbb{X}|\mathbb{X}^*, \mathbb{Z}; \widehat{\alpha})$ is used. At the third step, we approximate the outer integral of (5.53) using the Laplace approximation by treating the integrand as a function of u (Wolfinger 1993; Wolfinger and Lin 1997). The implementation details can be found in Li et al. (2004).

5.4.3 EM Algorithm

As an alternative to the three-stage estimation outlined in §5.4.2, the EM algorithm is employed for parameter estimation. The log-likelihood for the complete data $\{(Y_i, X_i, X_i^*, u_i, v_i) : i = 1, \dots, n\}$, given Z_i, is

$$\ell_{\rm c} = \sum_{i=1}^{n} \log\{f(y_i|u_i, x_i, z_i) + \log f(x_i^*|x_i, z_i) + \log f(x_i|z_i, v_i)$$
$$+ \log f(u_i) + \log f(v_i)\},$$

where $f(y_i|u_i, x_i, z_i)$ is given by model (5.43) with ξ_i replaced by (5.44), $f(x_i^*|x_i, z_i)$ is determined by (5.45), $f(x_i|z_i, v_i)$ is determined by (5.46), $f(u_i)$ and $f(v_i)$ represent the density functions of distributions $N(0, \Sigma_u)$ and $N(0, \Sigma_v)$, respectively, and the dependence on parameters is suppressed in the notation.

For iteration $(k + 1)$ at the E-step, we need to evaluate the conditional expectation of $\ell_{\rm c}$, $E(\ell_{\rm c}|Y_i, X_i^*, Z_i; \theta^{(k)}, \alpha^{(k)})$, where the conditional expectation is evaluated with respect to the model, $f(u_i, v_i, x_i|Y_i, X_i^*, Z_i; \theta^{(k)}, \alpha^{(k)})$, for the "missing" data $\{u_i, v_i, X_i\}$, given the observed data $\{Y_i, X_i^*, Z_i\}$, with the parameters evaluated at the estimates $\{\theta^{(k)}, \alpha^{(k)}\}$ of the model parameters at iteration k. At the M-step, one proceeds with maximization of the conditional expectation $E(\ell_{\rm c}|Y_i, X_i^*, Z_i; \theta^{(k)}, \alpha^{(k)})$ with respect to θ and α. However, this may be computationally difficult due to the nonlinear structure of function $g(\cdot)$.

To get around this problem, we use an approximation to simplify the conditional expectation $E(\ell_{\rm c}|Y_i, X_i^*, Z_i; \theta^{(k)}, \alpha^{(k)})$. The idea is to iteratively apply the EM algorithm to a *linear* mixed model which approximates the initial *nonlinear* mixed model. For the next iteration of the EM procedure, a first-order Taylor series expansion around the current estimates of the parameters and random effects estimates is used to approximate the initial nonlinear mixed model.

First, we write the two-step modeling of nonlinear mixed models (5.43) and (5.44), together with model (5.46), as a single equation

$$Y_{ij} = g_{ij}(\beta, \vartheta, u_i, v_i) + \sigma\epsilon_{ij}$$

for some nonlinear function $g_{ij}(\cdot)$ with the dependence on covariate Z_{ij} suppressed. Let $g_i = (g_{i1}, \ldots, g_{im_i})^{\rm T}$ and $\zeta = (\beta^{\rm T}, \vartheta)^{\rm T}$.

Let $\widetilde{\zeta}$ denote the current estimate of ζ obtained from the EM algorithm, and $(\widetilde{u}_i, \widetilde{v}_i)$ be the resulting empirical Bayesian estimates of (u_i, v_i). Calculate

$$\widetilde{g}_{i\zeta} = \frac{\partial g_i}{\partial \zeta^{\rm T}}; \ \widetilde{g}_{iu} = \frac{\partial g_i}{\partial u_i^{\rm T}}; \ \widetilde{g}_{iv} = \frac{\partial g_i}{\partial v_i^{\rm T}};$$

where $\{\zeta, u_i, v_i\}$ is replaced by the estimates $\{\widetilde{\zeta}, \widetilde{u}_i, \widetilde{v}_i\}$. Then around the current estimates $\{\widetilde{\zeta}, \widetilde{u}_i, \widetilde{v}_i\}$, we apply a Taylor series expansion to linearize nonlinear function $g_i(\zeta, u_i, v_i)$ approximately:

$$g_i(\zeta, u_i, v_i) \approx g_i(\widetilde{\zeta}, \widetilde{u}_i, \widetilde{v}_i) + \widetilde{g}_{i\zeta}(\zeta - \widetilde{\zeta}) + \widetilde{g}_{iu}(u_i - \widetilde{u}_i) + \widetilde{g}_{iv}(v_i - \widetilde{v}_i).$$

Define a *pseudo-response* as

$$\widetilde{Y}_i = Y_i - \{g_i(\widetilde{\zeta}, \widetilde{u}_i, \widetilde{v}_i) - \widetilde{g}_{i\zeta}\widetilde{\zeta} - \widetilde{g}_{iu}\widetilde{u}_i - \widetilde{g}_{iv}\widetilde{v}_i\}.$$

Then we obtain an approximate linear mixed model

$$\widetilde{Y}_i \approx \widetilde{g}_{i\zeta}\zeta + \widetilde{g}_{iu}u_i + \widetilde{g}_{iv}v_i + \sigma\epsilon_i. \qquad (5.54)$$

At the E-step of the next iteration, we calculate the conditional expectation of the complete log-likelihood obtained from the approximate response model (5.54) and measurement error model (5.45). Then this conditional expectation is maximized with respect to the model parameters at the M-step of the next iteration. Due to the assumption of normal distributions for all the relevant random variables, the updated estimates of the parameters for the next iteration are readily obtained. Detailed discussion and extension of this procedure were given by Wu (2002) and Liu and Wu (2007).

5.4.4 Remarks

In this section, we discuss likelihood-based methods for estimation of model parameters under nonlinear mixed measurement error models. Computation is a central issue for the implementation of the inferential procedures. There is a trade-off between computational feasibility and statistical validity when choosing a specific implementation algorithm. In §5.4.2 and §5.4.3, we describe two approximation schemes to ease computational difficulties which arise from handling high dimensional integrals with nonlinear integrands.

The discussion emphasizes how to find the point estimates for the model parameters. Variance estimates for the resulting estimators may be obtained based on the approximate models accordingly. For instance, for the EM algorithm employed for the approximate linear mixed model (5.54), one may apply the formula by Louis (1982) to calculate variance estimates for the resulting estimators, or alternatively, use the approximate formula discussed by McLachlan and Krishnan (1997) and Wu (2002).

Given a model setup, there may be multiple ways to introduce approximations to ease computation. Davidian and Giltinan (1995), Wolfinger and Lin (1997), and Wu (2009) provided some details on the comparisons of several approximate methods. No matter what method is used, it is important to recognize an issue: without additional sources of data (such as a validation subsample) being available to characterize the measurement error process, there is always the potential of running into the problem of nonidentifiability of model parameters. Discussion on this point is provided in §5.5.5.

5.5 Inference Methods in the Presence of Both Measurement Error and Missingness

Analysis of longitudinal error-prone data is often further complicated by the presence of missing observations. Although longitudinal studies are commonly designed to collect data at each assessment for every individual in the studies, missing observations occur. It is well known that indiscriminately ignoring missingness in the data analysis can result in seriously misleading results (e.g., Little and Rubin 2002;

Daniels and Hogan 2008). On the other hand, in §5.2, we show that ignoring measurement error can produce biased results. When both measurement error and missing values exist, the impact on inferences become even more complex due to the interplay of their effects. These effects depend on many factors, typically pertaining to the model structures of the response as well as the measurement error and missing data processes.

In this section, we discuss issues and methods for handling longitudinal data when both *covariate* measurement error and missing *response* observations exist. We start with a discussion on handling longitudinal data merely with missing response observations and then discuss longitudinal data with both features.

5.5.1 Missing Data and Inference Methods

We consider the situation where only the response variable Y_{ij} is subject to missingness. For $i = 1, \ldots, n$ and $j = 1, \ldots, m_i$, let R_{ij} be the missing data indicator, taking value 1 if Y_{ij} is observed, and 0 otherwise. Write $R_i = (R_{i1}, \ldots, R_{im_i})^{\mathrm{T}}$.

In handling longitudinal data with missing responses, several inference frameworks are available; differences in these frameworks are reflected in the way of modeling the response and missing data processes. In principle, valid inferences for data with missing values would involve modeling the joint distribution of the response and missing data indicator variables. Two general strategies may be considered: either a *parallel* or a *sequential* approach may be employed to characterize the relationship between the response and missing data processes.

The former method equally treats the response and missing data processes and uses a *parallel* manner to model both processes. In particular, Little (1995) discussed a unified framework for modeling the response and missing data processes simultaneously where random effects are shared by both processes and conditional independence, given random effects, is assumed for both processes. Vandenhende and Lambert (2002) described a method which postulates the response and missing data processes through a copula model.

Alternatively, modeling of the joint distribution of the response and missing data indicator variables may be realized using a *sequential* scheme. Little (1993) and Little and Rubin (2002) distinguished two classes of models with missing data: *selection models* and *pattern-mixture models*, based on the factorization form of the joint distribution $h(y_i, r_i|x_i, z_i)$ of the response vector Y_i and the missingness indicator vector R_i, given covariates X_i and Z_i.

In our discussion here, we consider the selection model which factorizes out the conditional model for the hypothetically complete responses, given the covariates, and then appends a model for the missing data indicators conditional on the responses and covariates:

$$h(y_i, r_i|x_i, z_i) = h(y_i|x_i, z_i)h(r_i|y_i, x_i, z_i), \tag{5.55}$$

where $h(y_i|x_i, z_i)$ and $h(r_i|y_i, x_i, z_i)$ are the conditional probability density or mass functions of Y_i given $\{X_i, Z_i\}$ and of R_i given $\{Y_i, X_i, Z_i\}$, respectively.

Factorization (5.55) explicitly spells out the response process $h(y_i|x_i, z_i)$ which is of primary interest. It also suggests a way to distinguish different missing data processes. Three missing data mechanisms are often classified for analysis of longitudinal data with missing responses. Given covariates $\{X_i, Z_i\}$,

- if $h(r_i|y_i, x_i, z_i)$ does not depend on the responses, i.e., $h(r_i|y_i, x_i, z_i) = h(r_i|x_i, z_i)$, then the missing data mechanism is called *missing completely at random* (MCAR);
- if $h(r_i|y_i, x_i, z_i) = h(r_i|y_i^{(o)}, x_i, z_i)$, then the mechanism is called *missing at random* (MAR), where $y_i^{(o)}$ represents the subvector of realizations for the observed components of Y_i;
- the *missing not at random* (MNAR) mechanism arises when $h(r_i|y_i, x_i, z_i)$ depends on the unobserved response components.

Such a classification is useful in differentiating varying effects of missingness on inferential procedures. Most statistical analyses, developed for scenarios with complete data, may be directly applied to the observed data and still yield consistent estimates under the MCAR mechanism; but they often give biased result if MNAR holds. With an MAR mechanism, however, missingness effects may be more related to the nature of the inference method. For example, usual likelihood methods, when applied to the observed data with the missing data process left unmodeled, can still lead to valid inference; whereas marginal methods, such as the GEE approach, may yield inconsistent estimates.

To see this, we consider a parametric model $\{f(y_i|x_i, z_i; \beta) : \beta \in \Theta_\beta\}$ for $h(y_i|x_i, z_i)$ and $\{f(r_i|y_i, x_i, z_i; \vartheta) : \vartheta \in \Theta_\vartheta\}$ for $h(r_i|y_i, x_i, z_i)$, where the parameters β and ϑ are assumed to be distinct, or functionally independent, respectively, taking values in the parameter space Θ_β and Θ_ϑ. We are interested in inference about β, which is, in principle, carried out based on the likelihood of the observed data. To be specific, we partition y_i into the observed response subvector $y_i^{(o)}$ and the subvector $y_i^{(m)}$ of missing components, then inference on β is conducted by integrating out $y_i^{(m)}$ from the joint model $f(y_i^{(o)}, y_i^{(m)}, r_i|x_i, z_i; \beta, \vartheta)$ for (5.55).

The observed likelihood contributed from the ith subject is

$$\begin{aligned} L_{oi} &= f(y_i^{(o)}, r_i|x_i, z_i; \beta, \vartheta) \\ &= \int f(r_i|y_i^{(o)}, y_i^{(m)}, x_i, z_i; \vartheta) f(y_i^{(o)}, y_i^{(m)}|x_i, z_i; \beta) d\eta(y_i^{(m)}). \quad (5.56) \end{aligned}$$

Under the MCAR and MAR mechanisms, $f(r_i|y_i^{(o)}, y_i^{(m)}, x_i, z_i; \vartheta)$ is assumed to be free of $y_i^{(m)}$, thus, yielding the log-likelihood for the observed data contributed from the ith subject

$$\log L_{oi} = \log f(r_i|x_i, z_i; \vartheta) + \log f(y_i^{(o)}|x_i, z_i; \beta)$$

and

$$\log L_{oi} = \log f(r_i|y_i^{(o)}, x_i, z_i; \vartheta) + \log f(y_i^{(o)}|x_i, z_i; \beta),$$

respectively. Since parameters ϑ and β are distinct, inference on response parameter β is then directly performed using the logarithm of the observed likelihood

$$\log f(y_i^{(o)}|x_i, z_i; \beta),$$

which is obtained from the response model alone with modeling of the missing data process ignored. Maximizing $\sum_{i=1}^{n} \log f(y_i^{(o)}|x_i, z_i; \beta)$ with respect to parameter β leads to the maximum likelihood estimate of β.

With MNAR, $\log f(y_i^{(o)}|x_i, z_i; \beta)$ is not *obviously* separated from the information on the missing data process by using (5.56), so modeling of the missing data process may be generally required. However, under the *composite likelihood* inference framework (Lindsay 1988; Lindsay, Yi and Sun 2011), the way of handling missing data processes or mechanisms may be different. These issues were discussed by Yi, Zeng and Cook (2011), He and Yi (2011), Li and Yi (2013a,b), and Li and Yi (2016).

If inference about β is not derived from the likelihood method but is based on the GEE method, the impact of ignoring the missing data process is different. With MCAR, applying the GEE method to the observed data still leads to a consistent estimator of β under regularity conditions, but biased results may arise if the missingness mechanism is MAR or MNAR. This is evident from the following illustrations.

Consider the GEE setup (5.4) which is developed for analysis of complete longitudinal data. When missing response measurements are present and if we directly apply this GEE formulation to the observed measurements, we would form the estimating function

$$U_i = D_i V_i^{-1} \text{diag}\left(R_{ij} : j = 1, \ldots, m_i\right)(Y_i - \mu_i)$$

for $i = 1, \ldots, n$.

However, such an estimating function does not guarantee to yield a consistent estimator for β since it is not unbiased. In fact,

$$\begin{aligned}
& E(U_i) - E_{Y_i|(X_i,Z_i)}\{E_{R_i|(Y_i,X_i,Z_i)}(U_i)\} \\
&= E_{Y_i|(X_i,Z_i)}\left[E_{R_i|(Y_i,X_i,Z_i)}\left\{D_i V_i^{-1} \text{diag}\left(R_{ij} : j = 1, \ldots, m_i\right)(Y_i - \mu_i)\right\}\right] \\
&= E_{Y_i|(X_i,Z_i)}\left[D_i V_i^{-1} \text{diag}\left\{P(R_{ij} = 1|Y_i, X_i, Z_i) : j - 1, \ldots, m_i\right\}(Y_i - \mu_i)\right] \\
&\neq E_{Y_i|(X_i,Z_i)}\left\{D_i V_i^{-1}(Y_i - \mu_i)\right\} \\
&= 0,
\end{aligned}$$

where the second last step is due to that under MAR or MNAR, the probability of missingness, $P(R_{ij} = 1|Y_i, X_i, Z_i)$, cannot be ignored when evaluating the expectation with respect to the model for the conditional distribution of Y_i, given $\{X_i, Z_i\}$.

Furthermore, this derivation suggests a way to adjust for missingness effects: *inverse probability weighting*. Let

$$U_i^* = D_i V_i^{-1} \text{diag}\left\{\frac{R_{ij}}{P(R_{ij} = 1|Y_i, X_i, Z_i)} : j = 1, \ldots, m_i\right\}(Y_i - \mu_i), \quad (5.57)$$

then U_i^* is an unbiased estimating function. As a result, inference about β may be carried out by solving

$$\sum_{i=1}^{n} U_i^* = 0$$

for β, where the missingness probabilities are replaced with their consistent estimates.

This inverse probability weighting strategy is often used in marginal analysis for longitudinal data with missing response measurements; it was initiated by Robins, Rotnitzky and Zhao (1995) for longitudinal data settings. Extensions were considered by Robins and Rotnitzky (2001), Yi and Cook (2002), Carpenter, Kenward and Vansteelandt (2006), Shardell and Miller (2008), Yi and He (2009), Yi, Cook and Chen (2010), Chen, Yi and Cook (2010b), and Chen et al. (2012), among many others.

In implementing the inverse probability weighting scheme, MAR is usually assumed for the sake of identifiability and estimability of the parameter associated with the missing data model. With MNAR, the inverse probability weighting method may be employed for sensitivity analysis (e.g., Yi, Ma and Carroll 2012). The validity of choosing suitable weights was discussed by Qu et al. (2011).

In summary, ignoring missing data has disparate effects on estimation of the response parameter for different inference methods. Using the likelihood method for the observed data is valid if MCAR or MAR holds while applying the GEE method to the observed data is only valid for the MCAR scenario. When MNAR arises, developing valid inferential procedures often calls for modeling of the missing data process, as evident from a large body of available work in the literature, although different perspectives may be taken as discussed by Yi, Zeng and Cook (2011) and He and Yi (2011).

These conclusions, however, do not hold when measurement error is involved. The preceding classification of missingness mechanisms is no longer useful to distinguish impacts of missingness on different inference methods. For instance, when X_i is error-prone and not observable, then the mechanism with $h(r_i|y_i, x_i, z_i) = h(r_i|x_i, z_i)$ (or $h(r_i|y_i, x_i, z_i) = h(r_i|y_i^{(o)}, x_i, z_i)$), initially termed MCAR (or MAR) for an error-free context, does not necessarily ensure the same advantage of the likelihood method over the GEE approach for which modeling of the missing data process can be ignored. Even when $h(r_i|y_i, x_i, z_i) = h(r_i|x_i, z_i)$, if there is measurement error in X_i, the missing data process cannot be left unattended to for the likelihood or GEE methods. Problem 5.12 sketches bias analysis for some settings where both missingness in responses and measurement error in covariates are present.

5.5.2 *Strategy of Correcting Measurement Error and Missingness Effects*

In addition to Y_{ij} being subject to missingness, suppose covariate X_i is error-contaminated and X_i^* is an observed version of X_i. Valid inference generally requires examining all the involved variables, $\{Y_i, X_i, Z_i, X_i^*, R_i\}$, jointly to untangle complex relationships among different processes. Frequently, this requirement is simplified to examining the joint distribution $h(y_i, x_i, x_i^*, r_i|z_i)$ by conditioning on the precisely measured covariate Z_i, where the distribution of Z_i is left unspecified. Such a strategy agrees with the common treatment in usual regression analysis where conditional analysis is used for inference about the response process with covariates fixed.

Because it is difficult to come up with a meaningful and realistic joint model for $\{Y_i, X_i, X_i^*, R_i\}$, we break modeling of the joint distribution of $\{Y_i, X_i, X_i^*, R_i\}$ (with Z_i kept fixed) into a sequence of conditional modeling steps by the probability multiplication rule. There is no unique way to do this, however. The choice of a particular method is mainly driven by the feature of data, the nature of questions, and the tractability and mathematical convenience of models as well as computation cost.

A useful scheme is to decompose the conditional distribution of $\{Y_i, X_i, X_i^*, R_i\}$, given Z_i, as follows:

$$h(y_i, x_i, x_i^*, r_i|z_i) = h(y_i|x_i, z_i)h(x_i, x_i^*|z_i)h(r_i|y_i, x_i, x_i^*, z_i), \tag{5.58}$$

where nondifferential measurement error is assumed. This factorization is compelling. It offers an explicit way to spell out the relationship between the response and the true covariates, which is of prime interest, and to separate measurement error and missingness processes, which are treated as a nuisance. Factorization (5.58) allows us to use modeling strategies for covariate measurement error to delineate the relationship between surrogate X_i^* and the true covariate X_i.

The only possible complication here is to handle the conditional probability $h(r_i|y_i, x_i, x_i^*, z_i)$ for the missing data indicators. In the presence of covariate measurement error, usual classification of missing data mechanisms, defined in §5.5.1, no longer provides clear insights into the missingness impact on inference methods. Therefore, we abandon the definition of missing data mechanisms classified for the error-free context, but take new perspectives to examine the nature of missingness.

The new perspectives place the emphasis on directly examining the relationship between the missing data indicator and error-prone covariate X_i and its surrogate X_i^*. We discuss two approaches to characterizing $h(r_i|y_i, x_i, x_i^*, z_i)$.

With the first approach, we take a measurement error viewpoint and feature the missing data process in terms of the underlying unobserved X_i. We differentiate missing data processes using the criterion whether or not

$$h(r_i|y_i, x_i, x_i^*, z_i) = h(r_i|y_i, x_i, z_i) \tag{5.59}$$

holds. This classification for the missing data indicator is somewhat analogous to the definition of the nondifferential or differential measurement error mechanism defined in §2.4. It says that the missingness probabilities do not depend on the surrogate value if the true covariates are controlled along with the response measurements.

For the second approach, we bypass a measurement error development entirely and simply characterize missing data processes directly in terms of the observed covariates together with the response measurements. In this case, we differentiate missing data processes according to whether or not the identity

$$h(r_i|y_i, x_i, x_i^*, z_i) = h(r_i|y_i, x_i^*, z_i) \tag{5.60}$$

holds. Identity (5.60) reflects that the missingness probabilities do not depend on the underlying true error-prone covariate X_i, once the surrogate X_i^* is controlled together with Y_i and Z_i.

These two strategies will be applied in the next two subsections. Identities (5.59) and (5.60) provide different ways to describe missing data processes. The mechanism of a missing data process is called the *true-covariate-driven missingness* if missing data satisfy (5.59). With true-covariate-driven missing data processes, we further divide those processes into three categories according to MCAR, MAR and MNAR mechanisms defined in §5.5.1, which gives the following mechanisms:

- If $h(r_i|y_i, x_i, z_i) = h(r_i|x_i, z_i)$ and (5.59) is true, then the missing data mechanism is called the *true-covariate-driven MCAR* mechanism.
- If $h(r_i|y_i, x_i, z_i) = h(r_i|y_i^{(o)}, x_i, z_i)$ and (5.59) is true, then the missing data mechanism is called the *true-covariate-driven MAR* mechanism.
- If $h(r_i|y_i, x_i, z_i)$ depends on unobserved $y_i^{(m)}$ and (5.59) is true, then the missing data mechanism is called the *true-covariate-driven MNAR* mechanism.

If a missing data possesses (5.60), then the missingness is called the *observed-covariate-driven missingness*. Among missing data with such a property, we further differentiate those processes according to their relationship with the response variables, which is done in a similar way to what is described in §5.5.1. Specifically, we describe $h(r_i|y_i, x_i^*, z_i)$ by the following three properties:

- If $h(r_i|y_i, x_i^*, z_i) = h(r_i|x_i^*, z_i)$ and (5.60) is true, then the missing data mechanism is called the *observed-covariate-driven MCAR* mechanism.
- If $h(r_i|y_i, x_i^*, z_i) = h(r_i|y_i^{(o)}, x_i^*, z_i)$ and (5.60) is true, then the missing data mechanism is called the *observed-covariate-driven MAR* mechanism.
- If $h(r_i|y_i, x_i^*, z_i)$ depends on unobserved $y_i^{(m)}$ and (5.60) is true, then the missing data mechanism is called the *observed-covariate-driven MNAR* mechanism.

Under the framework (5.58), inference methods may be classified as either *sequential* or *simultaneous* approaches, mainly determined by the model assumptions. If full distributional assumptions are made for the response, missing data and measurement error processes, then likelihood-based inference is naturally performed with measurement error and missingness effects *simultaneously* addressed. If interest centers around marginal features of the response process where only marginal models are assumed for responses, then *sequentially* accounting for measurement error effects and missingness effects is often possible. We elaborate on these methods in the next two subsections, which are mainly based on the development of Yi (2005, 2008), Yi, Ma and Carroll (2012) and Yi, Liu and Wu (2011).

5.5.3 Sequential Corrections

We discuss the marginal analysis of longitudinal data with response missing observations and covariate measurement error. The basic idea is to develop multiple steps for constructing an unbiased estimating function for estimation of the response model parameter, in which each step uses the available measurements to *sequentially* facilitate a particular feature of the data.

At the first step, we construct a set of unbiased estimating functions for the response model parameter under the ideal situation where neither missing responses nor covariate measurement error are present. This is accomplished by applying standard methods for the error-free and missingness-free context. For the next two steps, we modify the estimating functions obtained from the first step by sequentially incorporating the measurement error effects and missingness effects, where the order of correction mainly depends on the nature of the missing data process.

We elaborate on these ideas using subject-time-specific models. Suppose the response model is given as (5.3) and the measurement error model is given by

$$X_{ij}^* = X_{ij} + e_{ij}, \tag{5.61}$$

where the e_{ij} are independent of each other and of $\{X_{ij}, Z_{ij}, Y_{ij}\}$ for $i = 1, \ldots, n$ and $j = 1, \ldots, m_i$. We assume that e_{ij} follows a normal distribution $N(0, \Sigma_e)$ with known covariance matrix Σ_e for ease of discussion; however, this assumption may be relaxed.

In the error-free and missingness-free context, $U_{ij}(\beta; Y_{ij}, X_{ij}, Z_{ij})$, defined as (5.33), is used for estimation of parameter β. Depending on the property of the missing data process, one may choose different orders to correct for measurement error and missingness effects step by step. We discuss two scenarios of missing data processes: (1) missingness is observed-covariate-driven, and (2) missingness is true-covariate-driven.

Observed-Covariate-Driven MAR/MCAR

First, we consider missing data with the observed-covariate-driven MAR missingness. To reflect the dynamic nature of the observation process over time, we write

$$h(r_i|y_i, x_i^*, z_i) = \prod_{j=2}^{m_i} h(r_{ij}|\mathcal{H}_{ij}^{\mathrm{R}}, y_i, x_i^*, z_i),$$

where the conditional probability, $h(r_{i1}|y_i, x_i^*, z_i)$, of R_{i1} given $\{Y_i, X_i^*, Z_i\}$ is assumed to be 1; $\mathcal{H}_{ij}^{\mathrm{R}} = \{R_{i1}, \ldots, R_{i,j-1}\}$ is the history of the missing data indicator before time point j; $h(r_{ij}|\mathcal{H}_{ij}^{\mathrm{R}}, y_i, x_i^*, z_i)$ is the conditional probability $P(R_{ij} = r_{ij}|\mathcal{H}_{ij}^{\mathrm{R}}, Y_i, X_i^*, Z_i)$ for $j = 2, \ldots, m_i$; and $r_i = (r_{i1}, \ldots, r_{im_i})^{\mathrm{T}}$ is a realization of R_i.

Assume that

$$P(R_{ij} = 1|\mathcal{H}_{ij}^{\mathrm{R}}, Y_i, X_i^*, Z_i) = P(R_{ij} = 1|Y_i, X_i^*, Z_i)$$

for $j = 2, \ldots, m_i$, which says that given the responses and the observed covariates, the probability of being missing at a time point does not depend on missingness at previous assessment times. Since subjects are assessed sequentially over time, it is natural to consider missing data processes with the following type of observed-covariate-driven MAR (or MCAR) missingness:

$$P(R_{ij} = 1|Y_i, X_i^*, Z_i) = P(R_{ij} = 1|\mathcal{H}_{ij}^{Y(o)}, \mathcal{H}_{ij}^{X*}, \mathcal{H}_{ij}^{Z}),$$

where $\mathcal{H}_{ij}^{Y(o)}$ is the history of the observed response components before time j for subject i, $\mathcal{H}_{ij}^{X*} = \{X_{i1}^*, \ldots, X_{ij}^*\}$, $\mathcal{H}_{ij}^{Z} = \{Z_{i1}, \ldots, Z_{ij}\}$, and $j = 2, \ldots, m_i$.

Let $\tau_{ij} = P(R_{ij} = 1|\mathcal{H}_{ij}^{Y(o)}, \mathcal{H}_{ij}^{X*}, \mathcal{H}_{ij}^{Z})$ for $j = 2, \ldots, m_i$. We use a logistic regression model to posit this conditional probability:

$$\text{logit}\, \tau_{ij} = \vartheta^{\mathrm{T}} w_{ij},$$

where ϑ is the regression parameter and w_{ij} is a vector consisting of the information on the histories $\{\mathcal{H}_{ij}^{Y(o)}, \mathcal{H}_{ij}^{X*}, \mathcal{H}_{ij}^{Z}\}$.

Estimation of parameter ϑ proceeds using a likelihood-based method. Let

$$L_i(\vartheta) = \prod_{j=2}^{m_i} \tau_{ij}^{r_{ij}} (1 - \tau_{ij})^{1-r_{ij}}$$

be the likelihood contributed from subject i and $S_i(\vartheta) = \partial \log L_i(\vartheta)/\partial\vartheta$. Then solving

$$\sum_{i=1}^{n} S_i(\vartheta) = 0 \tag{5.62}$$

for ϑ leads to an estimate of ϑ. Let $\widehat{\vartheta}$ denote the corresponding estimator, which is a consistent estimator of ϑ under regularity conditions.

Next, we describe a sequential correction procedure to account for effects induced from measurement error and missingness. First, we use a strategy described in §5.3 to correct for measurement error effects, and let $U_{ij}^*(\beta; Y_{ij}, X_{ij}^*, Z_{ij})$ denote the resulting unbiased estimating function expressed in terms of the observed surrogate X_{ij}^* and $\{Z_{ij}, Y_{ij}\}$.

At the next step, we further modify function $U_{ij}^*(\beta; Y_{ij}, X_{ij}^*, Z_{ij})$ to correct for the effects caused from the missingness of the response measurements using the inverse probability weighting method. Let

$$\Phi_{ij}(\beta, \vartheta) = \frac{R_{ij}}{\tau_{ij}} U_{ij}^*(\beta; Y_{ij}, X_{ij}^*, Z_{ij}), \tag{5.63}$$

then $\Phi_{ij}(\beta, \vartheta)$ is unbiased by the definition of τ_{ij}.

As a side comment, we note that the unbiasedness of $\Phi_{ij}(\beta, \vartheta)$ allows us to create a class of unbiased estimating functions for β by an additive form

$$\frac{R_{ij}}{\tau_{ij}} U_{ij}^*(\beta; Y_{ij}, X_{ij}^*, Z_{ij}) + \frac{R_{ij} - \tau_{ij}}{\tau_{ij}} D(Y_{ij}, X_{ij}^*, Z_{ij}; \beta) \tag{5.64}$$

for some function $D(\cdot)$ which is free of the missing data indicator R_{ij}. When $U_{ij}^*(\beta; Y_{ij}, X_{ij}^*, Z_{ij})$ is linear in Y_{ij} with the form

$$U_{ij}^*(\beta; Y_{ij}, X_{ij}^*, Z_{ij}) = A(X_{ij}^*, Z_{ij}; \beta) Y_{ij} + B(X_{ij}^*, Z_{ij}; \beta)$$

for some functions $A(\cdot)$ and $B(\cdot)$, then setting

$$D(X_{ij}^*, Z_{ij}; \beta) = -B(X_{ij}^*, Z_{ij}; \beta)$$

shows that estimating function (5.64) is algebraically equivalent to replacing argument Y_{ij} with $(R_{ij}/\tau_{ij})Y_{ij}$ in $U_{ij}^*(\beta; Y_{ij}, X_{ij}^*, Z_{ij})$ and, hence, function

$$\Phi_{ij}^*(\beta, \vartheta) = U_{ij}^*\{\beta; (R_{ij}/\tau_{ij})Y_{ij}, X_{ij}^*, Z_{ij}\}$$

may be used for inference about β as well.

Finally, following the GMM method outlined in §5.3, we obtain an estimating equation for β by combining all the functions $\Phi_{ij}(\beta, \vartheta)$ in the same manner as that of formulating (5.34). Let $U_i^{**}(\beta, \vartheta)$ denote the resultant estimating function for β, and $\widehat{\beta}$ denote the corresponding estimator of β by solving $\sum_{i=1}^n U_i^{**}(\beta, \vartheta) = 0$ for β with ϑ replaced by its consistent estimate.

Under regularity conditions, $\sqrt{n}(\widehat{\beta} - \beta)$ has an asymptotic multivariate normal distribution with mean 0 and covariance matrix $\Gamma^{-1}\Sigma^{**}\Gamma^{-1\mathrm{T}}$, where $\Gamma = E\{\partial U_i^{**}(\beta, \vartheta)/\partial \beta^{\mathrm{T}}\}$, $\Sigma^{**} = E\{Q_i(\beta, \vartheta)Q_i^{\mathrm{T}}(\beta, \vartheta)\}$, and $Q_i(\beta, \vartheta) = U_i^{**}(\beta, \vartheta) - E\{\partial U_i^{**}(\beta, \vartheta)/\partial \vartheta^{\mathrm{T}}\}[E\{\partial S_i(\vartheta)/\partial \vartheta^{\mathrm{T}}\}]^{-1} S_i(\vartheta)$. Thus, inference on β is conducted based on replacing the asymptotic covariance matrix with its consistent estimate in the asymptotic distribution of $\widehat{\beta}$.

The following example illustrates the construction of function $\Phi_{ij}(\cdot)$.

Example 5.6. (*Logistic Regression with Missingness and Measurement Error*)

Suppose Y_{ij} is a binary response variable and $\{X_{ij}, Z_{ij}\}$ are the associated covariates where $i = 1, \ldots, n$ and $j = 1, \ldots, m_i$. The mean $\mu_{ij} = E(Y_{ij}|X_{ij}, Z_{ij})$ is described by the logistic regression model

$$\text{logit}\, \mu_{ij} = \beta_0 + \beta_x^{\mathrm{T}} X_{ij} + \beta_z^{\mathrm{T}} Z_{ij}, \tag{5.65}$$

where $\beta = (\beta_0, \beta_x^{\mathrm{T}}, \beta_z^{\mathrm{T}})^{\mathrm{T}}$ is the vector of regression parameters.

Suppose that X_{ij} is mismeasured as X_{ij}^* and they are linked by the model (5.61). Suppose that response variable Y_{ij} is subject to missingness and estimation of the parameter associated with the missing data model is based on (5.62).

First, we construct an estimating function for β merely using the response model assumptions. Specifically, we use the formulation of (5.33), which is an unbiased estimating function of β in the absence of measurement error or missingness:

$$U_{ij}(\beta; Y_{ij}, X_{ij}, Z_{ij}) = \left\{ Y_{ij} - \frac{\exp(\beta_0 + \beta_x^{\mathrm{T}} X_{ij} + \beta_z^{\mathrm{T}} Z_{ij})}{1 + \exp(\beta_0 + \beta_x^{\mathrm{T}} X_{ij} + \beta_z^{\mathrm{T}} Z_{ij})} \right\} \begin{pmatrix} 1 \\ X_{ij} \\ Z_{ij} \end{pmatrix}.$$

Next, we modify $U_{ij}(\beta; Y_{ij}, X_{ij}, Z_{ij})$ to incorporate measurement error effects. If using the insertion correction strategy to adjust for measurement error effects, we need to find an estimating function $U_{ij}^*(\beta; Y_{ij}, X_{ij}^*, Z_{ij})$ such that

$$\mathrm{E}\{U_{ij}^*(\beta; Y_{ij}, X_{ij}^*, Z_{ij})|Y_{ij}, X_{ij}, Z_{ij}\} = U_{ij}(\beta; Y_{ij}, X_{ij}, Z_{ij}), \tag{5.66}$$

where the expectation is taken with respect to the model for the conditional distribution of X_{ij}^*, given $\{Y_{ij}, X_{ij}, Z_{ij}\}$.

However, there is no analytical function $U_{ij}^*(\cdot)$ to match $U_{ij}(\cdot)$ such that (5.66) is met (Stefanski 1989). To get around this barrier, we modify $U_{ij}(\beta; Y_{ij}, X_{ij}, Z_{ij})$ by attaching it a weight function

$$w(\beta; X_{ij}, Z_{ij}) = 1 + \exp(\beta_0 + \beta_x^{\mathrm{T}} X_{ij} + \beta_z^{\mathrm{T}} Z_{ij}).$$

Define

$$U_{wij}(\beta; Y_{ij}, X_{ij}, Z_{ij}) = w(\beta; X_{ij}, Z_{ij}) U_{ij}(\beta; Y_{ij}, X_{ij}, Z_{ij}).$$

Then taking

$$\begin{aligned} U_{ij}^*(\beta; Y_{ij}, X_{ij}^*, Z_{ij}) = Y_{ij} &\begin{pmatrix} 1 \\ X_{ij}^* \\ Z_{ij} \end{pmatrix} + (Y_{ij} - 1) \begin{pmatrix} 1 \\ X_{ij}^* - \Sigma_e \beta_x \\ Z_{ij} \end{pmatrix} \\ &\cdot \exp\left(\beta_0 - \frac{\beta_x^{\mathrm{T}} \Sigma_e \beta_x}{2} + \beta_x^{\mathrm{T}} X_{ij}^* + \beta_z^{\mathrm{T}} Z_{ij} \right) \end{aligned}$$

gives us the identity

$$E\{U_{ij}^*(\beta; Y_{ij}, X_{ij}^*, Z_{ij}) | Y_{ij}, X_{ij}, Z_{ij}\} = U_{wij}(\beta; Y_{ij}, X_{ij}, Z_{ij}),$$

which ensures $U_{ij}^*(\beta; Y_{ij}, X_{ij}^*, Z_{ij})$ to be an unbiased estimating function.

Finally, to accommodate missingness effects, we follow (5.63) to construct function $\Phi_{ij}(\cdot)$.

True-Covariate-Driven MAR/MCAR

In contrast to the foregoing modeling strategy for the missing data process which is observed-covariate-driven, we examine the case where missing data processes are true-covariate-driven.

Suppose each subject may drop out before the study ends. That is, for $i = 1, \ldots, n$, $R_{ij} = 0$ implies $R_{ik} = 0$ for all $k > j$. Let $\widetilde{D}_i$ be the random drop-out time for subject i and d_i be a realization. Let $\tau_{ij} = P(R_{ij} = 1 | Y_i, X_i, Z_i)$ for $j = 2, \ldots, m_i$. Suppose that the drop-out process is true-covariate-driven MAR (or MCAR). Then

$$\begin{aligned} \tau_{ij} &= P(R_{ij} = 1 | Y_i^{(o)}, X_i, Z_i) \\ &= \prod_{l=2}^{j} P(R_{il} = 1 | R_{i,l-1} = 1, Y_i^{(o)}, X_i, Z_i), \end{aligned}$$

where we assume $P(R_{i1} = 1 | Y_i, X_i, Z_i) = 1$.

Let $\nu_{ij} = P(R_{ij} = 1 | R_{i,j-1} = 1, Y_i^{(o)}, X_i, Z_i)$ for $j = 2, \ldots, m_i$. Since logistic regression models are commonly used to model drop-out processes (e.g., Diggle and Kenward 1994; Robins, Rotnitzky and Zhao 1995), here we modulate ν_{ij} as

$$\operatorname{logit} \nu_{ij} = \vartheta^{\mathrm{T}} w_{ij}, \tag{5.67}$$

where w_{ij} is the vector consisting of the information of the covariates $\{X_i, Z_i\}$ and the observed responses $Y_i^{(o)}$, and ϑ is the regression parameter.

Then the likelihood contributed from subject i is

$$L_i(\vartheta) = (1 - \nu_{id_i}) \prod_{l=2}^{d_i - 1} \nu_{il}.$$

Let $S_i(\vartheta) = \partial \log L_i(\vartheta)/\partial\vartheta$ be the score function contributed from subject i. Denote $\theta = (\beta^{\mathrm{T}}, \vartheta^{\mathrm{T}})^{\mathrm{T}}$.

Now we describe a sequential method to incorporate measurement error and missingness effects into estimation procedures. We first account for missingness effects by modifying estimating functions $U_{ij}(\beta; Y_{ij}, X_{ij}, Z_{ij})$, where the inverse probability weighted generalized estimating equation (IPWGEE) method, discussed in §5.5.1, is employed. Similar to the construction of (5.57), for each time point j, define

$$U_{ij}^*(\beta, \vartheta) = \left(\frac{\partial \mu_{ij}}{\partial \beta}\right) v_{ij}^{-1} \left(\frac{R_{ij}}{\tau_{ij}}\right) (Y_{ij} - \mu_{ij}).$$

Let $U_i^*(\beta, \vartheta)$ be the combined estimating function of the $U_{ij}^*(\beta, \vartheta)$ using the GMM method as described for formulating (5.34). Define

$$H_i(\theta) = (U_i^{*\mathrm{T}}(\beta, \vartheta), S_i^{\mathrm{T}}(\vartheta))^{\mathrm{T}},$$

which satisfies $E\{H_i(\theta)\} = 0$ in the absence of measurement error.

Next, we correct for measurement error effects by working with $H(\theta)$. Strategies discussed in §5.3 may, in principle, be employed. However, depending on the complexity of the related models, those schemes may not be easily implemented in general. In such instances, we may use an approximate correction method, such as the SIMEX method or the regression calibration approach, to reduce measurement error effects following the implementation steps described in §2.5.3.

5.5.4 *Simultaneous Inference to Accommodating Missingness and Measurement Error Effects*

We discuss a strategy that simultaneously adjusts for effects induced from measurement error and missingness, which is accomplished using the likelihood-based methods. We consider the case where the response process is modeled as (5.9) and (5.10), which is denoted as $f(y_i|x_i, z_i, u_i; \beta)$ together with the model $f(u_i; \gamma)$ for random effects u_i. Here β and γ are the associated model parameters, and the dispersion parameter ϕ is treated as known for ease exposition.

For missing data processes, we consider the scenario where the process is true-covariate-driven and the missing data indicator R_i is independent of random effects u_i when $\{Y_i, X_i, X_i^*, Z_i\}$ is given, i.e.,

$$h(r_i|y_i, x_i, x_i^*, z_i, u_i) = h(r_i|y_i, x_i^*, x_i, z_i) = h(r_i|y_i, x_i, z_i). \tag{5.68}$$

We utilize the decomposition

$$h(r_i|y_i, x_i, z_i) = \prod_{j=2}^{m_i} h(r_{ij}|\mathcal{H}_{ij}^{\mathrm{R}}, y_i, x_i, z_i) \tag{5.69}$$

so that the missing data process can be determined by modeling a sequence of conditional distributions $h(r_{ij}|\mathcal{H}_{ij}^{\mathrm{R}}, y_i, x_i, z_i)$ for univariate variables R_{ij} given the history $\mathcal{H}_{ij}^{\mathrm{R}}$ and $\{Y_i, X_i.Z_i\}$, where $h(r_{i1}|y_i, x_i, z_i)$ is assumed to be 1.

For example, let $\nu_{ij} = P(R_{ij} = 1|\mathcal{H}_{ij}^{\mathrm{R}}, Y_i, X_i, Z_i)$, then a logistic regression model may be employed:

$$\text{logit } \nu_{ij} = \vartheta^{\mathrm{T}} w_{ij}, \tag{5.70}$$

where w_{ij} includes the information of the covariates and responses together with the history of the missing data indicator, and ϑ is the associated parameter.

To feature measurement error, we employ multiple regression model (2.29):

$$X_i = \alpha_0 + \Gamma_x X_i^* + \Gamma_z Z_i + e_i, \tag{5.71}$$

where the e_i are independent of $\{X_i^*, Z_i\}$ and the responses as well as random effects u_i; e_i has zero mean and follows a distribution $f(e_i; \alpha_e)$ with parameter vector α_e; and α_0, Γ_x and Γ_z are defined as for (2.28). Let α be the vector including all the parameters for model (5.71).

Let $\theta = (\beta^{\mathrm{T}}, \gamma^{\mathrm{T}}, \vartheta^{\mathrm{T}}, \alpha^{\mathrm{T}})^{\mathrm{T}}$ be the vector of all the parameters associated with the response, missing data and measurement error models. To conduct inference for θ, we employ an extended version of the EM algorithm, discussed in §2.5.1.

We assume that

$$h(y_i|x_i, x_i^*, z_i, u_i) = h(y_i|x_i, z_i, u_i)$$

and

$$h(u_i|x_i, x_i^*, z_i) = h(u_i), \tag{5.72}$$

where $h(\cdot|\cdot)$ and $h(\cdot)$ represent the conditional and marginal distributions for the variables indicated by the corresponding arguments.

Under the assumptions for the missing data process as well as (5.72), the logarithm of the complete data likelihood contributed from subject i is

$$\begin{aligned} \ell_{ci} = {} & \log f(r_i|y_i, x_i, z_i; \vartheta) + \log f(y_i|x_i, z_i, u_i; \beta) \\ & + \log f(u_i; \gamma) + \log f\left(x_i|x_i^*, z_i; \alpha\right), \end{aligned} \tag{5.73}$$

where $f(r_i|y_i, x_i, z_i; \vartheta)$ is the model for (5.69), determined by (5.70); and $f\left(x_i|x_i^*, z_i; \alpha\right)$ is determined by (5.71).

The E-step for iteration $(k + 1)$ gives

$$Q_i\left(\theta; \theta^{(k)}\right) = E\left\{\ell_{ci}|Y_i^{(o)}, R_i, X_i^*, Z_i; \theta^{(k)}\right\}$$

$$= \int\int\int \Big\{ \log f\left(r_i|y_i^{(o)}, y_i^{(m)}, x_i, z_i; \vartheta\right) + \log f\left(y_i^{(o)}, y_i^{(m)}|x_i, z_i, u_i; \beta\right)$$

$$+ \log f(u_i; \gamma) + \log f\left(x_i|x_i^*, z_i; \alpha\right) \Big\}$$

$$\cdot f\left(y_i^{(m)}, x_i, u_i|y_i^{(o)}, r_i, x_i^*, z_i; \theta^{(k)}\right) d\eta(y_i^{(m)})\, dx_i\, d\eta(u_i),$$

where $f(y_i^{(m)}, x_i, u_i|y_i^{(o)}, r_i, x_i^*, z_i; \theta^{(k)})$ is the model for the conditional distribution of the "missing" components $\{Y_i^{(m)}, X_i, u_i\}$, given the observed data $\{Y_i^{(o)}, R_i, X_i^*, Z_i\}$, evaluated at parameter value $\theta^{(k)}$ obtained from the kth iteration.

It is difficult to directly evaluate expectation $Q(\theta; \theta^{(k)})$ because the associated multiple integrals do not yield an analytically closed-form. Instead, we employ the Monte Carlo EM algorithm to encompass this problem. For each i, we generate a large number of samples from the distribution $f(y_i^{(m)}, x_i, u_i|y_i^{(o)}, r_i, x_i^*, z_i; \theta^{(k)})$ and use the sample information to approximate the integrals. Specifically, the Gibbs sampler technique is invoked to generate samples, where we iteratively sample from $f(y_i^{(m)}|x_i, u_i, y_i^{(o)}, r_i, x_i^*, z_i; \theta^{(k)})$, $f(x_i|u_i, y_i, r_i, x_i^*, z_i; \theta^{(k)})$, and $f(u_i|y_i, x_i, r_i, x_i^*, z_i; \theta^{(k)})$, using the decompositions:

$$f(y_i^{(m)}|x_i, u_i, y_i^{(o)}, r_i, x_i^*, z_i; \theta^{(k)}) = \frac{f(r_i, y_i|x_i, x_i^*, z_i, u_i; \theta^{(k)})}{f(r_i, y_i^{(o)}|x_i, x_i^*, z_i, u_i; \theta^{(k)})}$$

$$\propto f(r_i|x_i, y_i, z_i; \theta^{(k)}) f(y_i|x_i, u_i, z_i; \theta^{(k)});$$

$$f(x_i|u_i, y_i, r_i, x_i^*, z_i; \theta^{(k)}) = \frac{f(r_i, y_i, x_i|x_i^*, z_i, u_i; \theta^{(k)})}{f(r_i, y_i|x_i^*, z_i, u_i; \theta^{(k)})}$$

$$\propto f(r_i|x_i, y_i, z_i; \theta^{(k)}) f(y_i|x_i, u_i, z_i; \theta^{(k)}) f(x_i|x_i^*, z_i; \theta^{(k)});$$

$$f(u_i|x_i, y_i, r_i, x_i^*, z_i; \theta^{(k)}) = f(u_i|y_i, x_i, x_i^*, z_i; \theta^{(k)})$$

$$\propto f(y_i|x_i, u_i, z_i; \theta^{(k)}) f(u_i; \theta^{(k)});$$

where the assumptions for the missing data process and (5.72) are used.

At the kth iteration, for each i let

$$v_{il}^{(k)} = \{y_i^{(m)(l,k)}, x_i^{(l,k)}, u_i^{(l,k)}\}$$

denote the lth sample generated from distribution

$$f(y_i^{(m)}, x_i, u_i|y_i^{(o)}, r_i, x_i^*, z_i; \theta^{(k)}),$$

where $l = 1, \ldots, N_k$ and N_k is a given positive integer which may increase with the iteration number k to speed up the algorithm. Then we approximate $Q_i\left(\theta; \theta^{(k)}\right)$ with

$$\widehat{Q}_i\left(\theta; \theta^{(k)}\right) = \frac{1}{N_k} \sum_{l=1}^{N_k} \ell_{ci}(v_{il}^{(k)}; \theta^{(k)}),$$

where $\ell_{ci}(v_{il}^{(k)}; \theta^{(k)})$ is determined by (5.73) with $\{y^{(m)}, x_i, u_i\}$ replaced by $v_{il}^{(k)}$.

At the M-step, we maximize $\sum_{i=1}^{n} \widehat{Q}_i\left(\theta; \theta^{(k)}\right)$ with respect to θ using an optimization procedure and obtain an updated estimate $\theta^{(k+1)}$ for θ. Repeat through the E and M steps until convergence of $\theta^{(k+1)}$. Let $\widehat{\theta}$ denote the limit of estimates $\{\theta^{(k)} : k = 1, 2, \ldots\}$.

An estimate of the covariance matrix of $\widehat{\theta}$ may be obtained using the formula of Louis (1982) which requires computation of the second derivatives of ℓ_{ci}. Alternatively, one may employ the approximation formula of McLachlan and Krishnan (1997), as discussed by Liu and Wu (2007) and Yi, Liu and Wu (2011).

The preceding development is directed to true-covariate-driven missing data processes. It can be easily modified to accommodate missing data with the observed-covariate-driven mechanism. Our discussion here assumes a GLMM for the response process. Extensions to other response models, such as nonlinear mixed effects models, are carried out along the same lines.

5.5.5 Discussion

In the development of §5.5.3 and §5.5.4, we consider missing data with the true-covariate-driven or the observed-covariate-driven mechanism. With either mechanism, the sequential correction procedures can, at each step, fully adjust for one type of effects arising from measurement error in covariates or missingness in responses.

For general situations where missing data are neither true-covariate-driven nor observed-covariate-driven, it is difficult to *completely* sort out measurement error effects or missingness effects within a *single* step, although it is still possible to sequentially develop a valid inference method. In such instances, *simultaneously* addressing both measurement error effects and missingness effects may be more natural; factorization (5.58) provides a convenient way to develop likelihood-based methods.

The sequential methods, discussed in §5.5.3, are attractive in that the response model does not have to be fully specified; only the mean and variance structures are assumed for the response process. These methods usually require missing data to be MAR or MCAR together with (5.59) or (5.60) so that parameters associated with the missing data model are identifiable. If missing data are MNAR under (5.59) or (5.60), then these methods may only be employed for sensitivity analyses. On the other hand, the simultaneous procedures, discussed in §5.5.4, require full model assumptions, but they are flexible for accommodation of various types of missing data processes.

In this section, missingness arises from responses while measurement error comes from covariates. Other types of "imperfect" data, such as data with incomplete covariates or error-prone responses, may be handled following the same principles, although technical details are different. No matter what the specific technical details are, several important aspects need to be recognized.

In analyzing "imperfect" data which involve both missing observations and measurement error, usual classification of measurement error mechanisms for the missingness-free context and classification of missing data mechanisms for the error-free setting become less insightful. In a broad sense, when both missingness and measurement error are present, modeling of their processes, even though being a nuisance, is generally required. The feasibility of nuisance models is, however, often difficult to assess using standard model diagnostic techniques due to the unavailability of "perfect" data. To resolve this concern, sensitivity analyses serve as a viable strategy to evaluate inference results.

A second aspect is that model identifiability can be a serious concern when dealing with "imperfect" data. In analyzing data with measurement error alone, nonidentifiability is often an issue, which is normally overcome with use of an additional data source, such as a validation subsample, replicates, or instrumental variables (Carroll et al. 2006). On the other hand, in the error-free setting with MNAR incomplete data, model identifiability is commonly questionable due to the lack of information on the values of those unobserved variables (Verbeke and Molenberghs 2000).

The identifiability issue becomes more challenging when both missingness and measurement error are present. Empirically, if parameters are not identifiable, fast divergence occurs in numerical iterative procedures. For instance, the EM algorithm would diverge quickly if there is a nonidentifiability problem (Stubbendick and Ibrahim 2003). When model nonidentifiability arises, it is useful to conduct sensitivity analyses to evaluate how inference results may change for a series of given models and specified parameter values.

With sufficiently many repeated measurements of error-prone covariates, model parameters are more likely to be identified, especially when those within individual repeated measurements are conditionally independent, given other measurements. Parameter identification may also be possible for some highly structured models (Carroll et al. 2006, p. 189).

5.5.6 Simulation and Example

We conduct numerical studies to illustrate a sequential method discussed in Example 5.6. First, we run a simulation study where we set $n = 500$ and $m_i = 5$ for $i = 1, \ldots, n$, and generate 1000 simulated data sets for each parameter configuration. Response measurements Y_{ij} are generated independently from the logistic regression model (5.65) where the Z_{ij} are time-independent binary variables, denoted as Z_i, and take values 0 and 1 each with probability 0.5. Error-prone covariate $X_{ij} = (X_{ij1}, X_{ij2})^{\mathrm{T}}$ is, independent of Z_i, generated from $N(\mu_x, \Sigma_x)$ where $\mu_x = (\mu_{x1}, \mu_{x2})^{\mathrm{T}}$, and Σ_x has diagonal elements $\{\sigma_{x1}^2, \sigma_{x2}^2\}$ and off-diagonal elements $\rho_x \sigma_{x1} \sigma_{x2}$, with $\mu_{xk} = 0.5$ and $\sigma_{xk} = 1$ for $k = 1, 2$, and $\rho_x = 0.5$. We set $\beta_0 = -0.1$, $\beta_{x1} = 0.3$, $\beta_{x2} = 0.6$, and $\beta_z = 0.5$.

Surrogate $X_{ij}^* = (X_{ij1}^*, X_{ij2}^*)^{\mathrm{T}}$ and the true covariate X_{ij} are linked by the measurement error model (5.61), where covariance matrix Σ_e has diagonal elements $\{\sigma_{e1}^2, \sigma_{e2}^2\}$ and off-diagonal elements $\rho_e \sigma_{e1} \sigma_{e2}$. We consider the cases with $\rho_e = 0.5$ and $\sigma_{e1} = \sigma_{e2} = 0.15, 0.5, 0.75$, featuring minor, moderate and severe marginal measurement error; let σ_e denote common values of σ_{e1} and σ_{e2}.

Consider a drop-out scenario where the missing data indicator is generated from the model

$$\operatorname{logit} \tau_{ij} = \vartheta_0 + \vartheta_y Y_{i,j-1} + \vartheta_{x*} X_{i,j-1,1}^* + \vartheta_z Z_i$$

for $j = 2, \ldots, m_i$, where we set $\vartheta_0 = -0.3, \vartheta_y = 0.5, \vartheta_{x^*} = 0.2$, and $\vartheta_z = 0.2$. This yields approximately 47% missingness when $Y_{i,j-1} = 0, X_{i,j-1,1} = 1$, and $Z_i = 0$.

Four analyses are conducted. Analysis 1 is the naive analysis which ignores both covariate measurement error and response missingness, where the usual GEE method with an independence working matrix is employed; Analysis 2 modifies Analysis 1 with response missingness taken into account but covariate measurement error ignored; Analysis 3 modifies Analysis 1 with measurement error effects accommodated but missingness effects ignored; and Analysis 4 is carried out using the method described in Example 5.6 which corrects for the effects induced from both covariate measurement error and response missingness.

Fig. 5.1 plots the finite sample biases against the value of σ_e for the four analyses. As expected, the three analyses that do not accommodate measurement error or missingness produce strikingly biased results. The method accounting for both measurement error and missingness produces much smaller finite sample biases.

Next, we illustrate the method described in Example 5.6 by considering the data analyzed by Yi, Ma and Carroll (2012). The data set consists of repeated measurements for 1737 individuals with 24-hour recall food intake interviews taken on four different days. Information on age, vitamin A intake, vitamin C intake, total fat intake and total calorie intake is collected at each interview.

Let Y_{ij} be the binary response variable indicating whether or not the reported percentage of calories for individual i exceeds 35% at time point j. About 4% of the Y_{ij} measurements are missing. We study how the fat intake changes with age and how it is associated with the intake of vitamin A and vitamin C.

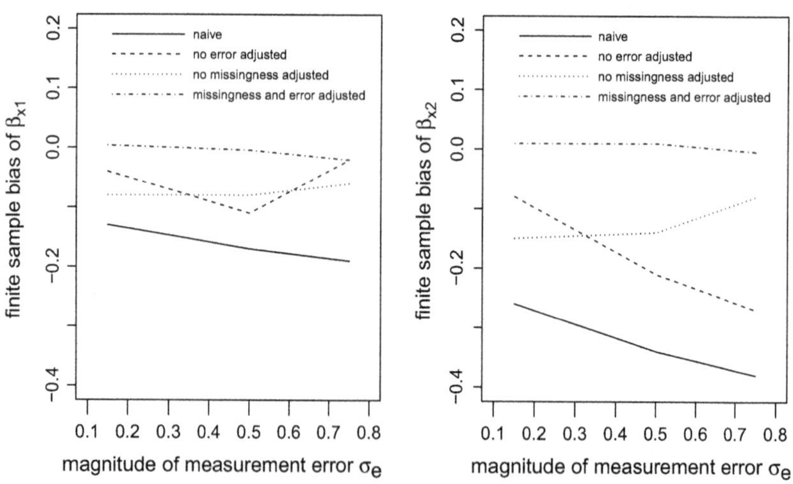

Fig. 5.1. *A Simulation Study for the Comparison of the Four Methods*

For subject i at interview j, let X_{ij1}^* be the logarithm of 0.005 plus the standardized reported vitamin A intake, X_{ij2}^* be similarly defined for reported vitamin C intake, and Z_i be the baseline age in years divided by 100. Yi, Ma and Carroll (2012) commented that such transformations allow us to reasonably use a normal distribution to approximate the measurement error process. Consider the logistic regression model

$$\text{logit } P(Y_{ij} = 1|X_i, Z_i) = \beta_0 + \beta_{x1} X_{ij1} + \beta_{x2} X_{ij2} + \beta_z Z_i$$

for $j = 1, \ldots, 4$ and $i = 1, \ldots, 1737$, where β_0, β_{x1}, β_{x2} and β_z are regression parameters.

Vitamins A and C are measured with substantial random error. However, the study does not have sufficient information for estimation of the covariance matrix of the measurement error directly. To obtain an approximate assessment, we first treat the four measurements of the vitamins A and C intake as repeated measurements of the long-term average intake value and obtain the sample variances, respectively, given by 0.90 and 0.84, and the sample correlation coefficient 0.36. Noticing that two sources of variability, the variability of the true vitamin intake near the time of the visits and the measurement error variability, are involved, and that no information is available for us to separate these two variabilities, we allocate half to each, so that the estimates of the measurement error variances are taken as $\widehat{\sigma}_{e1}^2 = 0.45$ and $\widehat{\sigma}_{e2}^2 = 0.42$.

Similar to the preceding simulation study, four analyses are performed. The results are reported in Table 5.1. The analyses show a significantly positive correlation between vitamin A intake and over-consumption of fat, while this association is negative for vitamin C. Considering that common sources of vitamin A are meat and animal organs while those of vitamin C are vegetables and fruits, these results are perhaps plausible. The consequence of ignoring the measurement error is attenuation towards zero while ignoring the missingness seems to result in slight overestimation of the covariate effects. A more detailed study on this data set was reported by Yi, Ma and Carroll (2012) where sensitivity analyses were performed to address different degrees of measurement error in the intake of vitamins A and C.

Table 5.1. *Analysis Results Reported by Yi, Ma and Carroll (2012)*

	Analysis 1			Analysis 2			Analysis 3			Analysis 4		
	EST	SE	p-value	EST	SE	p-value	EST	SE	p-value	EST	SE	p-value
β_0	0.21	0.14	0.14	0.21	0.15	0.14	0.31	0.15	0.04	0.26	0.16	0.09
β_{x1}	0.17	0.03	0.00	0.12	0.03	0.00	0.39	0.07	0.00	0.28	0.07	0.00
β_{x2}	−0.12	0.03	0.00	−0.13	0.03	0.00	−0.31	0.06	0.00	−0.31	0.07	0.00
β_z	0.41	0.39	0.29	0.42	0.39	0.29	0.60	0.40	0.13	0.57	0.41	0.16

5.6 Joint Modeling of Longitudinal and Survival Data with Measurement Error

In addition to collecting repeated measurements over a time period, many longitudinal studies also gather information on time-to-event of interest (often termed "survival time"), such as infection or death. As longitudinal and time-to-event outcomes are usually associated, marginal methods, which separately postulate the longitudinal and survival processes, become incapable of conducting inferences. In addition, longitudinal measurements cannot be observed after the event time, marginal methods often fail to incorporate this feature in the analysis.

A remedy to overcome the drawbacks of marginal methods is to combine the survival and longitudinal components and carry out inferences simultaneously within a likelihood-based framework. This approach enables us to mutually borrow information from each process and gain efficiency in estimation, besides correcting potential bias involved in the marginal analysis.

There has been increasing interest in joint modeling of longitudinal and survival data. Depending on research interest, longitudinal outcomes and the event time are handled with different schemes. Three categories divide the methods on joint modeling analysis, analogously to those for handling missing data outlined in §5.5.1. *Selection models* postulate the marginal distribution of the longitudinal measurements and the conditional distribution of the event time, given the longitudinal measurements (Diggle and Kenward 1994), while *pattern-mixture models* factorize the joint distribution into the marginal distribution of the event time and the distribution of the longitudinal measurements conditional on the event time (Little 1993). *Latent models*, on the other hand, assume an underlying latent process, and conditional on latent variables, repeated measurements and the event time are assumed independent (Wu and Carroll 1988; Wulfsohn and Tsiatis 1997).

In this section, we discuss some joint modeling methods with the focus on the selection model framework. To highlight the essence without being distracted by complex technical exposition, we consider the case where only a scalar covariate $X_i(t)$ contributes longitudinal measurements and other covariates Z_i are time-invariant. For the time-to-event process, we consider the same setup as in §3.1.5.

Consider the Cox proportional hazards model

$$\lambda(t|\mathcal{H}_{it}^{\mathrm{X}}, Z_i) = \lambda_0(t)\exp\{\beta_x X_i(t) + \beta_z^{\mathrm{T}} Z_i\}, \tag{5.74}$$

where $i = 1, \ldots, n$, $\mathcal{H}_{it}^{\mathrm{X}} = \{X_i(v) : 0 \le v \le t\}$ is the history of the time-dependent covariate up to and including time t for subject i, as defined on page 94; $\lambda(t|\mathcal{H}_{it}^{\mathrm{X}}, Z_i)$ is the hazard function at time t conditional on the covariate history; $\lambda_0(t)$ is the baseline hazard function; and $\beta = (\beta_x, \beta_z^{\mathrm{T}})^{\mathrm{T}}$ is the regression parameter.

The longitudinal process is usually not fully observed; it is measured intermittently at certain time points and with measurement error. In addition, in many studies, longitudinal covariate measurements terminate at censoring or the event time. Let $0 \le t_{i1} < \ldots < t_{im_i}$ be the observation times for subject i, where m_i is the number of longitudinal measurements for subject i, and the last observation time t_{im_i} is no bigger than t_i, the minimum of T_i and C_i.

It is customary to express the observed longitudinal measurements $X_i^*(t_{ij})$ for subject i at time t_{ij} as

$$X_i^*(t_{ij}) = X_i(t_{ij}) + e_{ij} \text{ for } j = 1, \ldots, m_i \text{ with } t_{im_i} \leq t_i, \tag{5.75}$$

where the e_{ij} are independent of each other and of $\{T_i, C_i, Z_i, X_i(t) : t \geq 0\}$ and follow a normal distribution $N(0, \sigma_e^2)$ with variance σ_e^2.

To complete the model setup, we describe modeling of the true covariate $X_i(t)$ process. To accommodate possible heterogeneity existing in different subjects, random effects models are used to describe the $X_i(t)$ process:

$$X_i(t) = u_i^{\mathrm{T}} \rho(t), \tag{5.76}$$

where u_i is a vector of random effects that are independent of the e_{ij} and $\{T_i, C_i, Z_i\}$, and $\rho(t)$ is a vector of functions in t. We write $X_i = \{X_i(t_{i1}), \ldots, X_i(t_{im_i})\}^{\mathrm{T}}$ and $X_i^* = \{X_i^*(t_{i1}), \ldots, X_i^*(t_{im_i})\}^{\mathrm{T}}$.

The linear structure of (5.76) is motivated from a viewpoint of functional data analysis, as discussed by Ding and Wang (2008). Model (5.76) is flexible to cover a broad class of random effects models by different specifications of $\rho(t)$. For example, setting $\rho(t) = (1, t, \ldots, t^{r-1})^{\mathrm{T}}$ leads to the polynomial growth-curve model that is often discussed in the literature (e.g., Wulfsohn and Tsiatis 1997; Tseng, Hsieh and Wang 2005), where r is a positive integer. If the trajectory of the $X_i(t)$ has a complex nonlinear form over time, other functional form of the $\rho(t)$ may be assumed. For instance, Tseng, Hsieh and Wang (2005) adopted the form of $\rho(t) = (\log t, t-1)^{\mathrm{T}}$ in their example for the egg-laying trajectories of the medfly data. Relaxation of model (5.76) to include fixed effects of covariates can be done readily; see Li, Hu and Greene (2009) for example. If there is little knowledge of choosing a suitable parametric form for $\rho(t)$, one may completely treat the elements of $\rho(t)$ as unknown smooth functions (Ding and Wang 2008).

For inferences, one needs to untangle the impact of the censoring and assessment processes on the response and covariate processes as well. As discussed in §3.1.4 and §4.1.3, modeling of the censoring and assessment processes is generally needed unless simplistic assumptions are made. To leave both processes unmodeled, we assume that the censoring and assessment processes are noninformative and independent of the future covariates and random effects u_i.

5.6.1 Likelihood-Based Methods

Assume that $f_{ui}(u; \sigma_u)$ is the model for the distribution of random effects u_i, where σ_u is the parameter and the function form $f_{ui}(\cdot)$ is given. Let $\theta = (\beta^{\mathrm{T}}, \lambda_0(\cdot), \sigma_e^{\mathrm{T}}, \sigma_u^{\mathrm{T}})^{\mathrm{T}}$ be the vector containing all the model parameters, where $\lambda_0(\cdot)$ is a function of time that involves additional parameters if modeled parametrically.

We assume that measurement error is nondifferential, as discussed in §3.2.2. Then the joint likelihood for the observed data is

$$L = \prod_{i=1}^{n} \int f_{\mathrm{s}i} f_{\mathrm{L}i} f_{ui} \, d\eta(u_i), \tag{5.77}$$

where $f_{\mathrm{s}i}$ denotes the probability density function which postulates the survival process, given by

$$\begin{aligned} f_{\mathrm{s}i} &= [\lambda_0(t_i) \exp\{\beta_x X_i(t_i) + \beta_z^{\mathrm{T}} Z_i\}]^{\delta_i} \\ &\quad \cdot \exp\left[- \int_0^{t_i} \lambda_0(v) \exp\{\beta_x X_i(v) + \beta_z^{\mathrm{T}} Z_i\} dv \right] \end{aligned}$$

with $X_i(t)$ replaced by model (5.76), $f_{\mathrm{L}i}$ represents the model for the longitudinal components

$$f_{\mathrm{L}i} = \frac{1}{(2\pi\sigma_e^2)^{m_i/2}} \exp\left[-\frac{1}{2\sigma_e^2} \sum_{j=1}^{m_i} \{X_i^*(t_{ij}) - X_i(t_{ij})\}^2 \right]$$

with $X_i(t_{ij})$ replaced by model (5.76), and the dependence on the parameter is supposed in the notation.

To use (5.77) for estimation, one needs to deal with the baseline hazard function $\lambda_0(t)$ in the survival model. One way is to take a nonparametric viewpoint by assuming that $\lambda_0(t)$ has masses at the observed survival times and regard these values as unknown parameters (e.g., Wulfsohn and Tsiatis 1997). Another approach is to assume that $\lambda_0(t)$ is a constant between two consecutive estimated baseline survival times, as considered by Tseng, Hsieh and Wang (2005). These methods create a set of additional parameters whose dimension is of the same order as the sample size n. While this growing dimension may not necessarily generate considerable computational complications, it does pose theoretical challenges which are pertinent to situations of infinitely many nuisance parameters, briefly described in §1.3.4.

As an alternative, one may handle $\lambda_0(t)$ using a weakly parametric approach, as described by (3.2), and apply standard likelihood theory to establish asymptotic properties of the resulting estimators. It should be noted, however, that this method essentially ignores variability induced from the specification of cut points for the pre-specified intervals, so it is viewed as a conditional analysis on a given set of cut points for modulating $\lambda_0(t)$.

With the baseline hazard function modeled, one may proceed with maximizing (5.77) with respect to the model parameter θ. As (5.77) does not have a closed-form, numerical approximations, such as the Monte Carlo algorithm, may be used to handle the integrals. When the dimension of random effects u_i is high, this method becomes infeasible.

Alternatively, one may employ the Monte Carlo EM algorithm which directly makes use of the joint likelihood for the complete data:

$$L_{\mathrm{C}}(\theta) = \prod_{i=1}^{n} f_{\mathrm{s}i} f_{\mathrm{L}i} f_{ui}.$$

At the E-step for iteration $(k+1)$, we need to evaluate the conditional expectation

$$E\{\log L_{\mathrm{C}}(\theta)|t_i, \delta_i, X_i^*, Z_i; \theta^{(k)}\},$$

where the expectation is taken with respect to the model for the conditional distribution of unobserved u_i, given the observed data $\{t_i, \delta_i, X_i^*, Z_i\}$, which is evaluated at the parameter estimate $\theta^{(k)}$ obtained at the kth iteration. Specifically, this conditional model is determined by

$$\begin{aligned} f(u_i|t_i, \delta_i, x_i^*, z_i; \theta) &= \frac{f(u_i, t_i, \delta_i|x_i^*, z_i; \theta)}{f(t_i, \delta_i|x_i^*, z_i; \theta)} \\ &= \frac{f_{\mathrm{si}}(u_i; \theta) f(u_i|x_i^*, z_i; \theta)}{\int f_{\mathrm{si}}(u_i; \theta) f(u_i|x_i^*, z_i; \theta) d\eta(u_i)}, \end{aligned} \tag{5.78}$$

where $f_{\mathrm{si}}(u_i; \theta)$ is f_{si} with $X_i(t)$ replaced by model (5.76), and the conditional model $f(u_i|x_i^*, z_i; \theta)$ is given by

$$f(u_i|x_i^*, z_i; \theta) = \frac{f_{\mathrm{Li}} f_{ui}}{\int f_{\mathrm{Li}} f_{ui} d\eta(u_i)}. \tag{5.79}$$

(5.79) assumes a simple form in some situations; it is a normal distribution if both f_{ui} for random effects u_i and f_{Li} for longitudinal measurements are assumed to be normal.

To evaluate $E\{\log L_{\mathrm{C}}(\theta)|t_i, \delta_i, X_i^*, Z_i; \theta^{(k)}\}$, it suffices to calculate

$$E\{g(u_i; \theta)|t_i, \delta_i, X_i^*, Z_i; \theta^{(k)}\}$$

for those functions $g(\cdot)$ of u_i which are involved in $\log L_{\mathrm{C}}(\theta)$. By (5.78), we write

$$\begin{aligned} E\{g(u_i; \theta)|t_i, \delta_i, X_i^*, Z_i; \theta^{(k)}\} &= \frac{\int g(u_i; \theta) f_{\mathrm{si}}(u_i; \theta^{(k)}) f(u_i|x_i^*, z_i; \theta^{(k)}) d\eta(u_i)}{\int f_{\mathrm{si}}(u_i; \theta^{(k)}) f(u_i|x_i^*, z_i; \theta^{(k)}) d\eta(u_i)} \\ &= \frac{E\{g(u_i; \theta) f_{\mathrm{si}}(u_i; \theta^{(k)})|X_i^*, Z_i; \theta^{(k)}\}}{E\{f_{\mathrm{si}}(u_i; \theta^{(k)})|X_i^*, Z_i; \theta^{(k)}\}}, \end{aligned} \tag{5.80}$$

where the expectations are evaluated with respect to (5.79) with parameter value $\theta^{(k)}$.

Consequently, (5.80) may be handled using the Monte Carlo method. For a large positive integer N, generate a sequence of values, say $\{u_i^1, \ldots, u_i^N\}$, from the conditional distribution (5.79) where θ is evaluated as $\theta^{(k)}$, then we approximate $E\{g(u_i; \theta)|t_i, \delta_i, X_i^*, Z_i; \theta^{(k)}\}$ by

$$\frac{\sum_{j=1}^N g(u_i^j; \theta) f_{\mathrm{si}}(u_i^j; \theta^{(k)})}{\sum_{j=1}^N f_{\mathrm{si}}(u_i^j; \theta^{(k)})}.$$

At the M-step, we maximize the resulting approximation of

$$E\{\log L_{\mathrm{C}}(\theta)|t_i, \delta_i, X_i^*, Z_i; \theta^{(k)}\}$$

with respect to θ and obtain an updated estimate $\theta^{(k+1)}$ of parameter θ. Repeat these steps until convergence of $\theta^{(k+1)}$; the estimate at convergence is taken as the point estimate, say $\widehat{\theta}$, of θ.

To calculate the variance estimate associated with $\widehat{\theta}$, we may utilize the formula of Louis (1982) based on the observed Fisher information matrix for parameter θ. However, this approach may become infeasible when the dimension of θ is huge. In this case, one may revert to the bootstrap procedure (Efron and Tibshirani 1993; Efron 1994) for an estimate of covariance matrix of $\widehat{\theta}$.

5.6.2 Conditional Score Method

In conducting likelihood-based methods outlined in §5.6.1, we impose a distributional assumption for random effects, which is not verifiable because random effects are never being observed. When distributional misspecification occurs in a likelihood formulation, biased results usually arise. In this section, we discuss an estimation method that requires no distributional assumption on random effects; this is the conditional score method explored by Tsiatis and Davidian (2001) and Song, Davidian and Tsiatis (2002); an outline of this method is given in §2.5.1.

First, for each subject i and a given time t, we derive an "estimator" of $X_i(t)$ by treating u_i in (5.76) to be a vector of parameters. This is carried out by combining (5.76) with (5.75) and using all the longitudinal measurements up to and including time point t from subject i.

Specifically, let $\mathcal{A}_i(t) = \{t_{ij} : t_{ij} \leq t \text{ for } j = 1, \ldots, m_i\}$ be the longitudinal assessment times for subject i up to and including time point t, and $m_i(t)$ be the number of measurements in $\mathcal{A}_i(t)$. In order to estimate $X_i(t)$ at time t, we must have $m_i(t) \geq r$, i.e., subject i must have at least r measurements up to time t, where r is the dimension of u_i. Define the at risk process

$$R_i(t) = I\{t_i \geq t;\ m_i(t) \geq r\}.$$

Let $\Psi_i(t) = [\rho(t_{i1}) \ldots \rho(t_{im_i(t)})]^{\mathrm{T}}$ be the $m_i(t) \times r$ matrix recording the changes for $X_i(t)$ by time t. Combining (5.75) and (5.76) yields

$$\mathcal{X}_i^*(t) = \Psi_i(t) u_i + e_i(t) \tag{5.81}$$

where $\mathcal{X}_i^*(t) = (X_i^*(t_{i1}), \ldots, X_i^*(t_{im_i(t)}))^{\mathrm{T}}$ and $e_i(t) = (e_{i1}, \ldots, e_{im_i(t)})^{\mathrm{T}}$.

Let $\mathcal{C}_i(t)$ denote the collection $\{R_i(t) = 1, u_i, Z_i, \mathcal{A}_i(t)\}$. Then conditional on $\mathcal{C}_i(t)$, we treat $\mathcal{X}_i^*(t)$ as a response vector with independent components, $\Psi_i(t)$ as the covariate matrix, and u_i as the parameter vector. Applying the least squares regression method to (5.81), we obtain an estimator, denoted by $\widehat{u}_i(t)$, of u_i, based on the measurements by time t:

$$\widehat{u}_i(t) = \{\Psi_i^{\mathrm{T}}(t)\Psi_i(t)\}^{-1}\Psi_i^{\mathrm{T}}(t)\mathcal{X}_i^*(t),$$

where the inverse matrix is assumed to exist.

Linear regression theory implies that conditional on $C_i(t)$, $\widehat{u}_i(t)$ has a normal distribution with mean u_i and covariance matrix $\Sigma_i(t)$, given by

$$\Sigma_i(t) = \sigma_e^2\{\Psi_i^{\mathrm{T}}(t)\Psi_i(t)\}^{-1}.$$

Let $\widehat{X}_i(t) = \widehat{u}_i^{\mathrm{T}}(t)\rho(t)$ be an "estimator" of $X_i(t)$. Then conditional on $C_i(t)$, $\widehat{X}_i(t)$ follows a normal distribution

$$\widehat{X}_i(t)|C_i(t) \sim N(X_i(t), \Sigma_{xi}(t)), \tag{5.82}$$

where $\Sigma_{xi}(t) = \rho^{\mathrm{T}}(t)\Sigma_i(t)\rho(t)$. As the estimation procedure is carried out for each subject separately, we further see that the $\widehat{X}_i(t)$ for $i = 1, \ldots, n$ are independent.

Define the counting process increment

$$dN_i(t) = I(t \le t_i < t + dt;\ \delta_i = 1;\ m_i(t) \ge r)$$

for a small time increment dt. Conditional on $C_i(t)$, $dN_i(t)$ and $\widehat{X}_i(t)$ are independent. Therefore, the conditional distribution of $\{dN_i(t) = l, \widehat{X}_i(t) = x\}$, given $C_i(t)$, is the product

$$P\{dN_i(t) = l|C_i(t)\}P\{\widehat{X}_i(t) = x|C_i(t)\},$$

where the first term is determined by a Bernoulli distribution with the probability determined by the proportional hazards model (5.74), given by

$$[\lambda_0(t)\exp\{\beta_x X_i(t) + \beta_z^{\mathrm{T}} Z_i\}dt]^l[1 - \lambda_0(t)\exp\{\beta_x X_i(t) + \beta_z^{\mathrm{T}} Z_i\}dt]^{1-l}$$

for $l = 0$ or 1, and the second term is, by (5.82), the probability density function

$$\frac{1}{\sqrt{2\pi\Sigma_{xi}(t)}}\exp\left[-\frac{\{x - X_i(t)\}^2}{2\Sigma_{xi}(t)}\right].$$

Thus, the conditional distribution of $\{dN_i(t), \widehat{X}_i(t)\}$, given $C_i(t)$, up to order dt, is

$$\begin{aligned}
&[\lambda_0(t)\exp\{\beta_x X_i(t) + \beta_z^{\mathrm{T}} Z_i\}dt]^{dN_i(t)}\frac{1}{\sqrt{2\pi\Sigma_{xi}(t)}}\exp\left[-\frac{\{\widehat{X}_i(t) - X_i(t)\}^2}{2\Sigma_{xi}(t)}\right]\\
&= \exp\left[X_i(t)\left\{\beta_x dN_i(t) + \frac{\widehat{X}_i(t)}{\Sigma_{xi}(t)}\right\}\right]\\
&\quad\cdot\frac{\{\lambda_0(t)\exp(\beta_z^{\mathrm{T}} Z_i)dt\}^{dN_i(t)}}{\sqrt{2\pi\Sigma_{xi}(t)}}\exp\left\{-\frac{\widehat{X}_i^2(t) + X_i^2(t)}{2\Sigma_{xi}(t)}\right\}.
\end{aligned} \tag{5.83}$$

Temporarily treating parameters σ_e^2 and β as known, replacing $X_i(t)$ with the multiplicative form (5.76) and then treating u_i as the parameters, we obtain that, by applying the property of the exponential family distribution to the representation (5.83),

$$\beta_x dN_i(t) + \frac{\widehat{X}_i(t)}{\Sigma_{xi}(t)}$$

or equivalently,

$$\Omega_i(t;\sigma_e^2,\beta_x) = \beta_x \Sigma_{xi}(t) dN_i(t) + \widehat{X}_i(t) \tag{5.84}$$

is a "sufficient statistic" for u_i, at each time t. This suggests that conditioning on $\Omega_i(t;\sigma_e^2,\beta_x)$ would remove the dependence on random effects u_i of the conditional distribution of $\{dN_i(t), \widehat{X}_i(t)\}$, given $\mathcal{C}_i(t)$.

This result offers us a simple way to perform inference about parameter β. Instead of directly working on the initial hazard function $\lambda(t|\mathcal{H}_{it}^{\mathrm{x}}, Z_i)$, given by (5.74), we may consider an alternative process by conditioning on $\Omega_i(t;\sigma_e^2,\beta_x)$ and $\{R_i(t) = 1, Z_i, \mathcal{A}_i(t)\}$. Let

$$\begin{aligned}&\lambda\{t|\Omega_i(t;\sigma_e^2,\beta_x), R_i(t) = 1, Z_i, \mathcal{A}_i(t)\}\\ &= \lim_{dt\to 0+} \frac{P\{dN_i(t) = 1|\Omega_i(t;\sigma_e^2,\beta_x), R_i(t) = 1, Z_i, \mathcal{A}_i(t)\}}{dt}.\end{aligned}$$

This conditional hazard function is equal, up to the order $o_p(dt)$, to

$$\lambda_0(t)\exp\{\beta_x\Omega_i(t;\sigma_e^2,\beta_x) - \beta_x^2\Sigma_{xi}(t)/2 + \beta_z^{\mathrm{T}} Z_i\}. \tag{5.85}$$

Let

$$\begin{aligned}G_{0i}(t;\sigma_e^2,\beta_x) &= R_i(t)\exp\{\beta_x\Omega_i(t;\sigma_e^2,\beta_x) - \beta_x^2\Sigma_{xi}(t)/2 + \beta_z^{\mathrm{T}} Z_i\};\\ G_{1i}(t;\sigma_e^2,\beta_x,\beta_z) &= \{\Omega_i(t;\sigma_e^2,\beta_x,\beta_z), Z_i^{\mathrm{T}}\}^{\mathrm{T}} G_{0i}(t;\sigma_e^2,\beta_x,\beta_z).\end{aligned}$$

Then by analogy with the derivation of the partial likelihood score function for the error-free setting (Tsiatis and Davidian 2001, §3), we obtain the estimating equation for parameter β:

$$\sum_{i=1}^{n} U_{i\beta} = 0, \tag{5.86}$$

where

$$U_{i\beta} = \int \left[\{\Omega_i(t;\sigma_e^2,\beta_x,\beta_z), Z_i^{\mathrm{T}}\}^{\mathrm{T}} - \frac{\sum_{j=1}^n G_{1j}(t;\sigma_e^2,\beta_x,\beta_z)}{\sum_{j=1}^n G_{0j}(t;\sigma_e^2,\beta_x,\beta_z)}\right] dN_i(t).$$

Combining the conditional hazard function (5.85) with (5.84) gives

$$\begin{aligned}&\lambda_0(t)\exp\{\beta_x\widehat{X}_i(t) + \beta_z^{\mathrm{T}} Z_i\}\\ &= \lambda\{t|\Omega_i(t;\sigma_e^2,\beta_x), R_i(t) = 1, Z_i, \mathcal{A}_i(t)\}\cdot\exp[-\beta_x^2\Sigma_x(t)\{dN_i(t) - 1/2\}] + o_p(dt).\end{aligned}$$

This identity reflects the difference of the hazard functions between the conditional method using (5.86) and the naive analysis based on the model (5.74) with $X_i(t)$ replaced by $\widehat{X}_i(t)$. It is clear that the difference is affected by the magnitude σ_e^2 of measurement error as well as the covariate effect β_x. The difference also depends on covariate $X_i(t)$ via function $\rho(\cdot)$. Under the extreme situation where $\sigma_e^2 = 0$ (i.e., there is no measurement error), (5.86) recovers the usual partial likelihood score function for the proportional hazards model.

Equation (5.86) may be used to estimate the response parameter β when the parameter σ_e^2 for the measurement error is known. If σ_e^2 is unknown, it must be estimated and the induced variability should be accounted for when developing the asymptotic distribution of the estimator $\widehat{\beta}$ of β.

We now describe a strategy of estimating σ_e^2 by applying the least squares fit to *all* the covariate measurements for those subjects i with $m_i > r$. This is different from the estimation of $X_i(t)$ where only the covariate measurements by time t for subject i are used.

Let $\Psi_i = [\rho(t_{i1}) \ \ldots \ \rho(t_{im_i})]^{\mathrm{T}}$ be the $m_i \times r$ matrix. Assume that Ψ_i has the rank r. Combining models (5.75) and (5.76) gives

$$X_i^* = \Psi_i u_i + e_i, \tag{5.87}$$

where $e_i = (e_{i1}, \ldots, e_{im_i})^{\mathrm{T}}$.

Conditional on $C_i(t_i)$, we think of X_i^* as a response vector with independent components, Ψ_i as the covariate matrix, and u_i as the parameter vector. Applying the least squares estimation procedure to (5.87) gives an estimator of u_i:

$$\widehat{u}_i = (\Psi_i^{\mathrm{T}} \Psi_i)^{-1} \Psi_i^{\mathrm{T}} X_i^*. \tag{5.88}$$

Let $\widehat{e}_i = X_i^* - \Psi_i \widehat{u}_i$. By (5.87) and (5.88), we obtain that

$$E\{I(m_i > r)\widehat{e}_i^{\mathrm{T}} \widehat{e}_i | C_i(t_i)\} = I(m_i > r) \cdot (m_i - r)\sigma_e^2. \tag{5.89}$$

Consequently, an unbiased estimating function of σ_e^2 is set as

$$U_{ie} = I(m_i > r)\{(X_i^* - \Psi_i \widehat{u}_i)^{\mathrm{T}} (X_i^* - \Psi_i \widehat{u}_i) - (m_i - r)\sigma_e^2\}.$$

Let $\theta = (\beta^{\mathrm{T}}, \sigma_e^2)^{\mathrm{T}}$ and $U_i(\theta) = (U_{i\beta}^{\mathrm{T}}, U_{ie})^{\mathrm{T}}$, then solving

$$\sum_{i=1}^{n} U_i(\theta) = 0$$

for θ yields an estimate of θ. Let $\widehat{\beta} = (\widehat{\beta}_x, \widehat{\beta}_z^{\mathrm{T}})^{\mathrm{T}}$ and $\widehat{\sigma}_e^2$, respectively, denote the corresponding estimators of β and σ_e^2.

Under regularity conditions, $\sqrt{n}(\widehat{\beta} - \beta)$ is asymptotically normally distributed with mean 0 and covariance matrix $\Gamma_\beta^{-1} \Sigma_\beta \Gamma_\beta^{-1\mathrm{T}}$, where

$$\Gamma_\beta = E\{(\partial/\partial\beta^{\mathrm{T}})U_{i\beta}\}, \ \Sigma_\beta = E(Q_i Q_i^{\mathrm{T}}),$$

and

$$Q_i = U_{i\beta} - E\left\{\partial U_{i\beta}/\partial(\sigma_e^2)\right\} \left[E\left\{\partial U_{ie}/\partial(\sigma_e^2)\right\}\right]^{-1} U_{ie}.$$

Empirical counterparts are employed to estimate Γ_β and Σ_β for inference of the parameters β.

The key idea of the conditional score method described here is to find "sufficient statistics" for random effects u_i first and then work on a new process by conditioning on the "sufficient statistics". The dependence of the original process on random effects is completely featured by the "sufficient statistics". This development uses the linearity form of (5.76) when deriving the "sufficient statistics" for random effects u_i. If there is a nonlinear relationship in (5.76), one may adapt the foregoing derivation by invoking a linear approximation of (5.76) first and then applying the delta method to obtain an asymptotic normal distribution of $\widehat{X}_i(t)$ (Song, Davidian and Tsiatis 2002). In the same lines, the preceding development may be extended to the case with multiple covariates as well. Details were provided by Song, Davidian and Tsiatis (2002).

5.7 Bibliographic Notes and Discussion

Measurement error in longitudinal studies has attracted substantial research interest (Carroll et al. 2006, Ch. 11; Wu 2009, Ch. 5). It is known that mismeasurement often distorts usual analysis methods for longitudinal data. With covariate measurement error, Chesher (1991) examined measurement error effects on changing the distributions of the responses and covariates. Wang et al. (1998) conducted bias analysis under generalized linear mixed models. Wang and Davidian (1996), Tosteson, Buonaccorsi and Demidenko (1998), and Ko and Davidian (2000) examined measurement error effects under nonlinear mixed effects models. With error in responses, Neuhaus (2002) investigated effects of misclassified binary response variables on analysis of longitudinal or clustered data.

To address measurement error effects, many authors explored inference methods under a variety of settings. To name a few, Higgins, Davidian and Giltinan (1997) proposed a two-stage estimation method for nonlinear mixed measurement error models. Zidek et al. (1998) discussed a nonlinear regression analysis method for clustered data. Assuming covariates are the regression parameters of random effects models, Wang, Wang and Wang (2000) compared estimators obtained from the pseudo-expected estimating equations, the regression calibration and the refined regression calibration approaches. Lin and Carroll (2000) used the SIMEX approach to correct for covariate measurement error effects under nonparametric regression models. Buonaccorsi, Demidenko and Tosteson (2000) discussed likelihood-based methods for estimation of both regression parameters and variance components in linear mixed models when a time-dependent covariate is subject to measurement error. Other work includes Palta and Lin (1999), Liang (2009), Zhou and Liang (2009), Xiao, Shao and Palta (2010), Yi, Chen and Wu (2017), and the references therein.

Analysis of longitudinal error-prone data is further challenged by the presence of other features, such as survival data with censoring or missing observations (Tsiatis, Degruttola and Wulfsohn 1995; Wulfsohn and Tsiatis 1997). An overview of joint modeling of survival and longitudinal data is available in Tsiatis and Davidian (2004), Wu (2009, Ch. 8), Rizopoulos (2012), Wu et al. (2012), and Gould et al. (2015). To jointly handle survival and longitudinal error-prone data, Tsiatis and Davidian (2001) developed an inference method by adapting the conditioning method on sufficient statistics discussed by Stefanski and Carroll (1987). Wu (2002) developed estimation methods to address censored data and error-prone covariates that are postulated by nonlinear mixed models. Tseng, Hsieh and Wang (2005) explored a joint modelling approach under the accelerated failure time model when covariates are assumed to follow a linear mixed effects model with measurement error. Ye, Lin and Taylor (2008) examined regression calibration methods to jointly model longitudinal and survival data using a semiparametric longitudinal model and a proportional hazards model. Xiong, He and Yi (2014) investigated joint modeling of survival and longitudinal data where the proportional odds model is employed to feature survival data and longitudinal covariates are postulated using measurement error models. Chen and Huang (2015) explored a Bayesian inferential procedure for semiparametric mixed effects joint models where skewed distributions are used to describe longitudinal measurements and the Cox proportional hazards model is adopted for modeling the event time process.

When both measurement error and missing observations are present, marginal and likelihood-based methods were developed by various authors. For example, Liang, Wang and Carroll (2007) explored estimation procedures for partially linear models where the response is subject to missingness and covariates are error-contaminated. Wang et al. (2008), Yi (2005, 2008), and Yi, Ma and Carroll (2012) proposed marginal methods to incorporate measurement error and missingness effects. Liu and Wu (2007) and Yi, Liu and Wu (2011) took a mixed model framework for the response process and developed likelihood-based inferential procedures. Other work can be found in the references therein.

5.8 Supplementary Problems

5.1. Consider the setup in §5.1.1.

(a) Assume that

$$E(Y_{ij}|X_i, Z_i) = E(Y_{ij}|X_{ij}, Z_{ij}) \tag{5.90}$$

holds for any $j = 1, \ldots, m_i$ and $i = 1, \ldots, n$. Show that estimating function $U_i(\beta)$ given by (5.4) is unbiased.

(b) Give a counterexample to show that the unbiasedness of $U_i(\beta)$ given by (5.4) breaks down if condition (5.90) does not hold.

(c) Assume that condition (5.90) is met and that there is a unique solution to the equation

$$\sum_{i=1}^{n} D_i V_i^{-1}(Y_i - \mu_i) = 0. \tag{5.91}$$

Let $\widehat{\beta}$ denote the corresponding estimator of β by solving (5.91) for β.

Show that under certain regularity conditions, $\widehat{\beta}$ is a consistent estimator of β. Discuss associated conditions.

(d) For the estimator obtained in (c), develop its asymptotic distribution.

(e) Let $V_i^* = B_i^{1/2} C_i^* B_i^{1/2}$, where C_i^* is a user-specified $m_i \times m_i$ matrix. Assume that the equation

$$\sum_{i=1}^{n} D_i V_i^{*-1}(Y_i - \mu_i) = 0$$

has a unique solution, and let $\widehat{\beta}^*$ denote the resulting estimator of β. Show that under condition (5.90) and certain regularity conditions, $\widehat{\beta}^*$ is a consistent estimator of β. Compare the efficiency between $\widehat{\beta}^*$ and $\widehat{\beta}$.

(f) Let C_i^{**} be a *diagonal* $m_i \times m_i$ matrix, $V_i^{**} = B_i^{1/2} C_i^{**} B_i^{1/2}$, and

$$U_i^* = D_i V_i^{**-1}(Y_i - \mu_i).$$

Show that U_i^* is unbiased even if condition (5.90) is not true.

(Pepe and Anderson 1994; Yi, Ma and Carroll 2012)

5.2. Consider the setting of Example 5.1.

(a) Show that

$$E(Y_{ij}|X_i) = E(Y_{ij}|X_{ij})$$

for $j = 1, \ldots, m$.

(b) If Σ_e is not diagonal and $\beta \neq 0$, show that the identity in (a) does not hold for the observed data. That is, $E(Y_{ij}|X_i^*) \neq E(Y_{ij}|X_{ij}^*)$ for $j = 1, \ldots, m$.

(Yi, Ma and Carroll 2012)

5.3. Prove the identities (5.19) in §5.2.1.

5.4.

(a) Repeat the discussion in Example 5.2 by replacing measurement error model (5.18) with

$$X_{ij} = \gamma_0 + \gamma_x X_{ij}^* + \gamma_z Z_{ij} + e_{ij},$$

where the e_{ij} are independent of $\{X_{ij}^*, Z_{ij}, \epsilon_{ij}\}$ and γ_0, γ_x and γ_z are regression coefficients.

Show that the relationship between β^* and β is

$$\beta_x^* = \gamma_x \beta_x;\ \beta_z^* = \beta_z + \gamma_z \beta_x;\ \beta_0^* = \beta_0 + \gamma_0 \beta_x.$$

(b) In the development in (a), suppose V_i in (5.4) is replaced by a working matrix that is not diagonal. Discuss the relationship between β^* and β.

5.5. *(Multivariate Normal Distributions)*

(a) Suppose that Y is an $n \times 1$ random vector which follows distribution $N(\mu, \Sigma)$, where μ is the mean vector and Σ is the covariance matrix. Partition Y into two subvectors $Y = (Y_1^{\mathrm{T}}, Y_2^{\mathrm{T}})^{\mathrm{T}}$, where Y_1 has dimension r and Y_2 has dimension $(n - r)$. Partition μ and Σ similarly so that $\mu = (\mu_1^{\mathrm{T}}, \mu_2^{\mathrm{T}})^{\mathrm{T}}$, and

$$\Sigma = \begin{pmatrix} \Sigma_{11} & \Sigma_{12} \\ \Sigma_{21} & \Sigma_{22} \end{pmatrix},$$

where μ_1 has dimension r, μ_2 has dimension $(n - r)$, Σ_{11} is an $r \times r$ matrix, Σ_{22} is an $(n - r) \times (n - r)$ matrix, Σ_{12} is an $r \times (n - r)$ matrix, and $\Sigma_{21} = \Sigma_{12}^{\mathrm{T}}$.

Show that the conditional distribution of Y_1 given $Y_2 = y_2$ is

$$N(\mu_{y_1|y_2}, \Sigma_{y_1|y_2}),$$

where

$$\mu_{y_1|y_2} = \mu_1 + \Sigma_{12}\Sigma_{22}^{-1}(y_2 - \mu_2),$$

and

$$\Sigma_{y_1|y_2} = \Sigma_{11} - \Sigma_{12}\Sigma_{22}^{-1}\Sigma_{21}.$$

(b) Let X and X^* be random vectors of the same dimension. Suppose that the marginal distribution of X is $N(\mu_x, \Sigma_x)$ and that the conditional distribution of X^*, given $X = x$, is $N(x, \Sigma_{x^*|x})$. Show that

(i) the joint distribution of X and X^* is

$$N\left(\begin{pmatrix} \mu_x \\ \mu_x \end{pmatrix}, \begin{pmatrix} \Sigma_x & \Sigma_x \\ \Sigma_x & \Sigma_x + \Sigma_{x^*|x} \end{pmatrix}\right);$$

(ii) the conditional distribution of X, given $X^* = x^*$, is $N(\mu_{x|x^*}, \Sigma_{x|x^*})$, where

$$\mu_{x|x^*} = \mu_x + \Sigma_x(\Sigma_x + \Sigma_{x^*|x})^{-1}(x^* - \mu_x),$$

and

$$\Sigma_{x|x^*} = \Sigma_x - \Sigma_x(\Sigma_x + \Sigma_{x^*|x})^{-1}\Sigma_x.$$

(c) Suppose that Y is an $n \times 1$ random vector, X and X^* are $p \times 1$ random vectors, and u is a $q \times 1$ random vector. Assume that the conditional model of Y, given X and u, is

$$Y = \mu_{y|xu} + AX + Bu + \epsilon,$$

where $\mu_{y|xu}$ is an $n \times 1$ vector of parameters, A is an $n \times p$ matrix of design characteristics, B is an $n \times q$ matrix featuring random effects u, and ϵ is an $n \times 1$ random vector.

Suppose that

$$X^* = X + e,$$

where e is a $p \times 1$ random vector. Further assume that
(1) random vectors X, u, ϵ and e are all independent of each other;
(2) they all have a normal distribution, given by

$$X \sim N(\mu_x, \Sigma_x);\ u \sim N(0, \Sigma_u);$$

$$\epsilon \sim N(0, \Sigma_{y|xu});\ e \sim N(0, \Sigma_{x^*|x});$$

(3) given $\{X, u\}$, Y and X^* are independent.

Prove the following results:

(i) The marginal distributions of Y and X^* are given by

$$Y \sim N(\mu_y, \Sigma_y) \text{ and } X^* \sim N(\mu_{x^*}, \Sigma_{x^*}),$$

respectively, where

$$\begin{aligned} \mu_y &= \mu_{y|xu} + A\mu_x; \\ \Sigma_y &= B\Sigma_u B^{\mathrm{T}} + A\Sigma_x A^{\mathrm{T}} + \Sigma_{y|xu}; \\ \mu_{x^*} &= \mu_x; \\ \Sigma_{x^*} &= \Sigma_x + \Sigma_{x^*|x}. \end{aligned}$$

(ii) The joint distribution of Y and X^* is given by

$$\left(\begin{pmatrix} \mu_y \\ \mu_{x^*} \end{pmatrix}, \begin{pmatrix} \Sigma_y & \Sigma_{yx^*} \\ \Sigma_{yx^*} & \Sigma_{x^*} \end{pmatrix} \right),$$

where $\Sigma_{yx^*} = A\Sigma_x$.

(iii) Conditional on $\{X^*, u\}$, Y can be expressed as

$$Y = \mu^*_{y|x^*u} + A^* X^* + Bu + \epsilon^*,$$

where

$$\mu^*_{y|x^*u} = \mu_{y|xu} + A\{I_n - \Sigma_x(\Sigma_{x^*|x} + \Sigma_x)^{-1}\}\mu_x;$$

$$A^* = A\Sigma_x(\Sigma_x + \Sigma_{x^*|x})^{-1};$$

the error term ϵ^* is normally distributed with mean 0 and covariance matrix

$$\operatorname{var}(\epsilon^*) = \Sigma_{y|xu} + A\Sigma_x A^{\mathrm{T}} - A\Sigma_x(\Sigma_x + \Sigma_{x^*|x})^{-1}\Sigma_x A^{\mathrm{T}};$$

and ϵ^* is independent of X^* and u.

(Tosteson, Buonaccorsi and Demidenko 1998)

5.6.

(a) Suppose that X and ϵ are independent continuous random variables with support $(-\infty, \infty)$ and that the marginal probability density function of ϵ is $f(\epsilon)$.

(i) Let

$$Y = \beta_0 + \beta_x X + \epsilon, \tag{5.92}$$

where β_0 and β_x are parameters. Show that the conditional probability density function of Y given $X = x$ is $f(y - \beta_0 - \beta_x x)$ for $-\infty < y < \infty$.

(ii) If Y is not necessarily linear in X as given by (5.92), but

$$Y = g(X; \beta) + \epsilon,$$

where β is a parameter, and $g(\cdot)$ is a real-valued function. Is the conditional probability density function of Y, given $X = x$, identical to $f(y - g(x; \beta))$?

(b) Suppose that X and Z are random variables and their joint distribution is a bivariate normal distribution.

(i) Let

$$Y = \beta_0 + \beta_x X + \beta_z Z, \tag{5.93}$$

where β_0, β_x and β_z are parameters. Show that X and Y are independent if and only if

$$\text{cov}(X, Y) = 0.$$

(ii) If Y is not linear in X as given by (5.93), is the result in (b)(i) still true?

5.7. Consider the model setup in §5.2.2, where we define

$$u_i^* = X_i - E(X_i | X_i^*, Z_i)$$

on page 208. Prove that

(a) $E(X_i | X_i^*, Z_i) = (I_{m_i} - \Omega_i)(\vartheta_0 1_{m_i} + \vartheta_z Z_i) + \Omega_i X_i^*$;
(b) $u_i^* = (I_{m_i} - \Omega_i)\epsilon_{xi} - \Omega_i e_i$;
(c) $u_i^* \sim N(0, (I_{m_i} - \Omega_i)\Sigma_{xi})$;
(d) Show that u_i^* is independent of u_i, X_i^* and Z_i.

(Wang et al. 1998)

5.8. Suppose the conditional probability density or mass function $h(y_i | x_i, z_i)$ of Y_i, given $\{X_i, Z_i\}$, is formulated through a two-stage modeling procedure as outlined in §5.1.2. That is, conditional on random effects u_i and $\{X_i, Z_i\}$, the

Y_{ij} are independent with the conditional distribution $h(y_{ij}|u_i, X_i, Z_i)$. Then the distribution of Y_i, given $\{X_i, Z_i\}$, is given by

$$h(y_i|x_i, z_i) = \prod_{j=1}^{m_i} \int h(y_{ij}|u_i, x_i, z_i)h(u_i)d\eta(u_i),$$

where $h(u_i)$ is the probability density or mass function of u_i.

Suppose X_i is measured with error and X_i^* is its surrogate measurement. Discuss the conditional distribution of Y_i, given $\{X_i^*, Z_i\}$. In particular, answer the following questions.

(a) Conditional on random effects u_i and $\{X_i^*, Z_i\}$, are the Y_{ij} independent? Can the conditional probability density or mass function $h(y_i|x_i^*, z_i)$ of Y_i, given $\{X_i^*, Z_i\}$, be written as

$$h(y_i|x_i^*, z_i) = \prod_{j=1}^{m_i} \int h^*(y_{ij}|u_i, x_i^*, z_i)h(u_i)d\eta(u_i)?$$

Here $h^*(y_{ij}|u_i, x_i^*, z_i)$ is obtained from $h(y_{ij}|u_i, x_i, z_i)$ with x_i replaced by x_i^*.

(b) Do there exist random effects $\widetilde{u}_i$ such that given $\widetilde{u}_i$ and $\{X_i^*, Z_i\}$, the Y_{ij} are conditionally independent, hence, yielding the conditional probability density or mass function of Y_i given $\{X_i^*, Z_i\}$

$$h(y_i|x_i^*, z_i) = \int \prod_{j=1}^{m_i} h(y_{ij}|x_i^*, z_i, \widetilde{u}_i)h(\widetilde{u}_i)d\eta(\widetilde{u}_i)?$$

Here $h(\widetilde{u}_i)$ represents the marginal probability density or mass function for $\widetilde{u}_i$, and $h(y_{ij}|x_i^*, z_i, \widetilde{u}_i)$ is the probability density or mass function of Y_{ij} given $\widetilde{u}_i$ and $\{X_i^*, Z_i\}$.

(c) If the answer in (b) is yes, are the random effects $\widetilde{u}_i$ unique? That is, suppose there exists another set of random effects $\widetilde{u}_i^*$ such that the Y_{ij} are conditionally independent, given $\{\widetilde{u}_i^*, X_i^*, Z_i\}$, hence leading to the conditional probability density or mass function Y_i given $\{X_i^*, Z_i\}$, given by

$$h(y_i|x_i^*, z_i) = \int \prod_{j=1}^{m_i} h(y_{ij}|x_i^*, z_i, \widetilde{u}_i^*)h(\widetilde{u}_i^*)d\eta(\widetilde{u}_i^*),$$

where $h(\widetilde{u}_i^*)$ represents the marginal probability density or mass function for $\widetilde{u}_i^*$, and $h(y_{ij}|x_i^*, z_i, \widetilde{u}_i^*)$ is the probability density or mass function of Y_{ij} given $\widetilde{u}_i^*$ and $\{X_i^*, Z_i\}$.

Do the random effects $\widetilde{u}_i^*$ have the same distribution as that of the random effects $\widetilde{u}_i$?

5.9. Suppose that for $i = 1, \ldots, n$ and $j = 1, \ldots, m_i$, the marginal distribution of the response component Y_{ij} is a Gamma distribution with the probability density function

$$f(y_{ij}) = \frac{\theta_{ij}^{\phi}}{\Gamma(\phi)} y_{ij}^{\phi-1} \exp(-\theta_{ij} y_{ij}),$$

where ϕ is known, and θ_{ij} is the canonical parameter which links the mean and variance of Y_{ij} via

$$\mu_{ij} = \phi \theta_{ij}^{-1} \text{ and } v_{ij} = \mu_{ij}^2 / \phi.$$

Consider the log-linear model with

$$\log \mu_{ij} = \beta_0 + \beta_x^{\mathrm{T}} X_{ij} + \beta_z^{\mathrm{T}} Z_{ij},$$

where X_{ij} and Z_{ij} are covariates for subject i at time point j and $\beta = (\beta_0, \beta_x^{\mathrm{T}}, \beta_z^{\mathrm{T}})^{\mathrm{T}}$ is the vector of regression coefficients.

(a) If both X_{ij} and Z_{ij} are precisely measured, discuss estimation of β by applying the GMM method to the estimating function (5.33):

$$U_{ij} = \left(\frac{\partial \mu_{ij}}{\partial \beta} \right) v_{ij}^{-1} (Y_{ij} - \mu_{ij})$$

for $i = 1, \ldots, n$ and $j = 1, \ldots, m_i$.

(b) Suppose that X_{ij} is mismeasured as X_{ij}^* and that X_{ij} and X_{ij}^* are linked by the model (5.41) where the e_{ij} have the moment generating function $M(\cdot)$. Applying the corrected estimating functions method outlined in §5.3.2, construct an unbiased estimating function U_{ij}^* based on the observed data $\{Y_{ij}, X_{ij}^*, Z_{ij}\}$ such that

$$E(U_{ij}^* | Y_{ij}, X_{ij}, Z_{ij}) = U_{ij},$$

where the expectation is evaluated with respect to the model for the conditional distribution of X_{ij}^* given $\{Y_{ij}, X_{ij}, Z_{ij}\}$.

(c) Discuss estimation of β by applying the GMM method, or using Theorem 1.8, to the estimating functions U_{ij}^* constructed in (b).

(d) Assume that e_{ij} in the model (5.41) is normally distributed and that conditional on Z_i, X_{ij} follows a normal distribution $N(\mu_x, \Sigma_x)$ with mean μ_x and variance Σ_x. Applying the expected estimating equations method outlined in §5.3.1, construct unbiased estimating functions U_{ij}^* which are obtained as $U_{ij}^* = E\{U_{ij} | Y_{ij}, X_{ij}^*, Z_{ij}\}$.

(f) Discuss estimation of β by applying the GMM method, or using Theorem 1.8, to the estimating functions U_{ij}^* constructed in (d).

(g) Suppose that the Y_{ij} are mutually independent. Under the assumptions of (d), develop an estimation procedure for β using the likelihood method.

(h) Compare the estimation methods developed in (c), (f) and (g).

5.10. Consider the following scenarios for §5.4:

(a) $n_i = 1$ and m_i is much bigger than 1 for $i = 1, \ldots, n$;
(b) $n_i = m_i$ for $i = 1, \ldots, n$.

Discuss how the inference procedures may be affected by the relationship between the observation times $\{t_{i1}, \ldots, t_{im_i}\}$ for the response variable $Y_i(t)$ and the observation times $\{t_{i1}^*, \ldots, t_{in_i}^*\}$ for the covariate $X_i(t)$. When do the procedures break down? When do the procedures work?

5.11.

(a) Verify that estimating function (5.63) is unbiased.
(b) Show that the estimating function (5.64) is unbiased regardless of whether or not $D(Y_{ij}, X_{ij}^*, Z_{ij}; \beta)$ is unbiased.

(Robins, Rotnitzky and Zhao 1994)

5.12. Consider the setup in §5.2.2. Suppose that conditional on random effects u_i and covariates $\{X_i, Z_i\}$, the responses Y_{ij} are independent and follow a linear mixed model

$$Y_{ij} = \beta_0 + \beta_x X_{ij} + \beta_z Z_{ij} + u_i + \epsilon_{ij}$$

for $j = 1, \ldots, m_i$ and $i = 1, \ldots, n$, where β_0, β_x and β_z are regression coefficients; the u_i are random effects; and the ϵ_{ij} are independent of each other and of $\{X_{ij}, Z_{ij}, u_i\}$ and have distribution $N(0, \sigma^2)$ with variance σ^2.

(a) Assume that u_i follows a normal distribution $N(0, \sigma_u^2)$ with variance σ_u^2. Show that the probability density function of Y_i given $\{X_i, Z_i\}$ is

$$f(y_i|x_i, z_i) = \frac{1}{(\sqrt{2\pi})^{m_i} \sigma^{m_i - 1} \sqrt{m_i \sigma_u^2 + \sigma^2}} \cdot \exp\left\{ -\frac{(m_i - 1)\sigma_u^2 + \sigma^2}{2\sigma^2(m_i \sigma_u^2 + \sigma^2)} \cdot \sum_{j=1}^{m_i} (y_{ij} - \mu_{ij})^2 + \frac{\sigma_u^2}{\sigma^2(m_i \sigma_u^2 + \sigma^2)} \cdot \sum_{j<k} (y_{ij} - \mu_{ij})(y_{ik} - \mu_{ik}) \right\},$$

where $\mu_{ij} = \beta_0 + \beta_x X_{ij} + \beta_z Z_{ij}$ is the marginal mean of Y_{ij}.

(b) Consider the case where the response variable Y_{ij} is subject to missingness, as described in §5.5. Let $\tau_{ij} = P(R_{ij} = 1|Y_i, X_i, Z_i)$ for $j = 1, \ldots, m_i$. Suppose that given $\{Y_i, X_i, Z_i\}$, the R_{ij} are independent, and the missing data process is modeled by

$$\text{logit } \tau_{ij} = \vartheta_0 + \vartheta_1 Y_{i,j-1} + \vartheta_2 Y_{ij} + \vartheta_3 X_{ij},$$

where $\vartheta = (\vartheta_0, \vartheta_1, \vartheta_2, \vartheta_3)^{\mathrm{T}}$ is the vector of regression parameters.

If we ignore the missingness feature and naively apply the result in (a) to the observed data to form a likelihood function L_o, then maximizing L_o with respect to the model parameters gives an estimator $\widehat{\beta}^*$ of β. Let β^* denote the limit to which $\widehat{\beta}^*$ converges in probability. Discuss the relationship between β^* and β.

(c) We further assume that X_{ij} is subject to measurement error with surrogate measurement X_{ij}^* and that (5.68) holds. Suppose the measurement error model is

$$X_{ij} = \gamma_0 + \gamma_x X_{ij}^* + \gamma_z Z_{ij} + e_{ij},$$

where $\gamma = (\gamma_0, \gamma_x, \gamma_z)^{\mathrm{T}}$ is the vector of parameters, and the e_{ij} are independent of each other and of $\{X_{ij}^*, Z_{ij}, Y_{ij}, e_{ij}\}$ and have distribution $N(0, \sigma_e^2)$ with variance σ_e^2.
If we perform a naive analysis with missingness and measurement error ignored, discuss the asymptotic bias for the resulting naive estimator of β.

(d) Develop an estimation method for β with missingness and measurement error incorporated. Discuss associated conditions.

(Yi, Liu and Wu 2011)

5.13. In contrast to the missing data scenarios (5.59) and (5.60) discussed in §5.5.2, we consider a special situation where

$$h(r_i|y_i, x_i, x_i^*, z_i) = h(r_i|y_i, z_i).$$

Assume that the measurement error model is given by (5.61). Discuss and compare the two sequential strategies of §5.5.3 for estimation of β of the following models.

(a) (*Inverse Gaussian Regression*)
Suppose that the marginal distribution of Y_{ij} is the inverse Gaussian distribution $IG(\mu_{ij}, 1)$ with the probability density function

$$f(y_{ij}; \mu_{ij}) = \sqrt{\frac{1}{2\pi y_{ij}^3}} \exp\left\{\frac{-(y_{ij} - \mu_{ij})^2}{2\mu_{ij}^2 y_{ij}}\right\} \quad \text{for } y_{ij} > 0,$$

where μ_{ij} is the mean of Y_{ij}. In this case, the variance of Y_{ij} is given by $v_{ij} = \mu_{ij}^3$. Consider the regression model

$$\mu_{ij}^{-2} = \beta_0 + \beta_x^{\mathrm{T}} X_{ij} + \beta_z^{\mathrm{T}} Z_{ij},$$

where $\beta = (\beta_0, \beta_x^{\mathrm{T}}, \beta_z^{\mathrm{T}})^{\mathrm{T}}$ is the vector of regression parameters.

(b) (*Poisson Regression Models*)
Suppose that the response component Y_{ij} is a count variable following a Poisson distribution with mean μ_{ij}. In this case, the variance of Y_{ij} is given by $v_{ij} = \mu_{ij}$. Consider the log-linear model

$$\log \mu_{ij} = \beta_0 + \beta_x^{\mathrm{T}} X_{ij} + \beta_z^{\mathrm{T}} Z_{ij},$$

where $\beta = (\beta_0, \beta_x^{\mathrm{T}}, \beta_z^{\mathrm{T}})^{\mathrm{T}}$ is the vector of regression parameters.

(Yi 2005)

5.14. Consider the setup in §5.6.2.

(a) Show that conditional on $C_i(t)$, $dN_i(t)$ and $\widehat{X}_i(t)$ are independent. Specify what assumptions made in §5.6 are used for this result.

(b) Prove the statement of (5.85).

(c) Verify (5.89).

(Tsiatis and Davidian 2001)

6

Multi-State Models with Error-Prone Data

Multi-state stochastic models are closely related to survival and longitudinal data analysis. They may be used to describe survival data from a perspective different from what is discussed in Chapter 3. They also provide a useful framework for analyzing longitudinal data when interest lies in dynamic aspects of the underlying process.

Often, multi-state event data may be distinguished according to the availability of state transition times. When subjects are observed continuously over a period of time, transitions between states can be observed. In contrast, when subjects are seen at discrete time points, exact transition times normally cannot be observed; only the state occupied at each assessment time is observed. An inference framework for analyzing multi-state data is formulated with the focus centered on either the transition intensity or transition probability among the states. A great number of methods, including parametric, semiparametric, and nonparametric ones, have been developed for analysis of such data in the error-free context.

Existing methods are, however, frequently distorted by error-contaminated data. Commonly, two types of error may arise from the analysis of data delineated by multi-state models: (1) covariates are subject to measurement error or misclassification, and (2) states are misclassified. This chapter discusses issues and inference procedures concerning multi-state model analysis with either type of measurement error. Similar to the preceding chapters, we begin with the discussion of the inference framework for the error-free situation, and then move on to various topics on error-related scenarios. We conclude this chapter with bibliographic notes and exercise problems.

G. Y. Yi, *Statistical Analysis with Measurement Error or Misclassification*, Springer Series in Statistics, DOI 10.1007/978-1-4939-6640-0_6

6.1 Framework of Multi-State Models

6.1.1 Notation and Setup

A *multi-state process* is a stochastic process $\{Y(t) : t \in \mathcal{T}\}$ with a finite *state space* $\mathcal{S} = \{1, \ldots, K\}$ and right-continuous sample paths: $Y(t^+) = Y(t)$, where $Y(t^+) = \lim_{\Delta t \to 0^+} Y(t + \Delta t)$, $Y(t)$ represents the state occupied at time t that takes value from the state space $\mathcal{S}$, and $\mathcal{T} = [0, \tau]$ with $\tau < +\infty$ or $\mathcal{T} = [0, +\infty)$ (Andersen and Keiding 2002). A multi-state model is often displayed using a diagram with boxes representing the states and arrows between the states representing possible transitions.

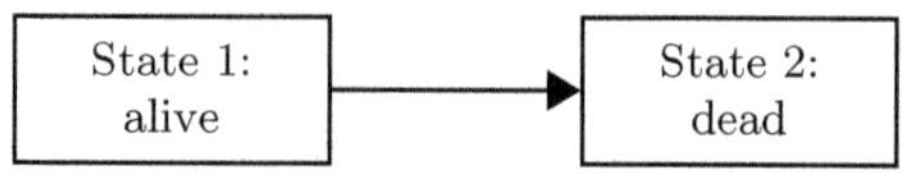

Fig. 6.1. *The Two-State Survival Model*

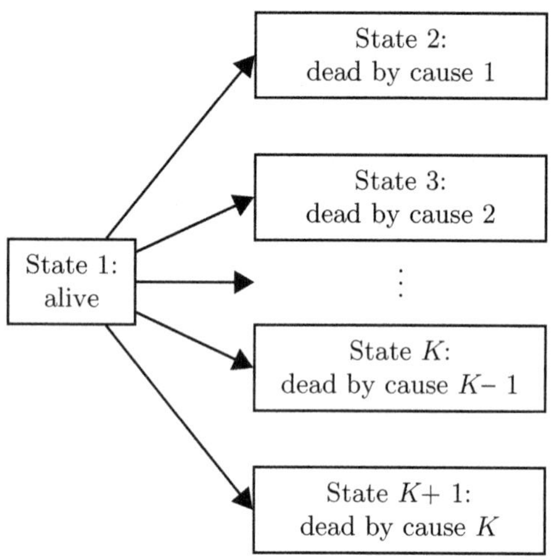

Fig. 6.2. *A Competing Risk Model with K Causes*

Fig. 6.1 presents the simplest multi-state model where only two states and a one-way transition are involved. Such a model may be used to describe survival data for which interest lies in describing the transition from the status of being alive to death. In some situations, one may be further interested in sorting out the causes of death; *competing risk models* are useful for this purpose (Kalbfleisch and Prentice 2002, §8.2). Fig. 6.2 displays such a model which shows K different causes related to the death of individuals. Another useful model for survival data is the *illness-death* model which has three states, indicated in Fig. 6.3.

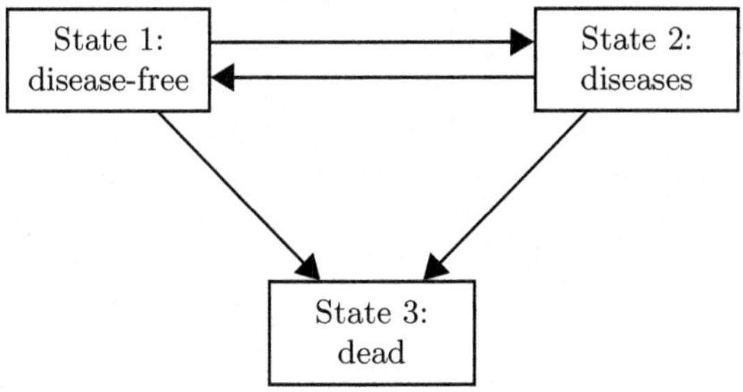

Fig. 6.3. *An Illness-Death Model*

These three examples show scenarios with at least one state from which transition out of it is impossible; such a state is called an *absorbing state*, discussed as follows. In application, not all models have an absorbing state as illustrated by Fig. 6.4.

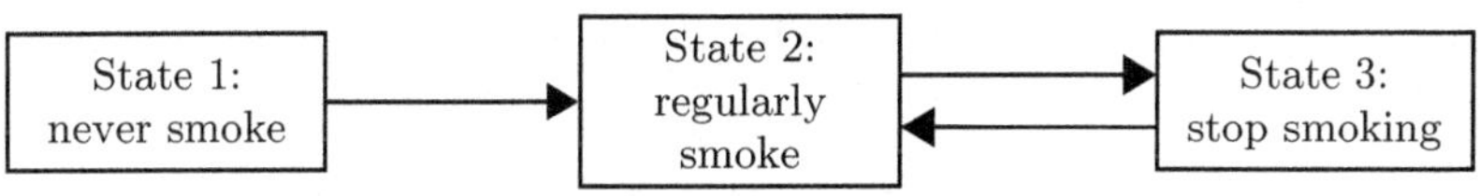

Fig. 6.4. *A Three-State Smoker Nonsmoker Model*

To portray a multi-state process, one often describes its *transition probabilities* or *transition intensities*, in conjunction with the *initial distribution*

$$\pi_j(0) = P(Y(0) = j) \text{ for } j \in \mathcal{S}.$$

Let

$$\mathcal{H}_t^{\mathrm{Y}} = \{Y(v) : 0 \leq v < t\}$$

be the history consisting of the observations of the process up to but not including time t. Relative to the process history, for $j, k \in \mathcal{S}$ and $s, t \in \mathcal{T}$ with $s \leq t$, we define the *transition probability* between time points s and t as

$$p_{jk}(s, t|\mathcal{H}_s^{\mathrm{Y}}) = P(Y(t) = k|Y(s) = j, \mathcal{H}_s^{\mathrm{Y}}).$$

At a given time point $t \in \mathcal{T}$, the *transition intensity* is defined as

$$\lambda_{jk}(t|\mathcal{H}_t^{\mathrm{Y}}) = \lim_{\Delta t \to 0+} \frac{p_{jk}(t, t + \Delta t|\mathcal{H}_t^{\mathrm{Y}})}{\Delta t}$$

for which we assume the limit exists. It is conventional to define

$$\lambda_{jj}(t|\mathcal{H}_t^{\mathrm{Y}}) = -\sum_{k \neq j} \lambda_{jk}(t|\mathcal{H}_t^{\mathrm{Y}})$$

for $j = 1, \ldots, K$, as discussed in §6.1.2.

A state j is called *absorbing* if for all $t \in \mathcal{T}$ and $k \in \mathcal{S}$ with $k \neq j$, we have

$$\lambda_{jk}(t|\mathcal{H}_t^{\mathrm{Y}}) = 0;$$

otherwise it is called *transient*. The *state probability* $\pi_j(t) = P(Y(t) = j)$ is given by

$$\pi_j(t) = \sum_{k \in \mathcal{S}} \pi_j(0) p_{jk}(0, t),$$

where $p_{jk}(0, t) = P(Y(t) = k|Y(0) = j)$.

The transition probabilities and transition intensities generally depend on the history of the process. In application, certain model assumptions are imposed to simplify the dependence on the process history. The following three scenarios are often considered in the literature.

- *Time Homogeneous Models:*
  For any states j and k, the transition intensities $\lambda_{jk}(t|\mathcal{H}_t^{\mathrm{Y}})$ are constant over time:
  $$\lambda_{jk}(t|\mathcal{H}_t^{\mathrm{Y}}) = \lambda_{jk}$$
  for any time t, where λ_{jk} is a constant that may be state-dependent but is free of time.

- *Markov Models:*
  For any states j and k, the intensities $\lambda_{jk}(t|\mathcal{H}_t^{\mathrm{Y}})$ depend on the history only through the state $Y(t) = j$ occupied at time t. In other words, transition probabilities have the property
  $$p_{jk}(s, t|\mathcal{H}_s^{\mathrm{Y}}) = P(Y(t) = k|Y(s) = j) \text{ for } s < t \text{ and } j, k \in \mathcal{S}.$$
  In this case the transition intensities and probabilities are denoted as $\lambda_{jk}(t)$ and $p_{jk}(s, t)$, respectively.

- *Semi-Markov Models:*
  For any states j and k, future evolution not only depends on the current state j, but also on the entry time into state j. Therefore, the intensity function is written as
  $$\begin{aligned}\lambda_{jk}(t|\mathcal{H}_t^{\mathrm{Y}}) &= \lim_{\Delta t \to 0+} \frac{P(Y(t + \Delta t) = k|Y(t) = j, \mathcal{H}_t^{\mathrm{Y}})}{\Delta t} \\ &= \lim_{\Delta t \to 0+} \frac{P(Y(t + \Delta t) = k|Y(t) = j, t_j)}{\Delta t}\end{aligned}$$
  to reflect such dependence, where t_j is the entry time into state j. We use $\lambda_{jk}(t|t_j)$ to denote such an intensity.

The Markov process is memoryless in that only the currently occupied state is relevant in specifying the transition intensities (Kalbfleisch and Prentice 2002, §8.3). Markov models are, perhaps, the most frequently used multi-state models due to their simplicity. Semi-Markov models are, sometimes, alternatively defined to be that the future of the process does not depend on the current time but rather on the duration in the current state, hence one may alternatively denote the transition intensities as $\lambda_{jk}(t|t-t_j)$ (Meira-Machado et al. 2009).

In application, different time scales, *clock forward* and *clock reset*, may be used to highlight distinct features of a process. By *clock forward*, time t refers to the time since the subject enters the *initial* state, and the clock keeps moving forward for the subject. For the *clock reset* scale, time t in $\lambda_{jk}(t|\mathcal{H}_t^Y)$ refers to the time since the entry in state j, and the clock is reset to 0 each time when the subject enters a new state. Discussion on the choice of a suitable time scale was given by Putter, Fiocco and Geskus (2007), among others. In this book, we use the clock-forward time scale unless otherwise indicated.

6.1.2 Continuous-Time Homogeneous Markov Processes

Under continuous-time homogeneous Markov processes, transition probabilities $p_{jk}(s,t) = P(Y(t) = k|Y(s) = j)$ are often written as $p_{jk}(t-s)$ to emphasize that the probabilities are independent of the starting time s but dependent on the elapsed time $(t-s)$. Over a small time interval with length Δt, transition probabilities and transition intensities are connected via

$$\begin{aligned} p_{jk}(\Delta t) &= \lambda_{jk}\Delta t + o(\Delta t); \\ p_{jj}(\Delta t) &= 1 + \lambda_{jj}\Delta t + o(\Delta t) \end{aligned} \tag{6.1}$$

for any $j = 1, \ldots, K$ and $k \neq j$, where $o(\Delta t)$ represents a term that is of smaller magnitude than Δt, i.e., $\lim_{\Delta t \to 0} o(\Delta t)/\Delta t = 0$.

Suppose that one of the states must be occupied at time $t + \Delta t$, given that a state j is occupied at time t. Since for each j, $\sum_{k=1}^{K} p_{jk}(\Delta t) = 1$, so identity (6.1) leads to

$$\lambda_{jj} + \sum_{k \neq j} \lambda_{jk} = 0$$

for $j = 1, \ldots, K$, which are the constraints commonly applied in modeling transition intensities (Kalbfleisch and Lawless 1985).

Relationship of Transition Intensity and Transition Probability

By definition and the probability property, we obtain that for any time points $s < t$ and states j and k,

$$p_{jk}(t) = \sum_{l=1}^{K} p_{jl}(s)p_{lk}(t-s);$$

this is called the *Chapman–Kolmogorov equation* (Cox and Miller 1965). Applying this equation and (6.1) yields that

$$p'_{jk}(t) = \sum_{l=1}^{K} p_{jl}(t)\lambda_{lk}, \tag{6.2}$$

where $p'_{jk}(t)$ is the derivative of $p_{jk}(t)$ taken with respect to t.

Let $P(t)$ be the $K \times K$ transition probability matrix with (j,k) element $p_{jk}(t)$ and Q be the $K \times K$ transition intensity matrix with (j,k) element λ_{jk} for $j,k \in \mathcal{S}$. Then (6.2) is presented in the matrix form

$$P'(t) = P(t)Q, \tag{6.3}$$

where $P'(t)$ is the $K \times K$ matrix with (j,k) element $p'_{jk}(t)$.

Analogously, working with

$$p_{jk}(t) = \sum_{l=1}^{K} p_{jl}(t-s)p_{lk}(s)$$

gives

$$P'(t) = QP(t). \tag{6.4}$$

Identities (6.3) and (6.4) are called the *forward equation* and the *backward equation*, respectively.

With an initial condition that $P(0) = I_K$, the solution to the forward or the backward equation (Cox and Miller 1965, Ch. 4) is given by

$$P(t) = \exp(Qt), \tag{6.5}$$

where $\exp(Qt)$ is defined to be

$$\exp(Qt) = \sum_{r=0}^{\infty} \frac{Q^r t^r}{r!}$$

with $Q^0 = I_K$.

To compute $P(t)$ using (6.5), one may use the matrix decomposition to re-write $P(t)$. Suppose Q has distinct eigenvalues $d_1, \ldots, d_K$, and let A be the $K \times K$ matrix whose jth column is a right eigenvector corresponding to d_j, then $Q = ADA^{-1}$, where $D = \text{diag}\{d_1, \ldots, d_K\}$. As a result, the transition probability matrix is

$$P(t) = A \cdot \text{diag}\{\exp(d_1 t), \ldots, \exp(d_K t)\} \cdot A^{-1}. \tag{6.6}$$

Expression (6.6) offers us a convenient way to calculate partial derivatives of $P(t)$ which are needed in inferential procedures (Kalbfleisch and Lawless 1985). Suppose that the transition intensity matrix Q contains parameter $\theta = (\theta_1, \ldots, \theta_p)^{\mathrm{T}}$, which, for example, arises from modeling the transition intensities λ_{jk} as discussed in §6.1.5.

Let $G^{(l)} = A^{-1}(\partial Q/\partial\theta_l)A$ and $g_{jk}^{(l)}$ be the (j,k) entry of $G^{(l)}$ for $l = 1,\ldots,p$. Define $V^{(l)} = [v_{jk}^{(l)}]$ to be the $K \times K$ matrix with (j,k) entry

$$v_{jk}^{(l)} = \begin{cases} \frac{g_{jk}^{(l)}\{\exp(d_j t)-\exp(d_k t)\}}{(d_j - d_k)}, & \text{if } j \neq k, \\ g_{jj}^{(l)} t \exp(d_j t), & \text{if } j = k, \end{cases}$$

then the partial derivatives of the transition probabilities are given by

$$\frac{\partial P(t)}{\partial\theta_l} = AV^{(l)}A^{-1} \tag{6.7}$$

for $l = 1,\ldots,p$.

Progressive Markov Model

A *progressive* continuous-time homogeneous Markov process is a continuous-time homogeneous Markov process for which individuals progress in one direction through K ordered states and the transition is irreversible, as shown in Fig. 6.5.

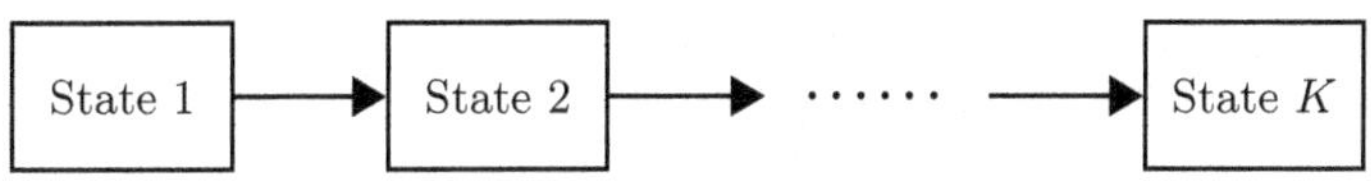

Fig. 6.5. *A K-State Progressive Model*

Since, under the progressive model, $\lambda_{jk} = 0$ if $k \neq j+1$, we simplify the notation and let λ_j denote the transition intensity from state j to state $(j+1)$ for $j = 1,\ldots,K-1$. Assume that $\lambda_1,\ldots,\lambda_{K-1}$ are distinct and let $\lambda = (\lambda_1,\ldots,\lambda_{K-1})^{\mathrm{T}}$. Then the transition probabilities are analytically expressed by transition intensities (Longini et al. 1989; Satten 1999):

$$p_{jk}(t) = \begin{cases} \sum_{l=j}^{k} C(j,l,k;\lambda)\exp(-\lambda_l t), & \text{if } j \leq k, \\ 0, & \text{if } j > k, \end{cases} \tag{6.8}$$

where the coefficients are given by

$$C(j,l,k;\lambda) = \frac{\prod_{i=j}^{k-1}\lambda_i}{\prod_{j\leq i\neq l\leq k}(\lambda_i - \lambda_l)}$$

for $j \leq l \leq k$, and $C(l,l,l;\lambda) = 1$ for $l = 1,\ldots,K-1$.

6.1.3 Continuous-Time Nonhomogeneous Markov Processes

Homogeneous Markov models are easy to use but may be too restrictive to describe many processes in application. It is necessary to develop models that are flexible while also preserving simplicity. A useful method is to partition the entire time period under the study into smaller intervals and to assume a constant intensity over each time interval. This gives Markov models with piecewise-constant intensities, defined by

$$\lambda_{jk}(t) = \lambda_{jkl} \text{ for } t \in A_l = (a_{l-1}, a_l],$$

where $0 = a_0 < a_1 < \ldots < a_{q-1} < a_q = \infty$ is a pre-specified sequence of constants for a given q, and the λ_{jkl} are positive constants for $j,k = 1,\ldots,K$ and $l = 1,\ldots,q$. This class of models can be viewed as nonhomogeneous models that are weakly parametrically postulated; detailed discussion on nonhomogeneous Markov processes was provided by Meira-Machado et al. (2009) and the references therein.

With a nonhomogeneous continuous-time Markov process, the relationship between transition probabilities and transition intensities cannot be expressed by (6.5) anymore. Instead, they are featured by the *product-integral.*

For $0 \le s \le t$, let $P(s,t)$ be the $K \times K$ transition probability matrix with entries $p_{jk}(s,t)$, and $\Lambda(u) = [\Lambda_{jk}(u)]$ be the cumulative transition intensity matrix with (j,k) element

$$\Lambda_{jk}(u) = \int_0^u \lambda_{jk}(v)dv \quad \text{for } j,k \in \mathcal{S}.$$

Then the transition probability matrix is expressed by the cumulative transition intensity matrix using the product-integral:

$$P(s,t) = \lim_{M\to\infty;\Delta u_l\to 0;l=1,\ldots,M} \prod_{l=1}^{M} \{I_K + \Lambda(u_l) - \Lambda(u_{l-1})\}$$

with $s = u_0 < u_1 < \ldots < u_M = t$, $\Delta u_l = u_l - u_{l-1}$ for $l = 1,\ldots,M$, and M is a positive integer which approaches infinity.

The cumulative transition intensity functions $\Lambda_{jk}(u)$ and the related transition probabilities $p_{jk}(s,t)$ can be empirically estimated using the sample data. Detailed discussion is available in Kalbfleisch and Prentice (2002, §8.3).

6.1.4 Discrete-Time Markov Models

For the discrete-time Markov model, there exists a set of ordered times $\mathcal{T} = \{t_l : l = 1,2,\ldots\}$ at which transitions occur, where $0 < t_1 < t_2 < \ldots$. For $l = 1,2,\ldots$, let P_l be the $K \times K$ matrix whose (j,k) element is the one-step transition probability, $P(Y(t_l) = k|Y(t_{l-1}) = j)$, from time t_{l-1} to time t_l, where $t_0 = 0$ and $j,k = 1,\ldots,K$. Let

$$p_{jk}^{(l)} = P(Y(t_l) = k|Y(0) = j)$$

be the l-step transition probability and $P^{(l)} = [p_{jk}^{(l)}]$ be the $K \times K$ matrix with (j,k) element $p_{jk}^{(l)}$.

Under Markov models, the l-step transition probabilities are expressed as the product of a sequence of one-step transition probabilities at different time points:

$$P^{(l)} = P_1 P_2 \ldots P_l$$

for $l = 1, 2, \ldots$. The order of multiplication matters since the matrices do not commute in general. If the chain, however, is homogeneous, then $P_l = P$ for a time-invariant matrix P, thus leading to

$$P^{(l)} = P^l$$

for $l = 1, 2, \ldots$.

6.1.5 Regression Models

Multi-state processes are usually correlated with covariates. It is interesting to describe the multi-state process by conditioning on the associated covariates. In this case, transition intensities and transition probabilities, discussed in the previous subsections, are modified by replacing the history $\mathcal{H}_t^{\mathrm{Y}}$ of states with an extended history which also includes the history of covariates.

Let $X(t)$ and $Z(t)$ be the covariates at time t, $\mathcal{H}_t^{\mathrm{X}} = \{X(v) : 0 \le v \le t\}$ and $\mathcal{H}_t^{\mathrm{Z}} = \{Z(v) : 0 \le v \le t\}$ be the respective history of $X(t)$ and $Z(t)$ up to and including time t, and $\mathcal{H}_t^{\mathrm{XZ}}$ be the union of $\mathcal{H}_t^{\mathrm{X}}$ and $\mathcal{H}_t^{\mathrm{Z}}$.

To accommodate the dependence on covariates of transition intensities or transition probabilities, we focus on the case with *endogenous covariates* where the covariates can be time-independent, or time-dependent so that the random development of the covariates is fully determined by the history of the process itself (e.g., Andersen and Keiding 2002). Typically, for $s < t$, we assume that

$$\begin{aligned} &P(Y(t) = y(t) | Y(s) = y(s), \mathcal{H}_s^{\mathrm{Y}}, \mathcal{H}^{\mathrm{XZ}}) \\ &= P(Y(t) = y(t) | Y(s) = y(s), \mathcal{H}_s^{\mathrm{Y}}, \mathcal{H}_s^{\mathrm{XZ}}), \end{aligned} \tag{6.9}$$

where $\mathcal{H}^{\mathrm{XZ}}$ is the union of $\mathcal{H}_t^{\mathrm{XZ}}$ for $t > 0$.

With endogenous covariates, inferences may be based only on modeling the conditional transition probabilities or transition intensities with the covariate process left unmodeled. If the model contains time-dependent covariates that are not endogenous, then a joint model for the multi-state process and the covariate process is often required, which is analogous to the discussion in §3.1.3 and §4.1.3.

For time points s and t with $s < t$, the transition probability and transition intensity are defined to be

$$p_{jk}(s, t | \mathcal{H}_s^{\mathrm{Y}}, \mathcal{H}_s^{\mathrm{XZ}}) = P(Y(t) = k | Y(s) = j, \mathcal{H}_s^{\mathrm{Y}}, \mathcal{H}_s^{\mathrm{XZ}})$$

and

$$\lambda_{jk}(t | \mathcal{H}_t^{\mathrm{Y}}, \mathcal{H}_t^{\mathrm{XZ}}) = \lim_{\Delta t \to 0+} \frac{p_{jk}(t, t + \Delta t | \mathcal{H}_t^{\mathrm{Y}}, \mathcal{H}_t^{\mathrm{XZ}})}{\Delta t},$$

respectively. The relationship between transition intensities $\lambda_{jk}(t | \mathcal{H}_t^{\mathrm{Y}}, \mathcal{H}_t^{\mathrm{XZ}})$ and transition probabilities $p_{jk}(s, t | \mathcal{H}_s^{\mathrm{Y}}, \mathcal{H}_s^{\mathrm{XZ}})$ may be established following the same lines of the previous subsections.

Parsimonious regression models are constantly used to characterize the dependence on covariates of transition intensities or transition probabilities. Here we briefly describe modeling of transition intensities but defer the discussion of transition probabilities to §6.1.7.

Assuming that

$$\lambda_{jk}(t|\mathcal{H}_t^{\text{Y}}, \mathcal{H}_t^{\text{XZ}}) = \lambda_{jk}(t|\mathcal{H}_t^{\text{XZ}}),$$

one may postulate transition intensities as

$$\lambda_{jk}(t|\mathcal{H}_t^{\text{Y}}, \mathcal{H}_t^{\text{XZ}}) = g(X(t), Z(t); \lambda_{0jk}(t), \beta_{jk})$$

for $j, k = 1, \ldots, K$, where $g(\cdot)$ is a given nonnegative function, $\lambda_{0jk}(t)$ represents the baseline transition intensity from state j to state k, and β_{jk} is the associated parameter which may be state-dependent. Here the dependence of transition intensities on the covariate history is indicated by the involvement of $X(t)$ and $Z(t)$ at current time point t.

A frequently used model is of a multiplicative form:

$$\lambda_{jk}(t|\mathcal{H}_t^{\text{Y}}, \mathcal{H}_t^{\text{XZ}}) = \lambda_{0jk}(t) \exp\{\beta_{xjk}^{\text{T}} X(t) + \beta_{zjk}^{\text{T}} Z(t)\},$$

where $\lambda_{0jk}(t)$ is the baseline intensity function and $\beta_{jk} = (\beta_{xjk}^{\text{T}}, \beta_{zjk}^{\text{T}})^{\text{T}}$ is the vector of regression coefficients related to the transition from state j to state k. The baseline intensity $\lambda_{0jk}(t)$ may be left completely unspecified as in the Cox proportional hazards model for survival analysis, or modeled parametrically or weakly parametrically, as discussed in §3.1.2. A more parsimonious model may be considered by assuming, for example, a common baseline transition intensity $\lambda_{0jk}(t) = \lambda_0(t)$ or common covariate effects among states with $\beta_{jk} = \beta$, where $\lambda_0(t)$ is a positive function and β is a vector of parameters.

Alternatively, an additive structure or time-dependent regression coefficients may be used to describe transition intensities. For instance, a nonparametric additive model may be considered:

$$\lambda_{jk}(t|\mathcal{H}_t^{\text{Y}}, \mathcal{H}_t^{\text{XZ}}) = \lambda_{0jk}(t) + \beta_{xjk}^{\text{T}}(t) X(t) + \beta_{zjk}^{\text{T}}(t) Z(t),$$

where we leave the baseline intensities $\lambda_{0jk}(t)$ and the regression functions $\{\beta_{xjk}(t), \beta_{zjk}(t)\}$ unspecified.

A detailed discussion on modeling of transition intensities was provided by Andersen et al. (1993), Andersen and Keiding (2002), and many others.

6.1.6 Likelihood Inference

Suppose that there is a random sample of n individuals and that subject i in the sample is observed at times $0 \le t_{i1} < \ldots < t_{im_i}$ for $i = 1, \ldots, n$, where m_i is a positive integer which may depend on i. In this subsection and the rest of this chapter, we add subscript i to show the dependence on a subject of the symbols corresponding to those defined in the previous subsections. For subject $i = 1, \ldots, n$, we observe the states $Y_i(t_{il}) = y_{il}$ occupied at these time points t_{il} for $l = 1, \ldots, m_i$; but the exact transition times are not available and they are *interval censored.*

The maximum likelihood method is a natural tool to conduct inference about regression parameters for multi-state models. Suppose the dependence of transition probabilities on covariates is described by regression models with parameter θ, and let $L_i(\theta)$ denote the product of conditional transition probabilities for the observed states of the ith individual. Assuming that being in the initial state at time t_{i1} carries no information about θ and that (6.9) holds, we may write $L_i(\theta)$ as

$$L_i(\theta) = \prod_{l=2}^{m_i} p_{y_{i,l-1}y_{il}}(t_{i,l-1}, t_{il}|\mathcal{H}^{\mathrm{Y}}_{t_{i,l-1}}, \mathcal{H}^{\mathrm{XZ}}_{it_{i,l-1}}),$$

where

$$\begin{aligned} & p_{y_{i,l-1}y_{il}}(t_{i,l-1}, t_{il}|\mathcal{H}^{\mathrm{Y}}_{t_{i,l-1}}, \mathcal{H}^{\mathrm{XZ}}_{it_{i,l-1}}) \\ &= P(Y_i(t_{il}) = y_{il}|Y_i(t_{i,l-1}) = y_{i,l-1}, \mathcal{H}^{\mathrm{Y}}_{it_{i,l-1}}, \mathcal{H}^{\mathrm{XZ}}_{it_{i,l-1}}) \end{aligned}$$

for $l = 2, \ldots, m_i$ and the dependence of the transition probabilities on the regression parameter θ is suppressed in the notation.

Conditional on individual i being in the initial state at time t_{i1}, the likelihood of θ is given as

$$L(\theta) = \prod_{i=1}^{n} L_i(\theta).$$

Maximizing $L(\theta)$ with respect to θ yields the maximum likelihood estimator of θ, provided regularity conditions.

If interest is not in modeling transition probabilities but in modeling transition intensities via regression models with parameter θ, then inference about the regression parameter θ may follow the same procedures but with an additional step included. In this case, working out the relationship between transition probabilities and transition intensities is needed. With a time-homogeneous Markov model, this may be done based on the discussion in §6.1.2.

Under certain scenarios, the maximum likelihood estimation procedure may be simplified. With time-homogeneous Markov models, Kalbfleisch and Lawless (1985) proposed a simple estimation procedure for transition intensity parameters. To highlight the idea, we consider a homogeneous population without covariates.

Suppose that the transition intensity matrix Q depends on parameter vector $\theta = (\theta_1, \ldots, \theta_p)^{\mathrm{T}}$ and that all the individuals are observed at the same time points with $m_i = m$ and $t_{il} = t_l$ for $i = 1, \ldots, n$ and $l = 1, \ldots, m$. Let n_{jkl} denote the number of individuals in state j at time t_{l-1} and in state k at time t_l. Write $p_{jk}(t_{l-1}, t_l) = P(Y_i(t_l) = k|Y_i(t_{l-1}) = j, \mathcal{H}^{\mathrm{Y}}_{it_{l-1}})$ for $l = 2, \ldots, m$. Conditional on the individuals being in their initial states at t_1, the likelihood function for θ is written as

$$L(\theta) = \prod_{l=2}^{m} \left[\prod_{j,k=1}^{K} \{p_{jk}(t_{l-1}, t_l)\}^{n_{jkl}} \right]. \tag{6.10}$$

For time-homogeneous processes, (6.10) gives the log-likelihood function:

$$\log L(\theta) = \sum_{l=2}^{m} \sum_{j,k=1}^{K} n_{jkl} \log p_{jk}(v_l),$$

where $p_{jk}(v_l) = p_{jk}(t_{l-1}, t_l)$ and $v_l = t_l - t_{l-1}$ for $l = 2, \ldots, m$.

Maximization of the log-likelihood with respect to θ may be carried out using a Newton–Raphson algorithm, which requires the evaluation of the first and second partial derivatives of the transition probabilities. To have a computationally efficient procedure, Kalbfleisch and Lawless (1985) developed a quasi Newton–Raphson procedure which requires evaluation of the first partial derivatives of $\log L(\theta)$ only.

For $u, v = 1, \ldots, p$, let

$$S_u(\theta) = \frac{\partial \log L(\theta)}{\partial \theta_u} \text{ and } M_{uv}(\theta) = E\left(- \frac{\partial^2 \log L}{\partial \theta_u \partial \theta_v} \right),$$

then

$$S_u(\theta) = \sum_{l=2}^{m} \sum_{j,k=1}^{K} \frac{n_{jkl}}{p_{jk}(v_l)} \left\{ \frac{\partial p_{jk}(v_l)}{\partial \theta_u} \right\}$$

and

$$M_{uv}(\theta) = \sum_{l=2}^{m} \sum_{j,k=1}^{K} \frac{E\{N_j(t_{l-1})\}}{p_{jk}(v_l)} \left\{ \frac{\partial p_{jk}(v_l)}{\partial \theta_u} \right\} \left\{ \frac{\partial p_{jk}(v_l)}{\partial \theta_v} \right\},$$

where $N_j(t_{l-1}) = \sum_{k=1}^{K} n_{jkl}$ represents the number of individuals in state j at time t_{l-1} for $l = 2, \ldots, m$.

Let $\widehat{M}_{uv}(\theta)$ be an estimate of $M_{uv}(\theta)$ where the expectation $E\{N_j(t_{l-1})\}$ is replaced by the raw count $N_j(t_{l-1})$. Let $S(\theta) = (S_1(\theta), \ldots, S_p(\theta))^{\mathrm{T}}$ and $\widehat{M}(\theta)$ be the $p \times p$ matrix with (u, v) entry $\widehat{M}_{uv}(\theta)$. Then an updated estimate of θ is obtained by the iterative equation

$$\theta^{(k+1)} = \theta^{(k)} + [\widehat{M}(\theta^{(k)})]^{-1} S(\theta^{(k)})$$

for $k = 1, 2, \ldots$, where $\theta^{(k)}$ is an estimate of θ at iteration k and $\widehat{M}(\theta^{(k)})$ is assumed nonsingular. The estimate of θ is then obtained as the limit of $\{\theta^{(k+1)} : k = 1, 2, \ldots\}$ as $k \to \infty$.

6.1.7 Transition Models

In this subsection, we discuss a useful extension of discrete-time Markov models: *transition models*. Suppose that there is a random sample of n individuals and that subject i in the sample is observed at times $0 \le t_{i1} < \ldots < t_{im_i}$ for $i = 1, \ldots, n$, where m_i is a positive integer which may depend on i. Let $Y_{ij} = Y_i(t_{ij})$ denote the response variable for subject i at time t_{ij} for $i = 1, \ldots, n$ and $j = 1, \ldots, m_i$. Unlike usual discrete-time multi-state models for which the Y_{ij} assume discrete values, here Y_{ij} can be either discrete or continuous. In addition to describing how the transition is associated with the response history, we are also interested in the dependence of transition on covariates which may be time-varying. Let X_{ij} and Z_{ij} be vectors of covariates for subject i at time t_{ij}. Here the components in X_{ij} are all time-dependent while Z_{ij} may include both time-dependent and time-independent covariates.

Write $X_i = (X_{i1}^{\mathrm{T}}, \ldots, X_{im_i}^{\mathrm{T}})^{\mathrm{T}}$ and $Z_i = (Z_{i1}^{\mathrm{T}}, \ldots, Z_{im_i}^{\mathrm{T}})^{\mathrm{T}}$. For positive integers q and r which are often much smaller the m_i, let $\mathcal{H}_{ij(q)}^{\mathrm{Y}} = \{Y_{i,j-1}, \ldots, Y_{i,j-q}\}$ for $j > q$, $\mathcal{H}_{ij(r)}^{\mathrm{X}} = \{X_{ij}, \ldots, X_{i,j-r+1}\}$, $\mathcal{H}_{ij(r)}^{\mathrm{Z}} = \{Z_{ij}, \ldots, Z_{i,j-r+1}\}$, and $\mathcal{H}_{ij(r)}^{\mathrm{XZ}}$ be the union of $\mathcal{H}_{ij(r)}^{\mathrm{X}}$ and $\mathcal{H}_{ij(r)}^{\mathrm{Z}}$ for $j > r$. Let $d = \max(r-1, q)$. We call the identity

$$h(y_{ij}|y_{i,j-1}, \ldots, y_{i1}, X_i, Z_i) = h(y_{ij}|\mathcal{H}_{ij(q)}^{\mathrm{Y}}, \mathcal{H}_{ij(r)}^{\mathrm{XZ}}) \text{ for } j > d \tag{6.11}$$

the (q, r)*-order Markov property*, where $h(y_{ij}|\mathcal{C})$ refers to the conditional probability density or mass function of Y_{ij}, given the set $\mathcal{C}$ of conditioning variables, and $\mathcal{C}$ is $\{Y_{i,j-1}, \ldots, Y_{i1}, X_i, Z_i\}$ or $\{\mathcal{H}_{ij(q)}^{\mathrm{Y}}, \mathcal{H}_{ij(r)}^{\mathrm{XZ}}\}$.

In transition models, the conditional distribution of Y_{ij}, given the outcome and covariate histories, is commonly modulated as a distribution from the exponential family with a (q, r)-order Markov property imposed for some positive integers q and r (Diggle et al. 2002, Ch. 10). To be specific, we define a (q, r)*-order transition model* to be the one for which the conditional probability density or mass function of Y_{ij}, given $\mathcal{H}_{ij(q)}^{\mathrm{Y}}$ and $\mathcal{H}_{ij(r)}^{\mathrm{XZ}}$, is

$$f(y_{ij}|\mathcal{H}_{ij(q)}^{\mathrm{Y}}, \mathcal{H}_{ij(r)}^{\mathrm{XZ}}) = \exp\left\{\frac{y_{ij}\xi_{ij} - b(\xi_{ij})}{a(\phi)} + c(\mathcal{H}_{ij(q)}^{\mathrm{Y}}; \phi)\right\}, \tag{6.12}$$

where ξ_{ij} is a canonical parameter, ϕ is a dispersion parameter, and $a(\cdot)$, $b(\cdot)$ and $c(\cdot)$ are specific functions associated with the exponential family distributions.

Since the conditional mean

$$\mu_{ij} = E(Y_{ij}|\mathcal{H}_{ij(q)}^{\mathrm{Y}}, \mathcal{H}_{ij(r)}^{\mathrm{XZ}})$$

equals $b'(\xi_{ij})$, a generalized linear model (McCullagh and Nelder 1989) is further employed to link the conditional mean μ_{ij} with the outcome and covariate histories:

$$\begin{aligned} g(\mu_{ij}) &= \xi_{ij} \\ &= \beta_0 + \sum_{k=1}^{q} \beta_{yk} y_{i,j-k} + \sum_{l=1}^{r} (\beta_{xl}^{\mathrm{T}} X_{i,j-l+1} + \beta_{zl}^{\mathrm{T}} Z_{i,j-l+1}), \end{aligned} \tag{6.13}$$

where $g(\cdot)$ is the canonical link function satisfying $g^{-1}(\cdot) = b'(\cdot)$ and β_0, β_{yk} ($k = 1, \ldots, q$), β_{xl}, and β_{zl} ($l = 1, \ldots, r$) are regression coefficients. When the Z covariates do not change with time, we would tacitly keep only one Z term in the regression model. Let $\beta = (\beta_0, \beta_{yk}, \beta_{xl}^{\mathrm{T}}, \beta_{zl}^{\mathrm{T}} : k = 1, \ldots, q; l = 1, \ldots, r)^{\mathrm{T}}$.

If the conditional distribution of $(Y_{i1}, \ldots, Y_{id})$, given $\{X_i, Z_i\}$, is modeled, then inference about β may be based on the model for the conditional distribution of $Y_i = (Y_{i1}, \ldots, Y_{im_i})^{\mathrm{T}}$ given covariates $\{X_i, Z_i\}$:

$$f(y_i|x_i, z_i) = \prod_{j=d+1}^{m_i} f(y_{ij}|\mathcal{H}_{ij(q)}^{\mathrm{Y}}, \mathcal{H}_{ij(r)}^{\mathrm{XZ}}) f(y_{i1}, \ldots, y_{id}|x_i, z_i),$$

where $f(y_{ij}|\mathcal{H}^{\mathrm{Y}}_{ij(q)}, \mathcal{H}^{\mathrm{XZ}}_{ij(r)})$ is determined by (6.12) together with (6.13) and $f(y_{i1}, \ldots, y_{id}|x_i, z_i)$ is the model for the conditional distribution of $(Y_{i1}, \ldots, Y_{id})$, given $\{X_i, Z_i\}$.

Alternatively, one may leave the conditional distribution of $(Y_{i1}, \ldots, Y_{id})$ unspecified by treating $(Y_{i1}, \ldots, Y_{id})$ as initial states and then conduct conditional analysis for parameter β using the conditional distribution

$$\prod_{j=d+1}^{m_i} f(y_{ij}|\mathcal{H}^{\mathrm{Y}}_{ij(q)}, \mathcal{H}^{\mathrm{XZ}}_{ij(r)}).$$

A useful transition model is the one with a normality assumption and $r = q = 1$ imposed:

$$Y_{ij} = \beta_0 + \beta_y Y_{i,j-1} + \beta_x^{\mathrm{T}} X_{ij} + \beta_z^{\mathrm{T}} Z_{ij} + \epsilon_{ij} \tag{6.14}$$

for $j = 2, \ldots, m_i$, where random errors ϵ_{ij} are assumed to be independent of each other and of the $\{X_{ij}, Z_{ij}\}$ and follow a common distribution $N(0, \sigma^2)$ with variance σ^2. At the baseline visit, the outcome may be solely modeled as a function of the covariates at the entry:

$$Y_{i1} = \widetilde{\beta}_0 + \widetilde{\beta}_x^{\mathrm{T}} X_{i1} + \widetilde{\beta}_z^{\mathrm{T}} Z_{i1} + \epsilon_{i1}, \tag{6.15}$$

where ϵ_{i1} is independent of $\{X_{i1}, Z_{i1}\}$ and follows distribution $N(0, \widetilde{\sigma}^2)$ with variance $\widetilde{\sigma}^2$. Here β_0, $\widetilde{\beta}_0$ and β_y are regression parameters, and β_x, $\widetilde{\beta}_x$, β_z and $\widetilde{\beta}_z$ are parameter vectors.

Transition models are also called *state dependence models*, *state-space models* (Anderson and Hsiao 1982), or *conditional autoregressive models* (Rosner et al. 1985; Rosner and Munoz 1992).

In addition to being an extension of discrete-time Markov models, transition models are also useful in modeling longitudinal data. As discussed in Chapter 5, featuring association structures for repeated outcome measurements is typical for longitudinal data analysis, as opposed to univariate data analysis. As a complement to the modeling strategies discussed in §5.1, transition models offer a convenient way to describe the dependence structure of the longitudinal response process. The interpretation of covariate effects in transition models, however, does not possess the marginal feature, such as that described in §5.1.1, because the covariate effects would change as the order q or r changes.

Some modified versions of transition models are available. For instance, one may replace the covariate history $\mathcal{H}^{\mathrm{XZ}}_{ij(r)}$ with the entire covariate vectors $\{X_i, Z_i\}$ when setting up (6.12) and (6.13); this modeling relaxes assumption (6.11) and emphasizes the dependence of the time-specific response on its own history. Azzalini (1994) introduced a Markov chain model which incorporates serial dependence and facilitates expression of covariate effects on marginal features. Heagerty and Zeger (2000) and Heagerty (2002) extended this work to the qth-order *marginalized transition* models. These models are formulated for analysis of binary data and do not deal with general categorical data. Chen, Yi and Cook (2009) described a method for modeling longitudinal categorical data based on a Markov model which accommodates regression modeling on marginal moments as well as on association structures.

6.2 Two-State Markov Models with Misclassified States

For subject i in a random sample of n individuals, suppose $\{Y_i(t) : t \geq 0\}$ is a two-state continuous-time Markov process, taking value 1 or 2. Assume that for $i = 1, \ldots, n$, subject i is assessed at times $0 \leq t_{i1} < \ldots < t_{im_i}$, and the true state $Y_i(t_{il})$, denoted as Y_{il}, is subject to misclassification with $Y_i^*(t_{il}) = Y_{il}^*$ denoting the observed state for $l = 2, \ldots, m_i$. Let

$$p_{jk}(t_{i,l-1}, t_{il}) = P\{Y_{il} = k | Y_{i,l-1} = j\}$$

be the transition probabilities for the underlying true process, where $j, k = 1, 2$; $i = 1, \ldots, n$; and $l = 2, \ldots, m_i$. Such a two-state model, shown in Fig. 6.6, is useful in describing problems with binary outcomes, such as diseased or disease-free, employed or unemployed, etc.

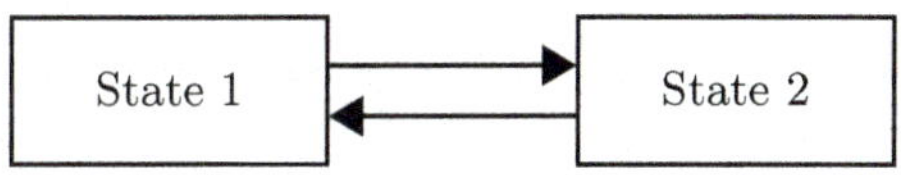

Fig. 6.6. *A Two-State Model*

Observed Transition Probability

Although the underlying true process has the Markov property, the observed process $\{Y_{il}^* : l = 1, \ldots, m_i\}$ does not necessarily retain this property. In fact, transition probabilities for the observed states may assume complex forms even when simplicity conditions are imposed. To see this, for $i = 1, \ldots, n$ and $l = 1, \ldots, m_i$, let

$$\gamma_{ijk} = P(Y_{il}^* = k | Y_{il} = j)$$

be the (mis)classification probabilities for subject i, where $j, k = 1, 2$; and we assume that (mis)classification probabilities are only state-dependent and are independent of time.

For $l = 2, \ldots, m_i$, let $\mathcal{H}_{il}^{Y*} = \{Y_{i1}^*, \ldots, Y_{i,l-1}^*\}$ denote the history of the observed states by time up to but not including t_{il}. Then the conditional probabilities for the observed states, given the history, is expressed in connection with the information of the true states, given by

$$\begin{aligned} & P(Y_{il}^* = 1 | \mathcal{H}_{il}^{Y*}) \\ =\ & P(Y_{il}^* = 1, Y_{il} = 1 | \mathcal{H}_{il}^{Y*}) + P(Y_{il}^* = 1, Y_{il} = 2 | \mathcal{H}_{il}^{Y*}) \\ =\ & \sum_{s=1,2} P(Y_{il}^* = 1 | Y_{il} = s, \mathcal{H}_{il}^{Y*}) P(Y_{il} = s | \mathcal{H}_{il}^{Y*}), \end{aligned} \quad (6.16)$$

where $l = 2, \ldots, m_i$.

The first conditional probability in each term of (6.16) is a (mis)classification probability if assuming

$$P(Y_{il}^* = 1|Y_{il} = s, \mathcal{H}_{il}^{Y*}) = P(Y_{il}^* = 1|Y_{il} = s) \tag{6.17}$$

for $l = 2, \ldots, m_i$ and $s = 1, 2$. This assumption is feasible for situations where misclassification of a state is merely governed by the state itself and not the history of the observed states.

The second conditional probability of each term in (6.16) can be expressed by spelling out its dependence on the history of the true state process:

$$\begin{aligned} & P(Y_{il} = s|\mathcal{H}_{il}^{Y*}) \\ &= P(Y_{il} = s, Y_{i,l-1} = 1|\mathcal{H}_{il}^{Y*}) + P(Y_{il} = s, Y_{i,l-1} = 2|\mathcal{H}_{il}^{Y*}) \\ &= \sum_{v=1,2} P(Y_{il} = s|Y_{i,l-1} = v, \mathcal{H}_{il}^{Y*}) P(Y_{i,l-1} = v|\mathcal{H}_{il}^{Y*}) \\ &= \sum_{v=1,2} P(Y_{il} = s|Y_{i,l-1} = v) P(Y_{i,l-1} = v|\mathcal{H}_{il}^{Y*}), \end{aligned} \tag{6.18}$$

where we assume that

$$P(Y_{il} = 1|Y_{i,l-1} = v, \mathcal{H}_{il}^{Y*}) = P(Y_{il} = 1|Y_{i,l-1} = v) \tag{6.19}$$

for $l = 2, \ldots, m_i$ and $v = 1, 2$. This assumption says that the transition probability from one state to another for the underlying true process depends only on that occupied state and not on the history of the observed surrogate states.

Define $\gamma_{i,l-1}^* = P(Y_{i,l-1} = 1|\mathcal{H}_{il}^{Y*})$ for $i = 1, \ldots, n$ and $l = 2, \ldots, m_i$, then combining (6.16) and (6.18) gives

$$\begin{aligned} & P(Y_{il}^* = 1|\mathcal{H}_{il}^{Y*}) \\ &= \gamma_{i11}\{(1 - \gamma_{i,l-1}^*) p_{21}(t_{i,l-1}, t_{il}) + \gamma_{i,l-1}^* p_{11}(t_{i,l-1}, t_{il})\} \\ &\quad + \gamma_{i21}\{(1 - \gamma_{i,l-1}^*) p_{22}(t_{i,l-1}, t_{il}) + \gamma_{i,l-1}^* p_{12}(t_{i,l-1}, t_{il})\}, \end{aligned} \tag{6.20}$$

where assumptions (6.17) and (6.19) are used. This expression shows how the conditional probability $P(Y_{il}^* = 1|\mathcal{H}_{il}^{Y*})$, $l = 2, \ldots, m_i$, for the observed states depends on the misclassification probabilities and the transition probabilities of the underlying true process.

The conditional probability γ_{il}^*, $l = 1, \ldots, m_i - 1$, is difficult to calculate directly, but can be recursively expressed in terms of the transition probabilities of the underlying true states and misclassification probabilities. For $j = 1, 2$ and $l = 2, \ldots, m_i - 1$, let

$$a_{ij}(y_{il}^*) = (2 - y_{il}^*)\gamma_{ij1} + (y_{il}^* - 1)\gamma_{ij2}$$

and

$$d_{ij}(t_{i,l-1}, t_{il}) = p_{1j}(t_{i,l-1}, t_{il}) - p_{2j}(t_{i,l-1}, t_{il}).$$

Then

$$\begin{aligned}
\gamma_{il}^* &= \frac{P(Y_{il}=1, Y_{il}^*=y_{il}^*, \mathcal{H}_{il}^{Y*})}{P(Y_{il}^*=y_{il}^*, \mathcal{H}_{il}^{Y*})} \\
&= \frac{P(Y_{il}^*=y_{il}^*|Y_{il}=1, \mathcal{H}_{il}^{Y*})P(Y_{il}=1|\mathcal{H}_{il}^{Y*})}{\sum_{v=1,2} P(Y_{il}^*=y_{il}^*|Y_{il}=v, \mathcal{H}_{il}^{Y*})P(Y_{il}=v|\mathcal{H}_{il}^{Y*})} \\
&= \frac{a_{i1}(y_{il}^*)\{p_{21}(t_{i,l-1}, t_{il}) + \gamma_{i,l-1}^* d_{i1}(t_{i,l-1}, t_{il})\}}{\sum_{j=1,2} a_{ij}(y_{il}^*)[p_{2j}(t_{i,l-1}, t_{il}) + \gamma_{i,l-1}^* d_{ij}(t_{i,l-1}, t_{il})]} \qquad (6.21)
\end{aligned}$$

with the starting value

$$\gamma_{i1}^* = \frac{a_{i1}(y_{i1}^*)P(Y_{i1}=1)}{a_{i2}(y_{i1}^*)\{1-P(Y_{i1}=1)\} + a_{i1}(y_{i1}^*)P(Y_{i1}=1)}.$$

The recursive identity (6.21) suggests that γ_{il}^* generally depends on the observed states $y_{i1}^*, \ldots, y_{il}^*$ for time point t_{il} with $l = 1, \ldots, m_i - 1$. As a result, (6.20) implies that the Markov property does not hold for the observed process $\{Y_{il}^* : l = 1, \ldots, m_i\}$, even though the underlying true process $\{Y_i(t) : t \geq 0\}$ is a Markov process.

Regression Model and Identifiability

Next, we examine how misclassification of states may affect estimation of regression parameters. We still consider a two-state Markov process but impose the time-homogeneous assumption for ease of discussion.

For $i = 1, \ldots, n$, let λ_{ijk} be the transition intensity from state j to state k for the process experienced by individual i. Then the transition probabilities may be analytically expressed as functions of the transition intensities:

$$p_{jk}(t_{i,l-1}, t_{il}) = \left(\frac{\lambda_{ijk}}{\lambda_{ijk} + \lambda_{ikj}}\right)[1 - \exp\{-v_{il}(\lambda_{ijk} + \lambda_{ikj})\}] \qquad (6.22)$$

for $j \neq k$ and $j, k = 1, 2$, where $v_{il} = t_{il} - t_{i,l-1}$ and $l = 2, \ldots, m_i$.

Suppose that transition intensities λ_{ijk} are associated with the subject-specific covariate vector, say Z_i, via regression models:

$$\lambda_{ijk} = g_{jk}(Z_i; \beta_{jk}) \qquad (6.23)$$

for $j \neq k$ and $j, k = 1, 2$, where $g_{jk}(\cdot)$ is a given positive function, and β_{jk} is the vector of regression coefficients corresponding to the transition from state j to state k. Let $\beta = (\beta_{12}^{\mathrm{T}}, \beta_{21}^{\mathrm{T}})^{\mathrm{T}}$ denote the vector of all the associated regression parameters.

Suppose the misclassification probabilities are reparameterized as regression functions of covariates:

$$\gamma_{ijk} = g(Z_i; \gamma_{jk}) \qquad (6.24)$$

for $j \neq k$ and $j, k = 1, 2$, where $g(\cdot)$ is a regression function and γ_{jk} denotes the associated parameter. Let $\gamma = (\gamma_{12}^{\mathrm{T}}, \gamma_{21}^{\mathrm{T}})^{\mathrm{T}}$ and $\theta = (\gamma^{\mathrm{T}}, \beta^{\mathrm{T}})^{\mathrm{T}}$.

Let $P(Y_{il}^* = y_{il}^* | \mathcal{H}_{il}^{Y*}, Z_i; \theta)$ be a modified version of (6.16) by including Z_i as an extra conditioning variable, which is determined by modifying (6.20) and (6.21) with covariate Z_i included as an additional conditioning variable, in combination with (6.22) and (6.23). We impose the assumptions which modify (6.17) and (6.19) by including Z_i as an additional conditioning variable.

Define

$$L_{oi}(\theta) = P(Y_{i1}^* = y_{i1}^* | Z_i; \theta) \prod_{l=2}^{m_i} P(Y_{il}^* = y_{il}^* | \mathcal{H}_{il}^{Y*}, Z_i; \theta)$$

to be the conditional probability of Y_i^*, given covariates Z_i, where $Y_i^* = (Y_{i1}^*, \ldots, Y_{im_i}^*)^{\mathrm{T}}$, y_{il}^* is the observed state for subject i at time t_{il} for $l = 1, \ldots, m_i$, and $P(Y_{i1}^* = y_{i1}^* | Z_i; \theta)$ is the probability at the initial state. Then the likelihood function of θ for the observed data is

$$L_o(\theta) = \prod_{i=1}^{n} L_{oi}(\theta). \tag{6.25}$$

Inference about θ is usually performed by maximizing likelihood function $L_o(\theta)$ with respect to θ. Standard likelihood theory gives the asymptotic properties of the resulting estimator under regular situations. In special instances, however, likelihood function $L_o(\theta)$ may not be suitable for inference about θ. For instance, in a misclassification case with $\gamma_{i12} + \gamma_{i21} = 1$, we have that, by the modified version of (6.20), $P(Y_{il}^* = 1 | \mathcal{H}_{il}^{Y*}, Z_i) = g(Z_i; \gamma_{21})$, which is a constant for any time point t_{il}. Hence, likelihood (6.25) is flat relative to the regression parameters θ, thus not suitable for estimation of θ.

The presence of state misclassification may not only alter the shape of the initial likelihood function obtained under the error-free setting but also change the nature of the model structure. Since modeling of the misclassification process is usually required for carrying out valid inferences, the parameter space is then enlarged with the parameter dimension increased, as opposed to the initial space for the response model parameters. Even if the original response model is well defined and identifiable, the inclusion of the misclassification model into the inference procedures may create nonidentifiability issues.

To see this, consider the case where model (6.23) for state transition intensities is given by

$$g_{jk}(Z_i; \beta_{jk}) = \exp(\beta_{jk}^{\mathrm{T}} Z_i) \tag{6.26}$$

for $j \neq k$ and $j, k = 1, 2$; and model (6.24) for the misclassification probabilities is the logistic regression model

$$\operatorname{logit} \gamma_{ijk} = \gamma_{jk0} + \gamma_{jkz}^{\mathrm{T}} Z_i, \tag{6.27}$$

where β_{jk}, γ_{jk0} and γ_{jkz} are regression parameters for $j \neq k$ and $j, k = 1, 2$. Write $\beta = (\beta_{12}^{\mathrm{T}}, \beta_{21}^{\mathrm{T}})^{\mathrm{T}}$ and $\gamma = (\gamma_{12}^{\mathrm{T}}, \gamma_{21}^{\mathrm{T}})^{\mathrm{T}}$, where $\gamma_{jk} = (\gamma_{jk0}, \gamma_{jkz}^{\mathrm{T}})^{\mathrm{T}}$ for $j \neq k$ and $j, k = 1, 2$.

Taking

$$\theta = (\gamma_{12}^{\mathrm{T}}, \gamma_{21}^{\mathrm{T}}, \beta_{12}^{\mathrm{T}}, \beta_{21}^{\mathrm{T}})^{\mathrm{T}} \text{ and } \theta^* = (-\gamma_{21}^{\mathrm{T}}, -\gamma_{12}^{\mathrm{T}}, \beta_{21}^{\mathrm{T}}, \beta_{12}^{\mathrm{T}})^{\mathrm{T}}$$

gives

$$L_{oi}(\theta) = L_{oi}(\theta^*),$$

which suggests that the model parameters are not identifiable. These parameter values reflect the model symmetry in the sense that the state labels are interchangeable. The permutation of state labels is a typical reason of nonidentifiability of *hidden Markov models* (MacDonald and Zucchini 1997; Rosychuk and Thompson 2004). In addition, it can be shown that these two sets of parameter values are the only distinct sets which yield the same distribution of Y_i^*, given Z_i (see Problem 6.6).

When nonindentifiability seems to be an issue, one may consider to change the model structure to attain model identifiability (e.g., Titman and Sharples 2010b). More common practice is, however, not to change the initial model structure but to reduce the parameter space by setting suitable constraints on the model parameters so that some parameter values are inadmissible. For example, to make $L_{oi}(\theta)$ be identifiable, we usually impose constraints that both γ_{i12} and γ_{i21} are smaller than 0.5, a reasonable assumption for misclassification probabilities.

Another approach is to call for additional data sources, as discussed in §2.4, to gain an understanding of the misclassification process so that the identifiability of the response model, which is established for the error-free setting, is preserved. In the lack of additional data sources, a general strategy for overcoming nonidentifiability is to conduct sensitivity analyses. This is normally done by specifying nuisance parameters to be certain representative values and then carrying out inference for parameters of interest to uncover how sensitive the results are to different magnitudes of nuisance parameters.

Essentially, these approaches reserve the initial response model structures but handle nuisance parameters differently. No matter what strategy is employed to overcome nonidentifiability caused by additional modeling of the mismeasurement process, a general principle is to reduce the *entire* parameter space to a *subspace* of the response model parameters (because its identifiability is well established for the context without mismeasurement) and to treat nuisance parameters in a way of reflecting a priori knowledge of mismeasurement or the availability of additional data sources.

6.3 Multi-State Models with Misclassified States

For subject i in a random sample of n individuals, suppose $\{Y_i(t) : t \geq 0\}$ is the true unobservable continuous-time process with K states and $\{Y_i^*(t) : t \geq 0\}$ is its observed process. Let $\lambda_{ijk}(t|\mathcal{H}_{it}^{\mathrm{Y}})$ be the transition intensities for the underlying true process $\{Y_i(t) : t \geq 0\}$, as defined in §6.1.1 with subject index i added. If the Markov property is imposed on the process $\{Y_i(t) : t \geq 0\}$, then $\lambda_{ijk}(t|\mathcal{H}_{it}^{\mathrm{Y}})$ is independent of the history $\mathcal{H}_{it}^{\mathrm{Y}}$ but dependent on the state at time t; and $\{Y_i(t) : t \geq 0\}$

is called a *hidden Markov process* or a *hidden Markov model* to reflect its unobservable feature (Cappé, Moulines and Rydén 2005). If the process $\{Y_i(t) : t \geq 0\}$ is assumed to be time-homogeneous, then $\lambda_{ijk}(t|\mathcal{H}_{it}^{Y})$ is independent of t and $\mathcal{H}_{it}^{Y}$, and it is thereby denoted as λ_{ijk}.

Strategies and Assumptions

Transitions of the underlying process $\{Y_i(t) : t \geq 0\}$ are usually associated with certain covariates. Let $Z_i(t)$ denote the associated covariate vector for subject i at time t. It is of interest to understand the relationship between $Y_i(t)$ and $Z_i(t)$. For $i = 1, \ldots, n$, assume that subject i is assessed at times $0 \leq t_{i1} < \ldots < t_{im_i}$, and let $Y_{il} = Y_i(t_{il})$ and $Y_{il}^* = Y_i^*(t_{il})$ denote the true and the observed states for subject i at time t_{il}, respectively, and $Z_{il} = Z_i(t_{il})$ for $l = 1, \ldots, m_i$. Write $Y_i = (Y_{i1}, \ldots, Y_{im_i})^{\mathrm{T}}$, $Y_i^* = (Y_{i1}^*, \ldots, Y_{im_i}^*)^{\mathrm{T}}$, and $Z_i = (Z_{i1}, \ldots, Z_{im_i})^{\mathrm{T}}$.

Since the surrogate version Y_i^* of Y_i is available, inference about the relationship between Y_i and Z_i typically roots from the joint distribution of all the associated random variables $\{Y_i, Y_i^*, Z_i\}$. Directly modeling this joint distribution is difficult to provide a transparent and meaningful description for each process, especially for the underlying true process which is of primary interest. Common practice is to first factorize the joint distribution as a product of a sequence of conditional distributions and a marginal distribution and then model the resulting distributions separately. This strategy has been constantly applied and illustrated in the previous chapters. It is known that such a factorization is not unique. Depending on the research focus, different formulations may be worked out to reflect varying modeling objectives. To elaborate on this, we describe two modeling schemes.

For $l = 2, \ldots, m_i$, let $\mathcal{H}_{il}^{Y*} = \{Y_{i1}^*, \ldots, Y_{i,l-1}^*\}$ and $\mathcal{H}_{il}^{Y} = \{Y_{i1}, \ldots, Y_{i,l-1}\}$ be the histories of $Y_i^*(t)$ and $Y_i(t)$ up to but not including time t_{il}, respectively, and $\mathcal{H}_{il}^{Z} = \{Z_{i1}, \ldots, Z_{i,l-1}, Z_{il}\}$ be the covariate history up to and including time t_{il}.

A strategy of modelling the joint distribution of $\{Y_i, Y_i^*, Z_i\}$ is to first separate the covariates from the response processes $Y_i(t)$ and $Y_i^*(t)$ using the conditioning principle, and then use the time order to form a sequence of models for the univariate conditional distributions, suggested as follows:

$$\begin{aligned}
& f(y_i, y_i^*, z_i) \\
&= f(y_i, y_i^*|z_i) f(z_i) \\
&\propto f(y_i, y_i^*|z_i) \\
&= f((y_{im_i}, y_{im_i}^*); \ldots; (y_{i2}, y_{i2}^*); (y_{i1}, y_{i1}^*)|z_i) \\
&= \left\{ \prod_{l=2}^{m_i} f(y_{il}^*|y_{il}, \mathcal{H}_{il}^{Y}, \mathcal{H}_{il}^{Y*}, z_i) f(y_{il}|\mathcal{H}_{il}^{Y}, \mathcal{H}_{il}^{Y*}, z_i) \right\} \\
&\quad \cdot f(y_{i1}^*|y_{i1}, z_i) f(y_{i1}|z_i), \qquad (6.28)
\end{aligned}$$

where $f(\cdot|\cdot)$ represents the model for the conditional distribution of the corresponding variables with the parameters suppressed in the notation, and we assume that the model for the marginal distribution of covariates Z_i carries no information about the parameter associated with the model of interest.

Alternatively, to describe the model for the joint distribution of $\{Y_i, Y_i^*, Z_i\}$, we treat all the variables Y_i, Y_i^* and Z_i equally and group them by the time points; then we use the time order to formulate a sequence of conditional models for each univariate variable, demonstrated as follows:

$$\begin{aligned}
& f(y_i, y_i^*, z_i) \\
&= f((y_{im_i}^*, y_{im_i}, z_{im_i}); \ldots; (y_{i2}^*, y_{i2}, z_{i2}); (y_{i1}, y_{i1}^*, z_{i1})) \\
&= \left\{ \prod_{l=2}^{m_i} f(y_{il}^* | y_{il}, \mathcal{H}_{il}^{Y}, \mathcal{H}_{il}^{Y*}, \mathcal{H}_{il}^{Z}) f(y_{il} | \mathcal{H}_{il}^{Y}, \mathcal{H}_{il}^{Y*}, \mathcal{H}_{il}^{Z}) \right. \\
& \quad \left. \cdot f(z_{il} | \mathcal{H}_{il}^{Y}, \mathcal{H}_{il}^{Y*}, \mathcal{H}_{i,l-1}^{Z}) \right\} f(y_{i1}^* | y_{i1}, z_{i1}) f(y_{i1} | z_{i1}) f(z_{i1}) \\
& \propto \left\{ \prod_{l=2}^{m_i} f(y_{il}^* | y_{il}, \mathcal{H}_{il}^{Y}, \mathcal{H}_{il}^{Y*}, \mathcal{H}_{il}^{Z}) f(y_{il} | \mathcal{H}_{il}^{Y}, \mathcal{H}_{il}^{Y*}, \mathcal{H}_{il}^{Z}) \right\} \\
& \quad \cdot f(y_{i1}^* | y_{i1}, z_{i1}) f(y_{i1} | z_{i1}),
\end{aligned} \tag{6.29}$$

where the product of the conditional models for time-specific covariates and the marginal model for Z_{i1} are assumed to carry no useful information about the parameter associated with the model of interest.

Factorization (6.28) focuses on the dynamic changes in the true and observed state processes by conditioning on the *entire covariate vector* over the course, while modeling scheme of (6.29) incorporates the dynamic change in covariates, in addition to those in the true and observed state processes, by conditioning on the *time-specific covariate* information.

To ease modeling, convenient assumptions are frequently made. With decomposition (6.28), it is often assumed that for $l = 2, \ldots, m_i$,

$$f(y_{il} | \mathcal{H}_{il}^{Y}, \mathcal{H}_{il}^{Y*}, z_i) = f(y_{il} | \mathcal{H}_{il}^{Y}, z_i) \tag{6.30}$$

and

$$f(y_{il}^* | y_{il}, \mathcal{H}_{il}^{Y}, \mathcal{H}_{il}^{Y*}, z_i) = f(y_{il}^* | y_{il}, \mathcal{H}_{il}^{Y*}, z_i); \tag{6.31}$$

while for factorization (6.29), one may assume

$$f(y_{il} | \mathcal{H}_{il}^{Y}, \mathcal{H}_{il}^{Y*}, \mathcal{H}_{il}^{Z}) = f(y_{il} | \mathcal{H}_{il}^{Y}, \mathcal{H}_{il}^{Z}) \tag{6.32}$$

and

$$f(y_{il}^* | y_{il}, \mathcal{H}_{il}^{Y}, \mathcal{H}_{il}^{Y*}, \mathcal{H}_{il}^{Z}) = f(y_{il}^* | y_{il}, \mathcal{H}_{il}^{Y*}, \mathcal{H}_{il}^{Z}). \tag{6.33}$$

In application, certain simplistic assumptions may be further imposed. For instance, a combined assumption of the Markov property and nondifferential misclassification:

$$f(y_{il} | \mathcal{H}_{il}^{Y}, \mathcal{H}_{il}^{Y*}, z_i) = f(y_{il} | y_{i,l-1}, z_i)$$

or

$$f(y_{il}|\mathcal{H}^{Y}_{il}, \mathcal{H}^{Y*}_{il}, \mathcal{H}^{Z}_{il}) = f(y_{il}|y_{i,l-1}, \mathcal{H}^{Z}_{il}), \tag{6.34}$$

may be imposed to replace (6.30) or (6.32), respectively.

Regarding the (mis)classification probabilities $f(y^*_{il}|y_{il}, \mathcal{H}^{Y*}_{il}, z_i)$ in (6.31) or $f(y^*_{il}|y_{il}, \mathcal{H}^{Y*}_{il}, \mathcal{H}^{Z}_{il})$ in (6.33), we sometimes assume that (mis)classification probabilities are homogeneous for all the subjects and time points and are independent of the misclassification history. In this case, the (mis)classification information may be simply summarized by a matrix with elements

$$P(Y^*_{il} = k|Y_{il} = j)$$

for $j, k = 1, \ldots, K; l = 1, \ldots, m_i$; and $i = 1, \ldots, n$.

With a factorization, such as (6.28) or (6.29), together with certain model assumptions, one can then proceed with modeling the true transition process and the misclassification process using standard techniques, followed by the development of estimation of associated model parameters. As illustrations, we next consider the decomposition (6.29) and discuss inferential procedures.

Regression Models

Under assumptions (6.33) and (6.34), for $i = 1, \ldots, n$ and $j \neq k$, we define

$$\gamma_{iljk} = P(Y^*_{il} = k|Y_{il} = j, \mathcal{H}^{Y*}_{il}, \mathcal{H}^{Z}_{il}) \text{ for } l = 1, \ldots, m_i$$

and

$$p_{iljk} = P(Y_{il} = k|Y_{i,l-1} = j, \mathcal{H}^{Z}_{il}) \text{ for } l = 2, \ldots, m_i,$$

where $\mathcal{H}^{Y*}_{i1}$ is null. To reflect the influence of the conditioning variables on these probabilities, we employ regression models. For $i = 1, \ldots, n$; $l = 1, \ldots, m_i$; and $j = 1, \ldots, K$, we consider multinomial logistic regression models for the misclassification probabilities γ_{iljk}:

$$\gamma_{iljk} = \frac{\exp(\gamma^{\mathrm{T}}_{jk} w_{il})}{1 + \sum_{s \neq j} \exp(\gamma^{\mathrm{T}}_{js} w_{il})} \text{ for } k \neq j;$$

where γ_{jk} represents the associated parameter vector for $j \neq k$ and $j, k = 1, \ldots, K$; and w_{il} is a subset of $\mathcal{H}^{Z}_{il}$ and $\mathcal{H}^{Y*}_{il}$.

Let $\gamma = (\gamma^{\mathrm{T}}_{jk} : j \neq k; j, k = 1, \ldots, K)^{\mathrm{T}}$. In certain applications, some of the γ_{iljk} are constrained to be a fixed constant or zero to reflect special features or a priori knowledge of data collection procedures. For example, the probability of misclassification may be negligibly small or even zero for nonadjacent states of certain disease and is then accommodated by choosing an appropriate form of w_{il} (e.g., Jackson et al. 2003).

On modeling the true state process $\{Y_i(t) : t \geq 0\}$, two approaches are often used. As discussed in §6.1, one may direct modeling attention to the transition intensities to describe the covariate effects on the process $\{Y_i(t) : t \geq 0\}$, and then express the transition probabilities p_{iljk} in terms of the transition intensities in order to formulate the likelihood function for inferences.

Alternatively, by analogy to the regression model for the misclassification process, one may directly model the transition probability p_{iljk}. Specifically, for $i = 1, \ldots, n$; $l = 2, \ldots, m_i$; and $j = 1, \ldots, K$, we consider the model

$$p_{iljk} = \frac{\exp(\beta_{jk}^{\mathrm{T}} z_{il})}{1 + \sum_{s \neq j} \exp(\beta_{js}^{\mathrm{T}} z_{is})} \quad \text{for } k \neq j,$$

where β_{jk} is the vector of regression parameters related to the transition from states j to k. Let $\beta = (\beta_{jk}^{\mathrm{T}} : j \neq k; j, k = 1, \ldots, K)^{\mathrm{T}}$.

To complete modeling, we express the model $f(y_{i1}|z_{i1})$ for the initial probability $P(Y_{i1} = y_{i1}|Z_{i1} = z_{i1})$ as logistic regression

$$P(Y_{i1} = j|Z_{i1} = z_{i1}) = \frac{\exp(\rho_j^{\mathrm{T}} z_{i1})}{1 + \sum_{s=1}^{K-1} \exp(\rho_s^{\mathrm{T}} z_{is})} \quad \text{for } j = 1, \ldots, K-1;$$

$$P(Y_{i1} = K|Z_{i1} = z_{i1}) = \frac{1}{1 + \sum_{l=1}^{K-1} \exp(\rho_s^{\mathrm{T}} z_{is})};$$

where $\rho = (\rho_1^{\mathrm{T}}, \ldots, \rho_{K-1}^{\mathrm{T}})^{\mathrm{T}}$ is the vector of regression parameters and $y_{i1} = 1, \ldots, K-1, K$.

As a result, corresponding to the factorization (6.29), the likelihood function for the complete data $\{y_i, y_i^*, z_i\}$ contributed from subject i is

$$L_{\mathrm{c}i}(\theta) = \left(\prod_{l=2}^{m_i} \gamma_{il y_{il} y_{il}^*} p_{il y_{i,l-1} y_{il}} \right) \gamma_{i1 y_{i1} y_{i1}^*} f(y_{i1}|z_{i1}), \tag{6.35}$$

leading to the observed likelihood function for the data $\{y_i^*, z_i\}$:

$$L_{\mathrm{o}i}(\theta) = \sum_{y_{i1}=1}^{K} \cdots \sum_{y_{im_i}=1}^{K} L_{\mathrm{c}i}(\theta) \tag{6.36}$$

where $\theta = (\gamma^{\mathrm{T}}, \beta^{\mathrm{T}}, \rho^{\mathrm{T}})^{\mathrm{T}}$ and the marginal distribution of Z_{i1} is assumed to carry no information about θ.

In principle, inference about θ may be based on the observed likelihood function for the entire sample:

$$L_{\mathrm{o}}(\theta) = \prod_{i=1}^{n} L_{\mathrm{o}i}(\theta)$$

by maximizing $L_{\mathrm{o}}(\theta)$ with respect to parameter θ. It is often necessary, however, to examine model identifiability before proceeding with estimation, as discussed in §6.2 and Problem 6.9. It is obvious that $L_{\mathrm{c}i}(\theta)$ in (6.35) is not identifiable if the number of parameters exceeds the dimension of the minimal sufficient statistic. For many applications, when the number of states or the number of assessment times is large or covariate Z_i assumes a large number of different values, model identifiability may likely be achieved.

EM Algorithm

An alternative approach to direct maximization of the observed likelihood is the EM algorithm, which places estimation of θ in the context with missing data, with the underlying true states Y_i regarded as "missing" data. Let

$$L_{\mathrm{C}}(\theta) = \prod_{i=1}^{n} L_{\mathrm{C}i}(\theta)$$

be the complete data likelihood. Then the logarithm of the complete data likelihood is the sum of three separate terms, each involving only one set of parameters corresponding to one process:

$$\ell_{\mathrm{C}}(\theta) = \log L_{\mathrm{C}}(\theta) = \ell_{\mathrm{M}}(\gamma) + \ell_{\mathrm{T}}(\beta) + \ell_{\mathrm{B}}(\rho),$$

where

$$\begin{aligned}
\ell_{\mathrm{M}}(\gamma) &= \sum_{i=1}^{n}\sum_{l=1}^{m_i} \log(\gamma_{ily_{il}y_{il}^*});\\
\ell_{\mathrm{T}}(\beta) &= \sum_{i=1}^{n}\sum_{l=2}^{m_i} \log(p_{ily_{i,l-1}y_{il}});\\
\ell_{\mathrm{B}}(\rho) &= \sum_{i=1}^{n} \log f(y_{i1}|z_{i1});
\end{aligned}$$

corresponding to the misclassification, the state transition, and the beginning information of the true state process, respectively.

At iteration $(k+1)$ of the E-step, we evaluate the conditional expectation, $E\{\ell_{\mathrm{C}}(\theta); \theta^{(k)}\}$, of $\ell_{\mathrm{C}}(\theta)$ with respect to the model, $f(y_i|y_i^*, z_i; \theta^{(k)})$, for the conditional distribution of Y_i given $\{Y_i^*, Z_i\}$, where realization y_i in $\ell_{\mathrm{C}}(\theta)$ is replaced by random variable Y_i when evaluating conditional expectations, $\theta^{(k)}$ represents the estimate of θ at iteration k, and $f(y_i|y_i^*, z_i; \theta^{(k)})$ is determined by

$$\frac{\left\{\prod_{l=1}^{m_i} \gamma_{ily_{il}y_{il}^*} \prod_{l=2}^{m_i} p_{ily_{i,l-1}y_{il}} f(y_{i1}|z_{i1})\right\}|_{\theta=\theta^{(k)}}}{\sum_{y_{i1}=1}^{K}\cdots\sum_{y_{im_i}=1}^{K}\left\{\prod_{l=1}^{m_i} \gamma_{ily_{il}y_{il}^*} \prod_{l=2}^{m_i} p_{ily_{i,l-1}y_{il}} f(y_{i1}|z_{i1})\right\}|_{\theta=\theta^{(k)}}}.$$

To evaluate $E\{\ell_{\mathrm{C}}(\theta); \theta^{(k)}\}$, it suffices to work out the conditional expectations

$$\begin{aligned}
w_{\mathrm{M}}^{il}(\gamma; \theta^{(k)}) &= E(\log \gamma_{ily_{il}y_{il}^*}; \theta^{(k)}) \text{ for } l = 1, \ldots, m_i;\\
w_{\mathrm{T}}^{il}(\beta; \theta^{(k)}) &= E(\log p_{ily_{i,l-1}y_{il}}; \theta^{(k)}) \text{ for } l = 2, \ldots, m_i;\\
w_{\mathrm{B}}^{i1}(\rho; \theta^{(k)}) &= E\{\log f(Y_{i1}|z_{i1}); \theta^{(k)}\};
\end{aligned}$$

which are calculated using the conditional model $f(y_i|y_i^*, z_i; \theta^{(k)})$.

Consequently, the conditional expectation $E\{\ell_{\mathrm{C}}(\theta);\theta^{(k)}\}$ is given by

$$E\{\ell_{\mathrm{C}}(\theta);\theta^{(k)}\} = E\{\ell_{\mathrm{M}}(\gamma);\theta^{(k)}\} + E\{\ell_{\mathrm{T}}(\beta);\theta^{(k)}\} + E\{\ell_{\mathrm{B}}(\rho);\theta^{(k)}\},$$

where

$$E\{\ell_{\mathrm{M}}(\gamma);\theta^{(k)}\} = \sum_{i=1}^{n}\sum_{l=1}^{m_i} w_{\mathrm{M}}^{il}(\gamma;\theta^{(k)});$$

$$E\{\ell_{\mathrm{T}}(\beta);\theta^{(k)}\} = \sum_{i=1}^{n}\sum_{l=2}^{m_i} w_{\mathrm{T}}^{il}(\beta;\theta^{(k)});$$

$$E\{\ell_{\mathrm{B}}(\rho);\theta^{(k)}\} = \sum_{i=1}^{n} w_{\mathrm{B}}^{i1}(\rho;\theta^{(k)}).$$

The M-step then follows with $E\{\ell_{\mathrm{C}}(\theta);\theta^{(k)}\}$ maximized with respect to θ, yielding an updated value $\theta^{(k+1)}$ for iteration $(k+1)$. Repeat this process until convergence of $\{\theta^{(k)} : k = 1, 2, \ldots\}$ as $k \to \infty$.

Implementation Note

A type of EM algorithm, known as the *Baum–Welch* or *forward-backward* algorithm, may be used for analysis of hidden Markov models in discrete-time (e.g., Albert 1999). A generalization of this algorithm for continuous-time models was described by Bureau, Hughes and Shiboski (2000). Implementation issues were briefly discussed by Jackson et al. (2003). An R package, *msm*, was written to fit continuous-time multi-state Markov models with or without misclassification in states. Details can be found in Jackson et al. (2003). Other discussions on software packages of handling multi-state data with or without measurement error were provided by Meira-Machado et al. (2009), and the references therein.

6.4 Markov Models with States Defined by Discretizing an Error-Prone Variable

In some applications, the state value is not directly measured; it is determined by the measurement of a biomarker or a covariate which is error-contaminated. For example, consider the human immunodeficiency virus (HIV) data analyzed by Satten and Longini (1996). Infection with HIV type-I (HIV-1), the virus that causes acquired immune deficiency syndrome (AIDS), is accompanied by a progressive decline in the CD4 cell count (the number of CD4 cells per microlitre), a type of white blood cell that plays a key role in the functioning of the immune system. To describe the HIV progression, CD4 cell counts are used as a covariate to determine the state status. Satten and Longini (1996) used a seven-state model to describe the progression to

AIDS in HIV-infected individuals. Six CD4-based states are defined using cut points $\infty, 900, 700, 500, 350, 200, 0$, and a seventh (absorbing) state is added for clinical AIDS. The progression to AIDS and transitions are displayed in Fig. 6.7.

Due to imperfectness of measurement procedures and biological variability of the variable, the collected measurements of CD4 counts are error-prone. If this aspect is ignored, then the inference results about the state process involve substantial biases, as illustrated by Satten and Longini (1996). Here we describe valid inference methods pertaining to such an error-involved situation.

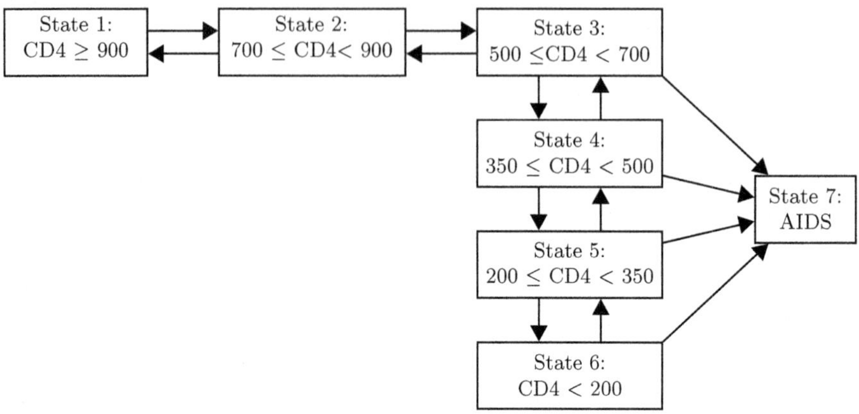

Fig. 6.7. *An AIDS Progression Model*

Suppose there is a sample of n individuals. For $i = 1, \ldots, n$, let $X_i(t)$ be the covariate for subject i at time t which defines the value of state $Y_i(t)$. Specifically, for any time t, covariate $X_i(t)$ is discretized into a finite number of nonoverlapped pre-specified intervals $[l_j, u_j)$ for $j = 1, \ldots, K$, and the state variable is defined to facilitate those categories:

$$Y_i(t) = j \text{ if } X_i(t) \in [l_j, u_j), \tag{6.37}$$

where $j = 1, \ldots, K$. Suppose subject i is observed at times $0 \le t_{i1} < \ldots < t_{im_i}$. However, the true value of $X_i(t)$ is not available, but a surrogate value $X_i^*(t)$ is observed. Write $Y_{il} = Y(t_{il})$, $X_{il} = X_i(t_{il})$, and $X_{il}^* = X_i^*(t_{il})$ for $l = 1, \ldots, m_i$. Let $Y_i = (Y_{i1}, \ldots, Y_{im_i})^{\mathrm{T}}$, $X_i = (X_{i1}, \ldots, X_{im_i})^{\mathrm{T}}$, and $X_i^* = (X_{i1}^*, \ldots, X_{im_i}^*)^{\mathrm{T}}$.

To develop valid inferences with measurement error accounted for, we begin with examining the joint distribution of all the relevant variables X_i^*, X_i and Y_i. Instead of directly modeling such a joint distribution, we employ a factorization to divide modeling into several steps using hierarchical structures:

$$h(x_i^*, x_i, y_i) = h(x_i^* | x_i, y_i) h(x_i | y_i) h(y_i),$$

where the notation $h(\cdot|\cdot)$ or $h(\cdot)$ stands for the conditional or marginal probability density or mass functions for the corresponding random variables. This decomposition explicitly spells out the distribution $h(y_i)$ of the response process $\{Y_i(t) : t \geq 0\}$.

It is often reasonable to assume the conditional independence between X_i^* and Y_i, given X_i:

$$h(x_i^*|x_i, y_i) = h(x_i^*|x_i).$$

This assumption says that the measurement error in X_i is nondifferentiable; the state value is solely determined by the true covariate value and not by its surrogate value. Therefore, we need only to model the conditional distributions $h(x_i^*|x_i)$ and $h(x_i|y_i)$, in addition to modeling of $h(y_i)$. To do so, we consider a hierarchical modeling strategy.

For $l = 1, \ldots, m_i$, let $\mathcal{H}_{il}^{\mathrm{Y}} = \{Y_{i1}, \ldots, Y_{i,l-1}\}$ be the history for the $Y_i(t)$ up to but not including time t_{il}. Let $\mathcal{H}_{il}^{\mathrm{X}} = \{X_{i1}, \ldots, X_{il}\}$ and $\mathcal{H}_{il}^{\mathrm{X}*} = \{X_{i1}^*, \ldots, X_{il}^*\}$ be the history for the $X_i(t)$ and $X_i^*(t)$ up to and including time t_{il}, respectively. We break the modeling of the distribution of X_i given Y_i (or of X_i^* given X_i) into a sequence of conditional models specified at each time point with Y_i (or X_i) held fixed:

$$X_i|Y_i \sim \prod_{l=1}^{m_i} f(x_{il}|\mathcal{H}_{i,l-1}^{\mathrm{X}}, Y_i; \vartheta) \tag{6.38}$$

or

$$X_i^*|X_i \sim \prod_{l=1}^{m_i} f(x_{il}^*|\mathcal{H}_{i,l-1}^{\mathrm{X}*}, X_i; \alpha), \tag{6.39}$$

where $\mathcal{H}_{i0}^{\mathrm{X}}$ and $\mathcal{H}_{i0}^{\mathrm{X}*}$ are null; ϑ is the parameter associated with the models $f(x_{il}|\mathcal{H}_{i,l-1}^{\mathrm{X}}, Y_i; \vartheta)$ for the conditional distribution of X_{il}, given $\{\mathcal{H}_{i,l-1}^{\mathrm{X}}, Y_i\}$; and α is the parameter associated with the models $f(x_{il}^*|\mathcal{H}_{i,l-1}^{\mathrm{X}*}, Y_i; \alpha)$ for the conditional distribution of X_{il}^*, given $\{\mathcal{H}_{i,l-1}^{\mathrm{X}*}, Y_i\}$.

To ease complexity of modeling and gain intuitive interpretation, additional assumptions are usually imposed:

$$\begin{aligned} f(x_{il}|\mathcal{H}_{i,l-1}^{\mathrm{X}}, Y_i; \vartheta) &= f(x_{il}|Y_i; \vartheta) \\ &= f(x_{il}|Y_{il}; \vartheta), \end{aligned}$$

which says that given the Y_i, X_{il} is independent of its history $\mathcal{H}_{i,l-1}^{\mathrm{X}}$, and that given Y_{il}, X_{il} is independent of $Y_{il'}$ for $l' \neq l$. Analogously, model (6.39) may proceed under the assumptions

$$\begin{aligned} f(x_{il}^*|\mathcal{H}_{i,l-1}^{\mathrm{X}*}, X_i; \alpha) &= f(x_{il}^*|X_i; \alpha) \\ &= f(x_{il}^*|X_{il}; \alpha). \end{aligned}$$

Detailed discussion on these assumptions was provided by Satten and Longini (1996) and Lai and Small (2007).

Let β denote the vector of parameters which are involved in the transition probability matrix and ρ represent the parameter associated with the initial probability of the process. Then the joint distribution of Y_i is modeled by the product

$$f(y_i;\rho,\beta) = f(y_{i1};\rho)\prod_{l=2}^{m_i} f(y_{il}|\mathcal{H}_{il}^{\mathrm{Y}};\beta), \tag{6.40}$$

where $f(\cdot)$ and $f(\cdot|\cdot)$, respectively, represent models for the marginal and conditional distributions for the corresponding variables.

To ease the presentation, in the following discussion we assume that the state process $\{Y(t) : t \geq 0\}$ is a homogeneous Markov process with

$$P(Y_{il} = y_{il}|\mathcal{H}_{il}^{\mathrm{Y}}) = P(Y_{il} = y_{il}|Y_{i,l-1} = y_{i,l-1})$$

for $l = 2,\ldots,m_i$.

Marginal Analysis

Let $\theta = (\beta^{\mathrm{T}},\vartheta^{\mathrm{T}},\alpha^{\mathrm{T}},\rho^{\mathrm{T}})^{\mathrm{T}}$ be the vector of all the associated model parameters. Because the state information about Y_i and the true covariate value of X_i are not observed, inference about θ can only proceed based on the marginal likelihood for the observed measurement X_i^*.

One way of obtaining such a marginal likelihood is to marginalize the joint distribution of X_i^* and X_i with respect to X_i. In this case, the marginal likelihood contributed from subject i is given by

$$f(x_i^*;\beta,\vartheta,\alpha,\rho) = \int f(x_i^*|x_i,\alpha)f(x_i;\rho,\beta,\vartheta)d\eta(x_i), \tag{6.41}$$

where the conditional model $f(x_i^*|x_i,\alpha)$ is given by (6.39), and the marginal model $f(x_i;\rho,\beta,\vartheta)$ for X_i is determined by (6.38) and (6.40):

$$f(x_i;\beta,\vartheta,\rho) = \sum_{y_{i1}}\cdots\sum_{y_{im_i}}\left\{\prod_{l=1}^{m_i} f(x_{il}|\mathcal{H}_{i,l-1}^{\mathrm{X}},y_i;\vartheta)f(y_i;\rho,\beta)\right\}. \tag{6.42}$$

Inference about parameter θ is then performed by the maximum likelihood method, i.e., maximizing

$$\prod_{i=1}^{n}\log f(x_i^*;\beta,\vartheta,\alpha,\rho)$$

with respect to θ yields the maximum likelihood estimator of θ.

This approach is conceptually straightforward but may be computationally intractable in some circumstances. The sum in (6.41) is evaluated over K^{m_i} product terms, and such a summation needs to be calculated for each individual when constructing the likelihood for the entire cohort. When the number of states and the number of observation times become large, computation burdens may become a central problem.

Alternatively, the marginal likelihood for the observed data X_i^* can be marginalized through the joint model for X_i^* and Y_i. Satten and Longini (1996) described a method under certain independence assumptions between X_i^* and Y_i. The marginal model for X_i^* is derived as follows:

$$\begin{aligned}
& f(x_i^*;\beta,\vartheta,\alpha,\rho) \\
&= \sum_{y_{i1}}\cdots\sum_{y_{im_i}}\left\{f(x_i^*|y_i;\vartheta,\alpha)f(y_i;\rho,\beta)\right\} \\
&= \sum_{y_{i1}}\cdots\sum_{y_{im_i}}\left\{\prod_{l=1}^{m_i} f(x_{il}^*|y_i;\vartheta,\alpha)\prod_{l=2}^{m_i} f(y_{il}|y_{i,l-1};\beta)f(y_{i1};\rho)\right\} \\
&= \sum_{y_{i1}}\cdots\sum_{y_{im_i}}\left\{f(x_{i1}^*|y_{i1};\vartheta,\alpha)f(y_{i1};\rho)\cdot f(x_{i2}^*|y_{i2};\vartheta,\alpha)f(y_{i2}|y_{i1};\beta)\right. \\
&\qquad \left.\ldots f(x_{im_i}^*|y_{im_i};\vartheta,\alpha)f(y_{im_i}|y_{i,m_i-1};\beta)\right\}, \qquad (6.43)
\end{aligned}$$

where the second equality is due to the Markov assumption for the state process, and the independence assumption that

$$f(x_i^*|y_i;\vartheta,\alpha)=\prod_{l=1}^{m_i} f(x_{il}^*|y_i;\vartheta,\alpha);$$

and the last step comes from the assumption that

$$f(x_{il}^*|y_i;\vartheta,\alpha)=f(x_{il}^*|y_{il};\vartheta,\alpha)\ \text{ for } l=1,\ldots,m_i.$$

This formulation leads to a matrix presentation:

$$f(x_i^*;\beta,\vartheta,\alpha,\rho)=V^{\mathrm{T}}(x_{i1}^*)\{T^{(2)}(x_{i2}^*)T^{(3)}(x_{i3}^*)\ldots T^{(m_i)}(x_{im_i}^*)\}1_K, \qquad (6.44)$$

where $V(x_{i1}^*)$ is the $K\times 1$ column vector with the jth component $V_j=f(x_{i1}^*|Y_{i1}=j;\vartheta,\alpha)f(Y_{i1}=j;\rho)$, and $T^{(l)}(x_{il}^*)$ is the $K\times K$ matrix with (j,k) element

$$T_{jk}^{(l)}(x_{il}^*)=f(x_{il}^*|Y_{il}=k;\vartheta,\alpha)P(Y_{il}=k|Y_{i,l-1}=j;\beta)$$

for $l=2,\ldots,m_i$.

To complete the discussion, we present the conditional probability density or mass function $f(x_{il}^*|Y_{il}=k;\vartheta,\alpha)$. Under the preceding assumptions, by the definition (6.37) of states, we obtain that

$$\begin{aligned}
& f(x_{il}^*|Y_{il}=k;\vartheta,\alpha) \\
&= \int_{l_k}^{u_k} f(x_{il}^*|X_{il}=x_{il};\alpha)f(X_{il}=x_{il}|Y_{il}=k;\vartheta)d\eta(x_{il}), \qquad (6.45)
\end{aligned}$$

where the conditional probability density or mass functions in the integral are models which are specified for determination of (6.39) and (6.38). Then inference about the parameter θ is again performed by maximizing $\prod_{i=1}^{n} \log f(x_i^*; \beta, \vartheta, \alpha, \rho)$ with respect to θ.

Both strategies of formulating (6.41) and (6.43) center around using the marginal likelihood for the observed measurements X_i^*. Although the formulations differ, both methods require modeling the conditional distributions of X_i given Y_i and of X_i^* given X_i, indicated by (6.38) and (6.39), respectively. For example, Satten and Longini (1996) used a uniform or log-normal distribution to feature the conditional probability density function of X_{il}, given Y_{il}, and an additive measurement error model to describe the conditional probability density function of X_{il}^*, given X_{il}. When using (6.43) for estimation of θ, the relationship (6.37) is explicitly reflected in the formulation (6.45); when using (6.41), however, the constraint (6.37) is implicitly imposed for the formulation (6.42).

6.5 Transition Models with Covariate Measurement Error

In this section, we consider inference methods for correcting covariate measurement error under transition models outlined in §6.1.7. Suppose that the response components are modulated by a (q, r)-order transition model (6.12) together with the regression model (6.13). Let $\theta = (\beta^{\mathrm{T}}, \phi)^{\mathrm{T}}$ be the associated parameter. Suppose X_{ij} is an error-prone covariate with an observed measurement X_{ij}^*. For ease of exposition, we consider the case where X_{ij}^* and X_{ij} are scalar. Let $X_i^* = (X_{i1}^*, \ldots, X_{im_i}^*)^{\mathrm{T}}$.

Suppose that the measurement error model is assumed to be additive:

$$X_i^* = X_i + e_i, \tag{6.46}$$

where $e_i = (e_{i1}, \ldots, e_{im_i})^{\mathrm{T}}$, and the e_{ij} are assumed to be independent of each other and of $\{X_i, Z_i, Y_i\}$ and marginally follow a normal distribution $N(0, \sigma_e^2)$ with variance σ_e^2. To focus on estimation of parameter θ, we assume that σ_e^2 is known.

We discuss two methods of adjusting for the effects incurred by the difference between the true covariate measurement X_i and surrogate version X_i^*. These methods mainly differ in the way of handling the true covariate X_i.

Structural Inference

The structural transition measurement error model is completed by specifying a conditional distribution of the unobserved covariate X_i, given the precisely observed covariate Z_i. One way for doing this parallels the modeling strategy for the response process. That is, we employ a transition model to portray the covariates X_{ij} with their serial correlation and the dependence on Z_i being reflected via a regression model. Specifically, consider the linear transition model with an $(s, 1)$-order dependence structure:

$$X_{ij} = \vartheta_0 + \sum_{l=1}^{s} \vartheta_{xl} X_{i,j-l} + \vartheta_z^{\mathrm{T}} Z_{ij} + \epsilon_{xij} \quad \text{for } j > s, \tag{6.47}$$

where $\vartheta = (\vartheta_0, \vartheta_{x1}, \ldots, \vartheta_{xs}, \vartheta_z^{\mathrm{T}})^{\mathrm{T}}$ is the vector of parameters; the ϵ_{xij} are independent of each other and of $\{e_i, Z_i, Y_i\}$ as well as of the history $\mathcal{H}_{i,j-1}^{\mathrm{X}}$; and the ϵ_{xij} are assumed to follow a distribution, say, a distribution from the exponential family. A normal distribution for ϵ_{xij} was considered by Pan, Lin and Zeng (2006).

To perform the likelihood inference, one may further specify a conditional distribution of $\{X_{i1}, \ldots, X_{is}\}$, given Z_i, and let ϑ_{B} denote the associated parameter. Combining this with model (6.47) gives the conditional model, $f(x_i|z_i; \vartheta, \vartheta_{\mathrm{B}})$, for X_i, given Z_i. Consequently, the joint likelihood for the observed data contributed from the ith subject is

$$L_{\mathrm{O}i}(\theta, \vartheta, \vartheta_{\mathrm{B}}) = \int f(y_i|x_i, z_i; \theta) f(x_i^*|x_i, z_i) f(x_i|z_i; \vartheta, \vartheta_{\mathrm{B}}) d\eta(x_i),$$

where the nondifferential measurement error mechanism is assumed, as suggested by the independence of e_i and $\{X_i, Z_i, Y_i\}$; $f(x_i^*|x_i, z_i)$ is given by (6.46); and $f(y_i|x_i, z_i; \theta)$ is the transition model determined by (6.12) and (6.13).

One may attempt to directly maximize the observed likelihood contributed from the sample, $\prod_{i=1}^n L_{\mathrm{O}i}(\theta, \vartheta, \vartheta_{\mathrm{B}})$, to perform estimation of the parameters. This strategy works well for some models, such as linear transition models. Alternatively, one may use the EM algorithm for estimation of the parameters, as described by Pan, Lin and Zeng (2006).

Pseudo Conditional Score Method

The structural method is conceptually easy to use but may be computationally intensive. Moreover, inference results are vulnerable to misspecification of the distribution of the X_i, even when the response and measurement error models are correctly specified. It is desirable to develop a functional method which does not require the distributional specification for the X_i.

Here we describe a *pseudo conditional score* method for estimation of θ, the method developed by Pan, Zeng and Lin (2009). The basic idea consists of two parts. First, assuming θ to be known and treating the X_{ij} as parameters, we derive "sufficient statistics" for the X_{ij}; secondly, using the "sufficient statistics", we construct a conditional distribution to get rid of the unobserved X_{ij}. This scheme parallels the classical *conditional score* approach proposed by Stefanski and Carroll (1987) with different technical details.

With the transition structure and possible nonlinearity of the link function $g(\cdot)$ in (6.13), it is difficult to use the joint model for $\{Y_i, X_i, X_i^*, Z_i\}$ to find "sufficient statistics" for the X_{ij}. Instead, we work with a sequence of conditional submodels, each specified for a time point. For $j \geq r$, let $\mathcal{H}_{ij(r)}^{\mathrm{X}*} = \{X_{ij}^*, \ldots, X_{i,j-r+1}^*\}$, and assume that measurement error is nondifferential with

$$f(y_{ij}, \mathcal{H}_{ij(r)}^{\mathrm{X}*}|\mathcal{H}_{ij}^{\mathrm{Y}}, X_i, Z_i) = f(y_{ij}|\mathcal{H}_{ij}^{\mathrm{Y}}, X_i, Z_i) f(\mathcal{H}_{ij(r)}^{\mathrm{X}*}|\mathcal{H}_{ij}^{\mathrm{Y}}, X_i, Z_i)$$

and

$$f(\mathcal{H}_{ij(r)}^{\mathrm{X}*}|\mathcal{H}_{ij}^{\mathrm{Y}}, X_i, Z_i) = f(\mathcal{H}_{ij(r)}^{\mathrm{X}*}|X_i, Z_i).$$

Combining these assumptions with the (q, r)-order transition models (6.12) and (6.13), we obtain the conditional model for $\{Y_{ij}, \mathcal{H}^{X*}_{ij(r)}\}$, given $\mathcal{H}^{Y}_{ij}$ and $\{X_i, Z_i\}$:

$$\begin{aligned} & f(y_{ij}, \mathcal{H}^{X*}_{ij(r)} | \mathcal{H}^{Y}_{ij}, X_i, Z_i) \\ &= f(y_{ij} | \mathcal{H}^{Y}_{ij}, X_i, Z_i) f(\mathcal{H}^{X*}_{ij(r)} | X_i, Z_i) \\ &= \exp\left[\frac{y_{ij} g(\mu_{ij})}{a(\phi)} - \frac{b\{g(\mu_{ij})\}}{a(\phi)} + c(\mathcal{H}^{Y}_{ij(q)}; \phi) \right. \\ & \quad \left. - \sum_{l=1}^{r} \frac{(X^*_{i,j-l+1} - X_{i,j-l+1})^2}{2\sigma_e^2} - r \log \sqrt{2\pi\sigma_e^2} \right]. \end{aligned} \tag{6.48}$$

Noting that (6.48) belongs to an exponential family and that the $X_{i,j-l+1}$ appear in the linear form in the regression model (6.13) for $g(\mu_{ij})$, we focus on the multiplication terms of the $X_{i,j-l+1}$ times other variables and then take

$$\Omega^{(j)}_{il} = \frac{\beta_{xl} Y_{ij}}{a(\phi)} + \frac{X^*_{i,j-l+1}}{\sigma_e^2}$$

as "sufficient statistics" for the $X_{i,j-l+1}$ with $l = 1, \ldots, r$. By the quotation marks attached to *sufficient statistic*, we mean to indicate the difference of this terminology from the usual definition of sufficient statistics. Here we temporally treat the authentic parameter θ as known and pretend the unobserved random variables X_{ij} are parameters.

The $\Omega^{(j)}_{il}$ are taken as "sufficient statistics" for the $X_{i,j-l+1}$ in the sense that by conditioning on the $\Omega^{(j)}_{il}$, one can come up with a distribution which is free of the $X_{i,j-l+1}$. Let $\mathcal{S}_{ij(r)} = \{\Omega^{(j)}_{i1}, \ldots, \Omega^{(j)}_{ir}\}$ and $\mathcal{V}_{ij}(\theta)$ be the collection of $\mathcal{H}^{Y}_{ij}$, $\mathcal{S}_{ij(r)}$ and $\{X_i, Z_i\}$. Define

$$\begin{aligned} B_{ij}(y_{ij}) &= \frac{y_{ij}(\beta_0 + \sum_{k=1}^{q} \beta_{yk} y_{i,j-k} + \sum_{l=1}^{r} \beta_{zl}^{\mathrm{T}} Z_{i,j-l+1})}{a(\phi)} \\ & \quad - \sum_{l=1}^{r} \frac{\sigma_e^2}{2} \left\{ \Omega^{(j)}_{il} - \frac{\beta_{xl} y_{ij}}{a(\phi)} \right\}^2. \end{aligned}$$

Then the conditional distribution of Y_{ij}, given $\mathcal{V}_{ij}(\theta)$, is modeled by

$$f(y_{ij} | \mathcal{V}_{ij}(\theta); \theta) = \frac{B_{ij}(y_{ij})}{\int B_{ij}(y_{ij}) d\eta(y_{ij})}, \tag{6.49}$$

which does not depend on X_i.

For $d = \min(q + 1, r)$, let

$$U_i(\theta) = \sum_{j=d}^{m_i} \frac{\partial}{\partial \theta} \log f(y_{ij} | \mathcal{V}_{ij}(\theta); \theta),$$

where calculations for the partial derivative $(\partial/\partial\theta) \log f(y_{ij} | \mathcal{V}_{ij}(\theta); \theta)$ are done by viewing $\mathcal{V}_{ij}(\theta)$ as fixed, say at v_{ij}, rather than as a function of θ. At the true value θ_0 of θ, $U_i(\theta)$ has zero mean in the sense that

$$
\begin{aligned}
& E_{\theta_0}\left(\left[\frac{\partial}{\partial\theta}\log f\{Y_{ij}|\mathcal{V}_{ij}(\theta_0);\theta\}\right]_{\theta=\theta_0}\right) \\
&= E_{\theta_0}\left[E_{\theta_0}\left\{\left[\frac{\partial}{\partial\theta}\log f\{Y_{ij}|\mathcal{V}_{ij}(\theta_0);\theta\}\right]_{\theta=\theta_0}\middle|\mathcal{V}_{ij}(\theta_0)\right\}\right] \\
&= 0,
\end{aligned} \tag{6.50}
$$

where the inner expectation is evaluated with respect to the model for the conditional distribution of Y_{ij} given $\mathcal{V}_{ij}(\theta_0)$, and the outer expectation stands for the marginal expectation taken with respect to the model for the marginal distribution of $\mathcal{V}_{ij}(\theta_0)$.

Then estimation of θ is carried out by solving

$$
\sum_{i=1}^{n} U_i(\theta) = 0 \tag{6.51}
$$

for θ. Under regularity conditions, including those in Pan, Zeng and Lin (2009), there exists a solution, say $\widehat{\theta}$, to (6.51) such that $\sqrt{n}(\widehat{\theta}-\theta_0)$ has the asymptotic normal distribution with mean zero and covariance matrix $\Gamma^{-1}\Sigma\Gamma^{-1\mathrm{T}}$, where $\Gamma = E_{\theta_0}\{(\partial/\partial\theta^{\mathrm{T}})U_i(\theta)|_{\theta=\theta_0}\}$, $\Sigma = E_{\theta_0}\{U_i(\theta_0)U_i^{\mathrm{T}}(\theta_0)\}$, and the expectation E_{θ_0} is evaluated in the sense of (6.50). Matrices Γ and Σ are consistently estimated by $\widehat{\Gamma} = n^{-1}\sum_{i=1}^{n}(\partial/\partial\theta^{\mathrm{T}})U_i(\theta)|_{\theta=\widehat{\theta}}$ and $\widehat{\Sigma} = n^{-1}\sum_{i=1}^{n}U_i(\widehat{\theta})U_i^{\mathrm{T}}(\widehat{\theta})$, respectively.

Example 6.1. Consider a logistic transition model with $r = q = 1$ for binary responses Y_{ij} which assumes value 0 or 1:

$$
\text{logit } P(Y_{ij} = 1|\mathcal{H}^{\mathrm{Y}}_{ij(q)}, \mathcal{H}^{\mathrm{XZ}}_{ij(r)}) = \beta_0 + \beta_y Y_{i,j-1} + \beta_x X_{ij} + \beta_z^{\mathrm{T}} Z_{ij},
$$

where $\theta = (\beta_0, \beta_y, \beta_x, \beta_z^{\mathrm{T}})^{\mathrm{T}}$ is the vector of regression coefficients and Y_{i0} is null. Applying the formulation (6.48) gives that

$$
\Omega_{i1}^{(j)} = \beta_x Y_{ij} + X_{ij}^{*}/\sigma_e^2
$$

is a "sufficient statistic" for X_{ij}.

Let

$$
\begin{aligned}
A_{ij} &= 1 + \exp\{(1/2 - Y_{ij})\beta_x^2\sigma_e^2 - \beta_x X_{ij}^{*} - (\beta_0 + \beta_z^{\mathrm{T}} Z_{ij} + \beta_y Y_{i,j-1})\}; \\
B_{ij}(y_{ij}) &= \exp\{-(\Omega_{i1}^{(j)} - y_{ij}\beta_x)^2\sigma_e^2/2 + y_{ij}(\beta_0 + \beta_y y_{i,j-1} + \beta_z^{\mathrm{T}} Z_{ij})\}.
\end{aligned}
$$

Then the conditional probability mass function of Y_{ij}, given $\mathcal{V}_{ij}(\theta)$, is modeled as

$$
\frac{B_{ij}(y_{ij})}{B_{ij}(y_{ij}=1) + B_{ij}(y_{ij}=0)},
$$

where $B_{ij}(y_{ij} = 1)$ and $B_{ij}(y_{ij} = 0)$ represent the expressions of $B_{ij}(y_{ij})$ with y_{ij} replaced by 1 and 0, respectively. Consequently, the pseudo conditional score equations for θ are given by

$$\sum_{i=1}^{n}\sum_{j=2}^{m_i}\begin{pmatrix}1\\ Y_{i,j-1}\\ Z_{ij}\end{pmatrix}(Y_{ij}-1/A_{ij})=0; \tag{6.52}$$

$$\sum_{i=1}^{n}\sum_{j=2}^{m_i}\{Y_{ij}X_{ij}^{*}-(Y_{ij}\beta_x+X_{ij}^{*}/\sigma_e^2-\beta_x)\sigma_e^2/A_{ij}\}=0. \tag{6.53}$$

In the preceding development, we assume that σ_e^2 is known. When σ_e^2 is estimated from an additional source of data, such as replications or a validation subsample, the induced variability needs to be accounted for, as indicated by (1.14) or (1.15). The discussion here focuses on the case with a scalar X_{ij}. Extensions to accommodating multiple covariates X_{ij} follow the same principle. Finally, one issue related to the developed methods is selection of transition orders q and r. When using the structural scheme for inference, usual model selection criteria, such as AIC or BIC, may be used to select suitable values of q and r because of the availability of the likelihood function. With the distribution of X_i unspecified, Pan, Zeng and Lin (2009) proposed heuristically to select q and r using the pseudo-likelihood function. For details, the readers are referred to Pan, Zeng and Lin (2009).

6.6 Transition Models with Measurement Error in Response and Covariates

In this section, we consider a problem which is related to, but different from, the one in §6.5. Here, both responses and covariates are subject to measurement error. We use the same notation as that in §6.5 with an additional symbol Y_{ij}^{*} to represent an observed measurement of Y_{ij} for $j = 1,\ldots,m_i$ and $i = 1,\ldots,n$, where the X_{ij} may be a vector.

Consider the $(1,1)$-order linear transition model

$$Y_{ij}=\beta_0+\beta_y Y_{i,j-1}+\beta_x^{\mathrm{T}}X_{ij}+\beta_z^{\mathrm{T}}Z_{ij}+\epsilon_{ij} \tag{6.54}$$

for $j = 2,\ldots,m_i$, where the ϵ_{ij} are independent of each other and of $\{X_{ij}, Z_{ij}\}$ and follow a normal distribution $N(0,\sigma^2)$ with variance σ^2; β_0 and β_y are regression parameters; β_x and β_z are $p_x \times 1$ and $p_z \times 1$ vectors of regression parameters, respectively; and p_x and p_z represent the dimension of β_x and β_z, respectively. At the baseline visit, the outcome is modeled as a function of the covariates at the entry:

$$Y_{i1}=\widetilde{\beta}_0+\widetilde{\beta}_x^{\mathrm{T}}X_{i1}+\widetilde{\beta}_z^{\mathrm{T}}Z_{i1}+\epsilon_{i1}, \tag{6.55}$$

where the ϵ_{i1} are random errors independent of each other and of the $\{X_{i1}, Z_{i1}\}$ and follow the distribution $N(0,\widetilde{\sigma}^2)$ with variance $\widetilde{\sigma}^2$; and $\widetilde{\beta}_0$, $\widetilde{\beta}_x$ and $\widetilde{\beta}_z$ are regression parameters, respectively, of the dimension of β_0, β_x and β_z.

Error-prone covariates X_{ij} are treated as stochastic quantities and modeled by

$$X_{ij} = \vartheta_0 + \vartheta_x X_{i,j-1} + \vartheta_z Z_{ij} + \epsilon_{xij} \text{ for } j = 2, \ldots, m_i;$$
$$X_{i1} = \widetilde{\vartheta}_0 + \widetilde{\vartheta}_z Z_{i1} + \epsilon_{xi1}; \tag{6.56}$$

where for $j = 2, \ldots, m_i$, the errors ϵ_{xij} and ϵ_{xi1} are independent of each other and of $\{\mathcal{H}^{\mathrm{X}}_{i,j-1}, Z_i\}$; $\epsilon_{xij} \sim N(0, \Sigma_x)$; $\epsilon_{xi1} \sim N(0, \widetilde{\Sigma}_x)$; and Σ_x and $\widetilde{\Sigma}_x$ are positive definite matrices. The model parameters are either vectors or matrices. Specifically, ϑ_0 and $\widetilde{\vartheta}_0$ are $p_x \times 1$ vectors, ϑ_x is a $p_x \times p_x$ matrix, and ϑ_z and $\widetilde{\vartheta}_z$ are $p_x \times p_z$ matrices.

Under the assumptions

$$f(x_{ij}|\mathcal{H}^{\mathrm{X}}_{i,j-1}, z_i) = f(x_{ij}|x_{i,j-1}, z_{ij})$$

and

$$f(x_{i1}|z_i) = f(x_{i1}|z_{i1}),$$

(6.56) determines the model for the conditional distribution of error-prone covariate X_i, given precisely observed covariate Z_i:

$$f(x_i|z_i) = \left\{\prod_{j=2}^{m_i} f(x_{ij}|x_{i,j-1}, z_{ij})\right\} f(x_{i1}|z_{i1}).$$

The preceding models for the response and covariate processes may be unified using the vector or matrix notation. Let $\widetilde{Y}_{ij} = (Y_{ij}, X_{ij}^{\mathrm{T}})^{\mathrm{T}}$ and $\widetilde{\epsilon}_{ij} = (\epsilon_{ij}, \epsilon_{xij}^{\mathrm{T}})^{\mathrm{T}}$ for $j = 2, \ldots, m_i$; $\widetilde{Y}_{i1} - Y_{i1}$; $\widetilde{\epsilon}_{i1} = (\epsilon_{i1}, \epsilon_{xi1}^{\mathrm{T}})^{\mathrm{T}}$; and $\widetilde{Z}_{ij} = (1, Z_{ij}^{\mathrm{T}})^{\mathrm{T}}$ for $j = 1, \ldots, m_i$, then (6.54), (6.55), and (6.56) are unified as

$$\widetilde{Y}_{ij} = P_y \widetilde{Y}_{i,j-1} + P_z \widetilde{Z}_{ij} + P_\epsilon \widetilde{\epsilon}_{ij} \text{ for } j = 2, \ldots, m_i; \tag{6.57}$$

$$\widetilde{Y}_{i1} = \widetilde{P}_z \widetilde{Z}_{i1} + \widetilde{P}_\epsilon \widetilde{\epsilon}_{i1}; \tag{6.58}$$

where $\widetilde{\epsilon}_{ij} \sim N(0_{1+p_x}, \widetilde{\Sigma})$ for $j = 2, \ldots, m_i$; $\widetilde{\epsilon}_{i1} \sim N(0_{1+p_x}, \widetilde{\Sigma}_1)$;

$$\widetilde{\Sigma} = \begin{pmatrix} \sigma^2 & 0_{p_x}^{\mathrm{T}} \\ 0_{p_x} & \Sigma_x \end{pmatrix}; \quad \widetilde{\Sigma}_1 = \begin{pmatrix} \widetilde{\sigma}^2 & 0_{p_x}^{\mathrm{T}} \\ 0_{p_x} & \widetilde{\Sigma}_x \end{pmatrix}; \quad P_y = \begin{pmatrix} \beta_y & \beta_x^{\mathrm{T}} \vartheta_x \\ 0_{p_x} & \vartheta_x \end{pmatrix};$$
$$P_z = \begin{pmatrix} \beta_0 + \beta_x^{\mathrm{T}} \vartheta_0 & \beta_x^{\mathrm{T}} \vartheta_z + \beta_z^{\mathrm{T}} \\ \vartheta_0 & \vartheta_z \end{pmatrix}; \quad P_\epsilon = \begin{pmatrix} 1 & \beta_x^{\mathrm{T}} \\ 0_{p_x} & I_{p_x \times p_x} \end{pmatrix};$$
$$\widetilde{P}_z = \left(\widetilde{\beta}_0 + \widetilde{\beta}_x^T \widetilde{\vartheta}_0 \;\; \widetilde{\beta}_x^{\mathrm{T}} \widetilde{\vartheta}_z + \widetilde{\beta}_z^{\mathrm{T}}\right); \text{ and } \widetilde{P}_\epsilon = \left(1 \;\; \widetilde{\beta}_x^{\mathrm{T}}\right).$$

As a result, the model for the conditional distribution of $\widetilde{Y}_i$, given Z_i, is given by

$$f(\widetilde{y}_i|z_i) = \left\{\prod_{j=2}^{m_i} f(\widetilde{y}_{ij}|\widetilde{y}_{i,j-1}, z_{ij})\right\} f(\widetilde{y}_{i1}|z_{i1}), \tag{6.59}$$

where $\widetilde{y}_i$ is a realization of $\widetilde{Y}_i = \left(\widetilde{Y}_{i1}^{\mathrm{T}}, \ldots, \widetilde{Y}_{im_i}^{\mathrm{T}}\right)^{\mathrm{T}}$, $f(\widetilde{y}_{ij}|\widetilde{y}_{i,j-1}, z_{ij})$ is determined by (6.57), and $f(\widetilde{y}_{i1}|z_{i1})$ is determined by (6.58), with the parameters suppressed.

To complete modeling, we specify measurement error models for the response and covariate processes. Let $\widetilde{Y}_{ij}^* = (Y_{ij}^*, X_{ij}^{*\mathrm{T}})^{\mathrm{T}}$ denote the surrogate version of $\widetilde{Y}_{ij}$ for $j = 1, \ldots, m_i$, $\widetilde{\widetilde{Y}}_{i1} = \left(Y_{i1}, X_{i1}^{\mathrm{T}}\right)^{\mathrm{T}}$, and $\widetilde{Y}_i^* = (\widetilde{Y}_{i1}^{*\mathrm{T}}, \ldots, \widetilde{Y}_{im_i}^{*\mathrm{T}})^{\mathrm{T}}$. Conditional on $\widetilde{Y}_i$ and Z_i, the distributions of $\widetilde{Y}_{ij}^*$ are modeled as

$$\begin{aligned}
\widetilde{Y}_{ij}^* &= \Lambda_y \widetilde{Y}_{ij} + \Lambda_z \widetilde{Z}_{ij} + e_{ij} \quad \text{for } j = 2, \ldots, m_i; \\
\widetilde{Y}_{i1}^* &= \widetilde{\Lambda}_y \widetilde{\widetilde{Y}}_{i1} + \widetilde{\Lambda}_z \widetilde{Z}_{i1} + e_{i1};
\end{aligned} \tag{6.60}$$

where for $j = 2, \ldots, m_i$, the e_{ij} and e_{i1} are independent of each other and of $\{\widetilde{Y}_{ij}, \widetilde{Z}_{ij}\}$ and $\{Y_{i1}, Z_{i1}\}$; $e_{ij} \sim N(0, \Sigma_e)$ with covariance matrix Σ_e; and $e_{i1} \sim N(0, \widetilde{\Sigma}_e)$ with variance $\widetilde{\Sigma}_e$. Here we assume that matrices Λ_y, Λ_z, $\widetilde{\Lambda}_y$, $\widetilde{\Lambda}_z$, Σ_e, and $\widetilde{\Sigma}_e$ are known.

Model (6.60) implicitly assumes

$$f(\widetilde{y}_{ij}^*|\widetilde{y}_i, z_i) = f(\widetilde{y}_{ij}^*|\widetilde{y}_{ij}, z_{ij}),$$

saying that the probability information of the surrogate measurements at time j depends only on the true measurements of response and covariate variables at that time point and not on those at other time points. Consequently, the model for the conditional distribution of $\widetilde{Y}_i^*$, given $\widetilde{Y}_i$ and Z_i, is given by

$$f(\widetilde{y}_i^*|\widetilde{y}_i, z_i) = \prod_{j=1}^{m_i} f(\widetilde{y}_{ij}^*|\widetilde{y}_{ij}, z_{ij}), \tag{6.61}$$

where the assumption $f(\widetilde{y}_{ij}^*|\widetilde{y}_{i,j-1}^*, \ldots, \widetilde{y}_{i1}^*, \widetilde{y}_i, z_i) = f(\widetilde{y}_{ij}^*|\widetilde{y}_i, z_i)$ is made for $j = 2, \ldots, m_i$.

Estimation Procedure

Let θ be the vector of parameters associated with the conditional model (6.59). Given the foregoing hierarchical modeling structures, the model for the conditional distribution of the observed data $\widetilde{Y}_i^*$, given Z_i, is

$$f(\widetilde{y}_i^*|z_i) = \int \sum_{y_i} f(\widetilde{y}_i^*, \widetilde{y}_i|z_i) d\eta(x_i) = \int \sum_{y_i} f(\widetilde{y}_i^*|\widetilde{y}_i, z_i) f(\widetilde{y}_i|z_i) d\eta(x_i),$$

where $f(\widetilde{y}_i|z_i)$ and $f(\widetilde{y}_i^*|\widetilde{y}_i, z_i)$ are determined by (6.59) and (6.61), respectively.

Inference about θ is then based on maximizing the observed likelihood

$$L_{\mathrm{o}}(\theta) = \prod_{i=1}^{n} f(\widetilde{y}_i^*|z_i)$$

with respect to parameter θ. Details were given by Schmid, Segal and Rosner (1994).

Alternatively, estimation of θ may be carried out using the EM algorithm, as developed by Schmid (1996). Given Z_i, the complete data likelihood for $\{\widetilde{Y}_i, \widetilde{Y}_i^*\}$ is

$$L_{\mathrm{c}}(\theta) = \prod_{i=1}^{n} L_{\mathrm{c}i}(\theta),$$

where

$$L_{\mathrm{c}i}(\theta) = f(\widetilde{y}_i^* | \widetilde{y}_i, z_i) f(\widetilde{y}_i | z_i).$$

Given the formulation of (6.59) and (6.61), the log-likelihood $\ell_{\mathrm{c}}(\theta) = \log L_{\mathrm{c}}(\theta)$ for the complete data is thus

$$\begin{aligned} \ell_{\mathrm{c}}(\theta) = -\frac{1}{2}\sum_{i=1}^{n}\Bigg\{ \sum_{j=2}^{m_i} \Bigg[& \log|P_\epsilon \widetilde{\Sigma} P_\epsilon^{\mathrm{T}}| + \log|\Sigma_e| \\ & + (\widetilde{y}_{ij} - P_y \widetilde{y}_{i,j-1} - P_z \widetilde{z}_{ij})^{\mathrm{T}} (P_\epsilon \widetilde{\Sigma} P_\epsilon^{\mathrm{T}})^{-1} (\widetilde{y}_{ij} - P_y \widetilde{y}_{i,j-1} - P_z \widetilde{z}_{ij}) \\ & + (\widetilde{y}_{ij}^* - \Lambda_y \widetilde{y}_{ij} - \Lambda_z \widetilde{z}_{ij})^{\mathrm{T}} \Sigma_e^{-1} (\widetilde{y}_{ij}^* - \Lambda_y \widetilde{y}_{ij} - \Lambda_z \widetilde{z}_{ij}) \Bigg] \\ & + (\widetilde{y}_{i1} - \widetilde{P}_z \widetilde{z}_{i1})^{\mathrm{T}} (\widetilde{P}_\epsilon \widetilde{\Sigma}_1 \widetilde{P}_\epsilon^{\mathrm{T}})^{-1} (\widetilde{y}_{i1} - \widetilde{P}_z \widetilde{z}_{i1}) \\ & + (\widetilde{y}_{i1}^* - \widetilde{\Lambda}_y \widetilde{\widetilde{y}}_{i1} - \widetilde{\Lambda}_z \widetilde{z}_{i1})^{\mathrm{T}} \Sigma_{e1}^{-1} (\widetilde{y}_{i1}^* - \widetilde{\Lambda}_y \widetilde{\widetilde{y}}_{i1} - \widetilde{\Lambda}_z \widetilde{z}_{i1}) \Bigg\} \\ & + \log|\widetilde{P}_\epsilon \widetilde{\Sigma}_1 \widetilde{P}_\epsilon^{\mathrm{T}}| + \log|\Sigma_{e1}|, \end{aligned} \tag{6.62}$$

where the constant is omitted.

At iteration $(k+1)$ of the E-step, we calculate the conditional expectation $E\{\ell_{\mathrm{c}}(\theta)|\widetilde{Y}_i^*, Z_i; \theta^{(k)}\}$, where the expectation is taken with respect to the conditional model, $f(\widetilde{y}_i|\widetilde{y}_i^*, z_i; \theta^{(k)})$, of the "missing" data $\widetilde{Y}_i$ given the observed data $\{\widetilde{Y}_i^*, Z_i\}$ with parameter θ evaluated at $\theta^{(k)}$, the estimate of θ obtained from iteration k. The conditional model $f(\widetilde{y}_i|\widetilde{y}_i^*, z_i; \theta)$ is determined by:

$$f(\widetilde{y}_i|\widetilde{y}_i^*, z_i; \theta) = \frac{L_{\mathrm{c}i}(\theta)}{\int \sum_{y_i} L_{\mathrm{c}i}(\theta) d\eta(x_i)}.$$

With the form (6.62), to evaluate $E\{\ell_{\mathrm{c}}(\theta)|\widetilde{Y}_i^*, Z_i; \theta^{(k)}\}$, we need only to calculate the conditional expectations of $\widetilde{Y}_{ij}$ and $\widetilde{Y}_{ij}^{\mathrm{T}}\widetilde{Y}_{ij}$ for $j \geq 1$ and of $\widetilde{Y}_{i,j-1}^{\mathrm{T}}\widetilde{Y}_{ij}$ for $j \geq 2$. Noting that $f(\widetilde{y}_i|\widetilde{y}_i^*, z_i)$ is the product of the conditional models at individual time points, we evaluate $E\{\widetilde{Y}_{ij}^{\mathrm{T}}\widetilde{Y}_{il}^{s}|\widetilde{Y}_i^*, Z_i; \theta^{(k)}\}$ sequentially using the conditional expectation at each time point, where $s = 0, 1; l = j-1, j$; and $j = 1, \ldots, m_i$ with $\widetilde{Y}_{i0}$ taken as null.

Let $\widetilde{\mathcal{H}}_{ij} = \{\widetilde{Y}_{i1}, \ldots, \widetilde{Y}_{i,j-1}; \widetilde{Y}_i^*, Z_i\}$ for $j = 2, \ldots, m_i$, then the conditional expectation is sequentially evaluated as

$$\begin{aligned}
&E\{\widetilde{Y}_{ij}^{\mathrm{T}}\widetilde{Y}_{il}^{s}|\widetilde{Y}_i^*, Z_i; \theta^{(k)}\}\\
&= E_{\widetilde{Y}_{i1}}(E_{\widetilde{Y}_{i2}|\widetilde{\mathcal{H}}_{i2}} \cdots [E_{\widetilde{Y}_{im_i}|\widetilde{\mathcal{H}}_{im_i}}\{\widetilde{Y}_{ij}^{\mathrm{T}}\widetilde{Y}_{il}^{s}; \theta^{(k)}\}])\\
&= E_{\widetilde{Y}_{i1}}(E_{\widetilde{Y}_{i2}|\widetilde{\mathcal{H}}_{i2}} \cdots [E_{\widetilde{Y}_{ij}|\widetilde{\mathcal{H}}_{ij}}\{\widetilde{Y}_{ij}^{\mathrm{T}}\widetilde{Y}_{il}^{s}; \theta^{(k)}\}])\\
&= E_{\widetilde{Y}_{i1}}(E_{\widetilde{Y}_{i2}|\widetilde{Y}_{i1}} \cdots [E_{\widetilde{Y}_{ij}|\widetilde{Y}_{i,j-1}}\{\widetilde{Y}_{ij}^{\mathrm{T}}\widetilde{Y}_{il}^{s}; \theta^{(k)}\}]),
\end{aligned} \tag{6.63}$$

where for $l = 2, \ldots, m_i$, $E_{\widetilde{Y}_{il}|\widetilde{\mathcal{H}}_{il}}$ and $E_{\widetilde{Y}_{il}|\widetilde{Y}_{i,l-1}}$ represent the conditional expectations taken with respect to the conditional model of $\widetilde{Y}_{il}$, given $\widetilde{\mathcal{H}}_{il}$, and the conditional model of $\widetilde{Y}_{il}$, given $\{\widetilde{Y}_{i,l-1}, \widetilde{Y}_i^*, Z_i\}$, respectively; and $E_{\widetilde{Y}_{i1}}$ represents the conditional expectation taken with respect to the conditional model of $\widetilde{Y}_{i1}$ given $\{\widetilde{Y}_i^*, Z_i\}$. The last identity is due to the structure of the response and covariate models.

The underlying conditional models in (6.63) are normal distributions, hence the conditional expectations in (6.63) are the first or second conditional moments of normal distributions, which have closed-forms (Schmid 1996). At the M step, we maximize the expected value $E\{\ell_{\mathrm{c}}(\theta)|\widetilde{Y}_i^*, Z_i; \theta^{(k)}\}$ with respect to θ using standard techniques for Gaussian data to obtain an updated value $\theta^{(k+1)}$ for iteration $(k + 1)$. Repeat the E and M steps for $k = 1, 2, \ldots$ until convergence of $\theta^{(k+1)}$. Let $\widehat{\theta}$ denote the resultant estimator of θ. Variance estimates of $\widehat{\theta}$ may be obtained using the formula of Louis (1982) or the bootstrap method.

In the preceding development we assume that the parameters of measurement error models (6.60) are known. This assumption allows us to confine attention to estimating the parameters associated with the response and covariate processes and prevents us from confronting potential problems of model nonidentifiability. The estimation procedures are useful for performing sensitivity analyses to assess the effects of different measurement error models on inferences about the parameters of interest (Schmid and Rosner 1993), where various model forms and associated parameters for the measurement error processes are specified by the user. In the instance where external data sources, such as a priori similar study or validation data, are available, the parameters for the measurement error models are estimated from these data, and the induced variability needs to be accounted for when describing the asymptotic properties of $\widehat{\theta}$.

6.7 Bibliographic Notes and Discussion

Continuous-time multi-state models are widely used to describe progression of chronic diseases. However, inference is difficult when the process is only observed at discrete time points where no information about the process between observation times is available, unless certain assumptions are made. The Markov assumption has been widely adopted in the literature (e.g., Kalbfleisch and Prentice 2002, §8.3), and goodness-of-fit for Markov models was developed by various authors. For instance, Aguirre-Hernández and Farewell (2002) proposed a Pearson-type test. Titman and Sharples (2008) generalized this test to the case with an absorbing state, and they extended the discussion to allow for hidden Markov models. A review of methods for diagnosing model fit for panel-observed continuous-time Markov models was given by Titman and Sharples (2010a). In the case where the Markov assumption is infeasible, alternative models have been proposed. These models include finite mixture models (e.g., Frydman 1984; Cook, Kalbfleisch and Yi 2002; Cook et al. 2004), semi-Markov models (e.g., Titman and Sharples 2010b), hidden Markov models (e.g., Bureau, Shiboski and Hughes 2003), random effects models (e.g., Satten 1999), and general regression models. A review of multi-state models was provided by Hougaard (1999), Andersen and Keiding (2002), Meira-Machado et al. (2009), and Cook and Lawless (2014), among many others.

The methods in this chapter mainly focus on addressing effects induced from misclassified states and mismeasured covariates, assuming that the underlying model assumptions for the multi-state models are plausible. The likelihood-based methods discussed in §6.4 modify the development by Satten and Longini (1996) and Sypsa et al. (2001). The EM algorithm discussed in §6.3 was employed by Pfeffermann, Skinner and Humphreys (1998) to handle problems in the context of survey sampling, where the modeling scheme (6.29) was used in combination with a proper incorporation of sampling weights. The EM algorithm was also employed by Albert, Hunsberger and Biro (1997) to address longitudinal ordinal data with diagnostic error under a latent Markov chain model. Using the EM algorithm, Hu and de Gruttola (2007) proposed a joint modeling method to incorporate the error-prone covariate process into the Cox proportional hazards model for failure times.

Other work on measurement error and misclassification problems under multi-state models includes Wolfe, Carlin and Patton (2003), Bureau, Shiboski and Hughes (2003), Jackson et al. (2003), Smith and Vounatsou (2003), Rosychuk and Thompson (2003, 2004), Chen and Sen (2007), Rosychuk and Islam (2009), He (2015), Yi, He and He (2017), and the references therein.

6.8 Supplementary Problems

6.1.

(a) Prove the identities (6.3) and (6.4).

(b) Consider a continuous-time Markov process. For $0 \leq s \leq t$ let $P(s,t)$ be the $K \times K$ transition probability matrix with entries $p_{jk}(s,t)$ and $Q(t)$ be the $K \times K$ transition intensity matrix with entries $\lambda_{jk}(t)$ for $j,k \in \mathcal{S}$. Show that the identities (6.3) and (6.4) for homogeneous models can be extended as

$$\frac{\partial P(s,t)}{\partial t} = P(s,t)Q(t)$$

and

$$-\frac{\partial P(s,t)}{\partial s} = Q(s)P(s,t),$$

respectively. These equations are called the *Kolmogorov differential equations*.

(Cox and Miller 1965, §4.5)

6.2. Consider a continuous-time homogeneous Markov process discussed in §6.1.2.

(a) Suppose that the transition matrix Q has K distinct eigenvalues. Prove the identity (6.7).

(b) If the transition matrix Q has repeated eigenvalues, derive a procedure to calculate the partial derivative matrix $\partial P(t)/\partial \theta_l$ of the transition probabilities for $l = 1, \ldots, p$.

(Kalbfleisch and Lawless 1985)

6.3. Consider the progressive homogeneous Markov model discussed in §6.1.2.

(a) Suppose the transition intensities $\lambda_1, \ldots, \lambda_{K-1}$ are distinct. Prove the identity (6.8).

(b) Suppose some of the transition intensities $\lambda_1, \ldots, \lambda_{K-1}$ are equal. Derive the expressions of the transition probabilities in terms of the transition intensities.

(Satten 1999; Longini et al. 1989)

6.4.

(a) Verify the recursive equation (6.21).

(b) Discuss the assumptions (6.17) and (6.19) which are made for the recursive equation (6.21).

(c) Derive a similar expression to (6.21) for a general case where the number of states, K, is larger than 2.

6.5. Suppose $\{Y(t) : t \geq 0\}$ is a continuous-time Markov process with K states. Let $\lambda_{jk}(t)$ be the transition intensity at time t from states j to k and $p_{jk}(s,t) = P(Y(t) = k|Y(s) = j)$ for $s < t$ and $j, k = 1, \ldots, K$.

(a) Suppose $K = 2$ and $\{Y(t) : t \geq 0\}$ is homogeneous with $\lambda_{jk}(t) = \lambda_{jk}$ for $t \geq 0$, $j \neq k$, and $j, k = 1, 2$. Show that the transition probabilities are

$$p_{jk}(s,t) = \left(\frac{\lambda_{jk}}{\lambda_{12} + \lambda_{21}}\right)[1 - \exp\{-(t-s)(\lambda_{12} + \lambda_{21})\}]$$

for $j \neq k$ and $j, k = 1, 2$.

(b) Consider a Markov model with three states as indicated by the illness-death model, shown by Fig. 6.3 in §6.1.1 except that the transition from states 2 to 1 is impossible, i.e., $\lambda_{21}(t) = 0$ for $t \geq 0$. Show that the transition probabilities have explicit expressions

$$p_{11}(s,t) = \exp[-\{\Lambda_{12}(s,t) + \Lambda_{13}(s,t)\}];$$
$$p_{22}(s,t) = \exp\{-\Lambda_{23}(s,t)\};$$
$$p_{12}(s,t) = \int_s^t p_{11}(s,v)\lambda_{12}(v)p_{22}(v,t)dv;$$

where $\Lambda_{jk}(s,t) = \int_s^t \lambda_{jk}(v)dv$ is the cumulative intensity from states j to k between time points s and t.

(c) Derive the expressions of the transition probabilities in terms of the transition intensities for the illness-death model of Fig. 6.3 in §6.1.1.

(Rosychuk and Thompson 2003; Meira-Machado et al. 2009)

6.6. Consider the transition intensity model (6.26) and the misclassification model (6.27) in §6.2. Let $L_{oi}(\theta)$ be defined as in (6.25). Let $\theta_1 = (\gamma_{12}^{\mathrm{T}}, \gamma_{21}^{\mathrm{T}}, \beta_{12}^{\mathrm{T}}, \beta_{21}^{\mathrm{T}})^{\mathrm{T}}$ and $\theta_2 = (-\gamma_{21}^{\mathrm{T}}, -\gamma_{12}^{\mathrm{T}}, \beta_{21}^{\mathrm{T}}, \beta_{12}^{\mathrm{T}})^{\mathrm{T}}$.

(a) Show that $L_{oi}(\theta_1) = L_{oi}(\theta_2)$.
(b) If there are two parameter values θ_1^* and θ_2^* such that $L_{oi}(\theta_1^*) = L_{oi}(\theta_2^*)$, then $\{\theta_1^*, \theta_2^*\} = \{\theta_1, \theta_2\}$.

(Rosychuk and Thompson 2004)

6.7. Consider a two-state continuous-time homogeneous Markov process in §6.2. For subject i, let Z_i be a discrete covariate assuming N different values and λ_{ijk} be the transition intensities from states j to k for the underlying true process $\{Y_i(t) : t \geq 0\}$, where $j \neq k$ and $j, k = 1, 2$. Consider the regression model

$$\log \lambda_{ijk} = \beta_{0jk} + \beta_z Z_i, \tag{6.64}$$

where β_{0jk} is the intercept that may be dependent on the transition from states j to k; β_z is the regression coefficient; $j \neq k$; and $j, k = 1, 2$. Let $\beta = (\beta_{012}, \beta_{021}, \beta_z)^{\mathrm{T}}$.

Assume that the (mis)classification probabilities $P(Y_{il}^* = k | Y_{il} = j, Z_i)$ depend only on the true underlying states and not on others, and let $\gamma_{jk} = P(Y_{il}^* = k | Y_{il} = j, Z_i)$ for all i, j, k, and l.

(a) Assume that the (mis)classification probabilities γ_{jk} are known. Derive an estimation procedure for β by respectively modifying
   (i) the observed likelihood formulation (6.25) in §6.2.
   (ii) the observed likelihood formulation (6.36) in §6.3.
   (iii) the EM algorithm in §6.3.
(b) Compare the formulations of (i) and (ii) in (a).
(c) If the (mis)classification probabilities γ_{jk} are unknown, can the procedures in (a) be carried through for estimation of β?
(d) Hairy leukoplakia (HL) is an oral lesion that is thought to have prognostic significance for the progression of HIV disease. Bureau, Shiboski and Hughes (2003) analyzed a data set concerning diagnosis of HL. Here we consider a modified subset with $n = 1254$ subjects who were assessed at most four times. Let Y_{il} denote the HL status, taking value 1 or 0, respectively, corresponding to having HL or HL free, at time point t_l for $l = 1, 2, 3, 4$ and $i = 1, \ldots, n$. Let Z_i represent CD4 counts for subject i that were categorized to be three levels, 1,2, and 3, corresponding to the range: CD4 count ≤ 200, $200 <$ CD4 count ≤ 500, and CD4 count > 500.

It is known that diagnosis of HL is subject to measurement error, and the false positive and false negative rates are about 3.40% and 24.2%, respectively. That is, $P(Y_{il}^* = 1|Y_{il} = 0) = 3.40\%$ and $P(Y_{il}^* = 0|Y_{il} = 1) = 24.2\%$ for $i = 1, \ldots, n$ and $l = 1, 2, 3, 4$, where Y_{il}^* represents the diagnostic value of HL. Table 6.1 records the frequencies of the observed value of HL for a subset of individuals classified by the CD4 counts, together with the frequencies of the observed diagnostic HL for a subset of individuals whose CD4 counts are unknown.

(i) Analyze this data set by modifying the methods in (a).
(ii) If the misclassification in HL is ignored by treating Y_{il}^* as Y_{il}, analyze this data set and compare the results to those obtained in (d) (i).

(Bureau, Shiboski and Hughes 2003)

Table 6.1. *HL Data (Bureau, Shiboski and Hughes 2003)*

HL status				CD4 count			No stratification
Y_{i1}^*	Y_{i2}^*	Y_{i3}^*	Y_{i4}^*	$Z_i = 1$	$Z_i = 2$	$Z_i = 3$	
1	0			10	6	5	18
1	1			17	23	6	39
0	0			45	101	100	207
0	1			7	9	4	18
1	1	0		2	4		6
1	1	1		6	12		26
1	0	0		7			12
1	0	1		2			4
0	1	0					8
0	1	1					6
0	0	0		23	59	76	184
0	0	1		5	2	2	8
1	1	1	0				8
1	1	1	1				18
0	0	0	0				153
0	0	0	1				6

6.8. Repeat the analysis in Problem 6.7 by replacing the regression model (6.64) for the transition intensities with

$$\text{logit}\, p_{ijk} = \beta_{0jk} + \beta_z Z_i,$$

where p_{ijk} is the transition probability from states j to k for subject i, β_{0jk} is the intercept that may be dependent on the transition from states j to k, and β_z is the regression coefficient.

(Bureau, Shiboski and Hughes 2003)

6.9. Consider the complete data likelihood function $L_{ci}(\theta)$ in (6.35) and the observed data likelihood function $L_{oi}(\theta)$ in (6.36) discussed in §6.3.

(a) Is $L_{ci}(\theta)$ identifiable when $m_i = 2$ and $K = 2$?
(b) Is $L_{ci}(\theta)$ identifiable if Z_i is a binary covariate?
(c) If $L_{ci}(\theta)$ is identifiable, is $L_{oi}(\theta)$ also identifiable?
(d) If $L_{oi}(\theta)$ is identifiable, is $L_{ci}(\theta, \alpha)$ also identifiable?

(Pfeffermann, Skinner and Humphreys 1998)

6.10. Consider the two sets of assumptions in §6.3.

(a) Show that the assumptions (6.30) and (6.31) for the factorization (6.28) are compatible. That is, there exists a joint model (6.28) so that the requirements (6.30) and (6.31) are satisfied for the response and misclassification models.
(b) Show that the assumptions (6.32) and (6.33) for the factorization (6.29) are compatible. That is, there exists a joint model (6.29) so that the requirements (6.32) and (6.33) are satisfied for the response and misclassification models.

6.11. Verify the matrix expression (6.44).

6.12. Assume the model assumptions in §6.5.

(a) Find the joint probability density or mass function for $\{Y_i, X_i, Z_i, X_i^*\}$. Show that this distribution does not necessarily belong to an exponential family.
(b) Prove (6.49).
(c) Verify the expressions (6.52) and (6.53) in Example 6.1.
(d) Can the development of the pseudo conditional score method in §6.5 go through if the measurement error model (6.46) is changed? Specifically, consider each of the following scenarios:
   (i) the independence assumption of the e_{ij} for (6.46) is not true;
   (ii) the normality assumption of the e_i for (6.46) is not true;
   (iii) the measurement error model is not (6.46) but a Berkson model.

(Pan, Zeng and Lin 2009)

6.13. Consider the $(1, 1)$-order transition model (6.14) with (6.15) in §6.1.7 where X_{ij} is a scalar covariate. Let $\theta = (\beta_0, \beta_y, \beta_x, \beta_z^{\mathrm{T}}, \sigma^2)^{\mathrm{T}}$. Suppose that covariate X_{ij} is subject to measurement error with observed version X_{ij}^*. Assume that the measurement error model is given by (6.46), and that the X_{ij} are modulated by (6.47) with $s = 1$ and $\epsilon_{xij} \sim N(0, \sigma_x^2)$. Assume that the parameters σ_e^2 and σ_x^2 are known.

(a) Discuss the asymptotic bias of the naive estimator for the response parameter vector θ which is obtained by replacing X_{ij} with X_{ij}^* in the linear transition model (6.14) and (6.15).
(b) Develop procedures for estimating θ using the pseudo conditional score method discussed in §6.5.
(c) Develop procedures for estimating θ using the EM algorithm discussed in §6.6.
(d) If the parameters σ_e^2 and σ_x^2 are unknown, can the EM algorithm be employed to estimate the parameter θ? Are there any potential issues that may be of concern?

(Pan, Lin and Zeng 2006; Pan, Zeng and Lin 2009)

6.14.

(a) Verify the matrix expressions (6.57) and (6.58) in §6.6.
(b) By analogy with (6.57) and (6.58), find the matrix expressions by extending the response model (6.54) to a $(q, 1)$-order linear model, and the covariate model (6.56) to an $(r, 1)$-order linear model, where q and r are positive integers greater than 1.
(c) Assume that the response, covariate and measurement error models are given as in §6.6. Find the model for the conditional distribution of Y_i^* given $\{X_i^*, Z_i\}$. Are there any assumptions for the measurement error process that you may make in order to find a simplified expression?
(d) Assume that the response, covariate and measurement error models are given as in §6.6. Can you develop an estimation method similar to the pseudo conditional score method discussed in §6.5?

(Schmid 1996)

7

Case–Control Studies with Measurement Error or Misclassification

In epidemiological research case–control studies provide an important method to investigate factors contributing to certain medical conditions, such as disease statuses. Case–control studies are quick and cheap to conduct. They enable us to study rare health outcomes without having to follow up a large number of subjects over a long period of time. Analysis of case–control studies dates back to Broders (1920) and Lane-Claypon (1926). Various statistical analysis methods for case–control data have been developed since the landmark paper by Cornfield (1951). Those methods are, however, vulnerable to measurement error and misclassification that commonly accompany case–control studies. This chapter deals with this topic and discusses inference methods for handling error-prone data arising from case–control studies.

This chapter differs from the foregoing development mainly in two aspects: measurement error mechanisms and sampling schemes. For observational or prospective studies, the nondifferential measurement error mechanism is almost ubiquitously assumed, but for case–control studies the differential measurement error or misclassification mechanism may be more feasible. In the discussion of the preceding chapters, the way of collecting data is often not regarded as an issue; a random sample is tacitly assumed to have been collected prospectively from the same framework that is used for the data analysis. On the other hand, when dealing with case–control data, the disparity between the disease development model and the retrospective sampling scheme becomes a concern.

The layout of this chapter aligns with the foregoing chapters. The first section outlines the basics of case–control studies in the error-free context. Misclassification effects are illustrated in the second section, followed by the sections which describe various inference methods of accounting for measurement error or misclassification effects. The chapter is closed with bibliographic notes and supplementary exercises.

G. Y. Yi, *Statistical Analysis with Measurement Error or Misclassification*,
Springer Series in Statistics, DOI 10.1007/978-1-4939-6640-0_7

7.1 Introduction of Case–Control Studies

7.1.1 Basic Concepts

The primary purpose of a case–control study is to study how risk factors are associated with the disease incidence. The study involves the comparison of cases (i.e., diseased individuals) with controls (i.e., disease-free individuals). Questions of interest usually include: (1) the degree of association between risk for developing a disease and the factors under study; (2) the extent to which the observed association may result from bias, confounding and/or chance; and (3) the extent to which the association may be described as causal (Breslow and Day 1980, Ch. 3).

A number of features make case–control studies different from usual prospective or observational studies discussed in the foregoing chapters. In subsequent subsections, we set forth a basic stage for case–control studies with basic issues briefly touched on. For comprehensive discussions, we refer the reader to Breslow and Day (1980) and Schlesselman (1982).

7.1.2 Unstratified Studies

Consider a simple case–control study with a single exposure variable and a binary disease status. Let $Y = 1$ if a subject is a case, and $Y = 0$ otherwise. Let $Z = 1$ if the subject is exposed to a condition of interest, and $Z = 0$ otherwise.

To describe the association between disease and exposure, the *relative risk* or *risk ratio*, defined to be

$$\phi_{\text{RR}} = \frac{P(Y = 1|Z = 1)}{P(Y = 1|Z = 0)},$$

is often used. This measure represents how many times more (or less) likely disease occurs in the presence of exposure versus unexposed. A difference of ϕ_{RR} from unity indicates that the exposure variable is associated with the risk of disease.

An alternative measure of associations is given by the ratio of the odds of disease in the exposed individuals relative to the unexposed subjects. The *odds ratio*, or *relative odds*, is defined as

$$\psi = \frac{P(Y = 1|Z = 1)/P(Y = 0|Z = 1)}{P(Y = 1|Z = 0)/P(Y = 0|Z = 0)}.$$

With a rare disease, the odds ratio ψ is nearly identical to the relative risk ϕ_{RR}. Although either a deviation of ϕ_{RR} from unity or a deviation of ψ from unity may suggest an association between exposure and disease, the odds ratio ψ is used more often than the relative risk ϕ_{RR} to describe the relation between exposure and disease. While the relative risk ϕ_{RR} is determined only from a prospective study, the odds ratio may be calculated from either a prospective study or a retrospective case–control study. In fact, the odds ratio calculated from the *exposure probabilities* (i.e., $P(Z = z|Y = y)$) is identical to the odds ratio of the *disease probabilities* (i.e., $P(Y = y|Z = z)$):

$$\psi = \frac{P(Z=1|Y=1)/P(Z=0|Y=1)}{P(Z=1|Y=0)/P(Z=0|Y=0)} = \frac{P(Y=1|Z=1)/P(Y=0|Z=1)}{P(Y=1|Z=0)/P(Y=0|Z=0)}. \tag{7.1}$$

Now we turn to discussing how the odds ratio is estimated from measurements of a sample. Suppose there are n patients in a case–control study. A 2×2 table, displayed by Table 7.1, summarizes the information of such a study, where for $i, j = 0, 1$, n_{ij} records the observed counts of individuals with $Y = i$ and $Z = j$, and n_{i+} and n_{+j} are the row and column totals, respectively.

Table 7.1. *A* 2 × 2 *Display for a Case–Control Study with a Binary Exposure Variable*

	Exposure status $Z = 1$	Exposure status $Z = 0$	Total
Disease status $Y = 1$	n_{11}	n_{10}	n_{1+}
Disease status $Y = 0$	n_{01}	n_{00}	n_{0+}
Total	n_{+1}	n_{+0}	n

An estimate of ψ is given by the sample odds ratio

$$\widehat{\psi} = \frac{n_{11}n_{00}}{n_{01}n_{10}}.$$

To avoid the constraint that $\psi > 0$, sometimes the log odds ratio, $\log \psi$, is used as a measure of association between exposure and disease. An estimate of the variance of $\log \widehat{\psi}$ is given by

$$\widehat{\mathrm{var}}(\log \widehat{\psi}) = \frac{1}{n_{01}} + \frac{1}{n_{00}} + \frac{1}{n_{11}} + \frac{1}{n_{10}}.$$

With a large sample, $\log \widehat{\psi}$ has an asymptotic normal distribution, and an approximate $(1-\alpha)100\%$ confidence interval for ψ is given by $(\widehat{\psi}_{\mathrm{L}}, \widehat{\psi}_{\mathrm{U}})$, where

$$\widehat{\psi}_{\mathrm{L}} = \widehat{\psi} \exp\left\{-z_{\alpha/2}\sqrt{\widehat{\mathrm{var}}(\log \widehat{\psi})}\right\},$$

$$\widehat{\psi}_{\mathrm{U}} = \widehat{\psi} \exp\left\{z_{\alpha/2}\sqrt{\widehat{\mathrm{var}}(\log \widehat{\psi})}\right\},$$

$z_{\alpha/2}$ is the critical value for the standard normal distribution such that the probability of exceeding this point is $\alpha/2$, and α is a value between 0 and 1 (Woolf 1955; Schlesselman 1982, Ch. 7).

Similar discussion may be carried out for unstratified studies displayed by $2 \times K$ tables, where K represents the levels of the discrete exposure variable Z and $K > 2$. Details were given by Breslow and Day (1980, §4.5).

We conclude this subsection with several comments. The sample odds ratio $\widehat{\psi}$ may be derived as a maximum likelihood estimate from different likelihood formulations. For $i, j = 1, 0$, let N_{ij} denote the number of individuals with $Y = i$ and $Z = j$. If regarding the cell counts $\{N_{01}, N_{00}, N_{11}, N_{10}\}$ as coming from a multinomial distribution with a total sample size fixed at n, we derive that the sample odds ratio $\widehat{\psi}$ is a maximum likelihood estimate of ψ.

Alternatively, $\widehat{\psi}$ may be obtained from the likelihood method by assuming that the sample sizes for cases and controls are fixed at n_{1+} and n_{0+}, respectively, and that simple random samples have been taken from theoretically infinite populations of cases and controls (or that random samples have been taken from finite populations with replacement). This method reflects the *retrospective sampling scheme* for case–control data for which study subjects are selected in light of the presence or absence of the disease under study. Under this sampling scheme, it is feasible to treat the marginal row totals n_{1+} and n_{0+} fixed by design, and hence the sampling distribution of the data $\{N_{ij} : i, j = 0, 1\}$ is the product of two binomial distributions, $\text{BIN}(n_{1+}, p_{11})$ and $\text{BIN}(n_{0+}, p_{01})$, where $p_{11} = P(Z = 1|Y = 1)$ and $p_{01} = P(Z = 1|Y = 0)$ are the conditional exposure probabilities for cases and controls, respectively.

In comparison, we contrast a different perspective taken for analysis of *prospective* studies. The major difference between a prospective study and a retrospective study is the selection of study subjects. In a case–control study, individuals with the disease are selected for comparison with disease-free individuals; the comparison focuses on existing or past attributes of exposures that are thought to be relevant to the development of the disease. A prospective study, however, selects individuals who are initially free of the disease and follows them over time (at least conceptually) to monitor the development of the disease in the presence or absence of exposure.

In the analysis of prospectively selected data, it is often assumed that study subjects are sampled at random from the exposed and unexposed subpopulations. Thus, the marginal column totals of n_{+1} exposed and n_{+0} unexposed subjects are regarded as fixed numbers, which are determined by the sample size requirements of the study design, and the *sampling distribution* of the data $\{N_{ij} : i, j = 0, 1\}$ is the product of two binomial distributions $\text{BIN}(n_{+1}, q_{11})$ and $\text{BIN}(n_{+0}, q_{01})$, where $q_{11} = P(Y = 1|Z = 1)$ and $q_{01} = P(Y = 1|Z = 0)$ are the probabilities of developing the disease for exposed and unexposed individuals, respectively.

7.1.3 Matching and Stratification

In this subsection, we outline strategies of *matching* and *stratification* to eliminate confounding effects on estimation of the odds ratio in case–control studies. Matching or stratifying the data provides an easy way to control for complex effects of confounding factors which would otherwise be difficult to perform because of their indeterminate nature. A comprehensive discussion on the issues of design, sampling, and analysis pertaining to various sources of bias was provided by Breslow and Day (1980, §3.4) and Schlesselman (1982, Ch. 4, Ch. 5).

Matched Design

Uncontrolled confounding may account for spurious effects of the exposure variable on the disease or mask the true underlying association. A *confounding* variable, or a *confounder*, refers to an extraneous variable that is correlated with both the disease and exposure variables and its association with the disease is *causal*. The exposure variable may, by its association with confounders, appear to elevate or reduce the risk of disease when in fact it has no effect, or oppositely, when it is actually associated with the disease, but such an association is not detected due to failing to control confounding effects. *Matching* the data provides a direct method to reduce the biased effect resulting from confounding. One or more controls are often paired or matched with each case according to their similarity or likeness in some characteristics, such as age, sex, race, marital status, occupation, weight, history of the disease, and so on.

Matched designs have an advantage of "balancing" the numbers of cases and controls on the basis of the matching variables. It is advisable that a matched design is accompanied by an analysis which accounts for the matching features. This avoids inefficiencies resulting from possibly a substantial imbalance of cases and controls, and more importantly, it retains the validity of the analysis. The estimate of the relative risk of disease associated with exposure may be biased for a matched design if an unmatched analysis is performed.

The simplest example of matched data occurs with a single binary exposure where there is 1:1 pair matching of cases with controls. One-to-one pair matching provides the most cost-effective design when cases and controls are equally "scarce". However, when control subjects are more readily obtained than cases, which is often true for studies of rare diseases, it may make sense to select two or more controls to match with each case. According to Ury (1975), the theoretical efficiency of a $1{:}M$ case–control ratio for estimating a relative risk, relative to having complete information on the control population ($M = \infty$), is $M/(M+1)$. Thus, one control per case is 50% efficient, while four per case is 80% efficient. However, increasing the number of controls beyond a large number, say 5 or bigger, brings rapidly diminishing returns.

Stratification

In addition to matching, *stratification* is another useful strategy for control of confounding. This method is to group the data into a series of subgroups or strata so that individuals within each stratum are relatively homogeneous with respect to the stratification factors. It is anticipated that separate calculations of the relative risk using the data from each stratum are free of bias arising from confounding.

We consider a case–control study with K strata. Let Y be the disease status and Z be the exposure variable; both are binary variables, taking value 0 or 1. Let $p_{k11} = P(Z = 1|Y = 1, \text{stratum } k)$ be the probability of exposure among cases in stratum k, and $p_{k01} = P(Z = 1|Y = 0, \text{stratum } k)$ be the exposure probability for controls in stratum k. For each stratum $k = 1, \ldots, K$, the odds ratio is defined to be

$$\psi_k = \frac{p_{k11}(1 - p_{k01})}{p_{k01}(1 - p_{k11})}.$$

The odds ratios ψ_k are estimated from the data in the corresponding stratum. Let n_{kij} denote the observed number of subjects with $Y = i$ and $Z = j$ in stratum k. Let n_{k1+} and n_{k0+} be the number of cases and controls in stratum k, respectively; and n_{k+1} and n_{k+0} be the number of exposed and unexposed individuals in stratum k, respectively. The data for stratum k are displayed in Table 7.2. The odds ratio for stratum k is estimated as

$$\widehat{\psi}_k = \frac{n_{k11} n_{k00}}{n_{k10} n_{k01}}.$$

Table 7.2. *Data Layout for Stratum k*

	Exposure ($Z = 1$)	Nonexposure ($Z = 0$)	Total
Case ($Y = 1$)	n_{k11}	n_{k10}	n_{k1+}
Control ($Y = 0$)	n_{k01}	n_{k00}	n_{k0+}
Total	n_{k+1}	n_{k+0}	

Although the odds ratios, for each stratum can be estimated separately using the data from the corresponding stratum, it is of interest to know whether the association between exposure and disease is constant from stratum to stratum. If ψ_k varies with k, it is important to understand how the ψ_k change with the levels of the factors used for stratification.

If the ψ_k are stratum-independent, a summary odds ratio is necessary. Mantel and Haenszel (1959) proposed an estimate of the common odds ratio, denoted as ψ, on the basis of adjusting for stratification effects. The estimate is a weighted average of the stratum-specific odds ratios, given by

$$\widehat{\psi}_{\text{MH}} = \frac{\sum_{k=1}^{K} w_k \widehat{\psi}_k}{\sum_{k=1}^{K} w_k}, \tag{7.2}$$

where $w_k = n_{k10} n_{k01} / n_{k++}$, $n_{k++} = n_{k1+} + n_{k0+}$, and $k = 1, \ldots, K$. With the numbers of cases and controls in each stratum being large, Hauck (1979) proposed an estimate of the variance of $\log \widehat{\psi}_{\text{MH}}$, given by

$$\widehat{\text{var}}(\log \widehat{\psi}_{\text{MH}}) = \frac{\sum_{k=1}^{K} w_k^2 \widehat{\text{var}}(\log \widehat{\psi}_k)}{(\sum_{k=1}^{K} w_k)^2},$$

where

$$\widehat{\text{var}}(\log \widehat{\psi}_k) = \frac{1}{n_{k11}} + \frac{1}{n_{k10}} + \frac{1}{n_{k01}} + \frac{1}{n_{k00}}$$

for $k = 1, \ldots, K$.

Alternatively, inference about the common odds ratio ψ may be based on the conditional distributions of the N_{k11}, given that all the marginal row totals are fixed at the observed outcomes for the strata, where N_{k11} represents the numbers of exposed cases in stratum k for $k = 1, \ldots, K$. Let $r_{k1} = \max(n_{k+1} - n_{k0+}, 0)$, and $r_{k2} = \min(n_{k+1}, n_{k1+})$. Assuming that the marginal row totals are fixed at the observed outcomes, the conditional probability of $N_{k11} = n_{k11}$ is given by

$$g_k(\psi) = \frac{\binom{n_{k1+}}{n_{k11}}\binom{n_{k0+}}{n_{k+1}-n_{k11}}\psi^{n_{k11}}}{\sum_{r=r_{k1}}^{r_{k2}}\binom{n_{k1+}}{r}\binom{n_{k0+}}{n_{k+1}-r}\psi^{r}}.$$

Assuming independence among the data across the strata, the likelihood function of ψ is

$$L(\psi) = \prod_{k=1}^{K} g_k(\psi).$$

Maximizing $L(\psi)$ with respect to ψ gives an estimate of ψ, which is called the *exact conditional estimate* and denoted as $\widehat{\psi}_{\mathrm{C}}$. In application, the Mantel–Haenszel estimate $\widehat{\psi}_{\mathrm{MH}}$ and the estimate $\widehat{\psi}_{\mathrm{C}}$ are often close in values (Schlesselman 1982, §7.2).

7.1.4 Regression Model

The preceding discussion focuses on the scenario where only a single exposure variable is available to characterize the disease information. In epidemiological studies, there are often multiple risk factors which may be either qualitative or quantitative or both. Using a table with odds ratios becomes inadequate to conduct inferences. It is necessary to assume a *model* to relate the disease incidence to risk factors or covariates. Let $Z = (Z_1, \ldots, Z_p)^{\mathrm{T}}$ denote the covariate vector of dimension p.

To describe an individual developing the disease during the study period, we frequently employ the logistic regression model

$$\operatorname{logit} P(Y = 1|Z) = \beta_0 + \beta_z^{\mathrm{T}} Z, \tag{7.3}$$

where β_0 and $\beta_z = (\beta_1, \ldots, \beta_p)^{\mathrm{T}}$ are regression coefficients. This formulation implies that the odds ratio for individuals having two different sets of values, $z = (z_1, \ldots, z_p)^{\mathrm{T}}$ and $\widetilde{z} = (\widetilde{z}_1, \ldots, \widetilde{z}_p)^{\mathrm{T}}$, of risk variables Z is

$$\begin{aligned}\psi(z, \widetilde{z}) &= \frac{P(Y = 1|Z = z)/P(Y = 0|Z = z)}{P(Y = 1|Z = \widetilde{z})/P(Y = 0|Z = \widetilde{z})} \\ &= \exp\left\{\sum_{j=1}^{p} \beta_j (z_j - \widetilde{z}_j)\right\}.\end{aligned} \tag{7.4}$$

Clearly, the intercept β_0 represents the log odds of disease risk for a person with a standard (i.e., $Z = 0$) set of regression variables, while $\exp(\beta_j)$ is the fraction by which this risk is increased (or decreased) for every unit change in Z_j with other components in Z held fixed, and $j = 1, \ldots, p$.

In case–control designs, an implicit assumption is commonly made that the sampling probabilities depend only on disease status and not on the risk factors, i.e., $P(R = 1|Y, Z) = P(R = 1|Y)$, where R is the indicator variable whether or not an individual is sampled, i.e., $R = I$(an individual is sampled). Let $\pi_1 = P(R = 1|Y = 1)$ be the probability that a diseased person is included in the study as a case and $\pi_0 = P(R = 1|Y = 0)$ be the probability of including a disease-free person in the study as a control. Then in combination with model (7.3), the conditional probability that an individual is diseased, given that this person has risk variables Z and that he/she is sampled for the study, is

$$\begin{aligned} &P(Y = 1|R = 1, Z) \\ &= \frac{P(R = 1|Y = 1, Z)P(Y = 1|Z)}{P(R = 1|Y = 0, Z)P(Y = 0|Z) + P(R = 1|Y = 1, Z)P(Y = 1|Z)} \\ &= \frac{\exp(\beta_0^* + \beta_z^{\mathrm{T}} Z)}{1 + \exp(\beta_0^* + \beta_z^{\mathrm{T}} Z)}, \end{aligned} \quad (7.5)$$

where $\beta_0^* = \beta_0 + \log(\pi_1/\pi_0)$.

Comparing model (7.5) to model (7.3) says that the risk factors Z have the same effects on the probability of developing the disease for subjects sampled into the study and subjects in the entire population, albeit a different value for the intercept in the model.

Finally, we comment that model (7.3) may be extended to accommodate stratified designs. For example, for each stratum $k = 1, \ldots, K$, consider the model

$$\text{logit } P(Y = 1|Z, \text{ stratum } k) = \beta_{k0} + \beta_z^{\mathrm{T}} Z,$$

where the intercept β_{k0} may be stratum-dependent and the regression vector β_z is common for all the strata. If none of the regression variables in Z are interaction terms involving the factors used for stratification, then this model implies that the odds ratios associated with the risk factors under study are constant over strata. By including interaction terms among the Z_j with $j = 1, \ldots, p$, one may model changes in the relative risk which accompany changes in the stratification variables (Breslow and Day 1980, §6.2).

7.1.5 Retrospective Sampling and Inference Strategy

When building the logistic regression model (7.3), covariates Z are regarded as fixed quantities while the response variable Y is random. This model reflects the nature of prospective studies where the disease status of the study subjects is unknown in advance, and the study subjects are selected based on their risk factors and then are followed up *prospectively* to monitor the development of the disease. To highlight this prospective sampling aspect, model (7.3) is called the *prospective logistic regression model*.

In contrast, in case–control studies, subjects are selected on the basis of their disease status, and their history of risk factors or exposures are determined by a *retrospective* interview or other means. Since case–control studies typically involve *separate samples* of fixed sizes from the diseased and disease-free populations, it is fairly reasonable to treat the disease status as fixed while regarding the risk factors as random. Consequently, it may be tempting to perform analysis of case–control data by specifying and fitting a statistical model, say $f_{Z|Y}(z|y)$, for the conditional distribution of Z given Y; this model is called a *retrospective model*.

However, starting with a retrospective model for inferences is not always plausible. When Z contains multiple continuous variables, such retrospective modeling often involves a large number of parameters and is unduly cumbersome, whereas a prospective model for the conditional distribution of Y given Z is much easier to handle. Furthermore, interpretation of risk factors' effects on the disease development is more transparent by using a prospective model. It is more intuitive to think of covariates as changing the disease status than to think of disease as altering the distribution of covariates or risk factors.

As a result, analysis of case–control data is typically pertinent to two aspects: (1) the model formulation is directed to a prospective regression model $f_{Y|Z}(y|z)$ for the conditional distribution of Y given Z, which clearly indicates the influence of risk factors on the disease development; and (2) inferential procedures are developed by using the retrospective model $f_{Z|Y}(z|y)$ for the conditional distribution of Z given Y, which naturally features the retrospectiveness of the data collection for case–control studies.

To relate these two aspects, it is necessary to express $f_{Z|Y}(z|y)$ in terms of the prospective model $f_{Y|Z}(y|z)$:

$$f_{Z|Y}(z|y) = \frac{f_{Y|Z}(y|z) f_Z(z)}{f_Y(y)}, \tag{7.6}$$

which says that in addition to the prospective model $f_{Y|Z}(y|z)$ of interest, inferences based on the retrospective model $f_{Z|Y}(z|y)$ typically involve the models, $f_Z(z)$ and $f_Y(y)$, for the marginal distribution of Z and of Y, respectively. Since Y is a binary variable, it is natural to take the probability $P(Y = 1)$ as a model parameter and then estimate this parameter together with the parameter, say β, of the prospective model $f_{Y|Z}(y|z)$. Probability $P(Y = 1)$ is called the *prevalence* or *point prevalence*.

To estimate β and $P(Y = 1)$ using the retrospective model (7.6), it remains to deal with the model $f_Z(z)$ for the marginal distribution of Z. One strategy is to treat $f_Z(z)$ as a nuisance and derive a suitable conditional likelihood by *eliminating* $f_Z(z)$, and then base estimation of the model parameters on this conditional likelihood. This strategy is used when the marginal distribution of Z is thought of as containing no information about parameter β, the quantity of prime interest. Examples were given by Prentice and Breslow (1978) and Breslow et al. (1978).

On the other hand, estimation of β may be obtained based on the joint likelihood by using the full form of (7.6). To this end, modeling the marginal distribution of Z is necessary, either parametrically or nonparametrically. If $f_Z(z)$ is specified parametrically, say, with parameter α, then it is straightforward to apply the parametric maximum likelihood method to (7.6) to jointly estimate β, α and $P(Y = 1)$. This method entails the most efficient estimate of β, provided that the model assumptions for $f_Z(z)$ are valid; otherwise, biased results may arise. An alternative to handling possible model misspecification is to treat $f_Z(z)$ nonparametrically. That is, we assume

$f_Z(z)$ to remain completely arbitrary, then proceed with a pseudo-likelihood method for estimation of parameter β. Details on this method are described in the next subsection.

7.1.6 Analysis of Case–Control Data with Prospective Logistic Model

The connection (7.6) shows that the prospective model $f_{Y|Z}(y|z)$ and the retrospective model $f_{Z|Y}(z|y)$ cannot be uniquely determined by each other. Identity (7.6) also suggests that the parameters of a prospective model may not be estimable from case–control data alone if no suitable model assumptions are made. However, if the prospective model $f_{Y|Z}(y|z)$ assumes a logistic regression form, this concern diminishes when the primary interest centers on the estimation of the odds ratio parameters. In this subsection, we elaborate on this point and discuss estimation issues of using the prospective logistic regression model for case–control data.

Model Connection

Although the prospective model $f_{Y|Z}(y|z)$ and the retrospective model $f_{Z|Y}(z|y)$ cannot determine each other, they can produce identical ratios in certain form. For any two values z and $\tilde{z}$ of Z and two values y and $\tilde{y}$ of Y, the conditional probability density or mass functions are linked by

$$\frac{f_{Y|Z}(y|z)/f_{Y|Z}(\tilde{y}|z)}{f_{Y|Z}(y|\tilde{z})/f_{Y|Z}(\tilde{y}|\tilde{z})} = \frac{f_{Z|Y}(z|y)/f_{Z|Y}(\tilde{z}|y)}{f_{Z|Y}(z|\tilde{y})/f_{Z|Y}(\tilde{z}|\tilde{y})}. \tag{7.7}$$

This identity generalizes (7.1) to accommodating the scenario where Z can be a vector of discrete or continuous covariates. The measure on the left-hand side is called the *prospective odds ratio* and the one on the right-hand side is called the *retrospective odds ratio*.

Assuming the prospective logistic regression model (7.3), we derive the retrospective model using the identity (7.7). Let $\tilde{z}$ be a reference value of Z, then model (7.3) gives the odds ratio (7.4) for individuals having the risk value $Z = z$ relative to the reference value $Z = \tilde{z}$. Let

$$\gamma(z) = \log\{f_{Z|Y}(z|0)/f_{Z|Y}(\tilde{z}|0)\}$$

for all z. Then combining (7.3), (7.4) and (7.7) gives the retrospective model

$$\begin{aligned} f_{Z|Y}(z|1) &= c_1 \exp\{\gamma(z) + \beta_z^{\mathrm{T}} z\}; \\ f_{Z|Y}(z|0) &= c_0 \exp\{\gamma(z)\}; \end{aligned} \tag{7.8}$$

where c_1 and c_0 are the normalizing constants, given by

$$\begin{aligned} c_1 &= f_{Z|Y}(\tilde{z}|1) \exp\{-\beta_z^{\mathrm{T}} \tilde{z}\}; \\ c_0 &= f_{Z|Y}(\tilde{z}|0). \end{aligned}$$

Conversely, if a retrospective model, such as given by (7.8), gives the odds ratio of the form (7.4) for individuals having the risk value $Z = z$ relative to the reference value $Z = \tilde{z}$, then we can recover the prospective logistic model (7.3) upon defining

$$\beta_0 = \log\{f_{Y|Z}(1|\tilde{z})/f_{Y|Z}(0|\tilde{z})\} - \beta_z^{\mathrm{T}}\tilde{z}.$$

The prospective logistic model (7.3) and the retrospective model (7.8) are equivalent in the sense that one model can derive the other, provided that β_z in (7.3) and the function $\gamma(z)$ in (7.8) are left unrestricted (Prentice and Pyke 1979). Both models produce the same odds ratio parameter β_z and differ only in the intercept.

Point Estimator

Suppose that n_{1+} cases and n_{0+} controls are randomly selected from their respective subpopulations. We are interested in using the data of those individuals to estimate parameter β_z of the prospective logistic model (7.3). Let $\{Y_{ij}, Z_{ij}\}$ denote the random variables for subject j in the group of cases with $Y_{1j} = 1$ or the group of controls with $Y_{0j} = 0$, where $Y_{ij} = i$ is the disease outcome and Z_{ij} is the vector of risk factors for subject j; $i = 0, 1$; and $j = 1, \ldots, n_{i+}$. Here we note a slightly different usage of subscripts from those in Chapters 5 and 6. The first subscript i of Y_{ij} appears somewhat unnecessary; attaching i to Y_{ij} merely makes clear the actual disease status of subject j when referring to the measurements of such a subject.

By the independence of selecting cases and controls, the retrospective likelihood function for the case–control data is

$$\prod_{i=0,1}\prod_{j=1}^{n_{i+}} f_{Z|Y}(z_{ij}|i), \tag{7.9}$$

where the conditional model $f_{Z|Y}(z_{ij}|i)$ is determined by (7.8).

We re-express (7.8) in combination with the data in order to contrast the prospective logistic model (7.3). Let $n = n_{0+} + n_{1+}$, $\alpha = \log\{c_1 n_{1+}/(c_0 n_{0+})\}$, and

$$q(z) = \exp\{\gamma(z)\}\{(n_{0+}/n)c_0 + (n_{1+}/n)c_1 \exp(\beta_z^{\mathrm{T}} z)\}. \tag{7.10}$$

Define

$$p_1(z) = \frac{\exp(\alpha + \beta_z^{\mathrm{T}} z)}{1 + \exp(\alpha + \beta_z^{\mathrm{T}} z)}$$

and

$$p_0(z) = \frac{1}{1 + \exp(\alpha + \beta_z^{\mathrm{T}} z)}. \tag{7.11}$$

Then the retrospective model (7.8) becomes

$$f_{Z|Y}(z|i) = p_i(z)q(z)\left(\frac{n}{n_{i+}}\right) \tag{7.12}$$

with the constraint

$$\frac{n_{i+}}{n} = \int p_i(z)q(z)d\eta(z) \tag{7.13}$$

for $i = 0, 1$.

We note that $q(z)$ is the marginal probability density or mass function for Z if the prevalence $P(Y = 1) = n_{1+}/n$, and that $p_1(z)$ differs from the prospective model (7.3) in the intercept only. Let $\theta = (\alpha, \beta_z^{\mathrm{T}})^{\mathrm{T}}$. If $q(z)$ and θ are treated arbitrarily without being constrained by (7.13), then by (7.9), estimation of θ may be carried out using (7.12) with $p_i(z)$ given by (7.11) for $i = 0, 1$.

Let $L_1 = \prod_{i=0,1}\prod_{j=1}^{n_{i+}} p_i(z_{ij})$ and $L_2 = \prod_{i=0,1}\prod_{j=1}^{n_{i+}} q(z_{ij})$. Then the likelihood function (7.9) is proportional to

$$L = L_1 L_2,$$

and the likelihood score functions for θ are

$$\begin{aligned}
\frac{\partial \log L_1}{\partial \alpha} &= n_{1+} - \sum_{i=0,1}\sum_{j=1}^{n_{i+}} p_1(z_{ij}); \\
\frac{\partial \log L_1}{\partial \beta_z} &= \sum_{j=1}^{n_{1+}} z_{1j} - \sum_{i=0,1}\sum_{j=1}^{n_{i+}} z_{ij}\, p_1(z_{ij}).
\end{aligned} \tag{7.14}$$

Solving

$$\frac{\partial \log L_1}{\partial \alpha} = 0 \text{ and } \frac{\partial \log L_1}{\partial \beta_z} = 0$$

for α and β_z gives the *unconstrained* maximum likelihood estimate, $\widehat{\theta} = (\widehat{\alpha}, \widehat{\beta}_z^{\mathrm{T}})^{\mathrm{T}}$, of θ. The corresponding *unconstrained* maximum likelihood estimate of the distribution $q(\cdot)$ is the empirical probability function, $\widehat{q}(\cdot)$, which assigns mass s/n to any value of z that is observed with multiplicity s and value zero elsewhere.

The likelihood function constrained by (7.13) can be at most as large as that evaluated at the unconstrained maximum likelihood estimates, $\widehat{\theta}$ and $\widehat{q}(\cdot)$. It happens that the constraint (7.13) is satisfied by $\widehat{\theta}$ and $\widehat{q}(\cdot)$, so the unconstrained maximum likelihood estimators for θ and $q(\cdot)$ are also the desired *constrained* maximum likelihood estimators. Therefore, if the prospective logistic model (7.3) were applied to the case–control data as if the data were collected with the prospective sampling, the likelihood score functions would be (7.14), leading to the maximum likelihood estimator of the odds ratio parameter β_z albeit the estimate of the intercept has a different meaning (Prentice and Pyke 1979).

Asymptotic Variance

We conclude this subsection with a comparison of the asymptotic variances induced from the prospective and retrospective models; the discussion here modifies that of Carroll, Wang and Wang (1995).

First, we examine estimation of θ using the retrospective model (7.12). To see the contribution from each individual, we define

$$S_{ij\alpha}(Y_{ij}, Z_{ij}; \theta) = Y_{ij} - p_1(Z_{ij}),$$
$$S_{ij\beta}(Y_{ij}, Z_{ij}; \theta) = \{Y_{ij} - p_1(Z_{ij})\}Z_{ij},$$

and

$$S_{ij}(Y_{ij}, Z_{ij}; \theta) = \{S_{ij\alpha}(Y_{ij}, Z_{ij}; \theta), S_{ij\beta}^{\mathrm{T}}(Y_{ij}, Z_{ij}; \theta)\}^{\mathrm{T}}$$

for $i = 0, 1$ and $j = 1, \ldots, n_{i+}$. Let $\mathbb{Z} = \{Z_{ij} : i = 0, 1; j = 1, \ldots, n_{i+}\}$ and $\mathbb{Y} = \{Y_{ij} : i = 0, 1; j = 1, \ldots, n_{i+}\}$.

Using (7.12), we obtain that

$$E\left\{\sum_{i=0,1}\sum_{j=1}^{n_{i+}} S_{ij}(Y_{ij}, Z_{ij}; \theta)\middle|\mathbb{Y}\right\} = 0,$$

where the conditional expectation is evaluated with respect to the retrospective model for the conditional distribution of $\mathbb{Z}$ given $\mathbb{Y}$. Consequently,

$$E\left\{\sum_{i=0,1}\sum_{j=1}^{n_{i+}} S_{ij}(Y_{ij}, Z_{ij}; \theta)\right\} = 0, \tag{7.15}$$

where the expectation is taken with respect to the model for the joint distribution of $\mathbb{Z}$ and $\mathbb{Y}$.

It is important to note that, although the zero-expectation (or unbiasedness) property (7.15) is true for *all* the case–control data, the zero-expectation property does not necessarily hold for *each* individual. That is, $E\{S_{ij}(Y_{ij}, Z_{ij}; \theta)\} = 0$ is not necessarily true for $i = 0, 1$ and $j = 1, \ldots, n_{i+}$, where the expectation is taken with respect to the model for the joint distribution of $\mathbb{Z}$ and $\mathbb{Y}$, or equivalently, the model for the joint distribution of Z_{ij} and Y_{ij}.

With the unbiasedness for the summation $\sum_{i=0,1}\sum_{j=1}^{n_{i+}} S_{ij}(Y_{ij}, Z_{ij}; \theta)$, we derive an estimator of θ by solving

$$\sum_{i=0,1}\sum_{j=1}^{n_{i+}} S_{ij}(y_{ij}, z_{ij}; \theta) = 0$$

for θ, and let $\widehat{\theta}$ denote the resulting estimator. Applying the Taylor series expansion to $\sum_{i=0,1}\sum_{j=1}^{n_{i+}} S_{ij}(Y_{ij}, Z_{ij}; \widehat{\theta})$ around the true value of θ, we can show that under regularity conditions and that $n_{i+}/n \to a_i$ for some constants $a_i > 0$ as $n \to \infty$ for $i = 0, 1$,

$$n^{1/2}(\widehat{\theta} - \theta) \xrightarrow{d} N\{0, \Gamma^{-1}(\theta)\Sigma(\theta)\Gamma^{-1\mathrm{T}}(\theta)\}, \tag{7.16}$$

where

$$\Sigma(\theta) = \lim_{n\to\infty}\left[\frac{1}{n}\mathrm{var}\left\{\sum_{i=0,1}\sum_{j=1}^{n_{i+}} S_{ij}(Y_{ij}, Z_{ij}; \theta)\right\}\right]$$

and

$$\Gamma(\theta) = \lim_{n\to\infty}\left[\frac{1}{n}\sum_{i=0,1}\sum_{j=1}^{n_{i+}} E\left\{\frac{\partial S_{ij}(Y_{ij}, Z_{ij};\theta)}{\partial\theta}\right\}\right],$$

which are assumed to exist; the expectation and covariance are taken with respect to the model for the joint distribution of $\mathbb{Z}$ and $\mathbb{Y}$.

By the independence among the $\{(Y_{ij}, Z_{ij}) : i = 0, 1; j = 1, \ldots, n_{i+}\}$, we express $\Sigma(\theta)$ as $C(\theta) - D(\theta)$, where

$$C(\theta) = \lim_{n\to\infty}\left[\frac{1}{n}\sum_{i=0,1}\sum_{j=1}^{n_{i+}} E\left\{S_{ij}(Y_{ij}, Z_{ij};\theta)S_{ij}^{\mathrm{T}}(Y_{ij}, Z_{ij};\theta)\right\}\right]$$

and

$$D(\theta) = \lim_{n\to\infty}\left[\frac{1}{n}\sum_{i=0,1}\sum_{j=1}^{n_{i+}} E\{S_{ij}(Y_{ij}, Z_{ij};\theta)\}E\{S_{ij}^{\mathrm{T}}(Y_{ij}, Z_{ij};\theta)\}\right],$$

which are assumed to exist; the expectations are taken with respect to the model for the joint distribution of $\mathbb{Z}$ and $\mathbb{Y}$.

As a result, the asymptotic covariance matrix of $\sqrt{n}(\widehat{\theta} - \theta)$ in (7.16) is also written as

$$\Gamma^{-1}(\theta)\{C(\theta) - D(\theta)\}\Gamma^{-1\mathrm{T}}(\theta). \tag{7.17}$$

On the other hand, if we pretend the data $\{(Y_{ij}, Z_{ij}) : i = 0, 1; j = 1, \ldots, n_{i+}\}$ were collected from the prospective sampling scheme and we fit the prospective logistic model (7.3), then the asymptotic covariance matrix would change.

To see this, let $\theta^* = (\beta_0, \beta_z^{\mathrm{T}})^{\mathrm{T}}$ denote the parameter of the prospective logistic model (7.3), then the prospective likelihood score function, calculated from (7.3), is $S_{ij}(Y_{ij}, Z_{ij};\theta^*)$ for the contribution from the subject with $\{Y_{ij}, Z_{ij}\}$. These prospective likelihood scores are identical to the retrospective likelihood scores in (7.15) except for the difference in the intercept. By the property for the likelihood score functions, we know that the unbiasedness property holds for the summation of the prospective likelihood score functions:

$$E\left\{\sum_{i=0,1}\sum_{j=1}^{n_{i+}} S_{ij}(Y_{ij}, Z_{ij};\theta^*)\middle|\mathbb{Z}\right\} = 0,$$

where the conditional expectation is taken with respect to the prospective model for the conditional distribution of $\mathbb{Y}$ given $\mathbb{Z}$. As a result, we obtain that

$$E\left\{\sum_{i=0,1}\sum_{j=1}^{n_{i+}} S_{ij}(Y_{ij}, Z_{ij};\theta^*)\right\} = 0,$$

where the expectation is evaluated with respect to the model for the joint distribution of $\mathbb{Y}$ and $\mathbb{Z}$.

Furthermore, unlike the retrospective setting, here the unbiasedness property holds *at the individual-level* as well:

$$E\{S_{ij}(Y_{ij}, Z_{ij}; \theta^*)\} = 0$$

for $i = 0, 1$ and $j = 1, \ldots, n_{i+}$. This key difference implies

$$\Sigma(\theta^*) = C(\theta^*).$$

Let $\widehat{\theta}^*$ correspond to the estimator of θ^* by solving the score equations obtained from the prospective logistic model (7.3)

$$\sum_{i=0,1} \sum_{j=1}^{n_{i+}} S_{ij}(y_{ij}, z_{ij}; \theta^*) = 0$$

for θ^*. Analogous to (7.16), the asymptotic covariance of $\sqrt{n}(\widehat{\theta}^* - \theta^*)$ is given by

$$\Gamma^{-1}(\theta^*) C(\theta^*) \Gamma^{-1\mathrm{T}}(\theta^*), \tag{7.18}$$

which equals $\Gamma^{-1}(\theta^*)$. Since $D(\theta)$ is nonnegative definite, the comparison between (7.17) and (7.18) indicates that in finite sample calculations, applying the prospective logistic model to fit case–control data tends to produce *conservative* variance estimates for the estimator of β_z.

7.2 Measurement Error Effects

To gain intuitive insights into measurement error effects on the analysis of case–control data, we consider a simplest situation where a binary exposure variable is subject to misclassification while the binary disease outcome is free of error. Let Y be the disease status with 1 indicating having the disease and 0 otherwise. Let X be the true exposure indicator with 1 being exposed and 0 otherwise, and X^* be an observed version of X.

Let $p_{11} = P(X = 1|Y = 1)$ be the true probability of exposure among cases, and $p_{01} = P(X = 1|Y = 0)$ be the exposure probability for controls. Then the true odds ratio is given by

$$\psi = \frac{p_{11}(1 - p_{01})}{p_{01}(1 - p_{11})}.$$

On the other hand, based on the observed exposure measurement X^*, one may calculate the "observed" odds ratio:

$$\psi^* = \frac{p_{11}^*(1 - p_{01}^*)}{p_{01}^*(1 - p_{11}^*)},$$

where $p_{11}^* = P(X^* = 1|Y = 1)$ is the probability of *observed* exposure among cases, and $p_{01}^* = P(X^* = 1|Y = 0)$ is the *observed* exposure probability for controls.

In general, the "observed" odds ratio ψ^* differs from the true odds ratio ψ. Suppose the exposure status has the same chance to be misclassified for diseased and disease-free subjects, i.e., the misclassification mechanism is nondifferential with

$$P(X^* = x^*|Y = y, X = x) = P(X^* = x^*|X = x)$$

for any given values x^*, x and y. Let π_{11} be the probability of (mis)classifying an exposed individual and π_{00} be the probability of (mis)classifying an unexposed person:

$$\begin{aligned} \pi_{11} &= P(X^* = 1|X = 1); \\ \pi_{00} &= P(X^* = 0|X = 0). \end{aligned}$$

Then the "observed" odds ratio is given by

$$\psi^* = \frac{(p_{11} + (1 - \pi_{00})/\widetilde{\pi})\{(1 - p_{01}) + (1 - \pi_{11})/\widetilde{\pi}\}}{(p_{01} + (1 - \pi_{00})/\widetilde{\pi})\{(1 - p_{11}) + (1 - \pi_{11})/\widetilde{\pi}\}}, \tag{7.19}$$

where $\widetilde{\pi} = \pi_{00} + \pi_{11} - 1$.

It is clear that ψ^* is not identical to ψ except for extreme situations, such as both π_{00} and π_{11} equal 1, i.e., no misclassification incurs in X. In the presence of misclassification, the "observed" odds ratio ψ^* may be bigger or smaller than the true odds ratio ψ, depending on the exposure probabilities p_{11} and p_{01} as well as the misclassification probabilities. Fig. 7.1 plots the ratio ψ^*/ψ versus (mis)classification probability π_{00} for different values of π_{11} and (p_{11}, p_{01}), where π_{11} is set as 1.0, 0.8 and 0.6; and (p_{11}, p_{01}) is taken as (0.9, 0.1) and (0.1, 0.9), respectively, corresponding to the left and right panels. Interestingly, misclassification effects may be, in some situations, counterintuitive, as shown in the left panel of Fig. 7.1, where the differences between ψ^* and ψ decrease as the misclassification probability $1 - \pi_{00}$ or $1 - \pi_{11}$ increases.

Stratified Designs

Effects of measurement error and misclassification are multiple. For instance, under stratified designs without mismeasurement, a common odds ratio may be shared for all strata, i.e., the odds ratio is stratum-independent. However, in the presence of measurement error or misclassification in covariates, the stratum-invariant odds ratio property often breaks down for the "observed" odds ratios.

With a stratified design with K strata, let

$$p_{k11} = P(X = 1|Y = 1, \text{stratum } k)$$

and

$$p_{k01} = P(X = 1|Y = 0, \text{stratum } k)$$

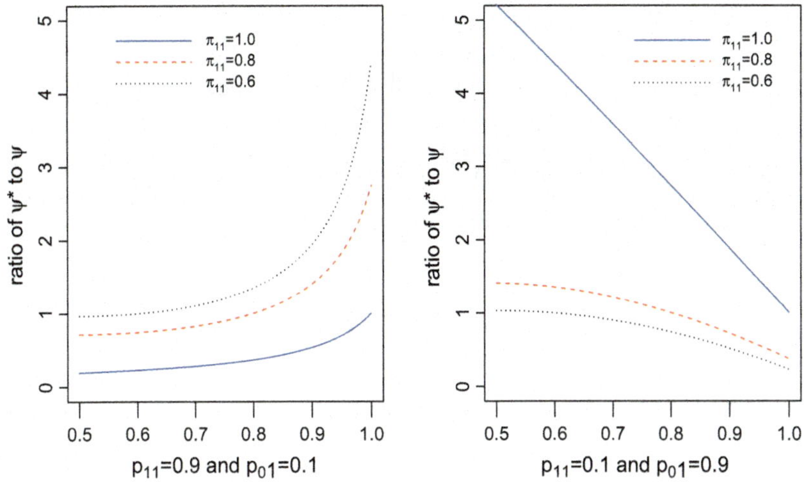

Fig. 7.1. *Comparison of the True Odds Ratio* ψ *and the Observed Odds Ratio* ψ^*

be the true probability of exposure for cases and controls in stratum k, respectively. Let ψ_k denote the true odds ratio constructed from stratum k:

$$\psi_k = \frac{p_{k11}(1 - p_{k01})}{p_{k01}(1 - p_{k11})}.$$

We assume that the ψ_k are identical for $k = 1, \ldots, K$, and let ψ denote such a common odds ratio.

When X is not available and only its surrogate value X^* is available, one may attempt to calculate the odds ratio using the observed data. Let

$$p_{k11}^* = P(X^* = 1|Y = 1, \text{stratum } k)$$

be the probability of observed exposure among cases in stratum k, and

$$p_{k01}^* = P(X^* = 1|Y = 0, \text{stratum } k)$$

be the observed exposure probability for controls in stratum k. Then the "observed" odds ratio constructed from the observed data of stratum k is given by

$$\psi_k^* = \frac{p_{k11}^*(1 - p_{k01}^*)}{p_{k01}^*(1 - p_{k11}^*)}.$$

Consider the setting where the misclassification probabilities are stratum-free but may be differential between cases and controls. That is, we assume that

$$\begin{aligned} & P(X^* = x^*|Y = y, X = x, \text{stratum } k) \\ &= P(X^* = x^*|Y = y, X = x) \end{aligned}$$

for $k = 1, \ldots, K$ and $x, y = 0, 1$. Let

$$\pi_{y11} = P(X^* = 1|Y = y, X = 1)$$

and

$$\pi_{y00} = P(X^* = 0|Y = y, X = 0)$$

be the (mis)classification probabilities for $y = 0, 1$. Then

$$\begin{aligned} p_{k11}^* &= p_{k11}\pi_{111} + (1 - p_{k11})(1 - \pi_{100}); \\ p_{k01}^* &= p_{k01}\pi_{011} + (1 - p_{k01})(1 - \pi_{000}). \end{aligned}$$

Let $a_{k1} = (1 - p_{k11})/p_{k11}$ be the odds of nonexposure for cases in stratum k, then the "observed" odds ratio defined by stratum k is connected with the true odds ratio ψ via the identity

$$\psi_k^* = \frac{\{\pi_{111} + a_{k1}(1 - \pi_{100})\}(1 - \pi_{011} + a_{k1}\pi_{000}\psi)}{(1 - \pi_{111} + a_{k1}\pi_{100})\{\pi_{011} + a_{k1}(1 - \pi_{000})\psi\}}. \tag{7.20}$$

This implies that even if the true odds ratios are identical for all the strata, this does not guarantee identical "observed" odds ratio for all the strata. The "observed" odds ratio for each stratum may attenuate or inflate the true odds ratio ψ, and this depends on the odds a_{k1} of nonexposure for cases in that stratum, misclassification rates as well as the value of ψ. In particular, if $\pi_{000} = \pi_{111} = \pi_{100} = 1$ but $0 < \pi_{011} < 1$, then ψ_k^* is always bigger than ψ. Problem 7.6 discusses the details.

7.3 Interacting Covariates Subject to Misclassification

Among many applications, case–control studies can also be used to study the synergism of gene and the environment in the etiology of rare and complex diseases (Zhang et al. 2008). It is of interest to understand how the gene-environment interaction may be associated with a disease. Such studies are often hampered by the presence of measurement error in gene expressions and environmental factors.

To shed light on this issue, we consider unmatched case–control studies with two binary covariates. Let X_e denote the environment exposure variable, with $X_e = 1$ for exposure and $X_e = 0$ for nonexposure; and X_g denote the binary genetic factor, with $X_g = 1$ and $X_g = 0$ for susceptible and nonsusceptible subjects, respectively. Both X_e and X_g are subject to misclassification, and they may interactively affect the disease status Y, where $Y = 1$ for a case, and $Y = 0$ for a control.

We start with discussion on inference methods for the error-free situation, and then describe methods which account for misclassification in covariates. The discussion here complements the foregoing development for which interactions among error-prone covariates are not being focused.

Unmatched Design without Misclassification

For $i, j, k = 0$ or 1, let

$$p_{ijk} = P(X_e = j, X_g = k | Y = i)$$

and

$$p_i = (p_{i00}, p_{i10}, p_{i01}, p_{i11}).$$

Taking the level $(X_e = 0, X_g = 0)$ as the baseline category, we let ψ_{jk} denote the odds ratio for cases versus controls with $(X_e = j, X_g = k)$:

$$\psi_{10} = \frac{P(X_e = 1, X_g = 0|Y = 1)/P(X_e = 0, X_g = 0|Y = 1)}{P(X_e = 1, X_g = 0|Y = 0)/P(X_e = 0, X_g = 0|Y = 0)};$$

$$\psi_{01} = \frac{P(X_e = 0, X_g = 1|Y = 1)/P(X_e = 0, X_g = 0|Y = 1)}{P(X_e = 0, X_g = 1|Y = 0)/P(X_e = 0, X_g = 0|Y = 0)};$$

$$\psi_{11} = \frac{P(X_e = 1, X_g = 1|Y = 1)/P(X_e = 0, X_g = 0|Y = 1)}{P(X_e = 1, X_g = 1|Y = 0)/P(X_e = 0, X_g = 0|Y = 0)};$$

where $(j, k) \neq (0, 0)$. Namely,

$$\psi_{jk} = \frac{p_{000}p_{1jk}}{p_{100}p_{0jk}} \quad \text{for } (j, k) \neq (0, 0).$$

Define

$$\psi = \frac{\psi_{11}}{\psi_{01}\psi_{10}}.$$

This measure may be used to reflect the association between the two binary covariates, such as the gene-environment association, which is classified by the subpopulations of cases and controls. It can be alternatively written as

$$\psi = \frac{\phi_1}{\phi_0},$$

where for $y = 0, 1$, ϕ_y is defined as

$$\phi_y = \frac{P(X_e = 0, X_g = 0|Y = y)P(X_e = 1, X_g = 1|Y = y)}{P(X_e = 0, X_g = 1|Y = y)P(X_e = 1, X_g = 0|Y = y)}.$$

The measure ψ is defined from the *retrospective* sampling viewpoint which directly reflects the nature of case–control designs. Equivalently, this measure has an equally interpretive feature in a prospective regression model.

Consider the logistic regression model with an interaction term between X_e and X_g:

$$\log\left\{\frac{P(Y = 1|X_e, X_g)}{P(Y = 0|X_e, X_g)}\right\} = \beta_0 + \beta_e X_e + \beta_g X_g + \beta_{eg} X_e X_g, \qquad (7.21)$$

where β_0, β_e, β_g and β_{eg} are the regression parameters. These parameters can be expressed in terms of the odds ratios defined for the retrospective sampling framework:

$$\beta_e = \log \psi_{10}, \ \beta_g = \log \psi_{01}, \text{ and } \beta_{eg} = \log \psi. \tag{7.22}$$

As pointed out in §7.1.5 and §7.1.6, the baseline parameter β_0 is not estimable from retrospectively collected data unless the prevalence $P(Y = 1)$ is known; but the coefficients $(\beta_e, \beta_g, \beta_{eg})$, or the odds ratios ψ_{jk}, are possible to be estimated from case–control data, which are collected retrospectively.

For $i, j, k = 0$ or 1, let n_{ijk} represent the number of subjects with $(Y = i, X_e = j, X_g = k)$, and $N_i = (n_{i00}, n_{i10}, n_{i01}, n_{i11})$. Table 7.3 displays the layout of data. Let n_{1++} and n_{0++} be the number of cases and controls, respectively. With the retrospective sampling scheme for case–control studies, these totals are treated as fixed, and multinomial distributions are often used to independently characterize the cell counts for the case and control subpopulations. Namely, N_0 and N_1 are assumed to be independent, marginally following a multinomial distribution with $N_i \sim \text{Multinomial}(n_{i++}, p_i)$ for $i = 0$ or 1.

Table 7.3. *Unmatched Case–Control Data with Binary Covariates X_e and X_g*

	$X_g = 0$		$X_g = 1$		
	$X_e = 0$	$X_e = 1$	$X_e = 0$	$X_e = 1$	Total
Case $(Y = 1)$	n_{100}	n_{110}	n_{101}	n_{111}	n_{1++}
Control $(Y = 0)$	n_{000}	n_{010}	n_{001}	n_{011}	n_{0++}

These distributional assumptions allow us to write the likelihood function for the cell probabilities p_{ijk} as

$$L = \prod_{i=0}^{1} \prod_{j=0}^{1} \prod_{k=0}^{1} p_{ijk}^{n_{ijk}}, \tag{7.23}$$

where the normalizing constant is omitted. In combination with the constraint $\sum_{j,k} p_{ijk} = 1$ for a given i, maximizing (7.23) with respect to the cell probabilities leads to the maximum likelihood estimator for the cell probabilities:

$$\widehat{p}_{ijk} = \frac{n_{ijk}}{n_{i++}}$$

for $i, j, k = 0$ or 1. Then using the invariance of maximum likelihood estimators gives an estimate of ψ_{jk}:

$$\widehat{\psi}_{jk} = \frac{n_{000} n_{1jk}}{n_{100} n_{0jk}}$$

for $j, k = 0$ or 1.

To calculate the asymptotic variance of the estimator $\widehat{\psi}_{jk}$ (as n_{1++} and n_{0++} both approach infinity), we equivalently consider the asymptotic variance of $\log \widehat{\psi}_{jk}$. For $i = 0$ or 1, the multinomial distribution $N_i \sim \text{Multinomial}(n_{i++}, p_i)$ yields the asymptotic distribution of $(\widehat{p}_{i00}, \widehat{p}_{i01}, \widehat{p}_{i10}, \widehat{p}_{i11})^{\mathrm{T}}$ (Serfling 1980, pp. 108–109):

$$\sqrt{n_{i++}} \left\{ \begin{pmatrix} \widehat{p}_{i00} \\ \widehat{p}_{i01} \\ \widehat{p}_{i10} \\ \widehat{p}_{i11} \end{pmatrix} - \begin{pmatrix} p_{i00} \\ p_{i01} \\ p_{i10} \\ p_{i11} \end{pmatrix} \right\} \xrightarrow{d} N(0, \Sigma_i) \tag{7.24}$$

as $n_{i++} \to \infty$, where

$$\Sigma_i = \begin{pmatrix} p_{i00}(1-p_{i00}) & -p_{i00}p_{i01} & -p_{i00}p_{i10} & -p_{i00}p_{i11} \\ -p_{i01}p_{i00} & p_{i01}(1-p_{i01}) & -p_{i01}p_{i10} & -p_{i01}p_{i11} \\ -p_{i10}p_{i00} & -p_{i10}p_{i01} & p_{i10}(1-p_{i10}) & -p_{i10}p_{i11} \\ -p_{i11}p_{i00} & -p_{i11}p_{i01} & -p_{i11}p_{i10} & p_{i11}(1-p_{i11}) \end{pmatrix}$$

with the constraints $\sum_{j,k} \widehat{p}_{ijk} = 1$ and $\sum_{j,k} p_{ijk} = 1$ imposed.

Using the delta method, we obtain estimates of the asymptotic variances

$$\widehat{\text{var}}\left\{\log\left(\frac{\widehat{p}_{ijk}}{\widehat{p}_{i00}}\right)\right\} = \frac{1}{n_{ijk}} + \frac{1}{n_{i00}}$$

and

$$\widehat{\text{var}}\left\{\log\left(\frac{\widehat{p}_{i11}\widehat{p}_{i00}}{\widehat{p}_{i01}\widehat{p}_{i10}}\right)\right\} = \frac{1}{n_{i11}} + \frac{1}{n_{i10}} + \frac{1}{n_{i01}} + \frac{1}{n_{i00}}.$$

Noticing that

$$\log \widehat{\psi}_{jk} = \log\left(\frac{\widehat{p}_{1jk}}{\widehat{p}_{100}}\right) - \log\left(\frac{\widehat{p}_{0jk}}{\widehat{p}_{000}}\right),$$

hence

$$\log \widehat{\psi} = \log\left(\frac{\widehat{p}_{111}\widehat{p}_{100}}{\widehat{p}_{101}\widehat{p}_{110}}\right) - \log\left(\frac{\widehat{p}_{011}\widehat{p}_{000}}{\widehat{p}_{001}\widehat{p}_{010}}\right),$$

and that the ratios $\widehat{p}_{1jk}/\widehat{p}_{100}$ and $\widehat{p}_{0jk}/\widehat{p}_{000}$ are independent, we obtain that

$$\text{var}(\log \widehat{\psi}_{jk}) = \text{var}\left\{\log\left(\frac{\widehat{p}_{1jk}}{\widehat{p}_{100}}\right)\right\} + \text{var}\left\{\log\left(\frac{\widehat{p}_{0jk}}{\widehat{p}_{000}}\right)\right\};$$

$$\text{var}(\log \widehat{\psi}) = \text{var}\left\{\log\left(\frac{\widehat{p}_{111}\widehat{p}_{100}}{\widehat{p}_{101}\widehat{p}_{110}}\right)\right\} + \text{var}\left\{\log\left(\frac{\widehat{p}_{011}\widehat{p}_{000}}{\widehat{p}_{001}\widehat{p}_{010}}\right)\right\}.$$

Hence, estimates of the asymptotic variances are

$$\widehat{\text{var}}(\log \widehat{\psi}_{jk}) = \frac{1}{n_{1jk}} + \frac{1}{n_{0jk}} + \frac{1}{n_{100}} + \frac{1}{n_{000}}$$

for $j, k = 0$ or 1, and

$$\widehat{\text{var}}(\log \widehat{\psi}) = \sum_{i=0}^{1}\sum_{j=0}^{1}\sum_{k=0}^{1} \frac{1}{n_{ijk}}. \tag{7.25}$$

Covariates with Misclassification

In the presence of misclassification of the binary covariates, let X_e^* and X_g^* be the observed values of X_e and X_g, respectively. Let

$$\pi_{ie11} = P(X_e^* = 1|X_e = 1, Y = i)$$

and

$$\pi_{ie00} = P(X_e^* = 0|X_e = 0, Y = i)$$

be, respectively, the *sensitivity* and *specificity* of X_e for the subpopulation with $Y = i$, and

$$\pi_{ig11} = P(X_g^* = 1|X_g = 1, Y = i)$$

and

$$\pi_{ig00} = P(X_g^* = 0|X_g = 0, Y = i)$$

be, respectively, the *sensitivity* and *specificity* of X_g for the subpopulation with $Y = i$. Define

$$\Pi_{ie} = \begin{pmatrix} \pi_{ie00} & 1 - \pi_{ie11} \\ 1 - \pi_{ie00} & \pi_{ie11} \end{pmatrix}$$

and

$$\Pi_{ig} = \begin{pmatrix} \pi_{ig00} & 1 - \pi_{ig00} \\ 1 - \pi_{ig11} & \pi_{ig11} \end{pmatrix}.$$

For $i, j, k = 0$ or 1, let

$$p_{ijk}^* = P(X_e^* = j, X_g^* = k|Y = i)$$

be the "observed" probabilities for the observed measurements of the exposure and genetic variables corresponding to the control or case subpopulation. Write $p_i^* = (p_{i00}^*, p_{i10}^*, p_{i01}^*, p_{i11}^*)$ for $i = 0$ or 1.

We assume that

$$\begin{aligned} P(X_e^* = j, X_g^* = k|X_e, X_g, Y) &= P(X_e^* = j|X_e, X_g, Y)P(X_g^* = k|X_e, X_g, Y); \\ P(X_e^* = j|X_e, X_g, Y) &= P(X_e^* = j|X_e, Y); \\ P(X_g^* = j|X_e, X_g, Y) &= P(X_g^* = j|X_g, Y). \end{aligned}$$

The first assumption says that the observed measurements X_e^* and X_g^* are conditionally independent, given the true values X_e and X_g and the disease status. The second and third conditions require that the misclassification probability of one variable does not depend on the true value of the other variable, given the true value of the variable itself and the disease status. Under these assumptions, we express the "observed" probabilities p_{ijk}^* using the true probabilities p_{ijk}:

$$\begin{pmatrix} p_{i00}^* & p_{i01}^* \\ p_{i10}^* & p_{i11}^* \end{pmatrix} = \Pi_{ie} \begin{pmatrix} p_{i00} & p_{i01} \\ p_{i10} & p_{i11} \end{pmatrix} \Pi_{ig}. \tag{7.26}$$

The identity (7.26) allows us to estimate the probability p_{ijk} using the estimates of p^*_{ijk} which are obtained from the observed counts. Let n^*_{ijk} represent the number of cases or controls with the observed measurement $(X^*_e = j, X^*_g = k)$ for $i, j, k = 0$ or 1. Table 7.4 displays the data format.

Table 7.4. *Observed Counts Parallel to Table 7.3*

	$X^*_g = 0$		$X^*_g = 1$		
	$X^*_e = 0$	$X^*_e = 1$	$X^*_e = 0$	$X^*_e = 1$	Total
Case ($Y = 1$)	n^*_{100}	n^*_{110}	n^*_{101}	n^*_{111}	n_{1++}
Control ($Y = 0$)	n^*_{000}	n^*_{010}	n^*_{001}	n^*_{011}	n_{0++}

Using the same reasoning as for (7.23), we obtain the likelihood based on the observed data

$$L_{\mathrm{O}} = \prod_{i=0}^{1} \prod_{j=0}^{1} \prod_{k=0}^{1} (p^*_{ijk})^{n^*_{ijk}}. \tag{7.27}$$

Maximizing the likelihood (7.27) with respect to the "observed" cell probabilities p^*_{ijk}, under the constraint

$$\sum_{j=0}^{1} \sum_{k=0}^{1} p^*_{ijk} = 1 \text{ for } i = 0 \text{ or } 1,$$

gives their estimators

$$\widehat{p}^*_{ijk} = \frac{n^*_{ijk}}{n_{i++}}$$

for $i, j, k = 0$ or 1. Then applying (7.26) gives the estimators for p_{ijk}:

$$\begin{pmatrix} \widehat{p}_{i00} & \widehat{p}_{i01} \\ \widehat{p}_{i10} & \widehat{p}_{i11} \end{pmatrix} = \Pi_{ie}^{-1} \begin{pmatrix} \widehat{p}^*_{i00} & \widehat{p}^*_{i01} \\ \widehat{p}^*_{i10} & \widehat{p}^*_{i11} \end{pmatrix} \Pi_{ig}^{-1}, \tag{7.28}$$

where the matrices Π_e and Π_g are assumed invertible.

To describe the asymptotic variance $\widehat{p}_{ijk}$, we apply the delta method to the asymptotic distribution of $(\widehat{p}^*_{i00}, \widehat{p}^*_{i01}, \widehat{p}^*_{i10}, \widehat{p}^*_{i11})^{\mathrm{T}}$ in combination of (7.28), where the asymptotic distribution of $(\widehat{p}^*_{i00}, \widehat{p}^*_{i01}, \widehat{p}^*_{i10}, \widehat{p}^*_{i11})^{\mathrm{T}}$ is of the same form as (7.24) except for replacing p_{ijk} and $\widehat{p}_{ijk}$ with p^*_{ijk} and $\widehat{p}^*_{ijk}$, respectively, for $i, j, k = 0$ or 1.

Example 7.1. Duffy, Rohan and Day (1989) described a case–control study of breast cancer. In the study, 451 breast cancer cases (coded as $Y = 1$) were compared with the same number of controls (coded as $Y = 0$) with respect to the risk factors: alcohol consumption and smoking, where alcohol consumption is defined as a binary variable by a threshold of 9.3 g ethanol/day, and the smoking variable is dichotomized by comparing the product of the number of cigarettes smoked per day and years of smoking to 300.

For any subject, let X_g be a binary variable indicating whether or not the product of the number of cigarettes smoked per day and years of smoking is more than 300, and X_e be a binary variable indicating whether or not alcohol consumption is more than 9.3 g ethanol/day ("yes" is coded as 1 and "no" is coded as 0). Table 7.5 records the data of the main study where one breast cancer case had missing values.

Since smoking and alcohol use are likely to be related to each other, and may each be associated with breast cancer risk, we use the logistic model (7.21) to analyze the data where the interaction term between X_e and X_g is included in the model in addition to individual terms X_e and X_g.

Table 7.5. *A Case–Control Study on Alcohol Consumption and Lifetime Cigarette-Years in a Study of Breast Cancer (Duffy, Rohan and Day 1989)*

	$X_g^* = 0$		$X_g^* = 1$		
	$X_e^* = 0$	$X_e^* = 1$	$X_e^* = 0$	$X_e^* = 1$	Total
$Y = 0$	305	70	56	20	451
$Y = 1$	268	82	61	39	450
Total	573	152	117	59	901

To understand how misclassification might affect the estimation of the response parameters, we perform a sensitivity analysis where the sensitivity and the specificity for X_e and X_g are set to be identical. Fig. 7.2 shows how estimation of covariate effects and their interaction, β_e, β_g and β_{eg}, may change with the different combinations of the sensitivity and the specificity.

The foregoing method assumes that the misclassification probabilities are known, hence is useful for conducting sensitivity analyses, as illustrated by Example 7.1, where plausible values of the sensitivity and specificity are specified to evaluate the misclassification effects on estimation of quantities of interest, such as odds ratios ψ_{jk} or cell probabilities p_{ijk}.

In some instances, the misclassification probabilities are unknown, and additional data sources are available for their estimation. Zhang et al. (2008) described an extension of the preceding method to accommodating the setting where an independent validation sample is available to feature the misclassification process. Yi and He (2017) considered the situation where an independent sample with two repeated covariate measurements is available and developed estimation methods to accommodate misclassification effects.

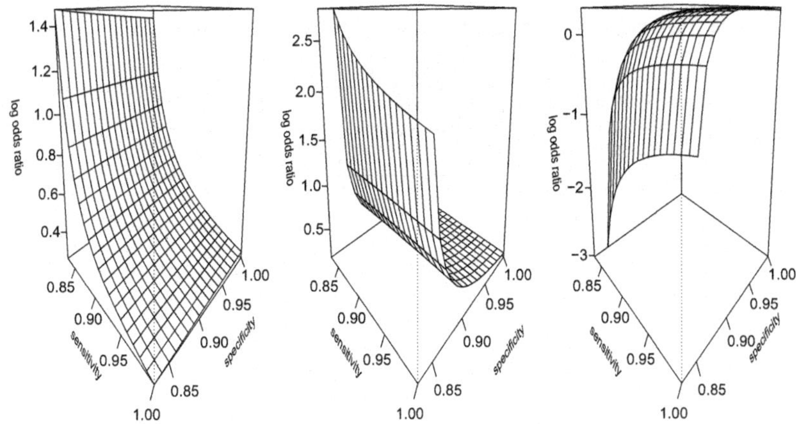

Fig. 7.2. *Sensitivity Analysis of Misclassification on Parameter Estimation: the First Graph Is for Estimation of β_e, the Second One Is for Estimation of β_g, and the Third One Is for Estimation of β_{eg}*

7.4 Retrospective Pseudo-Likelihood Method for Unmatched Designs

In this section, we describe an inference strategy for analyzing unmatched designs where covariates are error-prone and the disease status is error-free. For subject i, let Y_i be the binary disease status, taking value 1 if having the disease and 0 otherwise; let X_i^* be the surrogate measurement of the true covariate vector, X_i, which may have discrete or continuous components. We consider the scenario where an external validation sample is available in addition to the main study.

Let R_i be the indicator of selecting subject i into the study with value 1 being selected and 0 otherwise. Let V_i be the indicator whether or not subject i is included in the validation sample. Let $\mathcal{V} = \{i : V_i = 1\}$ be the index set for subjects in the validation sample and $\mathcal{M} = \{i : V_i = 0\}$ be the index set of subjects in the main study. That is, $\{Y_i, X_i, X_i^*\}$ is measured if $i \in \mathcal{V}$, and only $\{Y_i, X_i^*\}$ is observed if $i \in \mathcal{M}$. Suppose that the validation study consists of a random sample of n_{V1} cases and n_{V0} controls, and that the main study has n_{M1} cases and n_{M0} controls, where $P(Y_i = y|R_i = 1, V_i = 0, X_i) = P(Y_i = y|R_i = 1, V_i = 1, X_i)$ is assumed for $y = 0$ or 1. Define $n_{\text{V+}} = n_{\text{V0}} + n_{\text{V1}}$, $n_{\text{M+}} = n_{\text{M0}} + n_{\text{M1}}$, and $n = n_{\text{V+}} + n_{\text{M+}}$. The counts of cases and controls are displayed in Table 7.6.

Assume that selection of a subject into the validation sample is completely at random, and that the distribution of surrogates is the same for subjects in the validation sample and the main study, i.e.,

$$h(x_i^*|X_i = x, Y_i = y, V_i = v) = h(x_i^*|X_i = x, Y_i = y), \tag{7.29}$$

where $h(x_i^*|\cdot)$ represents the conditional distribution of X_i^* given the corresponding variables. Let $f_{\text{X}^*|\text{XY}}(x_i^*|x_i, y_i)$ denote the model for the conditional distribution of X_i^* given $X_i = x_i$ and $Y_i = y_i$.

Table 7.6. *Counts of Cases and Controls in the Validation Sample/Main Study*

	$V_i = 1$	$V_i = 0$
$Y_i = 1$	n_{V1}	n_{M1}
$Y_i = 0$	n_{V0}	n_{M0}
Total	n_{V+}	n_{M+}

As discussed in §7.1.4, we use the prospective model (7.3) to feature the relationship between Y_i and X_i:

$$P(Y_i = 1|X_i) = \frac{\exp(\beta_0 + \beta_x^{\mathrm{T}} X_i)}{1 + \exp(\beta_0 + \beta_x^{\mathrm{T}} X_i)},$$

where β_0 and β_x are the regression parameters. Analogous to (7.5), this model yields the prospective logistic model

$$P(Y_i = 1|X_i, V_i = v) = \frac{\exp(\beta_0^{(v)} + \beta_x^{\mathrm{T}} X_i)}{1 + \exp(\beta_0^{(v)} + \beta_x^{\mathrm{T}} X_i)}, \tag{7.30}$$

where by the argument similar to (7.5), the intercepts $\beta_0^{(0)}$ and $\beta_0^{(1)}$ are related via

$$\beta_0^{(0)} = \beta_0^{(1)} - \log\left\{\frac{\pi_1^{(0)}\pi_0^{(1)}}{\pi_0^{(0)}\pi_1^{(1)}}\right\}$$

with $\pi_y^{(v)} = P(R_i = 1|Y_i = y, X_i, V_i = v)$ for $y, v = 0$ or 1. Let $\beta = (\beta_0^{(1)}, \beta_x^{\mathrm{T}})^{\mathrm{T}}$.

For $v = 0$ or 1, define

$$H^{(v)}(x, y; \beta) = \frac{\exp\{y(\beta_0^{(v)} + \beta_x^{\mathrm{T}} x)\}}{1 + \exp(\beta_0^{(v)} + \beta_x^{\mathrm{T}} x)}.$$

Let $\delta_v = P(Y_i = 1|V_i = v)$ and $\delta = (\delta_1, \delta_0)^{\mathrm{T}}$. Parameter δ_v may be empirically estimated using the data in Table 7.6:

$$\widehat{\delta}_1 = \frac{n_{V1}}{n_{V+}} \text{ and } \widehat{\delta}_0 = \frac{n_{M1}}{n_{M+}}.$$

For $v = 0$ or 1, let $q_Y^{(v)}(y) = P(Y_i = y|V_i = v)$. Then $q_Y^{(v)}(y)$ is estimated by

$$\widehat{q}_Y^{(v)}(y) = \widehat{\delta}_v^{y}(1 - \widehat{\delta}_v)^{1-y}. \tag{7.31}$$

For $v = 0$ or 1, let $f_{X|Y}^{(v)}(x_i|y_i)$ represent the retrospective model for the conditional distribution of X_i given $Y_i = y_i$ and $V_i = v$, which may be expressed by means of the prospective response model:

$$f_{X|Y}^{(v)}(x_i|y_i) = \frac{H^{(v)}(x_i, y_i; \beta) q_X^{(v)}(x_i)}{q_Y^{(v)}(y_i)}, \tag{7.32}$$

where as illustrated for (7.6), the model $q_{\mathrm{X}}^{(v)}(x_i)$ for the conditional distribution of X_i given $V_i = v$ is involved.

To accommodate the sampling scheme for case–control studies, inferences are commonly based on the retrospective model. For the validation data with $V_i = 1$, the likelihood is proportional to

$$f^{(1)}_{\mathrm{XX^*|Y}}(x_i, x_i^*|y_i) = f^{(1)}_{\mathrm{X|Y}}(x_i|y_i) f_{\mathrm{X^*|XY}}(x_i^*|x_i, y_i); \tag{7.33}$$

while for the main study data with $V_i = 0$, the likelihood is proportional to

$$f^{(0)}_{\mathrm{X^*|Y}}(x_i^*|y_i) = \int f^{(0)}_{\mathrm{X|Y}}(x|y_i) f_{\mathrm{X^*|XY}}(x_i^*|x, y_i) d\eta(x), \tag{7.34}$$

where the assumption (7.29) is imposed, and $\eta(x)$ is the measure defined on page 55.

Consequently, inferences are performed using the retrospective likelihood

$$\left\{\prod_{i\in\mathcal{V}} f^{(1)}_{\mathrm{XX^*|Y}}(x_i, x_i^*|y_i)\right\}\left\{\prod_{i\in\mathcal{M}} f^{(0)}_{\mathrm{X^*|Y}}(x_i^*|y_i)\right\}, \tag{7.35}$$

where the terms are determined by (7.33) or (7.34). Therefore, in addition to the primarily interesting prospective model (7.30), using (7.35) to carry out inferences requires modeling the measurement error process as well as the covariate process. We discuss this in more details according to whether the X_i are discrete or continuous. To highlight the idea with a simple presentation, we focus the discussion on the case where the X_i are scalar.

Misclassified Discrete Covariate

First, we consider that X_i is a binary variable. Let

$$\pi_{yx^*x} = P(X_i^* = x^*|Y_i = y, X_i = x) \tag{7.36}$$

be the (mis)classification probabilities for $y, x = 0, 1$, and $\widetilde{\pi} = (\pi_{000}, \pi_{011}, \pi_{100}, \pi_{111})^{\mathrm{T}}$. Let

$$\lambda_v = P(X_i = 1|V_i = v) \quad \text{for } v = 0, 1,$$

and $\lambda = (\lambda_1, \lambda_0)^{\mathrm{T}}$.

Let $\theta = (\beta^{\mathrm{T}}, \widetilde{\pi}^{\mathrm{T}}, \lambda^{\mathrm{T}})^{\mathrm{T}}$. Define the pseudo-likelihood of θ to be the likelihood (7.35) with δ_v replaced by the empirical estimate $\widehat{\delta}_v$ for $v = 0, 1$:

$$\begin{aligned} L_{\mathrm{PS}}(\theta) &= \prod_{i\in\mathcal{V}}\left\{ f^{(1)}_{\mathrm{X|Y}}(x_i|y_i) f_{\mathrm{X^*|XY}}(x_i^*|x_i, y_i)\right\} \\ &\cdot \prod_{i\in\mathcal{M}}\left[\sum_x \{f^{(0)}_{\mathrm{X|Y}}(x|y_i) f_{\mathrm{X^*|XY}}(x_i^*|x_i, y_i)\}\right] \end{aligned} \tag{7.37}$$

where

$$
\begin{aligned}
& f_{X^*|XY}(x_i^*|x_i, y_i) \\
&= \{\pi_{111}^{x_i y_i}(1-\pi_{100})^{(1-x_i)y_i}\pi_{011}^{x_i(1-y_i)}(1-\pi_{000})^{(1-x_i)(1-y_i)}\}^{x_i^*} \\
&\cdot\{(1-\pi_{111})^{x_i y_i}\pi_{100}^{(1-x_i)y_i}(1-\pi_{011})^{x_i(1-y_i)}\pi_{000}^{(1-x_i)(1-y_i)}\}^{1-x_i^*},
\end{aligned}
$$

and $f_{X|Y}^{(v)}(x_i|y_i)$ is the retrospective conditional probability (7.32), given by

$$
\frac{H^{(v)}(x_i, y_i; \beta)\cdot\lambda_v^{x_i}(1-\lambda_v)^{1-x_i}}{\delta_v^{y_i}(1-\delta_v)^{1-y_i}}.
$$

Maximizing the pseudo-likelihood $L_{PS}(\theta)$ with respect to θ gives the estimator $\widehat{\theta}$ of θ. If n_{V+}/n and n_{M+}/n approach nonzero constants as $n \to \infty$, then under regularity conditions, $\sqrt{n}(\widehat{\theta}-\theta)$ has an asymptotic normal distribution with mean zero and a covariance matrix which is estimated by $J^{-1}(\widehat{\theta})$, where

$$
J(\theta) = -\frac{\partial^2 \log L_{PS}(\theta)}{\partial\theta\partial\theta^{T}}.
$$

Pseudo-Likelihood Estimation

When the X_i are discrete, the misclassification process and the covariate process of X_i can be directly indicated by a finite number of conditional probabilities which are treated as parameters, and maximizing (7.37) with respect to θ is computationally manageable. With continuous X_i, however, directly maximizing (7.35) becomes infeasible due to the involvement of integrals in (7.34); this is particularly troublesome when X_i has a high dimension. To handle this problem, Carroll, Gail and Lubin (1993) proposed a pseudo-likelihood method which aims to reduce the dimension of integrals with the marginal distribution of X_i replaced by its empirical estimate.

Suppose the measurement error process is modeled parametrically. Let

$$
\widetilde{\pi}(x^*|x, y; \alpha) = f_{X^*|XY}(x^*|X_i = x, Y_i = y)
$$

denote a parametric model for the conditional distribution of X_i^* given $X_i = x$ and $Y_i = y$, where α is the associated parameter. The dependence of this distribution on Y_i shows that measurement error may be differential. Nondifferential measurement error can also be accommodated by imposing certain constraints on the parameters. For instance, consider the measurement error model

$$
X_i^* = \alpha_0 + \alpha_x X_i + \alpha_y Y_i + e_i,
$$

where the e_i are independent of each other and of $\{X_i, Y_i\}$; and α_0, α_x and α_y are regression parameters. This model features both differential and nondifferential measurement error mechanisms by the value of α_y: $\alpha_y = 0$ gives nondifferential error while $\alpha_y \neq 0$ permits differential error.

For $v = 0$ or 1, let $Q_{\mathrm{X}}^{(v)}(x) = P(X_i \le x | V_i = v)$ be the conditional distribution function of X_i, given $V_i = v$. Then using (7.32), we express the likelihood (7.33) contributed from subject i in the validation sample as

$$f_{\mathrm{XX^*|Y}}^{(1)}(x_i, x_i^* | y_i) = \frac{q_{\mathrm{X}}^{(1)}(x_i) H^{(1)}(x_i, y_i; \beta) \widetilde{\pi}(x_i^* | x_i, y_i; \alpha)}{q_{\mathrm{Y}}^{(1)}(y_i)}, \tag{7.38}$$

and the likelihood (7.34) contributed from subject i in the main study as

$$f_{\mathrm{X^*|Y}}^{(0)}(x_i^* | y_i) = \frac{\int H^{(0)}(x, y_i; \beta) \widetilde{\pi}(x_i^* | x, y_i; \alpha) dQ_{\mathrm{X}}^{(0)}(x)}{q_{\mathrm{Y}}^{(0)}(y_i)}. \tag{7.39}$$

Let $\theta = (\beta^{\mathrm{T}}, \alpha^{\mathrm{T}})^{\mathrm{T}}$. If $q_{\mathrm{X}}^{(1)}(\cdot)$ and $q_{\mathrm{Y}}^{(1)}(\cdot)$ were known, then merely applying (7.38) to the validation sample may yield valid inference results about θ. However, the resulting estimator does not enjoy the efficiency as much as it can, because the main study data are not used at all. To use the measurements from the main study, we incorporate (7.39) into the estimation procedure and describe a two-stage estimation procedure. At the first stage, we use the validation data to estimate $Q_{\mathrm{X}}^{(0)}(\cdot)$, $q_{\mathrm{X}}^{(1)}(\cdot)$, $q_{\mathrm{Y}}^{(0)}(\cdot)$ and $q_{\mathrm{Y}}^{(1)}(\cdot)$, the quantities which are not of our interest but are relevant to estimation of θ. At the second stage, we estimate θ using the data from both the validation sample and the main study, and this is based on maximization of the pseudo-likelihood calculated from (7.38) and (7.39) by replacing $Q_{\mathrm{X}}^{(0)}(\cdot)$, $q_{\mathrm{X}}^{(1)}(\cdot)$, $q_{\mathrm{Y}}^{(0)}(\cdot)$ and $q_{\mathrm{Y}}^{(1)}(\cdot)$ with their estimates.

For $v = 0, 1$, let $F_{\mathrm{X|Y}}^{(v)}(x|y) = P(X_i \le x | Y_i = y, V_i = v)$ be the retrospective conditional distribution function of X_i, given $Y_i = y$ and $V_i = v$. Assuming that $F_{\mathrm{X|Y}}^{(1)}(x|y) = F_{\mathrm{X|Y}}^{(0)}(x|y)$, then the validation data may be used to estimate $F_{\mathrm{X|Y}}^{(v)}(x|y)$ empirically for $v = 0, 1$. Let $\widehat{F}_{\mathrm{X|Y}}(x|y)$ denote such a common estimate of $F_{\mathrm{X|Y}}^{(1)}(x|y)$ and $F_{\mathrm{X|Y}}^{(0)}(x|y)$, given by

$$\widehat{F}_{\mathrm{X|Y}}(x|y) = \sum_{i \in \mathcal{V}} \frac{I(X_i \le x, Y_i = y)}{n_{\mathrm{V}y}}.$$

Noting that for $v = 0, 1$,

$$Q_{\mathrm{X}}^{(v)}(x) = \sum_{y=0,1} F_{\mathrm{X|Y}}^{(v)}(x|y) q_{\mathrm{Y}}^{(v)}(y),$$

and that $q_{\mathrm{Y}}^{(v)}(y)$ is empirically estimated based on (7.31), we empirically estimate $Q_{\mathrm{X}}^{(1)}(x)$ and $Q_{\mathrm{X}}^{(0)}(x)$ by

$$\widehat{Q}_{\mathrm{X}}^{(1)}(x) = \sum_{y=0}^{1} \left\{ \left(\frac{n_{\mathrm{V}y}}{n_{\mathrm{V}+}} \right) \sum_{i \in \mathcal{V}} \frac{I(X_i \le x, Y_i = y)}{n_{\mathrm{V}y}} \right\}$$

and

$$\widehat{Q}_{\mathrm{X}}^{(0)}(x) = \sum_{y=0}^{1} \left\{ \left(\frac{n_{\mathrm{M}y}}{n_{\mathrm{M}+}} \right) \sum_{i \in \mathcal{V}} \frac{I(X_i \leq x, Y_i = y)}{n_{\mathrm{V}y}} \right\},$$

respectively.

Then combining (7.38) and (7.39) gives the pseudo-likelihood function:

$$\begin{aligned} L_{\mathrm{PS}}(\theta) &= \prod_{i \in \mathcal{V}} \left\{ \frac{\widehat{q}_{\mathrm{X}}^{(1)}(x_i)}{\widehat{q}_{\mathrm{Y}}^{(1)}(y_i)} H^{(1)}(x_i, y_i; \beta) \widetilde{\pi}(x_i^* | x_i, y_i; \alpha) \right\} \\ &\cdot \prod_{i \in \mathcal{M}} \left[\frac{1}{\widehat{q}_{\mathrm{Y}}^{(0)}(y_i)} \int H^{(0)}(x, y_i; \beta) \widetilde{\pi}(x_i^* | x, y_i; \alpha) d\widehat{Q}_{\mathrm{X}}^{(0)}(x) \right], \end{aligned} \quad (7.40)$$

where $\widehat{q}_{\mathrm{X}}^{(1)}(x_i)$ is the empirical estimate of $q_{\mathrm{X}}^{(1)}(x_i)$, or $d\widehat{Q}_{\mathrm{X}}^{(1)}(x_i)$.

The pseudo-likelihood score function is obtained by differentiating $L_{\mathrm{PS}}(\theta)$ with respect to parameter θ, and the Newton–Raphson approach may be invoked to solve the resulting equation to obtain the estimator for θ. This method is applicable to both discrete and continuous covariate X_i. Under regularity conditions, Carroll, Gail and Lubin (1993) showed that the pseudo-likelihood score function is asymptotically unbiased, leading to a consistent estimator $\widehat{\theta}$ for θ which, after a transformation, has an asymptotic normal distribution. As covariance estimates for $\widehat{\theta}$ require extensive computations, standard errors and confidence intervals may be alternatively obtained from bootstrap sampling. In particular, for the data with $Y_i = y$ in the validation sample, a bootstrap sample of size $n_{\mathrm{V}y}$ is obtained by sampling with replacement from the set $\{(X_i, X_i^*) : i \in \mathcal{V}, Y_i = y\}$. For the data with $Y_i = y$ in the main study, a bootstrap sample of size $n_{\mathrm{M}y}$ is obtained by sampling with replacement from the set $\{X_i^* : i \in \mathcal{M}, Y_i = y\}$. Details are referred to Carroll, Gail and Lubin (1993).

Example 7.2. Carroll, Gail and Lubin (1993) analyzed the HSV data of §2.7.5, respectively, using the formulations (7.37) and (7.40), called Analysis 1 and Analysis 2, respectively, where the prospective model (7.30) is used and differential and nondifferential misclassification mechanisms are compared.

Table 7.7 summarizes parameter estimates (EST), standard errors (SE) and 95% confidence intervals (CI), where $\pi_{x1} = P(X_i^* = 1 | X_i = x)$ is defined for $x = 0$ or 1 when misclassification is assumed to be nondifferntial, and π_{yxx} is given by (7.36) when the differential misclassification mechanism is considered.

Interestingly, estimation results for β_x are quite different under different assumptions of the misclassification mechanism, but are fairly comparable between different estimation methods (i.e., Analysis 1 and Analysis 2). It is unsurprising that standard errors associated with estimation of β_x are larger for both analyses when differential misclassification is employed than those obtained under the nondifferential misclassification mechanism, since the former case has two more parameters to estimate than the latter one. Under the same misclassification mechanism, variability associated with the two analyses does not seem to indicate one method is better than

Table 7.7. *Analysis Results of the HSV Data Using the Likelihood and Pseudo-Likelihood Methods (Carroll, Gail and Lubin 1993)*

	Analysis 1			Analysis 2		
	EST	SE	95% CI	EST	SE	95% CI
Differential						
β_x	0.609	0.350	$(-0.077, 1.295)$	0.622	0.355	$(-0.074, 1.318)$
$1-\pi_{000}$	0.311	0.055	$(0.203, 0.419)$	0.317	0.057	$(0.205, 0.429)$
$1-\pi_{011}$	0.189	0.085	$(0.022, 0.356)$	0.195	0.089	$(0.021, 0.369)$
π_{111}	0.784	0.068	$(0.651, 0.917)$	0.790	0.067	$(0.741, 0.839)$
π_{100}	0.578	0.067	$(0.447, 0.709)$	0.577	0.067	$(0.446, 0.708)$
Nondifferential						
β_x	0.958	0.237	$(0.493, 1.423)$	0.959	0.226	$(0.516, 1.402)$
π_{01}	0.257	0.043	$(0.173, 0.341)$	0.266	0.042	$(0.184, 0.348)$
π_{11}	0.679	0.041	$(0.599, 0.759)$	0.686	0.041	$(0.606, 0.766)$

the other. Finally, the analyses show evidence that misclassification probabilities are statistically significant, no matter what misclassification mechanism is adopted.

As a side note, if the true misclassification mechanism is differential but the nondifferential mechanism is assumed in the data analysis, then the resulting estimators for the model parameters are usually inconsistent. Some authors empirically investigated this problem, see, for instance, Carroll, Gail and Lubin (1993) and Yi and Cook (2005). Generally speaking, studies of impacts of misspecifying the misclassification or measurement error mechanism under various settings may be carried out using the theory of model misspecification discussed in §1.4.

7.5 Correction Method for Matched Designs

In this section, we describe a method of handling measurement error arising from matched case–control studies. Suppose the design is a $1{:}M$ matched case–control study with n strata. For subject j in stratum i, let X_{ij} be the error-prone covariate vector and Z_{ij} be the vector of error-free covariates; let Y_{ij} denote the binary disease outcome taking value 1 if subject j is a case and 0 otherwise, where $j = 0, 1, \ldots, M$ and $i = 1, \ldots, n$. This definition differs from that on page 311. Write $Y_i = (Y_{i0}, Y_{i1}, \ldots, Y_{iM})^{\mathrm{T}}$, $X_i = (X_{i0}^{\mathrm{T}}, X_{i1}^{\mathrm{T}}, \ldots, X_{iM}^{\mathrm{T}})^{\mathrm{T}}$ and $Z_i = (Z_{i0}^{\mathrm{T}}, Z_{i1}^{\mathrm{T}}, \ldots, Z_{iM}^{\mathrm{T}})^{\mathrm{T}}$. Let $y_i = (y_{i0}, y_{i1}, \ldots, y_{iM})^{\mathrm{T}}$ be a realized value of Y_i. For ease of notation, we let $j = 0$ be the subject index for a case and $j = 1, \ldots, M$ correspond to M controls. Namely, for the observed value y_{ij} of the outcome variable Y_{ij}, $y_{i0} = 1$ and $y_{ij} = 0$ for $j = 1, \ldots, M$.

For stratum i, a prospective logistic regression model

$$\operatorname{logit} P(Y_{ij} = 1 | X_{ij}, Z_{ij}) = \beta_{i0} + \beta_x^{\mathrm{T}} X_{ij} + \beta_z^{\mathrm{T}} Z_{ij}$$

is used for $j = 0, \ldots, M$, where β_{i0} is the intercept for stratum i, and $\beta = (\beta_x^{\mathrm{T}}, \beta_z^{\mathrm{T}})^{\mathrm{T}}$ is the vector of regression coefficients which is of dimension p. We are interested in estimation of β.

In the absence of covariate measurement error, we may, by analogy with the arguments in §7.1.6 or for (8.48) of Schlesselman (1982, p. 270), conduct estimation of β based on the prospective likelihood for $1 : M$ matching

$$L(\beta) = \prod_{i=1}^{n} \left[1 + \sum_{j=1}^{M} \exp\{\beta_x^{\mathrm{T}}(X_{ij} - X_{i0}) + \beta_z^{\mathrm{T}}(Z_{ij} - Z_{i0})\} \right]^{-1}. \quad (7.41)$$

In the presence of measurement error in X_{ij}, directly using (7.41) by replacing X_{ij} with its observed measurement may lead to biased results. It is necessary to account for measurement error effects in inferential procedures. Let X_{ij}^* be the observed version of X_{ij}. Assume that the measurement error model is

$$X_{ij}^* = X_{ij} + e_{ij} \quad (7.42)$$

for $i = 1, \ldots, n$ and $j = 0, 1, \ldots, M$, where the e_{ij} have a normal distribution with mean zero and covariance matrix Σ, and they are assumed to be independent of each other and of the $\{Y_{ij}, X_{ij}, Z_{ij}\}$. The independence assumption implies that the surrogate X_{ij}^* satisfy the nondifferential measurement error mechanism. We assume that Σ is known to highlight the discussion on the estimation of β.

To focus on the difference between a case and a matched control, for $i = 1, \ldots, n$ and $j = 1, \ldots, M$, we define $d_{ijx} = X_{ij} - X_{i0}$, $d_{ijz} = Z_{ij} - Z_{i0}$, $d_{ijx^*} = X_{ij}^* - X_{i0}^*$, and $d_{ije} = e_{ij} - e_{i0}$. Write $d_{ix} = (d_{i1x}^{\mathrm{T}}, \ldots, d_{iMx}^{\mathrm{T}})^{\mathrm{T}}$, $d_{iz} = (d_{i1z}^{\mathrm{T}}, \ldots, d_{iMz}^{\mathrm{T}})^{\mathrm{T}}$, $d_{ix^*} = (d_{i1x^*}^{\mathrm{T}}, \ldots, d_{iMx^*}^{\mathrm{T}})^{\mathrm{T}}$, and $d_{ie} = (d_{i1e}^{\mathrm{T}}, \ldots, d_{iMe}^{\mathrm{T}})^{\mathrm{T}}$. Then the measurement error model (7.42) leads to

$$d_{ix^*} = d_{ix} + d_{ie}. \quad (7.43)$$

Let $\Sigma_e = \mathrm{var}(d_{ie})$ be the covariance matrix of d_{ie}. Then Σ_e is a block matrix with block (j, k) being the covariance matrix $\Sigma_{ejk} = \mathrm{var}(e_{ij} - e_{i0}, e_{ik} - e_{i0})$, given by

$$\Sigma_{ejk} = \begin{cases} \Sigma, & j \neq k \\ 2\Sigma, & j = k \end{cases}.$$

Now we describe the method discussed by McShane et al. (2001). This is the conditional score method whose general idea is outlined in §2.5.1. By treating unobserved X_i as an unknown parameter and finding a "sufficient statistic" for X_i, we construct a conditional likelihood by conditioning on such a "sufficient statistic", and accordingly, obtain an unbiased score function which is expressed in terms of the parameters and the observed variables only.

Define $T_i = \sum_{j=0}^{M} Y_{ij}$ to be the total number of cases in stratum i. If $T_i = 1$, then by the definition where the observed case is designated as the subject indexed as 0 and controls are indexed from 1 to M, we have

$$\sum_{j=1}^{M} y_{ij}\{\beta_x^{\mathrm{T}}(X_{ij} - X_{i0}) + \beta_z^{\mathrm{T}}(Z_{ij} - Z_{i0})\} = 0.$$

Thus (7.41) is written as

$$L(\beta) = \prod_{i=1}^{n} P(Y_i = y_i | X_i, Z_i, T_i = 1),$$

where for $i = 1, \ldots, n$,

$$\begin{aligned} &P(Y_i = y_i | X_i, Z_i, T_i = 1) \\ &= \frac{\exp[\sum_{j=1}^{M} y_{ij} \{\beta_x^{\mathrm{T}}(X_{ij} - X_{i0}) + \beta_z^{\mathrm{T}}(Z_{ij} - Z_{i0})\}]}{1 + \sum_{j=1}^{M} \exp\{\beta_x^{\mathrm{T}}(X_{ij} - X_{i0}) + \beta_z^{\mathrm{T}}(Z_{ij} - Z_{i0})\}}. \end{aligned} \tag{7.44}$$

Define

$$B_{ix} = (Y_{i1}\beta_x^{\mathrm{T}}, \ldots, Y_{iM}\beta_x^{\mathrm{T}})^{\mathrm{T}}, \quad B_{iz} = (Y_{i1}\beta_z^{\mathrm{T}}, \ldots, Y_{iM}\beta_z^{\mathrm{T}})^{\mathrm{T}},$$

and

$$\{S_1(d_{ix}, d_{iz}; \beta)\}^{-1} = 1 + \sum_{j=1}^{M} \exp\{\beta_x^{\mathrm{T}} d_{ijx} + \beta_z^{\mathrm{T}} d_{ijz}\}.$$

Let

$$\mathcal{B}_{ix} = (y_{i1}\beta_x^{\mathrm{T}}, \ldots, y_{iM}\beta_x^{\mathrm{T}})^{\mathrm{T}} \text{ and } \mathcal{B}_{iz} = (y_{i1}\beta_z^{\mathrm{T}}, \ldots, y_{iM}\beta_z^{\mathrm{T}})^{\mathrm{T}}$$

for a realization y_i of Y_i. Then the conditional model (7.44) becomes

$$P(Y_i = y_i | d_{ix}, d_{iz}, T_i = 1) = S_1(d_{ix}, d_{iz}; \beta) \exp(\mathcal{B}_{ix}^{\mathrm{T}} d_{ix} + \mathcal{B}_{iz}^{\mathrm{T}} d_{iz}).$$

Therefore, under the Gaussian nondifferential measurement error model (7.43), the conditional model for the joint distribution of the surrogate d_{ix^*} and outcome Y_i, given $\{d_{ix}, d_{iz}, T_i = 1\}$, is

$$\begin{aligned} &P(Y_i = y_i | d_{ix}, d_{iz}, T_i = 1) f(d_{ix^*} | d_{ix}, d_{iz}, T_i = 1) \\ &= S_2(d_{ix}, d_{iz}; \beta) \\ &\quad \cdot \exp\{(d_{ix^*} + \Sigma_e \mathcal{B}_{ix})^{\mathrm{T}} \Sigma_e^{-1} d_{ix} + \mathcal{B}_{iz}^{\mathrm{T}} d_{iz} - \frac{1}{2} d_{ix^*}^{\mathrm{T}} \Sigma_e^{-1} d_{ix^*}\}, \end{aligned}$$

where $S_2(d_{ix}, d_{iz}; \beta)$ is $S_1(d_{ix}, d_{iz}; \beta) \exp(-\frac{1}{2} d_{ix}^{\mathrm{T}} \Sigma_e^{-1} d_{ix})$ times a constant, and $f(d_{ix^*} | d_{ix}, d_{iz}, T_i = 1)$ represents the model for the conditional distribution of d_{ix^*} given $\{d_{ix}, d_{iz}, T_i = 1\}$.

Define

$$\Omega_i = d_{ix^*} + \Sigma_e \mathcal{B}_{ix}$$

and let ω_i be its realization. Then given $\{d_{ix}, d_{iz}, T_i = 1\}$, the conditional model for the joint distribution of Y_i and Ω_i becomes

$$\begin{aligned} &f(y_i, \omega_i | d_{ix}, d_{iz}, T_i = 1) \\ &= S_2(d_{ix}, d_{iz}; \beta) \exp(\omega_i^{\mathrm{T}} \Sigma_e^{-1} d_{ix} - \frac{1}{2} \omega_i^{\mathrm{T}} \Sigma_e^{-1} \omega_i) \\ &\quad \cdot \exp(\mathcal{B}_{ix}^{\mathrm{T}} \omega_i + \mathcal{B}_{iz}^{\mathrm{T}} d_{iz} - \frac{1}{2} \mathcal{B}_{ix}^{\mathrm{T}} \Sigma_e \mathcal{B}_{ix}). \end{aligned}$$

Therefore, by canceling the first two terms which do not involve y_i, we obtain the model for the conditional probability function of Y_i, given $\{\Omega_i = \omega_i, d_{ix}, d_{iz}, T_i = 1\}$:

$$\begin{aligned} &P(Y_i = y_i | \Omega_i = \omega_i, d_{ix}, d_{iz}, T_i = 1) \\ &= \frac{\exp(\mathcal{B}_{ix}^{\mathrm{T}}\omega_i + \mathcal{B}_{iz}^{\mathrm{T}} d_{iz} - \frac{1}{2}\mathcal{B}_{ix}^{\mathrm{T}}\Sigma_e\mathcal{B}_{ix}\}}{\sum_{\widetilde{y}_i:\sum_{j=0}^{M}\widetilde{y}_{ij}=1}\exp(\widetilde{\mathcal{B}}_{ix}^{\mathrm{T}}\omega_i + \widetilde{\mathcal{B}}_{iz}^{\mathrm{T}} d_{iz} - \frac{1}{2}\widetilde{\mathcal{B}}_{ix}^{\mathrm{T}}\Sigma_e\widetilde{\mathcal{B}}_{ix}\}}, \end{aligned} \tag{7.45}$$

where in the denominator, $\widetilde{y}_i = (\widetilde{y}_{i0}, \ldots, \widetilde{y}_{iM})^{\mathrm{T}}$ represents any vector of possible binary values of Y_i which are constrained by $\sum_{j=0}^{M}\widetilde{y}_{ij} = 1$, and $\widetilde{\mathcal{B}}_{ix}$ and $\widetilde{\mathcal{B}}_{iz}$ are, respectively, $\mathcal{B}_{ix}$ and $\mathcal{B}_{iz}$ with y_{ij} replaced by $\widetilde{y}_{ij}$.

For $j = 1, \ldots, M$, let ω_{ij} denote the jth $p_x \times 1$ subvector of ω_i, where p_x is the dimension of β_x. Then the numerator of (7.45) equals

$$\exp\left\{\sum_{j=1}^{M} y_{ij}(\beta_x^{\mathrm{T}}\omega_{ij} + \beta_z^{\mathrm{T}} d_{ijz}) - \frac{1}{2}\sum_{j=1}^{M}\sum_{k=1}^{M} y_{ij}y_{ik}\beta_x^{\mathrm{T}}\Sigma_{ejk}\beta_x\right\},$$

which reduces to

$$\exp\left[\sum_{j=1}^{M} y_{ij}\{\beta_x^{\mathrm{T}}(\omega_{ij} - \Sigma\beta_x) + \beta_z^{\mathrm{T}} d_{ijz}\}\right]$$

because $y_{ij}y_{ik} = 0$ for $j \neq k$ and $y_{ij}y_{ik} = y_{ij}$ for $j = k$. Analogously, the denominator of (7.45) equals

$$1 + \sum_{j=1}^{M}\exp\{\beta_x^{\mathrm{T}}(\omega_{ij} - \Sigma\beta_x) + \beta_z^{\mathrm{T}} d_{ijz}\}.$$

Therefore, the conditional probability (7.45) simplifies to

$$\begin{aligned} &P(Y_i = y_i | \Omega_i = \omega_i, d_{ix}, d_{iz}, T_i = 1) \\ &= \frac{\exp[\sum_{j=1}^{M} y_{ij}\{\beta_x^{\mathrm{T}}(\omega_{ij} - \Sigma\beta_x) + \beta_z^{\mathrm{T}} d_{ijz}\}]}{1 + \sum_{j=1}^{M}\exp\{\beta_x^{\mathrm{T}}(\omega_{ij} - \Sigma\beta_x) + \beta_z^{\mathrm{T}} d_{ijz}\}}. \end{aligned} \tag{7.46}$$

This conditional probability function does not depend on d_{ix}, so we may treat Ω_i as a "sufficient statistic" for d_{ix} if the d_{ix} are pretended to be parameters and β is regarded as known. The conditional probability (7.46) may be further simplified for the observed data: $y_{i0} = 1$ and $y_{ij} = 0$ for $j = 1, \ldots, M$. At the observed values of Y_i, Ω_i takes value d_{ix*}, hence $\omega_{ij} = d_{ijx*}$. Then applying (7.46) to the entire sample gives the conditional likelihood:

$$\begin{aligned} &P(Y_1 = y_1, \ldots, Y_n = y_n | \{(\Omega_i = \omega_i, X_i, Z_i, T_i = 1) : i = 1, \ldots, n\}) \\ &= \prod_{i=1}^{n}\left\{1 + \sum_{j=1}^{M}\exp(\beta_x^{\mathrm{T}}\zeta_{ij} + \beta_z^{\mathrm{T}} d_{ijz})\right\}^{-1}, \end{aligned} \tag{7.47}$$

where $\zeta_{ij} = \omega_{ij} - \Sigma\beta_x$.

With $\{\Omega_i : i = 1, \ldots, n\}$ held fixed, or equivalently, treating the ζ_{ij} as if they were data, maximizing (7.47) with respect to β leads to a consistent estimator of β under regularity conditions. However, the ζ_{ij} involve the unknown parameter β, directly maximizing (7.47) with respect to β, with ζ_{ij} substituted by $d_{ijx*} - \Sigma\beta_x$, may not lead to the desired solution, as noted by Stefanski and Carroll (1987). Instead, iterative steps are recommended to find the solution.

Given an initial value $\beta^{(0)}$ of β, calculate $\zeta_{ij}^{(0)} = d_{ijx*} - \Sigma\beta_x^{(0)}$, then take $\zeta_{ij} = \zeta_{ij}^{(0)}$ to be the "data" (together with the d_{ijz}) and maximize (7.47) with respect to β; let $\beta^{(1)}$ denote the resulting maximizer. Repeat these steps and obtain a sequence of estimates, $\{\beta^{(k)} : k = 1, 2, \ldots\}$. Stop iterations until convergence of $\beta^{(k)}$ as k becomes large, and let $\widehat{\beta}$ denote the resultant estimator of β. This implementation may be realized using standard logistic regression software.

To obtain variance estimates of the components of estimator $\widehat{\beta}$, one may use the bootstrap or jackknife method. For instance, McShane et al. (2001) outlined the step based on the jackknife method. Let $\widehat{\beta}_{(i)}$ denote the estimate of β computed from the full data set minus the ith stratum. Then the jackknife covariance estimate for $\widehat{\beta}$ is calculated by

$$\widehat{\text{var}}_{\text{J}}(\widehat{\beta}) = \left(\frac{n-1}{n}\right)\sum_{i=1}^{n}\{\widehat{\beta}_{(i)} - \widehat{\beta}_{(+)}\}\{\widehat{\beta}_{(i)} - \widehat{\beta}_{(+)}\}^{\text{T}}, \tag{7.48}$$

where $\widehat{\beta}_{(+)} = n^{-1}\sum_{i=1}^{n}\widehat{\beta}_{(i)}$.

We conclude this section with comments. Introducing the difference-covariate vectors d_{ix} and d_{iz} to formulate the likelihood enables us to focus inferences on parameter β and ignore the nuisance intercepts β_{i0}. Building "sufficient statistics" Ω_i allows us to overpass the unavailability of the X_i when constructing an inference function. The foregoing development treats the measurement error covariance Σ as known; this is true when conducting sensitivity analyses to evaluate the impact of different degrees of measurement error on inference results for parameter β.

If the measurement error covariance Σ is estimated from other data sources, then the induced variability needs to be accommodated when developing variance estimates for estimator $\widehat{\beta}$. The following formula may be used for this purpose:

$$\text{var}(\widehat{\beta}_j) = \text{var}\{E(\widehat{\beta}_j|\widehat{\Sigma})\} + E\{\text{var}(\widehat{\beta}_j|\widehat{\Sigma})\}, \tag{7.49}$$

where $\widehat{\beta}_j$ is the jth element of $\widehat{\beta}$, and $\widehat{\Sigma}$ represents an estimator of the measurement error variance Σ.

Specifically, McShane et al. (2001) discussed a re-sampling procedure. Suppose that measurement error covariance matrix Σ is estimated from additional sources of data and that the asymptotic distribution of the resulting estimator is available. One may implement three steps to obtain variance estimates for the $\widehat{\beta}_j$. At Step 1, set a sufficiently large integer N, and then simulate N sets of measurement error covariance estimates from such an asymptotic distribution, Let $\widehat{\Sigma}^{(k)}$ denote these simulated versions for Σ, where $k = 1, \ldots, N$.

At Step 2, for $k = 1, \ldots, N$, set Σ to be $\widehat{\Sigma}^{(k)}$; then run the foregoing estimation method for the data to obtain an estimate of β, denoted as $\widehat{\beta}^{(k)}$; and then apply the jackknife procedure (7.48) to obtain a covariance estimate $\widehat{\mathrm{var}}_{\mathrm{J}}(\widehat{\beta}^{(k)})$.

At Step 3, let $\widehat{\beta}_j^{(k)}$ be the jth component of $\widehat{\beta}^{(k)}$ and $\widehat{\mathrm{var}}_{\mathrm{J}}(\widehat{\beta}_j^{(k)})$ be the jth diagonal element of $\widehat{\mathrm{var}}_{\mathrm{J}}(\widehat{\beta}^{(k)})$. Then calculate a standard error of $\widehat{\beta}_j$ using the square root of

$$\frac{\sum_{k=1}^{N}\{\widehat{\beta}_j^{(k)} - \widehat{\beta}_j^{(+)}\}^2}{N-1} + \frac{\sum_{k=1}^{N} \widehat{\mathrm{var}}_{\mathrm{J}}(\widehat{\beta}_j^{(k)})}{N},$$

as suggested by (7.49), where $\widehat{\beta}_j^{(+)} = N^{-1}\sum_{k=1}^{N} \widehat{\beta}_j^{(k)}$ for $j = 1, \ldots, p$.

7.6 Two-Phase Design with Misclassified Exposure Variable

When studying the relationship between the disease status Y and the exposure variable X, it is ideal to have error-free measurements of X. But in practice, measuring X may be expensive or time-consuming; instead, cheap, error-prone measurements X^* are readily obtained. Given a fixed budget or a constrained timeline, striving to obtain the precise measurement of X for every subject can be infeasible for us to recruit a sufficient number of individuals into the study, which is required for achieving a desirable statistical power. On the other hand, if attempting to include more subjects into the study and simply measure X^* to establish the disease-exposure relationship, biased results may be produced if naively disregarding the difference between X^* as X in the analysis. To deal with these issues, a two-phase study may be employed as a trade-off to balance the effectiveness of the data collection and the validity of inference results.

At the first phase, surrogate X^*, along with the disease status Y, is measured for *all the individuals* in the sample, while at the second phase, X is measured on the individuals in a *subsample* chosen from the first phase. Given a fixed budget, it is important to set a design so that statistical efficiency in estimation of interesting quantities, such as the log odds ratio linking Y and the exposure variable X, can be maximized from such a design.

In this section, we describe design issues, discussed by McNamee (2005), for two-phase case–control studies in which a binary exposure variable variable X is subject to misclassification. Let $X = 1$ if a subject is exposed and $X = 0$ otherwise, and X^* be a surrogate measurement of X.

Design Setup

We consider a two-phase case–control study with n subjects in total and the ratio of controls to cases being ω_0. At the first phase, suppose n_{1+} cases with $Y = 1$ and n_{0+} controls with $Y = 0$ are sampled independently of each other; and the surrogate measurement X^* is collected for every individual, giving n_{ij}^* subjects with $(Y = i, X^* = j)$; where $n_{1+} = n/(\omega_0 + 1)$, $n_{0+} = n\omega_0/(\omega_0 + 1)$, and $n_{i0}^* + n_{i1}^* = n_{i+}$ for $i = 0, 1$.

At the second phase of the study, a subsample of those n subjects from the first phase is randomly selected from each category of $\{(Y = i, X^* = j) : i, j = 0, 1\}$. Let ω_{ij} be the sampling fraction in the stratum with $(Y = i, X^* = j)$, and $m_{ij} = n_{i+}\omega_{ij}$ be the corresponding number of subjects sampled for $i, j = 0, 1$. The total second-phase size is then $m = \sum_{i,j} m_{ij}$, which is smaller than n; in costly studies, m is substantially smaller than n. Among those m subjects, the true exposure variable X is measured for everybody; let n_{ij} denote the number of truly exposed subjects (i.e., with $X = 1$) for the stratum with $(Y = i, X^* = j)$.

Variance Estimate

For $i = 0$ or 1, let $p_{i1} = P(X = 1|Y = i)$ be the (conditional) exposure probability for controls or cases. We are interested in estimating the log odds ratio of the relationship between Y and X, given by

$$\beta = \log \frac{p_{11}}{1 - p_{11}} - \log \frac{p_{01}}{1 - p_{01}}.$$

Although using the second-phase data may give us a reasonable estimate of β, this approach incurs efficiency loss. Especially when m is a lot smaller than n, the efficiency loss may be quite substantial. To increase statistical efficiency, it is viable to incorporate the measurements from the first-phase into the estimation of β.

For $i, j = 0$ or 1, let $p_{ij}^* = P(X^* = j|Y = i)$ be the "observed" exposure or nonexposure probability for controls or cases, and $\pi_{ij1}^* = P(X = 1|Y = i, X^* = j)$ be the (mis)classification probabilities. Then for $i = 0, 1$, the exposure probability is written as

$$p_{i1} = \sum_{j=0,1} p_{ij}^* \pi_{ij1}^*,$$

where $p_{i0}^* + p_{i1}^* = 1$. Since the probabilities p_{ij}^* and π_{ij1}^* are, respectively, estimated by the data collected from the first and second phases:

$$\widehat{p}_{ij}^* = \frac{n_{ij}^*}{n_{i+}} \text{ and } \widehat{\pi}_{ij1}^* = \frac{n_{ij}}{m_{ij}},$$

we may estimate p_{i1} by

$$\widehat{p}_{i1} = \sum_{j=0,1} \widehat{p}_{ij}^* \widehat{\pi}_{ij1}^*,$$

hence, leading to an estimate of β:

$$\widehat{\beta} = \log \frac{\widehat{p}_{11}}{1 - \widehat{p}_{11}} - \log \frac{\widehat{p}_{01}}{1 - \widehat{p}_{01}}.$$

The variance of $\widehat{p}_{i1}$ is given by (Cochran 1977; McNamee 2005):

$$\text{var}(\widehat{p}_{i1}) = \sum_{j=0,1} \frac{p_{ij}^{*2}\pi_{ij1}^{*}(1-\pi_{ij1}^{*})}{m_{ij}} + \frac{1}{n_{i+}}\left(\sum_{j=0,1} p_{ij}^{*}\pi_{ij1}^{*2} - p_{i1}^{2}\right).$$

When misclassification of X is differential, estimators $\widehat{p}_{11}$ and $\widehat{p}_{01}$ are independent, and the variance of $\widehat{\beta}$ is, therefore, the sum of the variances of estimators for the two log odds. By the delta method,

$$\text{var}\left\{\log\left(\frac{\widehat{p}_{i1}}{1-\widehat{p}_{i1}}\right)\right\} = \frac{1}{p_{i1}^{2}(1-p_{i1})^{2}}\text{var}(\widehat{p}_{i1}) \text{ for } i = 0, 1,$$

hence, we obtain

$$\text{var}(\widehat{\beta}) = \sum_{i=0,1}\sum_{j=0,1} \frac{p_{ij}^{*2}\pi_{ij1}^{*}(1-\pi_{ij1}^{*})}{m_{ij}p_{i1}^{2}(1-p_{i1})^{2}} + \sum_{i=0,1} \frac{\sum_{j=0,1} p_{ij}^{*}\pi_{ij1}^{*2} - p_{i1}^{2}}{n_{i+}p_{i1}^{2}(1-p_{i1})^{2}}.$$

This variance may also be expressed in terms of the sampling proportions:

$$\text{var}(\widehat{\beta}) = \frac{\omega_0+1}{n}\left\{\sum_{i=0,1}\sum_{j=0,1} \frac{p_{ij}^{*2}\pi_{ij1}^{*}(1-\pi_{ij1}^{*})}{\omega_i\omega_{ij}p_{i1}^{2}(1-p_{i1})^{2}} + \sum_{i=0,1}\frac{\rho_i^2}{\omega_i p_{i1}(1-p_{i1})}\right\}, \quad (7.50)$$

where $\omega_1 = 1$, and for $i = 0, 1$,

$$\rho_i^2 = \sum_{j=0,1} \frac{p_{ij}^{*}\pi_{ij1}^{*2} - p_{i1}^{2}}{p_{i1}(1-p_{i1})}.$$

Alternatively, the variance of $\widehat{\beta}$ may be expressed by using a dual way of describing the misclassification process. Let $\pi_{ij1} = P(X^* = 1|Y = i, X = j)$ for $i, j = 0, 1$. These probabilities may replace π_{ij1}^{*} to describe the variance $\text{var}(\widehat{\beta})$, leading to an alternative expression of (7.50), where we assume that $\pi_{i11} - \pi_{i01} \geq 0$ for the following development.

Optimal Design with Fixed Budget

Let the total budget for the study be B, and the costs of measuring X^* and X for each subject be c^* and c, respectively, with $c^* < c$. Assume that there are no other costs. Then the total cost of a two-phase study is $c^*\sum_i n_{i+} + c\sum_{i,j} m_{ij}$, which is constrained to be B. Consequently, as discussed by McNamee (2005), the choices of n, ω_0 and ω_{ij} must satisfy the budget constraint

$$\frac{n}{\omega_0+1}\left\{c^*(\omega_0+1) + c\sum_{i=0,1}\omega_i\sum_{j=0,1}p_{ij}^{*}\omega_{ij}\right\} = B. \quad (7.51)$$

Therefore, with a given total budget B, an optimal two-phase design may be constructed by minimizing $\text{var}(\widehat{\beta})$ under the constraint (7.51).

McNamee (2005) showed that the optimal values of ω_0 and ω_{ij} for a two-phase design are given by

$$\omega_0^{\text{OPT}} = \frac{f_0\rho_0}{f_1\rho_1}$$

and

$$\omega_{ij}^{\text{OPT}} = \begin{cases} \sqrt{\frac{c^*}{c}}\sqrt{\frac{(1-\pi_{i01})(1-\pi_{i11})}{\rho_i^2 p_{i0}^{*2}}}, & \text{if } j = 0, \\ \sqrt{\frac{c^*}{c}}\sqrt{\frac{\pi_{i01}\pi_{i11}}{\rho_i^2 p_{i1}^{*2}}}, & \text{if } j = 1, \end{cases}$$

where $f_i = 1/\sqrt{p_{i1}(1-p_{i1})}$ for $i = 0, 1$. Consequently, the optimal value of n is determined by substituting ω_0^{OPT} and ω_{ij}^{OPT} into (7.51).

In many case–control studies, additional constraints are imposed. For instance, the ratio ω_0 of controls to cases is fixed in advance. Commonly, ω_0 takes a value in the range of $[2, 8]$ to reflect the relative difficulty of finding cases. With this additional constraint together with (7.51), minimizing $\text{var}(\widehat{\beta})$ gives the constrained optimal sampling fractions

$$\widetilde{\omega}_{ij}^{\text{OPT}} = \omega_{ij}^{\text{OPT}}\sqrt{\frac{f_i^2\rho_i^2(\omega_0+1)}{\omega_i^2\sum_{k=0,1} f_k^2\rho_k^2/\omega_k}}$$

for $i, j = 0, 1$. Other optimal designs under different constraints were discussed by McNamee (2005) in detail.

7.7 Bibliographic Notes and Discussion

Measurement error and misclassification have long been a concern in epidemiological studies. Early work includes Bross (1954) and Goldberg (1975) who discussed misclassification effects for 2×2 tables. It has been well documented that odds ratio estimates can be seriously biased if misclassification and measurement error effects are not properly accounted for in the analysis (e.g., Barron 1977).

This chapter includes only a few methods of handling case–control data with measurement error or misclassification. More inference methods of correcting for measurement error or misclassification are available in the literature. For example, Breslow and Cain (1988) described a two-stage method for which misclassification probabilities are estimated from a validation subsample obtained from a second-stage design. Armstrong, Whittemore and Howe (1989) proposed a method for estimating odds ratios from case–control data with covariate measurement error, where the measurement error may contain both a random component and a systematic difference between cases and controls. Elton and Duffy (1983) and Drews, Flanders and Kosinski (1993) examined estimation methods when data are classified using two measurement schemes. Schill et al. (1993) suggested to jointly fit logistic models to both the main and validation samples. Wang and Carroll (1994) explored robust estimation for case–control studies with measurement error in covariates. Carroll, Wang and Wang (1995) proposed to ignore the design study aspect and base inference on a prospective formulation of estimating equations to handle case–control data with measurement error. Marinos, Tzonou and Karantzas (1995) studied epidemiological indices in case–control studies with nondifferential misclassification. With the retrospective logistic regression model, Forbes and Santner (1995) explored estimation procedures for the odds ratio and regression parameters for matched case–control studies. They considered the scenario where subject-specific covariates are subject to measurement error and covariance structures of the measurement error process may be different for cases and controls. Roeder, Carroll and Lindsay (1996) discussed a semiparametric approach under the prospective logistic model with a validation subsample. In their approach, they assumed a parametric model to characterize the measurement error process and imposed a nonparametric mixture model to describe the marginal distribution of the true covariates.

Morrissey and Spiegelman (1999) and Lyles (2002) discussed adjustment methods for exposure misclassification in case–control studies where a validation sample is available. Stürmer et al. (2002) carried out a simulation study to assess the performance of the regression calibration method in contrast to a semiparametric approach for case–control studies with internal validation data. Rice (2003) developed likelihood methods for analyzing case–control studies where a binary exposure is potentially misclassified and a variety of matching ratios may be present. Zheng and Tian (2005) studied the impact of diagnostic error on testing genetic association in case–control studies. Guolo (2008a) used prospective likelihood methods to analyze retrospective case–control data with error-contaminated covariates which are modeled with skew normal distributions. Chu et al. (2009) presented a likelihood-based approach for case–control studies with multiple non-gold standard exposure assessments. Lobach et al. (2008) explored a pseudo-score method to handle the data where some covariates are subject to measurement error and some covariates are subject to missingness.

Under the Bayesian framework, Müller and Roeder (1997) developed a nonparametric Bayes approach for case–control studies with measurement error. Gustafson, Le and Saskin (2001) studied the impact of misspecification of classification probabilities and demonstrated that even slight discrepancies between assumed and actual classification probabilities can result in seriously erroneous results. They suggested a Bayesian analysis by attaching a prior distribution to the classification probabilities to allow for uncertainty. Prescott and Garthwaite (2005) proposed methods for analyzing matched case–control studies in which a binary exposure variable is subject to misclassification. Mak, Best and Rushton (2015) studied sensitivity analysis for case–control studies subject to exposure misclassification. In terms of sample size determination, Stamey and Gerlach (2007) discussed a Bayesian simulation-based approach for case–control studies with misclassification.

Certain methods developed for observational studies may be readily adapted to handle case–control data, especially when nondifferential measurement error is assumed (e.g., Rosner, Willett and Spiegelman 1989). Thürigen et al. (2000) and Guolo (2008b) reviewed correction methods that are applicable to case–control studies and briefly discussed implementation procedures using available software packages.

7.8 Supplementary Problems

7.1. Let Y be a binary variable indicating the disease status with value 1 and 0 otherwise, and Z be a vector of covariates. Let $\phi = P(Y = 1)$ and $g(z)$ be the marginal probability density or mass function of Z. Suppose the conditional probability function of Y, given Z, is modeled as

$$P(Y = 1|Z = z) = \frac{\exp(\beta_0 + \beta_z^{\mathrm{T}} z)}{1 + \exp(\beta_0 + \beta_z^{\mathrm{T}} z)},$$

where β_0 and β_z are regression coefficients.

Suppose $(\beta_0, \beta_z, \phi, g)$ and $(\beta_0^*, \beta_z^*, \phi^*, g^*)$ are two sets of associated values for the conditional probability density or mass function, $f_{z|Y}(z|y)$, of Z given Y. Let

$$b(z) = \frac{1 + \exp(\beta_0^* + \beta_z^{\mathrm{T}} z)}{1 + \exp(\beta_0 + \beta_z^{\mathrm{T}} z)},$$

and

$$c(z) = \begin{cases} \frac{b(z)}{\sum_z b(z)g(z)}, & \text{if the } Z \text{ are discrete,} \\ \frac{b(z)}{\int b(z)g(z)dz}, & \text{if the } Z \text{ are continuous.} \end{cases}$$

Show that

$$f_{z|Y}(z|y; \beta_0, \beta_z, \phi, g) = f_{z|Y}(z|y; \beta_0^*, \beta_z^*, \phi^*, g^*)$$

if and only if
(a) $\beta_z = \beta_z^*$;
(b) $\beta_0^* = \beta_0 + \log\left\{\frac{\phi^*(1-\phi)}{(1-\phi^*)\phi}\right\}$;
(c) $g^*(z) = c(z)g(z)$.

This result implies that from the retrospective sample, only the parameter β_z is fully identifiable, while the marginal distribution of Z can be determined only up to an equivalence class of functions. But if the true population probability of disease, ϕ, is otherwise known, then β_0 and g are identifiable as well.

(Roeder, Carroll and Lindsay 1996)

7.2. Discuss the misclassification effect on the Mantel-Haenszel estimator (7.2) of ψ in §7.1.3 for stratified designs.

7.3.

(a) Verify the identity (7.12).
(b) Verify the identity (7.14).
(c) Verify the identity (7.15). Show that for each $i = 0, 1$ and $j = 1, \ldots, n_{i+}$, the expectation of $S_{ij}(Y_{ij}, Z_{ij}; \theta)$ is not necessarily zero.
(d) Generalize the development in §7.1.6 to the case where the disease outcome variable Y_{ij} assumes K different values, where K is an integer greater than 2.
(e) If the prospective model (7.3) is replaced by a probit model or a complementary log-log model, can the development in §7.1.6 go through?

(Prentice and Pyke 1979; Carroll, Wang and Wang 1995)

7.4.

(a) Suppose case–control data are collected from two clinics. Let Y denote a binary disease status, and X denote the presence ($X = 1$) or absence ($X = 0$) of a risk factor. In Clinic A, a sample of n_{1+} diseased patients (cases with $Y = 1$) includes n_{11} individuals who report $X = 1$, while in clinic B, a sample of n_{0+} asymptomatic patients (controls with $Y = 0$) includes n_{01} subjects who have $X = 1$.

In addition, a third group of y patients are interviewed in both clinics. In Clinic B, y_1 patients report $X = 1$ and y_0 patients report $X = 0$. Among those y_1 patients who report $X = 1$ in Clinic B, there are x_1 patients reporting $X = 1$ in Clinic A; and among those y_0 patients who report $X = 0$ in Clinic B, there are x_0 patients reporting $X = 0$ in Clinic A.

Assume that the measurements on the risk factor obtained in Clinic B are precise and the results reported in Clinic A are subject to misclassification. Let X^* denote a reported value of the risk factor from Clinic A. Define $p_{11} = P(X = 1|Y = 1)$ and $p_{01} = P(X = 1|Y = 0)$. Let ψ be the odds ratio

$$\psi = \frac{p_{11}(1 - p_{01})}{p_{01}(1 - p_{11})}.$$

Suppose the nondifferential misclassification mechanism

$$P(X^* = 1|X = x, Y = 1) = P(X^* = 1|X = x, Y = 0)$$

holds for $x = 0, 1$. Find a consistent estimator of ψ. Construct a $(1 - \alpha) \times 100\%$ confidence interval for ψ, where α is a constant between 0 and 1.

(b) Elton and Duffy (1983) reported the data coming from an epidemiological study of risk on breast cancer, where measurements were taken from two clinics. A diagnostic clinic, called Clinic A, had 236 confirmed cases while a screening clinic, called Clinic B, had 2962 asymptomatic controls. The records were also available for 167 women (mostly with benign

Table 7.8. *Case–Control Data on Breast Cancer (Elton and Duffy 1983)*

Case–control study data			Women attending both clinics		
	Clinic A Cases	Clinic B Controls	Clinic A Response	Clinic B Response	
				Married	Unmarried
Married	205	2288	yes	120	18
Unmarried	31	674	no	4	25

breast disease and therefore not qualifying for either the case or control groups), who had attended both clinics within a 6-month period.

It is interesting to assess the effect of the marital status on the development of breast cancer. The measurements for married individuals are given in Table 7.8. Measurements on marital status collected from Clinic A were regarded as error-prone whereas measurements from Clinic B were treated as correct. Apply the results obtained in (a) to analyze the data.

(Elton and Duffy 1983)

7.5. Consider the setup of §7.2.

(a) Suppose that X is subject to misclassification and that X^* is an observed value of X.

(i) Under the nondifferential misclassification mechanism, show that the "observed" odds ratio based on X^* and Y is given by (7.19).

(ii) Find an expression of the "observed" odds ratio based on X^* and Y for the setting where the misclassification mechanism is differential.

(iii) Let $\pi^*_{y1x} = P(X = x|Y = y, X^* = 1)$ and $\pi^*_{y0x} = P(X = x|Y = y, X^* = 0)$ be (mis)classification probabilities for $y = 0, 1$ and $x = 0, 1$. Using π^*_{y1x} and π^*_{y0x} together with p_{11} and p_{01}, derive the "observed" odds ratio for X^* and Y.

(b) If X is precisely classified, but Y is subject to misclassification with an observed surrogate Y^*. Derive the "observed" odds ratio based on X and Y^*.

(c) If both X and Y are subject to misclassification, and let X^* and Y^* be the observed value of X and Y, respectively. Derive the "observed" odds ratio based on X^* and Y^*.

7.6. Consider the setup of stratified designs in §7.2.

(a) Verify (7.20).

(b) Let $A_k = \pi_{111} + a_{k1}(1 - \pi_{100})$, $B_k = 1 - \pi_{111} + a_{k1}\pi_{100}$, and

$$D_k = (A_k a_{k1}\pi_{000} - B_k\pi_{011})^2 + 4A_k(1 - \pi_{011})B_k a_{k1}(1 - \pi_{000}).$$

Assume that $B_k a_{k1}(1 - \pi_{000}) > 0$. Define

$$C_k = \frac{(A_k a_{k1}\pi_{000} - B_k\pi_{011}) + \sqrt{D_k}}{2B_k a_{k1}(1 - \pi_{000})}.$$

Show that

(i) if the true odds ratio ψ takes a value smaller than C_k, then the "observed" odds ratio

$$\psi_k^* > \psi$$

for every stratum k;

(ii) if the true odds ratio ψ takes a value bigger than C_k, then the "observed" odds ratio

$$\psi_k^* < \psi$$

for every stratum k.

7.7.

(a) Verify the identity (7.22).
(b) Verify the identity (7.25).
(c) Verify the identity (7.26).

(Zhang et al. 2008)

7.8. Verify (7.30).

7.9. In a case–control study, let Y be the binary outcome variable taking values 0 and 1 and $\{X, Z\}$ be the risk factors. Suppose that Y is subject to misclassification and Y^* is its observed version. Assume that

$$P(Y^* = y^*|Y = y, X, Z) = P(Y^* = y^*|Y = y)$$

for $y^*, y = 0, 1$. Let

$$\gamma_{01} = P(Y^* = 1|Y = 0) \text{ and } \gamma_{10} = P(Y^* = 0|Y = 1)$$

be the misclassification probabilities. Consider a logistic regression model

$$P(Y = 1|X, Z) = \frac{\exp(\beta_0 + \beta_x^{\mathrm{T}} X + \beta_z^{\mathrm{T}} Z)}{1 + \exp(\beta_0 + \beta_x^{\mathrm{T}} X + \beta_z^{\mathrm{T}} Z)},$$

where β_0, β_z and β_x are regression coefficients.

(a) Show that the model for the misclassified outcome is

$$\begin{aligned} &P(Y^* = 1|X, Z) \\ &= \frac{\gamma_{01} + (1 - \gamma_{10}) \exp(\beta_0 + \beta_x^{\mathrm{T}} X + \beta_z^{\mathrm{T}} Z)}{1 + \exp(\beta_0 + \beta_x^{\mathrm{T}} X + \beta_z^{\mathrm{T}} Z)}. \end{aligned} \tag{7.52}$$

(b) Show that model (7.52) is unidentifiable if $\gamma_{01} + \gamma_{10} = 1$.
(c) If model (7.52) is unidentifiable, is $\gamma_{01} + \gamma_{10} = 1$ true?
(d) Find the retrospective model for the conditional distribution of $\{X, Z\}$ given Y^*. Discuss identifiability issues and relevant assumptions.
(e) Suppose that X is also subject to measurement error and X^* is an observed value of X. Derive a model for the conditional distribution of Y^* given $\{X^*, Z\}$. Discuss associated conditions and identifiability issues.

7.10. For any real value x, let

$$\phi(x) = \frac{1}{\sqrt{2\pi}} \exp\left(-\frac{x^2}{2}\right) \quad \text{and} \quad \Phi(x) = \int_{-\infty}^{x} \phi(v)dv.$$

(a) Show that

$$\int_{-\infty}^{\infty} \frac{1}{\sigma} \Phi(a+x)\phi\left(\frac{x}{\sigma}\right) dx = \Phi\left(\frac{a}{\sqrt{1+\sigma^2}}\right),$$

where a and σ are positive constants.

(b) Let Y be a binary response variable and X be a scalar covariate. Suppose Y and X are modulated by the probit regression model

$$P(Y = 1|X) = \Phi(\beta_0 + \beta_x X),$$

where β_0 and β_x are regression coefficients.

Assume that X is subject to measurement error, and let X^* be its observed value. The measurement error model is given by

$$X = X^* + e, \tag{7.53}$$

where e is independent of $\{X^*, Y\}$ and normally distributed with mean 0 and variance σ_e^2.

Show that the model for the conditional distribution of Y given X^* is also a probit regression model. That is, the conditional probability $P(Y = 1|X^*)$ can be written as

$$P(Y = 1|X^*) = \Phi(\beta_0^* + \beta_x^* X^*)$$

for some parameters β_0^* and β_x^*. Determine the relationship between the parameters (β_0^*, β_x^*) and (β_0, β_x).

(c) Suppose $\{(x_i^*, y_i) : i = 1, \ldots, n\}$ is a sample of realizations of (X^*, Y). Are β_0 and β_x estimable using the observations of the sample? What conditions do you need in order to estimate β_0 and β_x using the observations of the sample?

(d) Can you generalize the result in (b) to the setting where X is a vector of covariates? What assumptions do you need?

(e) If the measurement error model is not given by (7.53) but given by

$$X^* = X + e,$$

where e is independent of $\{X, Y\}$ and normally distributed with mean 0 and variance σ_e^2. Does the result in (b) still hold?

(Burr 1988)

7.11. Table 7.9 displays the layout of the data arising from a case–control study with n subjects, where Y is a binary outcome variable, X is a misclassification-prone binary exposure variable, and X^* is an observed version of X. In the validation sample $\mathcal{V}$, the counts for $\{Y = i, X^* = j, X = k\}$ are denoted as n_{ijk} for $i, j, k = 0, 1$; in the sample $\mathcal{M}$ of the main study, the counts for $\{Y = i, X^* = j\}$ are denoted as n_{ij}^* for $i, j = 0, 1$; and $\mathcal{V}$ is a subset of $\mathcal{M}$.

Table 7.9. *Data Layout for Study with Misclassified Exposure Data*

	Validation study				Main study		
	$Y=1$		$Y=0$				
X^*	$X=1$	$X=0$	$X=1$	$X=0$	Y	$X^*=1$	$X^*=0$
1	n_{111}	n_{110}	n_{011}	n_{010}	1	n_{11}^*	n_{10}^*
0	n_{101}	n_{100}	n_{001}	n_{000}	0	n_{01}^*	n_{00}^*

For $i = 0, 1$, let

$$\begin{aligned}
\pi_{i11} &= P(X^* = 1|Y = i, X = 1);\\
\pi_{i00} &= P(X^* = 0|Y = i, X = 0);\\
\pi_{i11}^* &= P(X = 1|Y = i, X^* = 1);\\
\pi_{i00}^* &= P(X = 0|Y = i, X^* = 0);\\
p_{i1}^* &= P(X^* = 1|Y = i);\\
p_{i1} &= P(X = 1|Y = i).
\end{aligned}$$

Define the log odds ratio of having the disease as

$$\beta = \log\left\{\frac{p_{11}(1-p_{01})}{(1-p_{11})p_{01}}\right\}. \tag{7.54}$$

Using the main study data alone, or both the validation and main studies, we estimate p_{i1}^*, respectively, by

$$\widetilde{p}_{11}^* = \frac{n_{11}^*}{n_{11}^* + n_{10}^*}; \quad \widetilde{p}_{01}^* = \frac{n_{01}^*}{n_{01}^* + n_{00}^*};$$

and

$$\widehat{p}_{11}^* = \frac{n_{11}^* + n_{11+}}{n_{11}^* + n_{10}^* + n_{1++}}; \quad \widehat{p}_{01}^* = \frac{n_{01}^* + n_{01+}}{n_{01}^* + n_{00}^* + n_{0++}};$$

where $n_{ij+} = n_{ij1} + n_{ij0}$ and $n_{i++} = n_{i1+} + n_{i0+}$ for $i, j = 0, 1$.

(a) Show that

$$\begin{pmatrix} p_{11} \\ 1-p_{11} \\ p_{01} \\ 1-p_{01} \end{pmatrix} = \begin{pmatrix} \pi_{111} & 1-\pi_{100} & 0 & 0 \\ 1-\pi_{111} & \pi_{100} & 0 & 0 \\ 0 & 0 & \pi_{011} & 1-\pi_{000} \\ 0 & 0 & 1-\pi_{011} & \pi_{000} \end{pmatrix}^{-1} \begin{pmatrix} p_{11}^* \\ 1-p_{11}^* \\ p_{01}^* \\ 1-p_{01}^* \end{pmatrix},$$

where the inverse matrix is assumed to exist.

(b) Using the validation study, we estimate π_{i11} and π_{i00} by

$$\widehat{\pi}_{i11} = \frac{n_{i11}}{n_{i+1}} \text{ and } \widehat{\pi}^*_{i00} = \frac{n_{i00}}{n_{i+0}},$$

respectively, where $n_{i+k} = n_{i1k} + n_{i0k}$ for $k = 0, 1$.

Let $\widetilde{\beta}_{\text{M}}$ and $\widehat{\beta}_{\text{M}}$ denote an estimator of β, determined by (7.54) in combination with the expression in (a), where p_{i1}^* is estimated by $\widetilde{p}_{i1}^*$ and $\widehat{p}_{i1}^*$, respectively. In both $\widetilde{\beta}_{\text{M}}$ and $\widehat{\beta}_{\text{M}}$, π_{i11} is estimated by $\widehat{\pi}_{i11}$ and π_{i00} is estimated by $\widehat{\pi}_{i00}$. Find the variance of $\widetilde{\beta}_{\text{M}}$ and $\widehat{\beta}_{\text{M}}$.

(c) Show that

$$\begin{pmatrix} p_{11} \\ 1-p_{11} \\ p_{01} \\ 1-p_{01} \end{pmatrix} = \begin{pmatrix} \pi^*_{111} & 1-\pi^*_{100} & 0 & 0 \\ 1-\pi^*_{111} & \pi^*_{100} & 0 & 0 \\ 0 & 0 & \pi^*_{011} & 1-\pi^*_{000} \\ 0 & 0 & 1-\pi^*_{011} & \pi^*_{000} \end{pmatrix} \begin{pmatrix} p_{11}^* \\ 1-p_{11}^* \\ p_{01}^* \\ 1-p_{01}^* \end{pmatrix}.$$

(d) Using the validation study, we estimate π^*_{i11} and π^*_{i00} by

$$\widehat{\pi}^*_{i11} = \frac{n_{i11}}{n_{i1+}} \text{ and } \widehat{\pi}^*_{i00} = \frac{n_{i00}}{n_{i0+}},$$

respectively. Let $\widetilde{\beta}_{\text{IM}}$ and $\widehat{\beta}_{\text{IM}}$ denote an estimator of β, determined by (7.54) in combination with the expression in (c), where p_{i1}^* is estimated by $\widetilde{p}_{i1}^*$ and $\widehat{p}_{i1}^*$, respectively. In both $\widetilde{\beta}_{\text{IM}}$ and $\widehat{\beta}_{\text{IM}}$, π^*_{i11} is estimated by $\widehat{\pi}^*_{i11}$, and π^*_{i00} is estimated by $\widehat{\pi}^*_{i00}$. Find the variance of $\widetilde{\beta}_{\text{IM}}$ and $\widehat{\beta}_{\text{IM}}$.

(e) Let $\theta = (p_{11}^*, p_{01}^*, \pi^*_{111}, \pi^*_{011}, \pi^*_{100}, \pi^*_{000})^{\text{T}}$. Construct a likelihood function of θ and derive the maximum likelihood estimator of θ. Develop an estimator of β accordingly.

(f) Consider that the conditional probabilities are parameterized as

$$\begin{aligned} P(X = 1|Y = 0) &= \alpha; \\ P(X = 1|Y = 1) &= \frac{\alpha \exp(\beta)}{1 - \alpha + \alpha \exp(\beta)}; \\ P(X^* = 1|Y = 0) &= \pi_{011}\alpha + (1 - \pi_{000})(1 - \alpha); \\ P(X^* = 1|Y = 1) &= \frac{\exp(\beta)\pi_{111}\alpha + (1 - \pi_{100})(1 - \alpha)}{1 - \alpha + \alpha \exp(\beta)}; \end{aligned}$$

$$P(X^* = x^*|X = x, Y = k) = \pi_{i11}^{xx^*}(1 - \pi_{i11})^{x(1-x^*)} \\ \pi_{i00}^{(1-x)(1-x^*)}(1 - \pi_{i00})^{(1-x)x^*}.$$

Let $\theta = (\beta, \alpha, \pi_{011}, \pi_{111}, \pi_{000}, \pi_{100})^{\mathrm{T}}$ be the parameter vector, and

$$L(\theta) = \prod_{l \in \mathcal{V}} \{P(X_l^* = x_l^*|X_l = x_l, Y_l = y_l)P(X_l = x_l|Y_l = y_l)\} \\ \cdot \prod_{l \in \mathcal{M} \setminus \mathcal{V}} P(X_l^* = x_l^*|Y_l = y_l)$$

be the "observed" retrospective likelihood, where $\{Y_l, X_l.X_l^*\}$ represents a copy of $\{Y, X, X^*\}$ for individual l. Develop an estimation procedure for θ.

(g) Discuss the efficiency among the estimators of β which are obtained in (b), (d), (e) and (f).

(h) Using the foregoing development, analyze the data arising from a case–control study on sudden infant death syndrome (SIDS) which were discussed by Chu, Gustafson and Le (2010). During investigation of a potential impact of maternal use of antibiotics during pregnancy on the occurrence of SIDS, surrogate exposure X^* was obtained from an interview question (yes=1, no=0). Information on antibiotic use from medical records, taken to be the actual exposure status X, was extracted for a subset of study patients. The data are displayed in Table 7.10.

Table 7.10. *Validation Study and Main Study of SIDS (Chu, Gustafson and Le 2010)*

	Validation sample				Main study		
	$Y = 1$		$Y = 0$				
X	$X^* = 1$	$X^* = 0$	$X^* = 1$	$X^* = 0$	Y	$X^* = 1$	$X^* = 0$
1	29	17	21	16	1	122	442
0	22	143	12	168	0	101	479

(Morrissey and Spiegelman 1999; Lyles 2002)
(Chu, Gustafson and Le 2010)

7.12. We consider data from a case–control study in which each subject has an underlying true, but unobserved, exposure X, coded as 1 for exposure and 0 for nonexposure. Exposure is assessed by applying two tests (standard and new tests) to each individual. Let X_1^* and X_2^* denote the measurements obtained from the two tests, which are coded as 1 for a positive result and 0 for a negative result. Let Y be the disease status, coded as 1 for a case and 0 for a control. Assume that each test nondifferentially misclassifies exposure. The data are summarized in Table 7.11.

Table 7.11. *Layout of Case–Control Data Obtained from Two Tests*

	Cases			Controls	
	$X_2^* = 1$	$X_2^* = 0$		$X_2^* = 1$	$X_2^* = 0$
$X_1^* = 1$	n_{111}	n_{110}	$X_1^* = 1$	n_{011}	n_{010}
$X_1^* = 0$	n_{101}	n_{100}	$X_1^* = 0$	n_{001}	n_{000}

For $j = 0, 1$, define

$$\alpha_j = P(X_2^* = j | X = j, X_1^* = j)$$

and

$$\beta_j = P(X_2^* = j | X = j, X_1^* = 1 - j).$$

To reflect the difference between α_j and β_j, we reparameterize them as

$$\alpha_j = \beta_j \phi_j \text{ for } j = 0, 1,$$

where ϕ_0 and ϕ_1 both taking value 1 represent that the two tests independently give measurements. Let $\theta = (\alpha_0, \alpha_1, \beta_0, \beta_1)^{\text{T}}$.

(a) Construct a retrospective likelihood for parameters θ, ϕ_0 and ϕ_1.
(b) Are parameters θ, ϕ_0 and ϕ_1 estimable by applying the formulation of (a) to the data in Table 7.11 ?
(c) Assuming that ϕ_0 and ϕ_1 are known, can you perform inference about θ using the EM algorithm?
(d) Assuming that ϕ_0 and ϕ_1 are known, can you perform inference about the odds ratio

$$\psi = \frac{P(X = 1|Y = 1)P(X = 0|Y = 0)}{P(X = 1|Y = 0)P(X = 0|Y = 1)}?$$

(e) Drews, Flanders and Kosinski (1993) considered data arising from a case–control study of sudden infant death syndrome (SIDS). The data include 213 SIDS victims (cases) and 216 controls. The exposure variable is defined to be the status of "maternal anemia during pregnancy". Exposure data are obtained from two sources: medical records and maternal interviews. Taking the interview data to represent test 1 results and medical records as test 2 measurements, we display the data in Table 7.12. Letting ϕ_0 and ϕ_1 assume various values between 0 and 1, conduct sensitivity analyses for this data set.

Table 7.12. *Case–Control Data of Sudden Infant Death Syndrome Collected from Medical Records and Interviews (Drews, Flanders and Kosinski 1993)*

	Cases			Controls	
	$X_2^* = 1$	$X_2^* = 0$		$X_2^* = 1$	$X_2^* = 0$
$X_1^* = 1$	24	49	$X_1^* = 1$	20	34
$X_1^* = 0$	15	125	$X_1^* = 0$	15	147

(Drews, Flanders and Kosinski 1993)

7.13. Prescott and Garthwaite (2005) discussed case–control data arising from a study of smoking and myocardial infarct. A case (disease present) is indicated by $Y = 1$ and a control (disease absent) by $Y = 0$. The information of smoking was obtained from the doctor's record and the patient's recall. The doctor's record (denoted as X) is treated as a gold standard measure and a patient's recall (denoted as X^*) is supposed to be potentially misclassified. The data are summarized in Tables 7.13 and 7.14, where the main study include 153 subjects and the internal validation subsample contains 100 subjects. Analyze this data set using a method discussed in this chapter.

Table 7.13. *Counts for the Validation Subsample Classified by the Smoking Exposure of the Doctor's Record and Patient's Recall (Prescott and Garthwaite 2005)*

	Cases ($Y = 1$)		Controls ($Y = 0$)	
X^*	$X = 1$	$X = 0$	$X = 1$	$X = 0$
1	27	1	14	4
0	2	20	3	29

(Prescott and Garthwaite 2005)

Table 7.14. *Counts for the Main Study Sample Classified by the Smoking Exposure of the Patient's Recall (Prescott and Garthwaite 2005)*

		Controls ($Y = 0$)	
		$X^* = 1$	$X^* = 0$
Cases	$X^* = 1$	12	26
($Y = 1$)	$X^* = 0$	5	10

7.14. Analyze the case–control data displayed in Table 2.4. Specifically, apply the regression calibration method, discussed in §2.5.2, to the retrospective model derived from one of the following prospective models for the relationship between Y and X; and compare the results:

(a) The logistic regression model

$$\text{logit}\, P(Y = 1|X) = \beta_0 + \beta_x X, \tag{7.55}$$

where β_0 and β_x are regression coefficients;

(b) Replace the logit link in (7.55) with the probit link function;

(c) Replace the logit link in (7.55) with the complementary log-log link function.

8

Analysis with Mismeasured Responses

In many settings, precise measurements of variables are difficult or expensive to obtain. Both response and covariate variables are equally likely to be mismeasured. Measurement error in covariates has received extensive research interest. A large body of analysis methods, as discussed in the aforementioned chapters, has been developed in the literature. Issues on mismeasured responses, on the other hand, have been relatively less explored.

With a continuous response variable described by a linear regression model, response measurement error, if assuming a linear form, may be ignored because this error may be featured in combination with the noise term in the model. Ignorance of measurement error in response is, however, not always reasonable. With nonlinear regression models for response processes or nonlinear error in response variables, error in response basically needs to be accounted for in order to conduct valid inferences. This chapter covers several inference procedures for handling response measurement error in different contexts. Both univariate and correlated data with error-prone responses are discussed. Methods of handling measurement error in both response and covariates are also explored briefly in this chapter.

8.1 Introduction

Let Y be the true response variable which may not be observed, and let Y^* be its observed measurement or surrogate version. As in the aforementioned chapters, we let Z denote error-free covariate vector and $h(\cdot|\cdot)$ denote the conditional distribution for the corresponding variables.

G. Y. Yi, *Statistical Analysis with Measurement Error or Misclassification*,
Springer Series in Statistics, DOI 10.1007/978-1-4939-6640-0_8

Surrogate variables are defined distinctively in different contexts. For instance, in the context without covariate measurement error, Prentice (1989) suggested a criterion for *outcome surrogacy* which requires that

$$h(y|y^*, z) = h(y|y^*). \tag{8.1}$$

This definition implies that the covariate effect of Z on the outcome Y would act solely through surrogate Y^*, hence allowing us to base inferences totally on surrogate outcome data.

This requirement is, however, restrictive and often difficult to verify in application (Pepe 1992). Our discussion on surrogate outcome data is somewhat different. We consider settings where Y^* and Y are correlated in the sense that

$$h(y^*|y, z) \neq h(y^*|z),$$

i.e., given covariate Z, Y^* and Y are not independent. To avoid confusion with the surrogacy defined by Prentice (1989), we use the *proxy* rather than the *surrogate outcome* to refer to Y^* throughout this chapter.

The discussion in this chapter includes two types of measurement error problems: (1) response measurement error only, and (2) both response and covariate variables are subject to measurement error. Such a development complements and extends the discussion in the preceding chapters.

In the instance where only the response variable is subject to measurement error or misclassification, inferences may proceed with the joint distribution of Y, Y^* and Z, which is factorized as

$$h(y, y^*, z) = h(y^*, y|z)h(z).$$

To study the relationship between Y and Z, we often focus on the conditional distribution $h(y^*, y|z)$ without modeling the distribution $h(z)$ of Z. The conditional distribution $h(y^*, y|z)$ is factorized as

$$h(y, y^*|z) = h(y^*|y, z)h(y|z),$$

where $h(y|z)$ is of interest to be modeled and $h(y^*|y, z)$ characterizes the response measurement error process.

If

$$h(y^*|y, z) = h(y^*|z),$$

or equivalently,

$$h(y|y^*, z) = h(y|z), \tag{8.2}$$

we call this *nondifferential response measurement error*, otherwise *differential response measurement error*. When Y is a discrete variable or vector, one may also refer to (8.2) as a *nondifferential response misclassification*, otherwise *differential response misclassification*. This definition is analogous to the covariate measurement error mechanisms described in §2.4. It says that if response measurement error is nondifferential, proxy Y^* does not carry additional information on explaining the relationship between Y and Z.

When both the response and covariate variables are subject to measurement error, inferences are more complicated. In addition to response variable Y, its proxy Y^*, and error-free covariate Z, we use symbol X to represent an error-contaminated covariate vector and X^* to be its observed version. The joint distribution of Y, Y^*, X, X^* and Z is written as

$$h(y, y^*, x, x^*, z) = h(y, y^*, x, x^*|z)h(z),$$

where the marginal distribution $h(z)$ of Z is often left unspecified.

Inferences are then carried out based on the conditional distribution $h(y, y^*, x, x^*|z)$. Although there are multiple ways to examine $h(y, y^*, x, x^*|z)$, it is convenient to write $h(y, y^*, x, x^*|z)$ as

$$h(y, y^*, x, x^*|z) = h(y|y^*, x, x^*, z)h(y^*, x, x^*|z) \tag{8.3}$$

or

$$h(y, y^*, x, x^*|z) = h(y^*|y, x, x^*, z)h(y, x, x^*|z). \tag{8.4}$$

These factorizations give us a basis to study the relationship between the response Y and true covariates $\{X, Z\}$. The choice of (8.3) or (8.4) is driven by the characteristics of measurement error. In the situation where

$$h(y|y^*, x, x^*, z) = h(y|x, z), \tag{8.5}$$

using factorization (8.3) enables us to directly perform inference on $h(y|x, z)$, where $h(y^*, x, x^*|z)$ is further factorized into conditional distributions pertinent to the response and covariate measurement error processes. Errors satisfying (8.5) are called *nondifferential errors-in-variables*, otherwise *differential errors-in-variables*.

On the other hand, factorization (8.4) allows us to invoke the strategies of handling covariate measurement error discussed in the previous chapters. In this instance, inference about $h(y|x, z)$ is conducted based on examining $h(y, x, x^*|z)$ which involves the covariate measurement error process, whereas $h(y^*|y, x, x^*, z)$ facilitates the response measurement error process. An example of using factorization (8.4) is provided in §8.2.2.

8.2 Effects of Misclassified Responses on Model Structures

In this section, we consider the situation where the response variable or vector is binary and subject to misclassification. The discussion focuses on how misclassification may change the model structure for response variables. Both cross-sectional data and correlated data are discussed.

8.2.1 Univariate Binary Response with Misclassification

For individual i, let Y_i be the univariate binary response, taking values 0 and 1; and Z_i be the vector of precisely measured covariates. We assume that conditional on Z_i, Y_i is postulated by a binary regression model falling in the class of generalized linear models with the probability mass function

$$f(y_i|z_i;\xi_i) = \exp\left[\{y_i\xi_i - b(\xi_i)\} + c(y_i)\right], \tag{8.6}$$

where ξ_i is the canonical parameter and $b(\cdot)$ and $c(\cdot)$ are known functions. This probability mass function immediately gives that the mean and variance of Y_i, given Z_i, are, respectively, the first and second derivatives of $b(\xi_i)$ with

$$E(Y_i|Z_i) = b'(\xi_i) \text{ and } \mathrm{var}(Y_i|Z_i) = b''(\xi_i).$$

To explicitly show the relationship between the response and covariate variables, we model the conditional mean response given covariates, $\mu_i = E(Y_i|Z_i)$, via a link function $g(\cdot)$:

$$g(\mu_i) = \eta_{zi},$$

where

$$\eta_{zi} = \beta_0 + \beta_z^{\mathrm{T}} Z_i$$

is the linear predictor, β_0 is the intercept, and the parameter vector β_z measures the covariate effects of Z_i. The link function is assumed to be strictly monotone and differentiable. Common choices of $g(\cdot)$ for binary data include the logistic, probit and complementary log-log functions (McCullagh and Nelder 1989, p. 31).

Suppose that Y_i is subject to misclassification and Y_i^* is an observed value of Y_i. Let

$$\gamma_{01}(Z_i) = P(Y_i^* = 1|Y_i = 0, Z_i) \text{ and } \gamma_{10}(Z_i) = P(Y_i^* = 0|Y_i = 1, Z_i)$$

denote the response misclassification probabilities. The probability $1 - \gamma_{10}(Z_i)$ is often called the *sensitivity* of the measurement Y_i^*, and $1 - \gamma_{01}(Z_i)$ is called the *specificity*. The conditional probability of the observed measurement Y_i^*, given Z_i, is linked with the conditional probability of the true response Y_i, given Z_i, via

$$P(Y_i^* = 1|Z_i) = \gamma_{01}(Z_i) + \{1 - \gamma_{01}(Z_i) - \gamma_{10}(Z_i)\}P(Y_i = 1|Z_i). \tag{8.7}$$

To see the structure difference between $P(Y_i = 1|Z_i)$ and $P(Y_i^* = 1|Z_i)$, we begin with a simple case where the misclassification probabilities are free of covariates:

$$\gamma_{01}(Z_i) = \gamma_{01} \text{ and } \gamma_{10}(Z_i) = \gamma_{10},$$

where γ_{01} and γ_{10} are nonnegative constants no greater than 1. This assumption in lines with the outcome surrogacy condition (8.1) discussed by Prentice (1989). Define $\mu_i^* = P(Y_i^* = 1|Z_i)$. Then (8.7) gives

$$\eta_{zi} = g\left(\frac{\mu_i^* - \gamma_{01}}{1 - \gamma_{01} - \gamma_{10}}\right),$$

implying that η_{zi} may be viewed as a function of μ_i^*, given the constancy assumption about γ_{01} and γ_{10}. Let $g^*(\cdot)$ denote such a function that

$$\eta_{zi} = g^*(\mu_i^*).$$

Differentiating the identity

$$g^*(\mu_i^*) = g\left(\frac{\mu_i^* - \gamma_{01}}{1 - \gamma_{01} - \gamma_{10}}\right)$$

with respect to μ_i^*, we obtain

$$\frac{\partial g^*(\mu_i^*)}{\partial \mu_i^*} = g'\left(\frac{\mu_i^* - \gamma_{01}}{1 - \gamma_{01} - \gamma_{10}}\right)\left(\frac{1}{1 - \gamma_{01} - \gamma_{10}}\right). \tag{8.8}$$

By the monotonicity of $g(\cdot)$ and the constancy assumption for γ_{01} and γ_{10}, $g^*(\cdot)$ is monotone. In particular, if $\gamma_{01} + \gamma_{10} < 1$, then $g^*(\cdot)$ and $g(\cdot)$ are both increasing or decreasing at the same time; otherwise, the monotonicity of $g^*(\cdot)$ and $g(\cdot)$ is opposite. The assumption $\gamma_{01} + \gamma_{10} < 1$ is often feasible, since both values of γ_{01} and of γ_{10} being larger than 0.5 would indicate that the measurement procedure of Y_i is useless: a chance operation, say, flipping a fair coin, would more likely yield a better measurement of Y_i than the actually measured value Y_i^*.

This derivation says that μ_i^* is linked with the linear predictor η_{zi} through a monotone, differential link function $g^*(\cdot)$:

$$g^*(\mu_i^*) = \eta_{zi},$$

thus the observed response Y_i^* still follows a generalized linear model. The only difference between the models of $P(Y_i = 1|Z_i)$ and $P(Y_i^* = 1|Z_i)$ is reflected by the difference in the link functions $g(\cdot)$ and $g^*(\cdot)$. Consequently, ignoring the feature of response misclassification in the analysis has the same effects as misspecifying the link function in the analysis for generalized linear models. These results are valid under the condition that the misclassification probabilities are constants.

For general situations where misclassification probability $\gamma_{01}(Z_i)$ or $\gamma_{10}(Z_i)$ depends on covariate Z_i, (8.8) does not hold anymore. The derivative $\partial g^*(\mu_i^*)/\partial \mu_i^*$ has a more complicated dependence on μ_i^*:

$$\frac{\partial g^*(\mu_i^*)}{\partial \mu_i^*} = g'\left\{\frac{\mu_i^* - \gamma_{01}(Z_i)}{1 - \gamma_{01}(Z_i) - \gamma_{10}(Z_i)}\right\}\left\{\frac{1 - D(Z_i)}{1 - \gamma_{01}(Z_i) - \gamma_{10}(Z_i)}\right\},$$

where

$$D(Z_i) = \frac{\partial \gamma_{01}(Z_i)}{\partial \mu_i^*} - \left\{\frac{\mu_i^* - \gamma_{01}(Z_i)}{1 - \gamma_{01}(Z_i) - \gamma_{10}(Z_i)}\right\}\left\{\frac{\partial \gamma_{01}(Z_i)}{\partial \mu_i^*} + \frac{\partial \gamma_{10}(Z_i)}{\partial \mu_i^*}\right\}.$$

Since the factor $D(Z_i)$ generally varies with the covariate values, the derivative $\partial g^*(\mu_i^*)/\partial \mu_i^*$ is not necessarily uniformly positive or negative, indicating that $g^*(\cdot)$ is not monotone anymore and that the model for $P(Y_i^* = 1|Z_i)$ does not necessarily fall in the family of the generalized linear models. A detailed discussion on this point was provided by Neuhaus (1999).

In summary, misclassification in the response variable may change the structure of the response model, and the change degree depends on the nature of the misclassification probabilities. If the model for Y_i given Z_i is a generalized linear model, then the model for the surrogate Y_i^* given Z_i can or cannot be a generalized linear model, depending on whether or not the misclassification probabilities are constants. In the case where the misclassification probabilities are constants, models for both $P(Y_i = 1|Z_i)$ and $P(Y_i^* = 1|Z_i)$ are generalized linear models, but the models may differ in the link function form.

8.2.2 Univariate Binary Data with Misclassification in Response and Measurement Error in Covariates

In addition to misclassification in response variable Y_i considered in §8.2.1, suppose some covariates are subject to measurement error. Let X_i denote the vector of error-prone covariates for individual i, X_i^* be the observed version of X_i, and Z_i be the vector of precisely measured covariates.

The conditional probability for the observed data may be written as

$$\begin{aligned} P(Y_i^* = 1|X_i^*, Z_i) = {} & P(Y_i^* = 1, Y_i = 0|X_i^*, Z_i) \\ & + P(Y_i^* = 1, Y_i = 1|X_i^*, Z_i), \end{aligned} \tag{8.9}$$

where for $y = 0, 1$, the probability $P(Y_i^* = 1, Y_i = y|X_i^*, Z_i)$ may be expressed as

$$\int P(Y_i^* = 1, Y_i = y|X_i = x, X_i^* = x_i^*, Z_i) f(x|x_i^*, Z_i) d\eta(x) \tag{8.10}$$

to reflect the role of the covariate measurement error process, featured by the model $f(x|x_i^*, Z_i)$ for the conditional distribution of X_i, given $\{X_i^*, Z_i\}$. Aligning with (8.4), one may further consider the factorization

$$\begin{aligned} & P(Y_i^* = 1, Y_i = y|X_i, X_i^*, Z_i) \\ = {} & P(Y_i^* = 1|Y_i = y, X_i, X_i^*, Z_i) P(Y_i = y|X_i, X_i^*, Z_i). \end{aligned} \tag{8.11}$$

If assuming the nondifferential covariate measurement error mechanism:

$$P(Y_i = y|X_i^*, X_i, Z_i) = P(Y_i = y|X_i, Z_i) \text{ for } y = 0, 1, \tag{8.12}$$

then combining (8.10) and (8.11) with (8.9) gives us a link between the conditional probability $P(Y_i^* = 1|X_i^*, Z_i)$ for the observed data and the conditional probability $P(Y_i = 1|X_i, Z_i)$ of interest. Moreover, these derivations show how models for the measurement error processes of the covariate and response variables, $f(x|x^*, z)$ and $P(Y_i^* = 1|Y_i, X_i, Z_i, X_i^*)$, may come into play when using the observed data to carry out inferences about $P(Y_i = 1|X_i, Z_i)$.

If $P(Y_i^* = 1|Y_i = y, X_i^*, X_i, Z_i)$ does not depend on X_i, then combining (8.10) and (8.11) with (8.9) gives that

$$
\begin{aligned}
&P(Y_i^* = 1|X_i^*, Z_i) = \gamma_{01}(X_i^*, Z_i) \\
&+\{1 - \gamma_{01}(X_i^*, Z_i) - \gamma_{10}(X_i^*, Z_i)\}E\{P(Y_i = 1|X_i, Z_i)|X_i^*, Z_i\}, \quad (8.13)
\end{aligned}
$$

where

$$
\begin{aligned}
\gamma_{01}(X_i^*, Z_i) &= P(Y_i^* = 1|Y_i = 0, X_i^*, Z_i), \\
\gamma_{10}(X_i^*, Z_i) &= P(Y_i^* = 0|Y_i = 1, X_i^*, Z_i),
\end{aligned}
$$

and the expectation is evaluated with respect to the model for the conditional distribution of X_i given $\{X_i^*, Z_i\}$.

Expression (8.13) illustrates that even under certain simplified assumptions, the conditional distribution $P(Y_i^* = 1|X_i^*, Z_i)$ for the observed data generally does not possess the same regression form as the conditional distribution $P(Y_i = 1|X_i, Z_i)$, the quantity of prime interest. In an extreme situation with

$$P(Y_i^* = 0|Y_i = 1, X_i^*, Z_i) = 1 - P(Y_i^* = 1|Y_i = 0, X_i^*, Z_i),$$

modeling the observed data $\{Y_i^*, X_i^*, Z_i\}$ is not helpful in conducting inference about the parameter associated with the model for $P(Y_i = 1|X_i, Z_i)$.

Comparing (8.13) to (8.7) in §8.2.1, we see that covariate measurement error adds through a conditional expectation of $P(Y_i = 1|X_i, Z_i)$,

$$E\{P(Y_i = 1|X_i, Z_i)|X_i^*, Z_i\},$$

whose structure is often quite different from that of $P(Y_i = 1|X_i, Z_i)$. This illustrates that in general, measurement error in both response and covariate variables has more complex effects on altering the model structure than measurement error in the response variable alone. This finding is not unexpected. However, in some special situations, as illustrated in the following example, the expectation $E\{P(Y_i = 1|X_i, Z_i)|X_i^*, Z_i\}$ and the probability $P(Y_i = 1|X_i, Z_i)$ share some similarity in the structure. In this case, the presence of covariate measurement error does not necessarily introduce additional complexity in contrast to the case where only the response variable is subject to measurement error.

Example 8.1. Suppose that the binary outcome is associated with the covariates through a regression model

$$P(Y_i = 1|X_i, Z_i) = \Phi^{-1}(\beta_0 + \beta_x X_i + \beta_z^{\mathrm{T}} Z_i),$$

where X_i is scalar and $\beta = (\beta_0, \beta_x, \beta_z^{\mathrm{T}})^{\mathrm{T}}$ is the vector of regression coefficients.

Suppose the (mis)classification probabilities for the response variable $P(Y_i^* = 1|Y_i = y, X_i^*, X_i, Z_i)$ do not depend on X_i and (8.12) holds. Assume that the conditional distribution of X_i, given $\{X_i^*, Z_i\}$, is the normal distribution $N(X_i^*, \Sigma_x)$ with variance Σ_x. Then

$$E\{P(Y_i = 1|X_i, Z_i)|X_i^*, Z_i\} = \Phi(\beta_0^* + \beta_x^* X_i^* + \beta_z^{*\mathrm{T}} Z_i), \tag{8.14}$$

where $\beta_0^* = \Lambda_x \beta_0, \beta_x^* = \Lambda_x \beta_x, \beta_z^* = \Lambda_x \beta_z$, and $\Lambda_x = \{1 + \beta_x^2 \Sigma_x\}^{-1/2}$.

Model (8.13) for the observed data then reduces to

$$\begin{aligned} P(Y_i^* = 1|X_i^*, Z_i) &= \gamma_{01}(X_i^*, Z_i) \\ &\quad + \{1 - \gamma_{01}(X_i^*, Z_i) - \gamma_{10}(X_i^*, Z_i)\}\Phi(\beta_0^* + \beta_x^* X_i^* + \beta_z^{*\mathrm{T}} Z_i), \end{aligned}$$

showing that the conditional probability for the observed data does not retain the same probit regression structure as that for the conditional probability $P(Y = 1|X, Z)$. However, if the misclassification probabilities $\gamma_{01}(X_i^*, Z_i)$ and $\gamma_{10}(X_i^*, Z_i)$ are constants, repeating the argument in §8.2.1 shows that ignoring measurement error in both response and covariate variables in the analysis can be regarded as misspecifying the probit link function of the model for $P(Y_i = 1|X_i, Z_i)$, the same effect as ignoring measurement error in the response variable alone.

8.2.3 Clustered Binary Data with Error in Responses

For individual i, let $Y_i = (Y_{i1}, \ldots, Y_{im_i})^{\mathrm{T}}$ be the binary response vector where m_i may be common or vary with i and $i = 1, \ldots, n$. With common m_i, Y_i may represent a multivariate response or a regularly assessed longitudinal vector for subject i, while a variable size m_i allows us to record clustered data or irregularly spaced longitudinal data by using Y_i. In the following discussion, we phase i as an index for a cluster and j for a subject for ease of terminology. Let Z_{ij} denote the covariate vector for cluster i and subject j for $j = 1, \ldots, m_i$ and $i = 1, \ldots, n$; and $Z_i = (Z_{i1}^{\mathrm{T}}, \ldots, Z_{im_i}^{\mathrm{T}})^{\mathrm{T}}$.

Suppose that we do not observe Y_{ij} but instead, observe an error-corrupted version Y_{ij}^*. In principle, misclassification probabilities may depend on all the true responses and covariates in a cluster. For ease of modeling, however, we assume that for all i and j,

$$P(Y_{ij}^* = 1|Y_i, Z_i) = P(Y_{ij}^* = 1|Y_{ij}, Z_i) = P(Y_{ij}^* = 1|Y_{ij}, Z_{ij}). \tag{8.15}$$

These assumptions are reasonable in describing situations, such as applying a common diagnostic test procedure to patients, where error-prone results for one subject do not depend on the results of others.

For $i = 1, \ldots, n$ and $j = 1, \ldots, m_i$, let

$$\gamma_{01}(Z_i) = P(Y_{ij}^* = 1|Y_{ij} = 0, Z_i) \text{ and } \gamma_{10}(Z_i) = P(Y_{ij}^* = 0|Y_{ij} = 1, Z_i)$$

denote the misclassification probabilities. Following the discussion of Neuhaus (2002), we examine misclassification effects on two estimation approaches based on model settings discussed in §5.1.

Population-Average Approach: GEE

The population-average approach stresses modeling the first two moments for the response components Y_{ij}. Marginally, the probability mass function of Y_{ij} is described by (8.6); the conditional mean of Y_{ij} relates to the covariate vector Z_{ij} through the link function $g(\cdot)$ with

$$g\{E(Y_{ij}|Z_{ij})\} = \eta_{zij}, \tag{8.16}$$

where $\eta_{zij} = \beta_0 + \beta_z^{\mathrm{T}} Z_{ij}$ is the linear predictor, the parameter vector β_z measures the covariate effects of Z_{ij}, and β_0 is the intercept. Let $\beta = (\beta_0, \beta_z^{\mathrm{T}})^{\mathrm{T}}$.

Define $\mu_{ij}^* = P(Y_{ij}^* = 1|Z_{ij})$. As shown in §8.2.1, if misclassification probabilities $\gamma_{01}(Z_i)$ and $\gamma_{10}(Z_i)$ are constants, then μ_{ij}^* is connected with the linear predictor η_{zij} via a monotone, differential link function $g^*(\cdot)$:

$$g^*(\mu_{ij}^*) = \eta_{zij}. \tag{8.17}$$

This suggests that the marginal structure of the Y_{ij}^* can still be featured using a generalized linear model with a link different from (8.16).

To examine the covariance structure among the observed components of Y_i^*, we make assumptions for paired components of the misclassification process:

$$\begin{aligned}
&P(Y_{ij}^* = 1, Y_{ik}^* = 1|Y_{ij}, Y_{ik}, Z_i)\\
&= P(Y_{ij}^* = 1|Y_{ij}, Y_{ik}, Z_i)P(Y_{ik}^* = 1|Y_{ij}, Y_{ik}, Z_i)\\
&= P(Y_{ij}^* = 1|Y_{ij}, Z_i)P(Y_{ik}^* = 1|Y_{ik}, Z_i).
\end{aligned}$$

Under these assumptions, we obtain that

$$\mathrm{cov}(Y_{ij}^*, Y_{ik}^*|Z_i) = \{1 - \gamma_{01}(Z_i) - \gamma_{10}(Z_i)\}^2 \mathrm{cov}(Y_{ij}, Y_{ik}|Z_i), \tag{8.18}$$

which says that the conditional covariance structures of the surrogate vector Y_i^* and the true response vector Y_i, given Z_i, differ only by a multiplicative factor $\{1 - \gamma_{01}(Z_i) - \gamma_{10}(Z_i)\}^2$.

Given these comparisons for the mean and covariance structures between Y_i and Y_i^*, we now examine estimation procedures of applying the GEE approach to Y_i or Y_i^*. Specifically, we employ the GEE formulation (5.4) to Y_i or Y_i^* for estimation of β, where

$$P(Y_{ij} = y_{ij}|Z_i) = P(Y_{ij} = y_{ij}|Z_{ij}) \tag{8.19}$$

is assumed, as discussed in §5.1.1, for $j = 1, \ldots, m_i$ and $y_{ij} = 0, 1$. It is easily seen that assumptions (8.15) and (8.19) yield that

$$P(Y_{ij}^* = y_{ij}^*|Z_i) = P(Y_{ij}^* = y_{ij}^*|Z_{ij})$$

for $j = 1, \ldots, m_i$ and $y_{ij}^* = 0, 1$.

Consequently, comparing the structures of μ_{ij}^* and $E(Y_{ij}|Z_{ij})$ based on (8.16) and (8.17), and using (8.18), we obtain an interesting property of the GEE approach.

When the misclassification probabilities $\gamma_{01}(Z_i)$ and $\gamma_{10}(Z_i)$ are constants, applying the precise measurements Y_{ij} to the GEE formulation (5.4) with link function $g(\cdot)$ and covariance matrix V_i is equivalent to using the surrogate responses Y_{ij}^* for the GEE approach with a different link function but the same covariance matrix V_i, because the constant factor $\{1-\gamma_{01}(Z_i)-\gamma_{10}(Z_i)\}$ in (8.18) can be ignored when solving the resulting equations.

Generalized Linear Mixed Model (GLMM)

In contrast to the marginal approach based on the GEE formulation, we discuss the modeling of Y_i by a GLMM outlined in §5.1.2. Conditional on random effects u_i and covariate Z_i, the Y_{ij} are assumed to be independent, each following a model

$$g\{P(Y_{ij}=1|u_i,Z_i)\} = \beta_0 + \beta_z^{\mathrm{T}} Z_{ij} + u_i^{\mathrm{T}} S_{ij}, \tag{8.20}$$

where $\beta = (\beta_0, \beta_z^{\mathrm{T}})^{\mathrm{T}}$ is the parameter vector, $g(\cdot)$ is a link function, and S_{ij} is a covariate vector which may be a subset of Z_i.

We consider the case where the misclassification probabilities do not depend on the random effects u_i and are free of covariates:

$$P(Y_{ij}^*=1|Y_{ij}=0,u_i,Z_i)=\gamma_{01} \text{ and } P(Y_{ij}^*=0|Y_{ij}=1,u_i,Z_i)=\gamma_{10},$$

where γ_{01} and γ_{10} are nonnegative constants no greater than 1. Then the conditional model for the observed responses is

$$P(Y_{ij}^*=1|Z_i,u_i)=\gamma_{01}+(1-\gamma_{01}-\gamma_{10})g^{-1}(\beta_0+\beta_z^{\mathrm{T}} Z_{ij}+u_i^{\mathrm{T}} S_{ij}).$$

Following the arguments in §8.2.1, we can show that if conditional on random effects u_i and covariate Z_i, the marginal model of Y_{ij} follows the GLMM (8.20) with link function $g(\cdot)$, then conditional on the same random effects u_i and covariate Z_i, the observed responses Y_{ij}^* may also be featured by a GLMM with a different link function $g^*(\cdot)$.

Assuming that conditional on random effects u_i and covariate Z_i, the misclassification process possesses the property

$$\begin{aligned} &P(Y_{ij}^*=1,Y_{ik}^*=1|Y_{ij},Y_{ik},u_i,Z_i)\\ &=P(Y_{ij}^*=1|Y_{ij},Y_{ik},u_i,Z_i)P(Y_{ik}^*=1|Y_{ij},Y_{ik},u_i,Z_i)\\ &=P(Y_{ij}^*=1|Y_{ij},Z_i)P(Y_{ik}^*=1|Y_{ik},Z_i),\end{aligned}$$

we obtain that

$$\mathrm{cov}(Y_{ij}^*,Y_{ik}^*|u_i,Z_i)=(1-\gamma_{01}-\gamma_{10})^2\mathrm{cov}(Y_{ij},Y_{ik}|u_i,Z_i). \tag{8.21}$$

Since given u_i and Z_i, the Y_{ij} are conditionally independent, identity (8.21) implies that conditional on u_i and Z_i, Y_{ij}^* and Y_{ik}^* are uncorrelated. Because Y_{ij}^* and Y_{ik}^* are binary, we conclude that Y_{ij}^* and Y_{ik}^* conditionally independent, given u_i and Z_i (see Problem 8.2). These derivations show that given the random effects u_i and covariate Z_i, the conditional *pairwise* independence of the response components Y_{ij}

is not changed when the Y_{ij} are replaced by their proxy measurements Y_{ij}^*. However, the conditional independence among all the response components Y_{ij} is not necessarily retained when the Y_{ij} are replaced by their observed measurements Y_{ij}^* (see Problem 8.2). Finally, compared to the discussion in §5.2.2, we see that response measurement error has different effects on altering the structure of GLMMs than covariate measure error does.

8.3 Methods for Univariate Error-Prone Response

Let Y be the response variable which is subject to measurement error, and Z be an associated covariate vector which is precisely measured. Let Y^* be an observed version of Y. The interest here is focused on estimation of parameter β in the regression model $f(y|z;\beta)$ which postulates the relationship between the response variable Y and covariate Z.

We consider settings where an internal validation sample, indexed by $\mathcal{V}$, is randomly selected from the main study subjects, indexed by $\mathcal{M}$. Let n be the number of subjects in $\mathcal{M}$ and $\{Y_i, Y_i^*, Z_i\}$ denote independent and identically distributed copies of $\{Y, Y^*, Z\}$ for $i = 1, \ldots, n$. When $i \in \mathcal{V}$, measurements of $\{Y_i, Y_i^*, Z_i\}$ are available whereas when $i \in \mathcal{M} \setminus \mathcal{V}$, only measurements for $\{Y_i^*, Z_i\}$ are available.

Likelihood Method

When parametric modeling is used to describe the associated processes, inferences may be based on the likelihood function for the observed data:

$$L = \left\{\prod_{i\in\mathcal{V}} f(y_i, y_i^*|z_i)\right\} \left\{\prod_{i\in\mathcal{M}\setminus\mathcal{V}} f(y_i^*|z_i)\right\}, \tag{8.22}$$

where the contributions of the subjects in the validation sample are reflected by model $f(y_i, y_i^*|z_i)$ for the conditional distribution of $\{Y_i, Y_i^*\}$ given Z_i, while the subjects in the main study contribute via model $f(y_i^*|z_i)$ for the conditional distribution of Y_i^* given Z_i. The dependence on the associated parameter is suppressed in the notation.

In addition to the conditional distribution of Y given Z being postulated by model $f(y|z;\beta)$, suppose the conditional distribution of Y^* given $\{Y, Z\}$ is modeled by $f(y^*|y,z;\gamma)$, where γ is the associated parameter. Then the likelihood (8.22) may be further expressed as

$$\begin{aligned} L(\beta,\gamma) = &\left\{\prod_{i\in\mathcal{V}} f(y_i|z_i;\beta) f(y_i^*|y_i,z_i;\gamma)\right\} \\ &\cdot\left\{\prod_{i\in\mathcal{M}\setminus\mathcal{V}} \int f(y|z_i;\beta) f(y_i^*|y,z_i;\gamma) d\eta(y)\right\}, \end{aligned} \tag{8.23}$$

where similar to measure $d\eta(x)$ defined on page 55, measure $d\eta(y)$ facilitates the two cases for the Y_i: $d\eta(y) = dy$ if the Y_i are continuous, and the integral is replaced with the summation if the Y_i are discrete.

Maximization of the likelihood (8.23) with respect to β and γ gives us consistent estimators of β and γ under regularity conditions. The implementation of the maximum likelihood method is conceptually straightforward and is computationally manageable in certain situations. For instance, with discrete Y_i, the terms in (8.23) are often tractable; when Y_i is continuous with a convenient distributional form such as a normal distribution, the evaluation of the integrals in (8.23) is possible with standard numerical integration techniques (e.g., Problem 8.3).

Mean Score Method

When directly calculating or approximating the integrals in (8.23) is difficult, one may consider an alternative, such as the EM algorithm, to get around the problem. In these instances, we write the log-likelihood for complete data based on the model for $\{Y, Y^*\}$ given Z:

$$\ell_{\mathrm{C}}(\beta,\gamma) = \ell_{\mathrm{CV}}(\beta,\gamma) + \ell_{\mathrm{CM}}(\beta,\gamma)$$

where $\ell_{\mathrm{CV}}(\beta,\gamma) = \sum_{i\in\mathcal{V}} \ell_{\mathrm{C}i}(\beta,\gamma)$, $\ell_{\mathrm{CM}}(\beta,\gamma) = \sum_{i\in\mathcal{M}\setminus\mathcal{V}} \ell_{\mathrm{C}i}(\beta,\gamma)$, and

$$\ell_{\mathrm{C}i}(\beta,\gamma) = \log f(y_i|z_i;\beta) + \log f(y_i^*|y_i,z_i;\gamma).$$

Since the measurements involved in $\ell_{\mathrm{CV}}(\beta,\gamma)$ are all available from the validation sample, when implementing the E-step for the log-likelihood $\ell_{\mathrm{C}}(\beta,\gamma)$, it is only necessary to evaluate the conditional expectation of $\ell_{\mathrm{CM}}(\beta,\gamma)$ with respect to the model for the "missing" data, Y_i, given the observed data $\{Y_i^*, Z_i\}$, evaluated at the estimated parameter values of the previous iteration.

To be specific, for $k = 0, 1, \ldots$, at iteration $(k+1)$ of the E-step, we calculate

$$Q(\beta,\gamma;\beta^{(k)},\gamma^{(k)}) = \ell_{\mathrm{CV}}(\beta,\gamma) + \sum_{i\in\mathcal{M}\setminus\mathcal{V}} E\{\ell_{\mathrm{C}i}(\beta,\gamma)|Y_i^*, Z_i;\beta^{(k)},\gamma^{(k)}\},$$

where the conditional expectation is taken with respect to the model

$$f(y_i|y_i^*,z_i;\beta,\gamma) = \frac{f(y_i^*|y_i,z_i;\gamma)f(y_i|z_i;\beta)}{\int f(y_i^*|y,z_i;\gamma)f(y|z_i;\beta)d\eta(y)} \tag{8.24}$$

for the conditional distribution of Y_i given $\{Y_i^*, Z_i\}$, with β and γ, respectively, replaced by their estimates at the kth iteration, $\beta^{(k)}$ and $\gamma^{(k)}$.

The M-step is consequently invoked to maximize $Q(\beta,\gamma;\beta^{(k)},\gamma^{(k)})$ with respect to β and γ to produce their updated values for iteration $(k+1)$. Under suitable regularity conditions, including the exchangeability between the operations of expectation and differentiation, the maximization is equivalent to finding the solution of the partial derivatives of $Q(\beta,\gamma;\beta^{(k)},\gamma^{(k)})$ with respect to β and γ.

This equivalence motivates the so-called *mean score method* proposed by Pepe, Reilly and Fleming (1994). If parameters β and γ are functionally independent, estimation of β may proceed with finding the solution of the partial derivative of $Q(\beta, \gamma; \beta, \gamma)$ with respect to β:

$$\sum_{i \in \mathcal{V}} \frac{\partial \log f(y_i|z_i;\beta)}{\partial \beta} + \sum_{i \in \mathcal{M} \setminus \mathcal{V}} E\left\{ \left. \frac{\partial \log f(Y_i|Z_i;\beta)}{\partial \beta} \right| Y_i^*, Z_i \right\} = 0, \quad (8.25)$$

where the conditional expectation is evaluated with respect to the model, $f(y_i|y_i^*, z_i)$, for Y_i given Y_i^* and Z_i.

The validity of this method may be justified from the viewpoint of estimating function theory. It is easily seen that the estimating functions in (8.25) have zero mean, i.e., are unbiased, thus under regularity conditions, solving (8.25) for β yields a consistent estimator of β (see §1.3.2).

The evaluation of the expectation in (8.25) generally requires the knowledge of model $f(y_i|y_i^*, z_i)$ for the conditional distribution of Y_i, given Y_i^* and Z_i. This may be done based on using (8.24) if one is willing to use a parametric model for $f(y_i^*|y_i, z_i)$. On the other hand, one may replace the conditional expectation $E\{\partial \log f(Y_i|Z_i;\beta)/\partial\beta | Y_i^*, Z_i\}$ with a nonparametric estimate and then proceed with estimation of β using (8.25).

With low dimensional and discrete Y_i^* and Z_i, Pepe, Reilly and Fleming (1994) suggested using the validation data to estimate the expectation $E\{\partial \log f(Y_i|Z_i;\beta)/\partial\beta | Y_i^*, Z_i\}$ by

$$\sum_{k \in \mathcal{V}(y_i^*, z_i)} \frac{\partial \log f(y_k|z_k;\beta)}{\partial \beta} \cdot \frac{1}{n_{\mathrm{v}}(y_i^*, z_i)},$$

where $\mathcal{V}(y_i^*, z_i)$ denotes the index set for the subjects in the validation sample whose values of (Y^*, Z) equal (y_i^*, z_i), and $n_{\mathrm{v}}(y_i^*, z_i)$ denotes the number of subjects in $\mathcal{V}(y_i^*, z_i)$. Then substitute this estimate into (8.25), and solve

$$\sum_{i \in \mathcal{V}} \frac{\partial \log f(y_i|z_i;\beta)}{\partial \beta} + \sum_{i \in \mathcal{M} \setminus \mathcal{V}} \left\{ \sum_{k \in \mathcal{V}(y_i^*, z_i)} \frac{\partial \log f(y_k|z_k;\beta)}{\partial \beta} \cdot \frac{1}{n_{\mathrm{v}}(y_i^*, z_i)} \right\} = 0 \quad (8.26)$$

for β.

Let $\widehat{\beta}$ denote the resultant estimator of β. Under suitable regularity conditions, $\widehat{\beta}$ is a consistent estimator for β and $\sqrt{n}(\widehat{\beta} - \beta)$ has the asymptotic normal distribution with mean zero. Details may be found in Pepe, Reilly and Fleming (1994).

Semiparametric Method

The mean score method based on (8.26) is a semiparametric approach where the conditional distribution of Y_i given Z_i is modeled parametrically, but no structure is placed on the model $f(y_i^*|y_i, z_i)$ for the measurement error process. Although this method typically applies when Y_i^* and Z_i are discrete and their dimensions are low, it can be extended to more general settings, as discussed by Pepe (1992). We now elaborate on the extensions.

To facilitate various dependence of proxy Y_i^* on the covariates, we let S_i denote the subvector of Z_i which is thought to be informative with respect to the association between Y_i^* and Y_i. That is,

$$f(y_i^*|y_i, z_i) = f(y_i^*|y_i, s_i),$$

where $f(\cdot|\cdot)$ represents the model for the conditional distribution of the corresponding variables. In extreme situations, if Y_i^* is conditionally independent of the covariates, given Y_i, S_i is null; taking S_i to be Z_i gives an opposite scenario where the entire covariate vector is related to the surrogate Y_i^* even after conditioning on Y_i.

Write

$$f(y_i^*|z_i; \beta) = \int f(y|z_i; \beta) f(y_i^*|y, s_i) d\eta(y), \tag{8.27}$$

where $f(y_i^*|y_i, s_i)$ is given by

$$f(y_i^*|y_i, s_i) = \frac{f(y_i^*, y_i, s_i)}{f(y_i, s_i)}, \tag{8.28}$$

$f(y_i^*, y_i, s_i)$ is the model for the joint distribution of $\{Y_i^*, Y_i, S_i\}$, and $f(y_i, s_i)$ is the model for the joint distribution of $\{Y_i, S_i\}$.

The idea here is to place no specific model structure on $f(y_i^*|y_i, s_i)$ to avoid potential misspecification of the measurement error process. This is virtually equivalent to regarding $f(y_i^*|y_i, s_i)$ as an infinite-dimensional parameter. Without loss of generality, it is plausible to assume that $f(y_i^*|y_i, s_i)$ is functionally independent of β. Consequently, inference about β is based on the likelihood

$$L(\beta) = \left\{ \prod_{i \in \mathcal{V}} f(y_i|z_i; \beta) \right\} \left\{ \prod_{i \in \mathcal{M} \setminus \mathcal{V}} f(y_i^*|z_i; \beta) \right\}, \tag{8.29}$$

which comes from (8.22) with the terms $f(y_i^*|y_i, s_i)$ dropped from the first product. Thereby, it suffices to characterize $f(y_i^*|z_i; \beta)$ for the main study data, which is, by (8.27) and (8.28), determined by $f(y_i^*, y_i, s_i)$ and $f(y_i, s_i)$, together with $f(y|z_i; \beta)$.

To avoid strong modeling assumptions, we estimate function forms $f(y^*, y, s)$ and $f(y, s)$ nonparametrically using the validation sample. Let $\widehat{f}(y^*, y, s)$ and $\widehat{f}(y, s)$ denote their estimates, respectively. Then (8.28) leads to an estimate of $f(y^*|y, s)$:

$$\widehat{f}(y^*|y,s) = \frac{\widehat{f}(y^*,y,s)}{\widehat{f}(y,s)},$$

hence by (8.29), yielding the *estimated* likelihood

$$\widehat{L}(\beta) = \left\{ \prod_{i\in\mathcal{V}} f(y_i|z_i;\beta) \right\} \left\{ \prod_{i\in\mathcal{M}\setminus\mathcal{V}} \widehat{f}(y_i^*|z_i;\beta) \right\}, \tag{8.30}$$

where $\widehat{f}(y_i^*|z_i;\beta) = \int f(y|z_i;\beta)\widehat{f}(y_i^*|y,s_i)d\eta(y)$ for $i \in \mathcal{M}\setminus\mathcal{V}$.

An estimate of β may be obtained by maximizing the estimated likelihood $\widehat{L}(\beta)$ with respect to β. This is often implemented by using the Newton–Raphson iteration scheme. Let $\widehat{\beta}^{(k)}$ denote the estimate of β at the kth iteration, then at iteration $(k+1)$, the estimate is given by

$$\widehat{\beta}^{(k+1)} = \widehat{\beta}^{(k)} + \widehat{I}^{-1}(\widehat{\beta}^{(k)})\widehat{S}(\widehat{\beta}^{(k)}),$$

where $\widehat{S}(\beta) = \partial \log \widehat{L}(\beta)/\partial\beta$, $\widehat{I}(\beta) = -\partial^2 \log \widehat{L}(\beta)/\partial\beta\partial\beta^{\mathrm{T}}$, and $k = 0, 1, \ldots$. Let $\widehat{\beta}$ denote the estimate of β, which is taken as the limit of $\{\beta^{(k)} : k = 0, 1, \ldots\}$ as $k \to \infty$.

The procedure applies to situations with either discrete or continuous variables. With different types of variables, estimates of $f(y^*, y, s)$ and $f(y, s)$ may assume varying forms. For instance, when Y_i^*, Y_i, and S_i are all discrete, $f(y^*, y, s)$ and $f(y, s)$ are, respectively, estimated by the empirical counterparts:

$$\widehat{f}(y^*,y,s) = \frac{1}{n_{\mathrm{V}}} \sum_{i\in\mathcal{V}} I(Y_i^* = y^*, Y_i = y, S_i = s);$$

$$\widehat{f}(y,s) = \frac{1}{n_{\mathrm{V}}} \sum_{i\in\mathcal{V}} I(Y_i = y, S_i = s);$$

where n_{V} is the number of subjects in the validation sample $\mathcal{V}$.

If some components of Y_i^*, Y_i, and S_i are continuous, then kernel functions may be used to replace the empirical counts. For instance, if Y_i^* is continuous and $\{Y_i, S_i\}$ are discrete, then function $f(y^*, y, s)$ may be estimated by

$$\widehat{f}(y^*,y,s) = \frac{1}{n_{\mathrm{V}}} \sum_{i\in\mathcal{V}} \left\{ I(Y_i = y, S_i = s)\frac{1}{b}K\left(\frac{y_i^* - y^*}{b}\right) \right\},$$

where $K(\cdot)$ is a kernel function and b is a bandwidth.

Under regularity conditions on the models and the bandwidth, if the validation sample fraction n_{V}/n has a nonzero limit as $n \to \infty$, then, asymptotically, $\sqrt{n}(\widehat{\beta}-\beta)$ has a normal distribution with mean zero and a covariance matrix whose expression was given by Pepe (1992). Discussions on using this asymptotic distribution to perform inference about β, such as calculating confidence intervals or conducting hypothesis testing, were provided by Pepe (1992) in detail.

8.4 Logistic Regression Model with Measurement Error in Response and Covariates

For subject i, let Y_i be a misclassification-prone binary response variable taking value 0 or 1, X_i be a vector of error-prone covariates, and Z_i be a vector of error-free covariates. Let

$$\mu_i = P(Y_i = 1|X_i, Z_i)$$

be the mean of the response variable Y_i, given covariates $\{X_i, Z_i\}$. Assume that the binary outcome is associated with the covariates through the regression model:

$$g(\mu_i) = \beta_0 + \beta_x^{\mathrm{T}} X_i + \beta_z^{\mathrm{T}} Z_i, \tag{8.31}$$

where $g(\cdot)$ is a link function, such as the logit, probit or complementary log-log function, and $\beta = (\beta_0, \beta_x^{\mathrm{T}}, \beta_z^{\mathrm{T}})^{\mathrm{T}}$ is the vector of regression coefficients.

Let Y_i^* and X_i^* be the observed measurements of Y_i and X_i, respectively. Assume that

$$h(y_i|x_i, x_i^*, z_i) = h(y_i|x_i, z_i) \tag{8.32}$$

and

$$h(y_i^*|y_i, x_i, x_i^*, z_i) = h(y_i^*|y_i, x_i^*, z_i), \tag{8.33}$$

where the symbol $h(\cdot|\cdot)$ represents the conditional probability mass function for the random variables corresponding to the arguments. These assumptions require that Y_i and X_i^* are conditionally independent, given the true covariates $\{X_i, Z_i\}$; and that Y_i^* and X_i are conditionally independent, given $\{Y_i, X_i^*, Z_i\}$. Let

$$\gamma_{10}(X_i^*, Z_i) = P(Y_i^* = 0|Y_i = 1, X_i^*, Z_i)$$

and

$$\gamma_{01}(X_i^*, Z_i) = P(Y_i^* = 1|Y_i = 0, X_i^*, Z_i)$$

be the misclassification probabilities for the response variable.

We consider settings where an internal validation sample, indexed by $\mathcal{V}$, is randomly selected from the main study subjects, indexed by $\mathcal{M}$. When $i \in \mathcal{V}$, measurements of $\{Y_i, Y_i^*, X_i, X_i^*, Z_i\}$ are available whereas when $i \in \mathcal{M} \setminus \mathcal{V}$, only measurements for $\{Y_i^*, X_i^*, Z_i\}$ are available. Let n and n_{v} be the size of $\mathcal{M}$ and $\mathcal{V}$, respectively.

Our primary interest is in inference about response parameter β. A simple way is to directly base estimation of β on the validation sample because this sample contains the measurements of Y_i and X_i in addition to those of Z_i. This scheme is easy to implement using a standard analysis method but incurs efficiency loss, especially when the size of the validation sample is small. To improve estimation efficiency, a common method is to capitalize on the available information from both the validation sample and the main study. Here we describe two strategies for estimation of β.

Likelihood Method

First, we describe likelihood-based methods for estimating β. For this purpose, we postulate the misclassification and measurement error processes. Misclassification for the response variable is modeled by, say, logistic regression models:

$$\text{logit } \gamma_{01}(X_i^*, Z_i) = g_0(X_i^*, Z_i; \gamma_y);$$
$$\text{logit } \gamma_{10}(X_i^*, Z_i) = g_1(X_i^*, Z_i; \gamma_y);$$

where $g_0(\cdot)$ and $g_1(\cdot)$ are specified functions, such as the linear and quadratic functions, and γ_y is a vector of unknown regression coefficients.

Regarding the covariate measurement error process, we employ a modeling scheme discussed in Chapter 2. Let $f_{\mathrm{X|X^*}}(x_i|x_i^*, z_i; \gamma_x)$ denote the model for the conditional distribution of X_i, given $\{X_i^*, Z_i\}$, where the function form of $f(\cdot|\cdot)$ is specified but parameter γ_x is left unknown. Let $\gamma = (\gamma_x^{\mathrm{T}}, \gamma_y^{\mathrm{T}})^{\mathrm{T}}$.

Let $\theta = (\beta^{\mathrm{T}}, \gamma^{\mathrm{T}})^{\mathrm{T}}$ denote the vector of all involved parameters. Then inference about θ may be based on the likelihood function for the observed data

$$L^*(\theta) = \left\{ \prod_{i \in \mathcal{V}} f(y_i, y_i^* | x_i, x_i^*, z_i) \right\} \left\{ \prod_{i \in \mathcal{M} \setminus \mathcal{V}} f(y_i^* | x_i^*, z_i) \right\},$$

where the contributions of the subjects in the validation sample are reflected by the model $f(y_i, y_i^*|x_i, x_i^*, z_i)$ for the conditional distribution of $\{Y_i, Y_i^*\}$, given $\{X_i, X_i^*, Z_i\}$; and the subjects in the main study contribute via the model, $f(y_i^*|x_i^*, z_i)$, for the conditional distribution of Y_i^*, given $\{X_i^*, Z_i\}$. The dependence on θ is suppressed in the notation.

Let $\mu_i^* = P(Y_i^* = 1|X_i^*, Z_i)$ be the mean for the observed data, which is determined by (8.13). Then the likelihood for $L^*(\theta)$ becomes

$$L^*(\theta) = \prod_{i \in \mathcal{V}} \{\mu_i^{y_i}(1-\mu_i)^{1-y_i} \{a_1(y_i^*, x_i^*)\}^{y_i} \{a_0(y_i^*, x_i^*)\}^{1-y_i} f(x_i|x_i^*, z_i; \gamma_x)\}$$
$$\cdot \prod_{i \in \mathcal{M} \setminus \mathcal{V}} \left\{ \mu_i^{*y_i^*}(1-\mu_i^*)^{1-y_i^*} \right\}, \tag{8.34}$$

where for $k = 0$ and 1, $a_k(y_i^*, x_i^*) = P(Y_i^* = y_i^*|Y_i = k, X_i^*, Z_i)$, which is given by

$$a_0(y_i^*, x_i^*) = \gamma_{01}(X_i^*, Z_i)^{y_i^*}\{1 - \gamma_{01}(X_i^*, Z_i)\}^{1-y_i^*};$$
$$a_1(y_i^*, x_i^*) = \gamma_{10}(X_i^*, Z_i)^{1-y_i^*}\{1 - \gamma_{10}(X_i^*, Z_i)\}^{y_i^*}.$$

Let

$$S_i(\beta) = \left\{ \frac{y_i - \mu_i}{\mu_i(1-\mu_i)} \right\} \left(\frac{\partial \mu_i}{\partial \beta} \right); \tag{8.35}$$

$$S_i(\gamma_x) = \frac{\partial \log f(x_i|x_i^*, z_i; \gamma_x)}{\partial \gamma_x};$$

$$S_i(\gamma_y) = \left\{\frac{y_i}{a_1(y_i^*, x_i^*)}\right\}\left\{\frac{\partial a_1(y_i^*, x_i^*)}{\partial \gamma_y}\right\} + \left\{\frac{1-y_i}{a_0(y_i^*, x_i^*)}\right\}\left\{\frac{\partial a_0(y_i^*, x_i^*)}{\partial \gamma_y}\right\};$$

and $S_i(\theta; y_i, x_i, y_i^*, x_i^*, z_i) = (S_i^{\mathrm{T}}(\beta), S_i^{\mathrm{T}}(\gamma_x), S_i^{\mathrm{T}}(\gamma_y))^{\mathrm{T}}$. Then the likelihood score function $\partial \log L^*(\theta)/\partial\theta$ gives the likelihood score equation

$$\sum_{i\in\mathcal{V}} S_i(\theta; y_i, x_i, y_i^*, x_i^*, z_i) + \sum_{i\in\mathcal{M}\setminus\mathcal{V}} S_i^*(\theta; y_i^*, x_i^*, z_i) = 0, \tag{8.36}$$

where

$$S_i^*(\theta; y_i^*, x_i^*, z_i) = \left\{\frac{y_i^* - \mu_i^*}{\mu_i^*(1-\mu_i^*)}\right\}\left(\frac{\partial \mu_i^*}{\partial\theta}\right). \tag{8.37}$$

We now examine the expression (8.37) in terms of the misclassification probabilities and the model for the response process. For ease of exposition, let

$$d(x_i^*, z_i; \beta) = E(\mu_i|X_i^* = x_i^*, Z_i = z_i);$$

$$r(y_i^*, x_i^*; \beta) = \frac{1}{a_1(y_i^*, x_i^*)d(x_i^*, z_i; \beta) + a_0(y_i^*, x_i^*)\{1 - d(x_i^*, z_i; \beta)\}};$$

$$R(y_i^*, x_i^*; \beta) = \frac{a_1(y_i^*, x_i^*) - a_0(y_i^*, x_i^*)}{a_1(y_i^*, x_i^*)d(x_i^*, z_i; \beta) + a_0(y_i^*, x_i^*)\{1 - d(x_i^*, z_i; \beta)\}};$$

where the expectation is evaluated with respect to the model for the conditional distribution of X_i, given $\{X_i^*, Z_i\}$; and the dependence on parameters γ_x and γ_y is suppressed in the notation.

Assuming that the operations of integration and differentiation are exchangeable and using model (8.13), we express $S_i^*(\theta; y_i^*, x_i^*, z_i)$ as

$$S_i^*(\theta; y_i^*, x_i^*, z_i) = (S_i^{*\mathrm{T}}(\beta; y_i^*, x_i^*, z_i), S_i^{*\mathrm{T}}(\gamma_x; y_i^*, x_i^*, z_i), S_i^{*\mathrm{T}}(\gamma_y; y_i^*, x_i^*, z_i))^{\mathrm{T}},$$

where

$$S_i^*(\beta; y_i^*, x_i^*, z_i) = R(y_i^*, x_i^*; \beta)\left(\frac{\partial d(x_i^*, z_i; \beta)}{\partial\beta}\right), \tag{8.38}$$

$$S_i^*(\gamma_x; y_i^*, x_i^*) = R(y_i^*, x_i^*; \beta)\left(\frac{\partial d(x_i^*, z_i; \beta)}{\partial\gamma_x}\right),$$

and

$$\begin{aligned} S_i^*(\gamma_y; y_i^*, x_i^*) &= r(y_i^*, x_i^*; \beta)(-1)^{y_i^*+1} \\ &\cdot \left[\frac{\partial\gamma_{01}(x_i^*, z_i)}{\partial\gamma_y} - \left\{\frac{\partial\gamma_{10}(x_i^*, z_i)}{\partial\gamma_y} + \frac{\partial\gamma_{01}(x_i^*, z_i)}{\partial\gamma_y}\right\} d(x_i^*, z_i; \beta)\right]. \end{aligned} \tag{8.39}$$

Consequently, maximizing (8.34) with respect to θ, or under regularity conditions, solving (8.36) for θ, leads to the maximum likelihood estimate for θ. Let $\widehat{\theta} = (\widehat{\beta}^{\mathrm{T}}, \widehat{\gamma}^{\mathrm{T}})^{\mathrm{T}}$ denote the resulting estimator for θ. Under regularity conditions, $\sqrt{n}(\widehat{\theta} - \theta)$ has an asymptotic normal distribution with mean zero.

This estimation procedure simultaneously estimates nuisance parameter γ and parameter β of interest and typically requires numerical approximations to integrals. Depending on the complexity of models for the covariate measurement error and the response misclassification processes, computation intensity may vary considerably. In many situations, simultaneously estimating γ and β is rather challenging. To get around this, one may alternatively employ a two-stage algorithm which treats estimation of β and γ differently. At the first stage, the maximum likelihood method is applied to estimate nuisance parameter γ merely using the validation sample. At the second stage, estimation of β is carried out by solving (8.36) for β where nuisance parameter γ is replaced by the estimate obtained from the first stage.

Semiparametric Method

Likelihood-based methods require modeling the response process as well as the misclassification and measurement error processes. If a model is misspecified, the results may incur biases and be misleading. To produce robust results, we describe a semiparametric approach based on a two-stage procedure. The idea is to treat the response process differently from the misclassification and measurement error processes; the response process is modeled parametrically by (8.31) while the misclassification and measurement error processes are handled nonparametrically.

At the first stage, we utilize the validation sample to estimate relevant quantities nonparametrically using the kernel method. Let $K(v)$ be a dth order kernel function and $b = b_n$ be a bandwidth satisfying $b \to 0$, $nb^{2p} \to \infty$ and $nb^{2d} \to 0$ as $n \to \infty$, where p is the dimension of $(X_i^{\mathrm{T}}, Z_i^{\mathrm{T}})^{\mathrm{T}}$, d is an integer greater than p, and the bandwidth b_n depends on n. Write $K_b(v) = b^{-1}K(v/b)$.

Let $W_i^* = (X_i^{*\mathrm{T}}, Z_i^{\mathrm{T}})^{\mathrm{T}}$. Using the measurements in the validation sample, we estimate the misclassification probabilities by

$$\widehat{\gamma}_{10}(w^*) = \frac{\sum_{i \in \mathcal{V}} K_b(w^* - w_i^*) y_i (1 - y_i^*)}{\sum_{i \in \mathcal{V}} K_b(w^* - w_i^*) y_i}$$

and

$$\widehat{\gamma}_{01}(w^*) = \frac{\sum_{i \in \mathcal{V}} K_b(w^* - w_i^*)(1 - y_i) y_i^*}{\sum_{i \in \mathcal{V}} K_b(w^* - w_i^*)(1 - y_i)}.$$

Let $\Psi(x, z; \beta)$ denote $g^{-1}(\beta_0 + \beta_x^{\mathrm{T}} x + \beta_z^{\mathrm{T}} z)$ or $(\partial/\partial\beta) g^{-1}(\beta_0 + \beta_x^{\mathrm{T}} x + \beta_z^{\mathrm{T}} z)$, the conditional expectation $E\{\Psi(X, Z; \beta) | W^* = w^*\}$ is estimated by

$$\widehat{\Psi}(w^*; \beta) = \frac{\sum_{i \in \mathcal{V}} K_b(w^* - w_i^*) \Psi(x^*, z; \beta)}{\sum_{i \in \mathcal{V}} K_b(w^* - w_i^*)},$$

where $w^* = (x^{*\mathrm{T}}, z^{*\mathrm{T}})^{\mathrm{T}}$.

At the second stage, we construct the *pseudo-likelihood score function* by modifying the likelihood score function (8.36) as:

$$\sum_{i\in\mathcal{V}} S_i(\beta; y_i, x_i, z_i) + \sum_{i\in\mathcal{M}\setminus\mathcal{V}} S_i^*(\beta; y_i^*, x_i^*, z_i) = 0, \tag{8.40}$$

where $S_i(\beta; y_i, x_i, z_i)$ is given by (8.35); $S_i^*(\beta; y_i^*, x_i^*, z_i)$ has the form of (8.38) in which the $\gamma_{k,1-k}(x_i^*, z_i)$ contained in $a_k(y_i^*, x_i^*)$ are replaced by their nonparametric estimates $\widehat{\gamma}_{k,1-k}(w_i^*)$ for $k = 0, 1$; and $E\{\Psi(X, Z; \beta)|W^* = w^*\}$ is replaced by $\widehat{\Psi}(w^*; \beta)$. Then estimation of β is carried out by solving (8.40) for β. Let $\widehat{\beta}_{\text{PS}}$ denote the resulting estimator of β.

Under the conditions of Cheng and Hsueh (2003), $\sqrt{n}\,(\widehat{\beta}_{\text{PS}} - \beta)$ has an asymptotic normal distribution with mean zero and a covariance matrix whose expression was given by Cheng and Hsueh (2003).

8.5 Least Squares Methods with Measurement Error in Response and Covariates

In contrast to a discrete response variable being considered in §8.4, we discuss the case where a continuous response variable is error-contaminated together with error-prone covariates. Let Y be the response variable and X be an associated $p \times 1$ covariate vector. Let Y^* and X^* be the observed measurements of Y and X, respectively.

Suppose that Y and X are postulated by the regression model

$$Y = g(X; \beta) + \epsilon, \tag{8.41}$$

where $g(\cdot)$ is a linear or nonlinear function whose form is known, β is a vector of regression parameters, and the error term ϵ has $E(\epsilon|X) = 0$ and a constant conditional variance $\sigma^2 = \text{var}(\epsilon|X)$.

For subject i, let $\{Y_i, X_i, Y_i^*, X_i^*\}$ denote a copy of $\{Y, X, Y^*, X^*\}$. We consider settings where the study subjects are divided into three disjoint groups. In the main study group, denoted by $\mathcal{M} = \{i : (Y_i^*, X_i^*) \text{ are available}\}$, subjects are only measured with response and covariate surrogates; the other two groups consist of subjects with precise measurements on X_i or Y_i, and are random validation subsamples, denoted by $\mathcal{V}_{\text{X}} = \{i : (X_i, X_i^*) \text{ are available}\}$ and $\mathcal{V}_{\text{Y}} = \{i : (X_i^*, Y_i, Y_i^*) \text{ are available}\}$. Let n, n_{X} and n_{Y} be the size of $\mathcal{M}$, $\mathcal{V}_{\text{X}}$, and $\mathcal{V}_{\text{Y}}$, respectively.

Least Squares Projection without Measurement Error

To develop estimation procedures for β, we start with an ideal situation where X and Y were error-free. In this case, we have only the main study data $\{(Y_i, X_i) : i \in \mathcal{M}\}$ where $Y_i^* = Y_i$ and $X_i^* = X_i$ for $i \in \mathcal{M}$.

To ease the exposition of the following development, we use the matrix form analogous to what is often adopted in regression analysis. Let $\mathbb{Y} = (Y_i : i \in \mathcal{M})^{\mathrm{T}}$ denote the $n \times 1$ vector of the true response variables, and $\mathbb{X} = (X_i : i \in \mathcal{M})^{\mathrm{T}}$ stand for the $n \times p$ matrix of the true covariate variables. Let $\mathbb{G}(\mathbb{X}; \beta) = \{g(X_i; \beta) : i \in \mathcal{M}\}^{\mathrm{T}}$ be an $n \times 1$ vector.

In the absence of measurement error in X and Y, the usual least squares method can be used to estimate β by minimizing

$$\{\mathbb{Y} - \mathbb{G}(\mathbb{X}; \beta)\}^{\mathrm{T}}\{\mathbb{Y} - \mathbb{G}(\mathbb{X}; \beta)\}$$

with respect to β. However, in the presence of measurement error, not all X_i and Y_i are observed, and we need to modify the least squares method in order to properly use available surrogate measurements X_i^* or Y_i^*.

Least Squares Projection with Covariate Error Only

To highlight the idea, we first look at a simplified case where only covariates are subject to measurement error and the response variable is treated as error-free. In this instance, the data include the measurements $\{(X_i, X_i^*) : i \in \mathcal{V}_{\mathrm{X}}\}$ of the validation sample and the measurements $\{(Y_i, X_i^*) : i \in \mathcal{M}\}$ of the main study where $Y_i^* = Y_i$.

Since X in model (8.41) is not observed, directly working on model (8.41) is not possible for estimating β. A natural way is to work with a modified version of model (8.41) by evaluating the conditional expectation of $g(X; \beta)$ with respect to the observed surrogate variable X^*:

$$E(Y|X^*) = E\{g(X; \beta)|X^*\} + E(\epsilon|X^*).$$

Letting $\epsilon^{**} = Y - E(Y|X^*)$, we write

$$Y = E\{g(X; \beta)|X^*\} + \epsilon^*, \tag{8.42}$$

where $\epsilon^* = E(\epsilon|X^*) + \epsilon^{**}$.

Under the nondifferential measurement error mechanism with $h(y|x, x^*) = h(y|x)$, it is seen that $E(\epsilon^*|X^*) = 0$ and ϵ^* is uncorrelated with any function of X^*. Estimation of β is then carried out by applying the nonlinear least squares method to model (8.42). Namely, using the main study data, we minimize

$$\sum_{i \in \mathcal{M}} [Y_i - E\{g(X_i; \beta)|X_i^*\}]^2$$

with respect to β.

This algorithm is feasible only if the function form $E\{g(X; \beta)|X^*\}$ is known except for the value of β. When $E\{g(X; \beta)|X^*\}$ is unknown, one may follow the lines of §8.4 and use the nonparametric kernel regression estimate based on the validation data to estimate it. Let $m(X_i^*; \beta)$ be the kernel regression estimate of

$E\{g(X_i;\beta)|X_i^*\}$; discussion on such an estimate may be found in Carroll and Wand (1991), Sepanski and Carroll (1993), and Sepanski, Knickerbocker and Carroll (1994). Then minimizing

$$\sum_{i\in\mathcal{M}}\{y_i - m(X_i^*;\beta)\}^2$$

with respect to β gives an estimate of β.

Those nonparametric methods are generally computationally demanding and involve the issue of bandwidth selection. Here we discuss an alternative which is computationally simpler; this method originates from the projection idea and was explored by Lee and Sepanski (1995).

The idea is to view $E\{g(X;\beta)|X^*\}$ as an element in an infinite-dimensional functional space, and then approximate it by an element of a finite-dimensional subspace spanned by some functions of X^*, such as linear, quadratic or other polynomials of X^*. Let $\widetilde{X}^*$ denote the $q\times 1$ vector of those functions of X^*, where q denotes the dimension of $\widetilde{X}^*$. Suppose $E(\widetilde{X}^*\widetilde{X}^{*\mathrm{T}})$ is nonsingular and $E\{g(X;\beta)|X^*\}$ is square integrable.

Within the finite-dimensional subspace spanned by $\widetilde{X}^*$, $E\{g(X;\beta)|X^*\}$ is approximated by the least squares projection

$$\Psi^{\mathrm{T}}(\beta)\widetilde{X}^*,$$

where $\Psi(\beta) = \{E(\widetilde{X}^*\widetilde{X}^{*\mathrm{T}})\}^{-1}E\{\widetilde{X}^*g(X;\beta)\}$ (Tsiatis 2006, §2.4) and the expectations are evaluated with respect to the model for the joint distribution of $\{X, X^*\}$.

Let

$$R_x(\widetilde{X}^*;\beta) = E\{g(X;\beta)|X^*\} - \Psi^{\mathrm{T}}(\beta)\widetilde{X}^*$$

denote the corresponding residual. Then $R_x(\widetilde{X}^*;\beta)$ has mean zero and is orthogonal to $\Psi^{\mathrm{T}}(\beta)\widetilde{X}^*$ with

$$E[\{\Psi^{\mathrm{T}}(\beta)\widetilde{X}^*\}\cdot R_x^{\mathrm{T}}(\widetilde{X}^*;\beta)] = 0. \tag{8.43}$$

Therefore, $E\{g(X;\beta)|X^*\}$ is decomposed as the sum of two orthogonal terms:

$$E\{g(X;\beta)|X^*\} = \Psi^{\mathrm{T}}(\beta)\widetilde{X}^* + R_x(\widetilde{X}^*;\beta).$$

Consequently, model (8.42) is decomposed as

$$Y = \Psi^{\mathrm{T}}(\beta)\widetilde{X}^* + \epsilon_x^* \tag{8.44}$$

so that the error term $\epsilon_x^* = \epsilon^* + R_x(\widetilde{X}^*;\beta)$ has mean zero and is orthogonal to $\Psi^{\mathrm{T}}(\beta)\widetilde{X}^*$ with $E[\{\Psi^{\mathrm{T}}(\beta)\widetilde{X}^*\}\cdot\epsilon_x^*] = 0$.

Form (8.44) suggests the feasibility of using the least squares method to estimate β with the suitable use of the validation sample $\mathcal{V}_{\mathrm{x}}$ and the main study data: the data in the validation sample $\mathcal{V}_{\mathrm{x}}$ is used to estimate the function form $\Psi(\cdot)$, and the main study data are used to fit the model for estimation of β. Specifically, for subject i, let $\widetilde{X}_i^*$ denote the ith copy of $\widetilde{X}^*$, $\widetilde{\mathbb{X}}_{\mathrm{v}}^* = (\widetilde{X}_i^* : i \in \mathcal{V}_{\mathrm{x}})^{\mathrm{T}}$ denote the

$n_{\mathrm{x}} \times q$ matrix for the validation sample $\mathcal{V}_{\mathrm{x}}$, and $\widetilde{\mathbb{X}}^* = (\widetilde{X}_i^* : i \in \mathcal{M})^{\mathrm{T}}$ denote the $n \times q$ matrix for all the main study subjects. Let $\mathbb{H}_{\mathrm{v}}(\beta) = (\widetilde{\mathbb{X}}_{\mathrm{v}}^{*\mathrm{T}}\widetilde{\mathbb{X}}_{\mathrm{v}}^*)^{-1}\widetilde{\mathbb{X}}_{\mathrm{v}}^{*\mathrm{T}}\mathbb{G}(\mathbb{X}_{\mathrm{v}};\beta)$ where $\mathbb{G}(\mathbb{X}_{\mathrm{v}};\beta) = \{g(X_i;\beta) : i \in \mathcal{V}_{\mathrm{x}}\}$ is an $n_{\mathrm{x}} \times 1$ vector, then β is estimated by minimizing

$$\{\mathbb{Y} - \widetilde{\mathbb{X}}^*\mathbb{H}_{\mathrm{v}}(\beta)\}^{\mathrm{T}}\{\mathbb{Y} - \widetilde{\mathbb{X}}^*\mathbb{H}_{\mathrm{v}}(\beta)\}$$

with respect to β.

Measurement Error in Response and Covariate Variables

We extend the preceding method to further accommodate measurement error in response. The idea again stems from the least squares projection method. Using the working model (8.44), we first assess the difference of the proxy response variable from the true response:

$$\begin{aligned} Y^* &= Y + (Y^* - Y) \\ &= \{\Psi^{\mathrm{T}}(\beta)\widetilde{X}^* + \epsilon_x^*\} + (Y^* - Y). \end{aligned} \tag{8.45}$$

Because the difference $Y^* - Y$ may be correlated with the regressor $\widetilde{X}^*$ as well as Y^*, we further decompose it as the sum of orthogonal terms. Let $W = (Y^*, \widetilde{X}^{*\mathrm{T}})^{\mathrm{T}}$. Then write $Y^* - Y$ as

$$Y^* - Y = E(Y^* - Y|W) + e, \tag{8.46}$$

where the error term $e = (Y^* - Y) - E(Y^* - Y|W)$ has mean zero and is orthogonal to $E(Y^* - Y|W)$.

We further project $E(Y^* - Y|W)$ onto the subspace spanned by linear functions of W and obtain the decomposition

$$E(Y^* - Y|W) = \Psi_y^{\mathrm{T}}W + R_y(W), \tag{8.47}$$

where $\Psi_y = \{E(WW^{\mathrm{T}})\}^{-1}E\{W(Y^* - Y)\}$ and $R_y(W) = E(Y^* - Y|W) - \Psi_y^{\mathrm{T}}W$ is the residual. It is known that the residual $R_y(W)$ has mean zero and is orthogonal to the projection $\Psi_y^{\mathrm{T}}W$, i.e., $R_y(W)$ and $\Psi_y^{\mathrm{T}}W$ are uncorrelated. Therefore, combining (8.45), (8.46) and (8.47) gives

$$Y^* - \Psi_y^{\mathrm{T}}W = \Psi^{\mathrm{T}}(\beta)\widetilde{X}^* + \epsilon_y^*, \tag{8.48}$$

where $\epsilon_y^* = \epsilon_x^* + R_y(W) + e$. It is easily seen that $E(\epsilon_y^*) = 0$ and that ϵ_y^* is orthogonal to $\Psi^{\mathrm{T}}(\beta)\widetilde{X}^*$ due to the orthogonality of $\Psi^{\mathrm{T}}(\beta)\widetilde{X}^*$to individual terms in ϵ_y^*.

As a result, (8.48) may be regarded as a usual nonlinear regression model by treating $Y^* - \Psi_y^{\mathrm{T}}W$ as the response and $\widetilde{X}^*$ as covariates. Thus, the nonlinear least squares method is used to estimate β after Ψ_y and $\Psi(\cdot)$ are estimated using the validation data.

Let $\mathbb{X}_{\mathrm{v}} = (X_i : i \in \mathcal{V}_{\mathrm{x}})^{\mathrm{T}}$ denote the $n_{\mathrm{x}} \times p$ matrix of the true covariate variables from the validation sample $\mathcal{V}_{\mathrm{x}}$. Let $\mathbb{Y}_{\mathrm{v}} = (Y_i : i \in \mathcal{V}_{\mathrm{Y}})^{\mathrm{T}}$ and $\mathbb{Y}_{\mathrm{v}}^* = (Y_i^* : i \in \mathcal{V}_{\mathrm{Y}})^{\mathrm{T}}$

be the $n_Y \times 1$ vectors of the measurements from the validation sample $\mathcal{V}_Y$, and $\mathbb{Y}^* = (Y_i^* : i \in \mathcal{M})^T$ be the $n \times 1$ vector of the measurements from the main study. Let $\mathbb{W}_V = \{(Y_i^*, \widetilde{X}_i^{*T})^T : i \in \mathcal{V}_Y\}^T$ be the $n_Y \times (1+q)$ matrix corresponding to the measurements in the validation sample $\mathcal{V}_Y$, and $\mathbb{W} = \{(Y_i^*, \widetilde{X}_i^{*T})^T : i \in \mathcal{M}\}^T$ be the $n \times (1+q)$ matrix corresponding to the measurements of all the main study subjects.

Define

$$\mathbb{P}_V = (\mathbb{W}_V^T \mathbb{W}_V)^{-1} \mathbb{W}_V^T (\mathbb{Y}_V^* - \mathbb{Y}_V)$$

and

$$\mathbb{H}_V(\beta) = (\widetilde{\mathbb{X}}_V^{*T} \widetilde{\mathbb{X}}_V^*)^{-1} \widetilde{\mathbb{X}}_V^{*T} \mathbb{G}(\mathbb{X}_V; \beta),$$

then minimizing

$$\{(\mathbb{Y}^* - \mathbb{W}\mathbb{P}_V) - \widetilde{\mathbb{X}}^* \mathbb{H}_V(\beta)\}^T \{(\mathbb{Y}^* - \mathbb{W}\mathbb{P}_V) - \widetilde{\mathbb{X}}^* \mathbb{H}_V(\beta)\}$$

with respect to β gives an estimate of β. Let $\widehat{\beta}$ denote the resulting estimator of β.

Under the regularity conditions of Lee and Sepanski (1995), the estimator $\widehat{\beta}$ is consistent for β. The asymptotic distribution of $\sqrt{n}(\widehat{\beta} - \beta)$ has a complicated form and can be found in Lee and Sepanski (1995).

We comment that one may replace Y^* by its function when forming W for the projection space. The choice of functions of X^* or Y^* for the projection space remains arbitrary. Under relevant identification conditions, all of them provide consistent estimators. Limited numerical studies suggest that polynomials with small orders are good enough even for highly nonlinear functions (Lee and Sepanski 1995). The least squares projection methods are computationally and analytically simpler than a nonparametric or semiparametric method. This method relies on neither distributional assumptions nor the specification of the model relating the measured variables with the true variables.

8.6 Correlated Binary Data with Diagnostic Error

In biomedical studies, measurement error in response arises often in a form of diagnostic error (e.g., Hui and Zhou 1998). For example, a binary disease outcome may be measured repeatedly in time or space or be assessed by multiple raters, and misclassification may occur. Unlike univariate data, repeated measurements are associated and their analysis typically requires care of handling association structures. In this section, we discuss a modeling scheme for correlated binary data measured with diagnostic error.

For $i = 1, \ldots, n$ and $j = 1, \ldots, m_i$, let Y_{ij} be the true binary response for subject i at time j, and Z_{ij} be the associated vector of covariates. Write $Y_i = (Y_{i1}, \ldots, Y_{im_i})^T$ and $Z_i = (Z_{i1}^T, \ldots, Z_{im_i}^T)^T$. To facilitate the correlation among the measurements within subjects and the dependence of the observed outcomes on the true underlying responses, we use a shared random effect framework to unify the response and misclassification processes (e.g., Shih and Albert 1999). We consider the random effects framework outlined in §8.2.3 with a slightly different exposition.

Given random effects u_i and the covariates, we assume that the Y_{ij} are conditionally independent and

$$P(Y_{ij} = 1|Z_i, u_i) = P(Y_{ij} = 1|Z_{ij}, u_i)$$

for $j = 1, \ldots, m_i$ and $i = 1, \ldots, n$. Let $\mu_{uij} = P(Y_{ij} = 1|Z_{ij}, u_i)$ be the conditional mean which is modeled as

$$g(\mu_{uij}) = \beta_0 + \beta_z^{\mathrm{T}} Z_{ij} + u_i,$$

where $g(\cdot)$ is a given link function and $\beta = (\beta_0, \beta_z^{\mathrm{T}})^{\mathrm{T}}$ is the vector of parameters. We assume that random effects u_i are modeled by $f(u_i; \vartheta)$ with parameter ϑ.

Suppose at each visit a study subject is assessed by m raters; let Y_{ijk}^* denote the measurement of Y_{ij} assessed by rater k, where $k = 1, \ldots, m$, $i = 1, \ldots, n$, and $j = 1, \ldots, m_i$. Given random effects u_i and the true response and covariates, the Y_{ijk}^* are assumed to be independent and satisfy

$$P(Y_{ijk}^* = 1|Y_i, Z_i, u_i) = P(Y_{ijk}^* = 1|Y_{ij}, Z_{ij}, u_i).$$

Assume that given $\{Y_{ij}, Z_{ij}, u_i\}$, all the raters have the same (mis)classification probability, and let $\gamma_{uij} = P(Y_{ijk}^* = 1|Y_{ij}, Z_{ij}, u_i)$ denote the (mis)classification probability with the dependence on the values of $\{Y_{ij}, Z_{ij}\}$ suppressed in the notation γ_{uij}.

Consider the regression model

$$g_u(\gamma_{uij}) = \gamma_0 + \gamma_y Y_{ij} + \gamma_z^{\mathrm{T}} Z_{ij} + u_i,$$

where $g_u(\cdot)$ is a given link function that may or may not differ from $g(\cdot)$ and $\gamma = (\gamma_0, \gamma_y, \gamma_z^{\mathrm{T}})^{\mathrm{T}}$ is the vector of parameters.

Let $\theta = (\beta^{\mathrm{T}}, \gamma^{\mathrm{T}}, \vartheta^{\mathrm{T}})^{\mathrm{T}}$. Estimation of θ may be carried out using the likelihood approach. The observed likelihood contributed from subject i is given by

$$\begin{aligned} L_{\mathrm{o}i}(\theta) &= \int \sum_{y_i} f(y_i|u_i, z_i) f(y_i^*|y_i, u_i, z_i) f(u_i) d\eta(u_i) \\ &= \int \sum_{y_{i1}, \ldots, y_{im_i}} \left\{ \prod_{j=1}^{m_i} \mu_{uij}^{y_{ij}} (1 - \mu_{uij})^{(1-y_{ij})} \gamma_{uij}^{y_{ij+}^*} (1 - \gamma_{uij})^{(m - y_{ij+}^*)} \right\} f(u_i) d\eta(u_i), \end{aligned}$$

where $y_{ij+}^* = \sum_{k=1}^m y_{ijk}^*$ and $f(\cdot|\cdot)$ and $f(\cdot)$ represent models for the corresponding variables.

Maximizing likelihood $L_{\mathrm{o}}(\theta) = \prod_{i=1}^n L_{\mathrm{o}i}(\theta)$ with respect to θ results in the maximum likelihood estimator, $\widehat{\theta}$. Under regularity conditions, $\sqrt{n}(\widehat{\theta} - \theta)$ has the asymptotic normal distribution with mean zero and the covariance matrix that is determined by the inverse of the information matrix.

Alternatively, estimation of θ may be carried out using the EM algorithm. Specifically, the log-likelihood for the complete data contributed from subject i is

$$\begin{aligned}\ell_{ci}(\theta) = &\sum_{j=1}^{m_i}\{y_{ij}\log\mu_{uij} + (1-y_{ij})\log(1-\mu_{uij})\\ &+y_{ij+}^*\log\gamma_{uij} + (m-y_{ij+}^*)\log(1-\gamma_{uij})\} + \log f(u_i).\end{aligned}$$

At the E-step of iteration $(k+1)$, we calculate the conditional expectation of $\ell_{ci}(\theta)$ where y_{ij} is replaced by random variable Y_{ij}:

$$\begin{aligned}Q_i(\theta;\theta^{(k)}) = &E_{c,\theta^{(k)}}\left\{\left(\sum_{j=1}^{m_i} Y_{ij}\right)\log\left(\frac{\mu_{uij}}{1-\mu_{uij}}\right) + \sum_{j=1}^{m_i}\log(1-\mu_{uij})\right\}\\ &+\sum_{j=1}^{m_i} y_{ij+}^* E_{c,\theta^{(k)}}(\log\gamma_{uij}) + \sum_{j=1}^{m_i}(m-y_{ij+}^*)E_{c,\theta^{(k)}}\{\log(1-\gamma_{uij})\}\\ &+E_{c,\theta^{(k)}}\{\log f(u_i)\},\end{aligned}$$

where $\theta^{(k)}$ is the estimated value of θ at iteration k for $k = 0, 1, \ldots$, and the conditional expectation $E_{c,\theta^{(k)}}$ is evaluated with respect to the model, $f(y_i, u_i|y_i^*, z_i; \theta^{(k)})$, for the conditional distribution of $\{Y_i, u_i\}$ given the observed data $\{Y_i^*, Z_i\}$ with the parameter value $\theta^{(k)}$. The conditional model $f(y_i, u_i|y_i^*, z_i; \theta)$ is determined by

$$f(y_i, u_i|y_i^*, z_i; \theta) = \frac{\exp\{\ell_{ci}(\theta)\}}{L_{oi}(\theta)}.$$

At the M-step of iteration $(k+1)$, maximizing $\sum_{i=1}^n Q_i(\theta;\theta^{(k)})$ with respect to θ gives an updated value $\theta^{(k+1)}$. Repeat the E and M steps until convergence of $\{\theta^{(k+1)} : k = 0, 1, \ldots\}$ as $k \to \infty$.

The EM algorithm may be carried out directly if the conditional expectations are easy to compute or approximate. In many cases, it is necessary to employ the Monte Carlo EM algorithm to update values of θ and approximate the associated expectations involved in $Q_i(\theta;\theta^{(k)})$. Variance estimates for the resulting estimator of θ may be obtained by using the method of Louis (1982) or the bootstrap procedure.

8.7 Marginal Method for Clustered Binary Data with Misclassification in Responses

8.7.1 Models and Method

In contrast to the likelihood-based methods described in §8.6, we discuss marginal methods developed by Chen, Yi and Wu (2011) for clustered binary data with misclassification in responses. For $i = 1, \ldots, n$ and $j = 1, \ldots, m_i$, let Y_{ij}, Z_{ij}, Y_i, and Z_i be defined as in §8.6. Let

$$\mu_{ij} = E(Y_{ij}|Z_i) \text{ and } v_{ij} = \text{var}(Y_{ij}|Z_i)$$

which are related via $v_{ij} = \mu_{ij}(1 - \mu_{ij})$.

A generalized linear regression model is used to link μ_{ij} to the covariates:

$$g(\mu_{ij}) = \beta_0 + \beta_z^{\mathrm{T}} Z_{ij},$$

where $\beta = (\beta_0, \beta_z^{\mathrm{T}})^{\mathrm{T}}$ is a vector of regression parameters, and $g(\cdot)$ is a monotone link function, such as the logit, probit, or complementary log-log function. An implicit assumption

$$E(Y_{ij}|Z_i) = E(Y_{ij}|Z_{ij}) \tag{8.49}$$

is made here (e.g., Pepe and Anderson 1994); see §5.1.1 for discussion on this assumption.

We assume that Y_{ij} and $Y_{i'k}$ are independent when $i \neq i'$ but Y_{ij} and Y_{ik} may be correlated for $j \neq k$. To facilitate inference for association parameters that may be of interest in clustered data analysis, we use odds ratios to reflect correlation among binary data within clusters. For $j < k$ and $i = 1, \ldots, n$, the odds ratio for Y_{ij} and Y_{ik} is defined as

$$\psi_{ijk} = \frac{P(Y_{ij} = 1, Y_{ik} = 1|Z_i)P(Y_{ij} = 0, Y_{ik} = 0|Z_i)}{P(Y_{ij} = 1, Y_{ik} = 0|Z_i)P(Y_{ij} = 0, Y_{ik} = 1|Z_i)}.$$

The odds ratios are customarily modeled as

$$\log \psi_{ijk} = \phi^{\mathrm{T}} u_{ijk}, \tag{8.50}$$

where ϕ is the vector of regression coefficients, and u_{ijk} is a set of pair-specific covariates featuring various association structures, such as autoregressive or exchangeable structure between Y_{ij} and Y_{ik}. As opposed to the assumption (8.49), a pairwise assumption

$$P(Y_{ij} = y_{ij}, Y_{ik} = y_{ik}|Z_i) = P(Y_{ij} = y_{ij}, Y_{ik} = y_{ik}|Z_{ij}, Z_{ik})$$

is often implicitly made.

For $i = 1, \ldots, n$ and $j < k$, let $\widetilde{\mu}_{ijk} = E(Y_{ij}Y_{ik}|Z_i)$. The relationship between $\widetilde{\mu}_{ijk}$ and ψ_{ijk} is given by (e.g., Lipsitz, Laird and Harrington 1991; Yi and Cook 2002):

$$\widetilde{\mu}_{ijk} = \begin{cases} \frac{a_{ijk} - \sqrt{a_{ijk}^2 - 4(\psi_{ijk} - 1)\psi_{ijk}\mu_{ij}\mu_{ik}}}{2(\psi_{ijk} - 1)}, & \text{if } \psi_{ijk} \neq 1, \\ \mu_{ij}\mu_{ik}, & \text{if } \psi_{ijk} = 1, \end{cases} \tag{8.51}$$

where $a_{ijk} = 1 - (1 - \psi_{ijk})(\mu_{ij} + \mu_{ik})$.

Estimating Equations in the Absence of Error

Given the model setup for the mean and association structures, it is natural to employ two sets of generalized estimating equations to perform estimation of the mean and association parameters $\theta = (\beta^{\mathrm{T}}, \phi^{\mathrm{T}})^{\mathrm{T}}$.

When the response variable is free of misclassification, an estimate of mean parameter β may be obtained by solving a first-order estimating equation, as discussed in §5.1.1. Let $\mu_i = (\mu_{i1}, \ldots, \mu_{im_i})^{\mathrm{T}}$, $D_{1i} = \partial\mu_i^{\mathrm{T}}/\partial\beta$, $B_{1i} = \mathrm{diag}(v_{i1}, \ldots, v_{im_i})$, and $V_{1i} = \mathrm{cov}(Y_i|Z_i) = B_{1i}^{1/2} C_{1i} B_{1i}^{1/2}$ where C_{1i} is the correlation matrix of Y_i with diagonal entries 1 and off-diagonal entries $(\widetilde{\mu}_{ijk} - \mu_{ij}\mu_{ik})/\sqrt{v_{ij}v_{ik}}$ for $j \neq k$. Define

$$U_{1i}(\theta) = D_{1i}V_{1i}^{-1}(Y_i - \mu_i),$$

then estimation of β may be based on the first-order estimating equation

$$\sum_{i=1}^{n} U_{1i}(\theta) = 0. \tag{8.52}$$

To estimate the association parameter ϕ, using the same idea of formulating $U_{1i}(\theta)$, we construct a second-order estimating equation (Prentice 1988). For $j < k$ and $i = 1, \ldots, n$, define

$$\widetilde{Y}_{ijk} = Y_{ij}Y_{ik}$$

to be the pairwise products for components of Y_i. Let $\widetilde{Y}_i = (\widetilde{Y}_{ijk} : j < k)^{\mathrm{T}}$, $\widetilde{\mu}_i = (\widetilde{\mu}_{ijk} : j < k)^{\mathrm{T}}$, and $D_{2i} = \partial\widetilde{\mu}_i^{\mathrm{T}}/\partial\phi$. Define

$$U_{2i}(\theta) = D_{2i}V_{2i}^{-1}(\widetilde{Y}_i - \widetilde{\mu}_i),$$

where V_{2i} is the conditional covariance matrix of $\widetilde{Y}_i$ given the covariates. Then estimation of association parameter ϕ is based on the second-order estimating equation

$$\sum_{i=1}^{n} U_{2i}(\theta) = 0. \tag{8.53}$$

Working with (8.53) requires care of V_{2i}. Matrix V_{2i} involves the conditional third and fourth moments of Y_i, given Z_i, which are often not modeled in application. Common practice is to replace V_{2i} with a working covariance matrix, for example, an independence matrix $\mathrm{diag}\left\{\widetilde{\mu}_{ijk}(1 - \widetilde{\mu}_{ijk}) : j < k\right\}$, when using (8.53). Although choosing an independence working matrix for (8.53) may incur efficiency loss, this method has the appeal of not modeling the conditional third and fourth moments of the response variables, given Z_i; and it still retains the unbiasedness of estimating functions $U_{1i}(\theta)$ and $U_{2i}(\theta)$, which ensures a consistent estimator of θ under regularity conditions (Prentice 1988; Yi and Cook 2002).

Let $U_i(\theta) = \{U_{1i}^{\mathrm{T}}(\theta), U_{2i}^{\mathrm{T}}(\theta)\}^{\mathrm{T}}$. Solving

$$\sum_{i=1}^{n} U_i(\theta) = 0$$

for θ gives an estimate of θ. Let $\widehat{\theta}$ denote the resulting estimator of θ.

Under regularity conditions, $\widehat{\theta}$ is a consistent estimator of θ and $\sqrt{n}(\widehat{\theta}-\theta)$ has an asymptotic distribution with mean zero and covariance matrix $\Gamma^{-1}(\theta)\Sigma(\theta)\Gamma^{-1\mathrm{T}}(\theta)$, where $\Gamma(\theta) = E\{\partial U_i^{\mathrm{T}}(\theta)/\partial\theta\}$ and $\Sigma(\theta) = E\{U_i(\theta)U_i^{\mathrm{T}}(\theta)\}$.

Misclassification Model

Suppose Y_{ij} is subject to misclassification and a proxy for Y_{ij}, denoted as Y_{ij}^*, is observed. Write $Y_i^* = (Y_{i1}^*, \ldots, Y_{im_i}^*)^{\mathrm{T}}$. Instead of imposing certain independence assumptions to simplify the modeling of the misclassification process as in the previous sections, here we consider a modeling scheme for the misclassification process to feature possible pairwise dependence among the components of Y_i^*. We use a slightly different way to indicate misclassification in response. Instead of directly modeling the conditional probability of measurement Y_{ij}^* given the true response variable Y_{ij} and covariates as before, we use a binary indicator to display the discrepancy between the true and observed variables. Let $R_{ij} = I(Y_{ij}^* = Y_{ij})$ be the misclassification indicator variable and $R_i = (R_{i1}, \ldots, R_{im_i})^{\mathrm{T}}$.

The marginal probability of misclassifying Y_{ij} is assumed to depend only on the true outcome Y_{ij} itself, given the covariates in cluster i:

$$P(R_{ij} = 1|Y_i, Z_i) = P(R_{ij} = 1|Y_{ij}, Z_i).$$

Let $\gamma_{0ij} = P(R_{ij} = 1|Y_{ij} = 0, Z_i)$ and $\gamma_{1ij} = P(R_{ij} = 1|Y_{ij} = 1, Z_i)$, where the dependence on Z_i is suppressed in the notation γ_{lij} for $l = 0, 1$.

The marginal (mis)classification probabilities are postulated by logistic regression models

$$\text{logit}\,\gamma_{0ij} = \gamma_0^{\mathrm{T}} w_{0ij}; \quad \text{logit}\,\gamma_{1ij} = \gamma_1^{\mathrm{T}} w_{1ij}; \tag{8.54}$$

where γ_0 and γ_1 are vectors of regression parameters, and w_{0ij} and w_{1ij} are covariates that reflect various misclassification mechanisms and may contain constant 1. Covariates w_{0ij} and w_{1ij} may contain the entire covariate vector Z_i in some situations; while in extreme cases, they can be 1 so that two parameters γ_0 and γ_1 are sufficient to describe the misclassification mechanism. The latter scenario corresponds to homogeneous misclassification across all observations and clusters, with (mis)classification probabilities independent of covariates and outcomes. Let $\gamma = (\gamma_0^{\mathrm{T}}, \gamma_1^{\mathrm{T}})^{\mathrm{T}}$.

To describe possible dependence between R_{ij} and R_{ik} for any $j < k$ and $i = 1, \ldots, n$, we invoke the odds ratios

$$\psi_{ijk}^*(y_{ij}, y_{ik}) = \frac{P(R_{ij} = 1, R_{ik} = 1|Y_i = y_i, Z_i)P(R_{ij} = 0, R_{ik} = 0|Y_i = y_i, Z_i)}{P(R_{ij} = 1, R_{ik} = 0|Y_i = y_i, Z_i)P(R_{ij} = 0, R_{ik} = 1|Y_i = y_i, Z_i)},$$

where

$$\begin{aligned} &P(R_{ij} = r_{ij}, R_{ik} = r_{ik}|Y_i = y_i, Z_i) \\ &= P(R_{ij} = r_{ij}, R_{ik} = r_{ik}|Y_{ij} = y_{ij}, Y_{ik} = y_{ik}, Z_i) \end{aligned}$$

is assumed for $r_{ij}, r_{ik}, y_{ij}, y_{ik} = 0, 1$ and any realization y_i of Y_i. The odds ratio $\psi^*_{ijk}(y_{ij}, y_{ik})$ is described by the log-linear model

$$\log\left\{\psi^*_{ijk}(y_{ij}, y_{ik})\right\} = \phi^{*\mathrm{T}} u^*_{ijk}, \tag{8.55}$$

where u^*_{ijk} is a vector of covariates which may contain constant 1, and ϕ^* is a vector of regression coefficients.

Let $\vartheta = (\gamma^{\mathrm{T}}, \phi^{*\mathrm{T}})^{\mathrm{T}}$. For $i = 1, \ldots, n$ and $j < k$, let $\widetilde{R}_{ijk} = R_{ij} R_{ik}$, $\widetilde{R}_i = (\widetilde{R}_{ijk}, j < k)^{\mathrm{T}}$, $\xi^*_{ijk}(y_{ij}, y_{ik}) = E(\widetilde{R}_{ijk}|Y_{ij} = y_{ij}, Y_{ik} = y_{ik}, Z_i)$, and $\xi^*_i = E(\widetilde{R}_i|Y_i, Z_i)$. Analogous to (8.51), $\xi^*_{ijk}(y_{ij}, y_{ik})$ may be expressed in terms of $\psi^*_{ijk}(y_{ij}, y_{ik})$ together with (8.54).

Estimating Equations for Misclassified Responses

Let $\mu^*_{ij} = E(Y^*_{ij}|Z_i)$, $\widetilde{Y}^*_{ijk} = Y^*_{ij} Y^*_{ik}$, and $\widetilde{\mu}^*_{ijk} = E(\widetilde{Y}^*_{ijk}|Z_i)$. Following the discussion in §8.2, it can be shown that

$$\mu^*_{ij} \neq \mu_{ij} \text{ and } \widetilde{\mu}^*_{ijk} \neq \widetilde{\mu}_{ijk}.$$

As a consequence, the naive analysis with Y_{ij} and $\widetilde{Y}_{ijk}$, respectively, replaced by Y^*_{ij} and $\widetilde{Y}^*_{ijk}$ in (8.52) and (8.53) distorts the unbiasedness of the estimating functions, hence the resulting estimators of β and ϕ may no longer be consistent (Yi and Reid 2010).

To conduct valid inference, one must correct the bias due to misclassification. There are several strategies to do so. One scheme is to replace the true estimating functions $U_{1i}(\theta)$ and $U_{2i}(\theta)$ with their conditional expectations $E\{U_{1i}(\theta)|Y^*_i, Z_i\}$ and $E\{U_{2i}(\theta)|Y^*_i, Z_i\}$, which are unbiased and expressed in terms of the parameters and the observed data. This is the expectation correction strategy discussed in §2.5.2, which basically requires the knowledge of the conditional distribution of Y_i, given $\{Y^*_i, Z_i\}$.

Alternatively, we consider the insertion correction strategy, outlined in §2.5.2. We construct estimating functions, say U^*_{1i} and U^*_{2i}, using the observed data $\{Y^*_i, Z_i\}$ so that their conditional expectations recover the estimating functions in (8.52) and (8.53):

$$E\{U^*_{1i}|Y_i, Z_i\} = U_{1i}(\theta); \quad E\{U^*_{2i}|Y_i, Z_i\} = U_{2i}(\theta); \tag{8.56}$$

where the expectations are evaluated with respect to the model for the conditional distribution of Y^*_i given $\{Y_i, Z_i\}$. The unbiasedness of U^*_{li} follows from that of $U_{li}(\theta)$ for $l = 1, 2$.

Recognizing that response components in $U_{1i}(\theta)$ and $U_{2i}(\theta)$ appear merely through the linear term Y_{ij} and pairwise product $\widetilde{Y}_{ijk}$, the construction of U^*_{1i} and U^*_{2i} is possible merely based on the marginal and association models (8.54) and (8.55), with the full conditional distribution of Y^*_i given $\{Y_i, Z_i\}$ left unspecified.

We construct unbiased proxy variables for Y_{ij} and $\widetilde{Y}_{ijk}$, given by

$$Y_{ij}^{**} = \frac{Y_{ij}^* - 1 + \gamma_{0ij}}{\gamma_{0ij} + \gamma_{1ij} - 1} \quad \text{and} \quad \widetilde{Y}_{ijk}^{**} = \frac{a_0 + (Y_{ij}^* - a_1)(Y_{ik}^* - a_2)}{a_3},$$

respectively, where

$$a_0 = (1 - a_1)\gamma_{0ik} + (1 - a_2)\gamma_{0ij} - \xi_{ijk}^*(0,0) - (1 - a_1)(1 - a_2);$$

$$a_1 = \frac{\gamma_{0ij} + \gamma_{0ik} + \gamma_{1ik} - 1 - \xi_{ijk}^*(0,1) - \xi_{ijk}^*(0,0)}{\gamma_{1ik} + \gamma_{0ik} - 1};$$

$$a_2 = \frac{\gamma_{0ik} + \gamma_{0ij} + \gamma_{1ij} - 1 - \xi_{ijk}^*(1,0) - \xi_{ijk}^*(0,0)}{\gamma_{1ij} + \gamma_{0ij} - 1};$$

$$a_3 = \sum_{s=0,1} \sum_{t=0,1} \xi_{ijk}^*(s,t) - \sum_{l=0,1} \gamma_{lij} - \sum_{l=0,1} \gamma_{lik} + 1.$$

It is readily shown that

$$E(Y_{ij}^{**}|Y_i, Z_i) = Y_{ij} \text{ and } E(\widetilde{Y}_{ijk}^{**}|Y_i, Z_i) = \widetilde{Y}_{ijk} \tag{8.57}$$

for $j < k$ and $i = 1, \ldots, n$.

Let $Y_i^{**} = (Y_{i1}^{**}, \ldots, Y_{im_i}^{**})^{\mathrm{T}}$ and $\widetilde{Y}_i^{**} = (\widetilde{Y}_{ijk}^{**} : j < k)^{\mathrm{T}}$. Define

$$U_{1i}^*(\theta, \vartheta) = D_{1i} V_{1i}^{-1}(Y_i^{**} - \mu_i),$$

$$U_{2i}^*(\theta, \vartheta) = D_{2i} V_{2i}^{-1}(\widetilde{Y}_i^{**} - \widetilde{\mu}_i),$$

and $U_i^*(\theta, \vartheta) = \{U_{1i}^{*\mathrm{T}}(\theta, \vartheta), U_{2i}^{*\mathrm{T}}(\theta, \vartheta)\}^{\mathrm{T}}$, where parameter ϑ comes into play through the involvement in Y_i^{**} and $\widetilde{Y}_i^{**}$.

Because Y_i^{**} and $\widetilde{Y}_i^{**}$ are, respectively, unbiased proxy variables of Y_i and $\widetilde{Y}_i$ satisfying (8.57), estimating functions $U_{1i}^*(\theta, \vartheta)$ and $U_{2i}^*(\theta, \vartheta)$ satisfy (8.56), thus are unbiased.

If the value of parameter ϑ is known, then solving

$$\sum_{i=1}^{n} U_i^*(\theta, \vartheta) = 0 \tag{8.58}$$

for θ leads to an estimate of θ. Let $\widehat{\theta}$ be the resulting estimator for θ. Under suitable regularity conditions, $\widehat{\theta}$ is a consistent estimator of θ and $\sqrt{n}(\widehat{\theta} - \theta)$ has an asymptotic normal distribution with mean 0 and covariance matrix $\Gamma^{*-1}\Sigma^*(\Gamma^{*-1})^{\mathrm{T}}$, where $\Gamma^* = E\{\partial U_i^{*\mathrm{T}}(\theta, \vartheta)/\partial\theta\}$ and $\Sigma^* = E\{U_i^*(\theta, \vartheta)U_i^{*\mathrm{T}}(\theta, \vartheta)\}$.

When ϑ is unknown, it may be estimated if there is an additional data source, such as a validation sample or replicate observed measurements of Y_{ij}. Estimation of ϑ is often based on constructing an unbiased estimating function for ϑ using the additional data information. Then combining this estimating function with $U_i^*(\theta, \vartheta)$, we perform inference about θ following the discussion in §1.3.4. The details of estimation procedures for these scenarios were given by Chen, Yi and Wu (2011).

In situations where no knowledge of the misclassification process is avaiable, estimating equation (8.58) may be employed for conducting sensitivity analyses. In this instance, a sequence of values are specified for ϑ to reflect different misclassification scenarios, and (8.58) is used to estimate θ to assess how the estimates are affected by different values of ϑ.

8.7.2 An Example: CCHS Data

Chen, Yi and Wu (2011) applied the method described in §8.7.1 to analyze a data set arising from the Canadian Community Health Survey (CCHS) cycle 3.1 which was conducted in 2005. This is a large scale on-going survey targeting individuals aged 12 and older in the Canadian population. The design of the survey is fairly complex, with three sampling frames being used to sample households: an area frame, a list frame of telephone numbers, and a random digit dialing sampling frame. For each sampled household, an individual aged 12 and older was randomly chosen for the interview.

It is of interest to study the relationship between obesity and certain risk factors, including age, sex, and physical activity index. There are three levels of physical activity index: active, moderate (taken as a reference category), and inactive.

A sample of 2699 respondents aged 18 and older in Toronto health region was analyzed. These respondents were from 435 clusters based on postal codes with size varying from 2 to 15. Among them, 150 were included by randomization as a validation subsample for which body mass index was accurately measured, and the resultant obesity status was regarded as the precise response value for each subject in this subsample. For other individuals, the obesity status was determined by the self-reported information, and therefore was subject to misclassification.

Let Y_{ij} denote the binary obesity status for subject j in cluster i. We assume Y_{ij} follows the logistic model

$$\text{logit}\,\mu_{ij} = \beta_0 + \beta_1 X_{ij1} + \beta_2 X_{ij2} + \beta_3 X_{ij3} + \beta_4 X_{ij4},$$

where for subject j in cluster i, X_{ij1} is the subject's age, X_{ij2} is 1 if the subject is male and 0 otherwise, X_{ij3} is 1 if physical activity index is active and 0 otherwise, and X_{ij4} is 1 if physical activity index is inactive and 0 otherwise. The association between Y_{ij} and Y_{ik}, measured by odds ratio ψ_{ijk}, is modelled by (8.50) where u_{ijk} is specified as 1. Because the proxy responses are obtained from self-reporting, misclassification in obesity is treated independent for different individuals and clusters.

Assuming that misclassification probabilities are covariate-independent and common for all subjects in all clusters, i.e., $\gamma_{0ij} = \gamma_0$ and $\gamma_{1ij} = \gamma_1$ for some constants γ_0 and γ_1, Chen, Yi and Wu (2011) applied the method in §8.7.1 to analyze the data in contrast to the naive analysis which ignores misclassification. The results are displayed in Table 8.1. Although the two methods yield different estimates and standard errors, they reveal the same nature of the covariate effects. There is evidence that age is statistically significant; people tend to be more likely to develop obesity as they get older. The probability of developing obesity is not significantly different between males and females. There is some evidence that active individuals have a smaller chance of developing obesity than individuals who are moderately active. In contrast, individuals in the inactive group are more likely to develop obesity than those in the other two groups. Association parameter ϕ is not statistically significant. While there is no evidence to show significance of misclassification probability γ_0, there is strong evidence that (mis)classification probability γ_1 is statistically significant. More detailed analyses were provided by Chen, Yi and Wu (2011) with different models being assumed for the misclassification process.

Table 8.1. *Analyses of the CCHS Data (Chen, Yi and Wu 2011)*

		Naive method			Method of §8.7.1		
		EST	SE	p-value	EST	SE	p-value
Response model							
Intercept		−2.798	0.225	<0.001	−2.652	0.372	<0.001
Age		0.014	0.003	<0.001	0.016	0.005	<0.001
Sex		0.006	0.124	0.958	0.003	0.152	0.982
Activity	Active	−0.421	0.191	0.027	−0.550	0.265	0.038
	Inactive	0.345	0.153	0.025	0.427	0.189	0.024
Association (ϕ)		0.073	0.114	0.521	0.106	0.170	0.532
Misclassification model							
γ_0		–	–	–	0.984	0.712	0.076
γ_1		–	–	–	0.667	0.408	<0.001

8.8 Bibliographic Notes and Discussion

While covariate mismeasurement has attracted extensive research interest, response measurement error has received much less attention in the statistical literature. In addition to the references discussed in this chapter, here we briefly review some recent work on measurement error in response.

Existing work on measurement error in response may be classified according to whether the response variable is discrete or continuous. While misclassification of discrete response variables may arise from case–control studies (discussed in Chapter 7) and multi-state models (discussed in Chapter 6), misclassified response models are also considered for regression analysis. Under generalized linear models or generalized linear mixed models, Neuhaus (1999, 2002) studied the bias and efficiency issues for misclassified binary response variables. Luan et al. (2005)

conducted simulation studies to assess the trade-off between the reduced biases and increased mean squared errors when misclassification is taken into account for the logistic regression model. Hausman, Abrevaya and Scott-Morton (1998) proposed a semiparametric approach to handle misclassified response models.

With continuous response variables subject to measurement error, Yanez, Kronmal and Shemanski (1998) discussed a moment method for estimation and hypothesis testing for the linear regression model, and Sepanski (2001) described a method of moments for repeated response variable under a linear mixed model. With the linear model, Buonaccorsi (1996) explored estimation methods for a class of measurement error models, including linear and nonlinear response error models.

For the case where both the response and covariate variables are subject to mismeasurement, Ganse, Amemiya and Fuller (1983) discussed prediction for the situation where the parameters of the estimation population differ from those of the prediction population. Spiegelman (1986) illustrated that standard regression diagnostics may fail to detect model departures for the measurement error model. Reilman and Gunst (1985) and Reilman, Gunst and Lakshminarayanan (1986) compared the asymptotic properties for the maximum likelihood estimators and the least squares estimators for linear structural models. Cheng and Van Ness (1994) discussed construction of confidence regions for the linear regression models when both response and covariate variables are observed with measurement error. Wong (1989) explored likelihood estimation for the simple linear regression model, while Roy, Banerjee and Maiti (2005) and Roy and Banerjee (2009) discussed a likelihood method for binary data. McGlothlin, Stamey and Seaman (2008) considered a Bayesian analysis for modeling a binary response that is subject to misclassification and covariates that involve measurement error. Chen, Yi and Wu (2014) proposed a marginal analysis method for handling longitudinal ordinal data with misclassification in both the response and covariate variables.

Early work on errors-in-variables includes Wald (1940), Reiersøl (1950), and Madansky (1959), among many others. Other relevant work on response measurement error includes Breslow and Day (1980), Green (1983), Lakshminarayanan and Gunst (1984), Chua and Fuller (1987), Cheng and Van Ness (1994), Palta and Lin (1999), Bollinger and David (1997, 2001), Chen (2010), and the references therein.

8.9 Supplementary Problems

8.1. Verify (8.14).

(Roy, Banerjee and Maiti 2005)

8.2.

(a) Verify the covariance identity (8.18).

(b) Suppose U and V are two binary variables. If U and V are uncorrelated, show that U and V are independent.

(c) Suppose U, V and W are three binary variables. If they are pairwise independent, are they necessarily independent?

(d) Suppose U, V and W are three random variables.
   (i) If U and V are conditionally independent, given W, is it true that U and V are unconditionally independent?
   (ii) If U and V are independent, is it true that U and V are also conditionally independent, given W?

8.3. Consider the setting in §8.3 where Z_i is scalar. Suppose response Y_i and covariate Z_i are linked by the simple linear regression model

$$Y_i = \beta_0 + \beta_z Z_i + \epsilon_i$$

for $i = 1, \ldots, n$, where $\beta = (\beta_0, \beta_z)^{\mathrm{T}}$ is the vector of regression coefficients, ϵ_i is independent of Z_i, and $\epsilon_i \sim N(0, \sigma^2)$ with variance σ^2.

Assume that conditional on $\{Y_i, Z_i\}$, Y_i^* follows the model

$$Y_i^* = \alpha_0 + \alpha_y Y_i + \alpha_z Z_i + e_i,$$

where $\alpha = (\alpha_0, \alpha_y, \alpha_z)^{\mathrm{T}}$ is the vector of regression coefficients, e_i is independent of $\{Y_i, Z_i\}$, and $e_i \sim N(0, \sigma_e^2)$ with variance σ_e^2.

(a) Show that conditional on Z_i, Y_i^* follows a simple linear regression model

$$Y_i^* = (\alpha_0 + \alpha_y \beta_0) + (\beta_z \alpha_y + \alpha_z) Z_i + e_i^*,$$

where e_i^* is independent of Z_i and $e_i^* \sim N(0, \sigma_e^2 + \alpha_y^2 \sigma^2)$.

(b) Work out the expression of the likelihood (8.23).

(c) Perform inference about β using the result in (b).

8.4. For the setup of Problem 8.3, we assume that σ^2 and σ_e^2 are known, and that Y_i, Z_i and Y_i^* are centered so that $\beta_0 = \alpha_0 = 0$.

(a) Using the validation subsample $\mathcal{V}$ alone, perform the likelihood method for estimation of β_z.

(b) Using both the validation and the main study data, perform estimation of β_z using the *estimated* likelihood function described in §8.3.

(c) Let $\widetilde{\beta}_z$ and $\widehat{\beta}_z$ denote the estimators obtained from (a) and (b), respectively. Find the conditions that $\widetilde{\beta}_z$ is more efficient than $\widehat{\beta}_z$.

(Pepe 1992)

8.5. Consider the setting in §8.4, and suppose that assumptions (8.32) and (8.33) hold. Prove the following results.

(a) For any $y_i, y_i^* = 0, 1$,

$$\begin{aligned} &P(Y_i^* = y_i^* | Y_i = y_i, X_i^*, Z_i) E\{P(Y_i = y_i | X_i, Z_i) | X_i^*, Z_i\} \\ &= P(Y_i^* = y_i^*, Y_i = y_i | X_i^*, Z_i). \end{aligned}$$

(b)

$$\frac{(Y_i^* - \mu_i^*)\{1 - \gamma_{01}(X_i^*, Z_i) - \gamma_{10}(X_i^*, Z_i)\}}{\mu_i^*(1 - \mu_i^*)} = \frac{E(Y_i|Y_i^*, X_i^*, Z_i) - E(\mu_i|X_i^*, Z_i)}{E(\mu_i|X_i^*, Z_i)E(1 - \mu_i|X_i^*, Z_i)}.$$

(c) Prove (8.38) and (8.39).

(Cheng and Hsueh 2003)

8.6. Suppose $(X_1, Y_1), \ldots, (X_n, Y_n)$ are independently and identically distributed. Consider the simple linear regression model

$$Y_i = \beta_0 + \beta_x X_i + \epsilon_i, \tag{8.59}$$

where $\beta = (\beta_0, \beta_x)^{\mathrm{T}}$ is the vector of regression coefficients, the ϵ_i are independent of each other and of the X_i, $\epsilon_i \sim N(0, \sigma^2)$ with variance σ^2, and $i = 1, \ldots, n$.

Suppose that both Y_i and X_i cannot be observed directly. Instead, we observe Y_i^* and X_i^* which are related to Y_i and X_i as follows:

$$Y_i^* = Y_i + e_{yi}; \quad X_i^* = X_i + e_{xi};$$

where the e_{yi} and the e_{xi} are independent of each other and of the $\{X_i, Y_i\}$; $e_{yi} \sim N(0, \sigma_{ye}^2)$ with variance σ_{ye}^2; $e_{xi} \sim N(0, \sigma_{xe}^2)$ with variance σ_{xe}^2; $X_i \sim N(\mu_x, \sigma_x^2)$ with mean μ_x and variance σ_x^2; and $i = 1, \ldots, n$.

In the following questions (b)-(f), assume that σ_{ye}^2 and σ_{xe}^2 are known and identical, and let σ_0^2 denote this common variance.

(a) If both σ_{ye}^2 and σ_{xe}^2 are unknown, is β_x identifiable?
(b) Run the least squares regression analysis by naively replacing Y_i with Y_i^* and X_i with X_i^* in model (8.59), and let $\widehat{\beta}^* = (\widehat{\beta}_0^*, \widehat{\beta}_x^*)^{\mathrm{T}}$ be the resulting estimator for β. Determine the limit to which the naive estimator $\widehat{\beta}^*$ converges in probability as $n \to \infty$.
(c) Show that (X_i^*, Y_i^*) has a bivariate normal distribution. Identify the mean vector and the covariance matrix.
(d) Let $\theta = (\mu_x, \sigma_x^2, \sigma^2, \beta_0, \beta_x)^{\mathrm{T}}$. Can you estimate θ using the likelihood method?
(e) Consider the following reparameterization

$$\alpha_0 = \mu_x; \; \alpha_1 = \beta_0 + \beta_x\mu_x; \; \alpha_2 = \sigma_x^2(\beta_x^2 + 1) + \sigma_0^2.$$

Let $\alpha = (\alpha_0, \alpha_1, \alpha_2, \sigma^2, \beta_x)^{\mathrm{T}}$. Can you estimate α using the likelihood method?
(f) Compare the estimators of β_x obtained in (d) and (e).

Wong (1989)

8.7. Sposto et al. (1992) and Roy, Banerjee and Maiti (2005) discussed a cohort study which assesses the effect of radiation exposure on cancer mortality. Individual radiation exposures were estimated by using DS86 dosimetry; let X^* denote the resulting dose measurement. The true dose for a person is represented by the absorbed radiation, X, measured in Gray (Gy), to his/her intestine at the time of exposure. Assume that given the surrogate X^*, the distribution of the true dose X is normal with mean X^* and variance $0.5X^{*2}$.

The autopsy program reported that the cause of death recorded on the death certificate was subject to misclassification. Let Y be the binary variable indicating the true death cause, with $Y = 1$ for true cancer death and 0 otherwise; and Y^* be the cause based on death certificate diagnosis. Sposto et al. (1992) found that the overall crude misclassification rate of cancer deaths is 22% and of noncancer deaths is 3.5%, i.e., $P(Y^* = 0|Y = 1) = 22\%$ and $P(Y^* = 1|Y = 0) = 3.5\%$. Assume these are the common misclassification rates among different dose categories.

Table 8.2. *Radiation Doses X^* and Death Counts for Cancer and Noncancer Individuals Based on Death Certificate Diagnosis (Sposto et al. 1992)*

Dose X^*	Cancer deaths	Noncancer deaths
0.000	2784	10, 201
0.018	2105	7451
0.072	439	1509
0.137	523	1701
0.324	586	1785
0.693	339	826
1.350	204	369
2.350	57	86
3.520	21	51
4.430	13	23

Table 8.2 shows the number of cancer and noncancer deaths grouped by the death certificate corresponding to different dose values X^*. The data are viewed as contaminated with both measurement error in covariate and misclassification error in response. Analyze the data to uncover how cancer-death is associated with the true radiation exposure amount X by the following four schemes and compare the analysis results:

(a) Ignoring both measurement error in X and misclassification in Y;
(b) Ignoring measurement error in X but accounting for misclassification in Y;
(c) Ignoring misclassification in Y but accounting for error in X;
(d) Accounting for both error in X and misclassification in Y.

(Roy, Banerjee and Maiti 2005)

8.8.

(a) For model (8.42) in §8.5, assume the nondifferential measurement error mechanism with $h(y|x, x^*) = h(y|x)$, where $h(\cdot|\cdot)$ represents the conditional distribution for the corresponding variables. Prove that $E(\epsilon^*|X^*) = 0$ and that ϵ^* is uncorrelated with any function of X^*.

(b) Prove (8.43).

(c) Prove that in (8.46), e is orthogonal to $E(Y^* - Y|W)$.

(Lee and Sepanski 1995)

8.9. Consider the nonlinear model (8.41) in §8.5 where Y is the response variable and X is the covariate vector.

(a) Suppose Y is subject to measurement error and X is precisely observed. Assume the validation sample $\mathcal{V}_y$ is available where $X_i^* = X_i$, along with the main study data $\{(Y_i^*, X_i) : i = 1, \ldots, n\}$. Develop an estimation procedure for β using the least squares projection method.

(b) Suppose both Y and X are subject to measurement error. Instead of having two independent validation samples $\mathcal{V}_x$ and $\mathcal{V}_y$ available as in §8.5, there is a common validation sample $\mathcal{V}$ for which $\{(X_i, Y_i, X_i^*, Y_i^*) : i \in \mathcal{V}\}$ is available, in addition to the availability of the main study data $\{(X_i^*, Y_i^*) : i = 1, \ldots, n\}$. Develop an estimation procedure for β using the least squares projection method. Comment on the differences between this procedure and that described in §8.5?

8.10.

(a) Verify (8.57).

(b) Instead of using (8.58) for estimation of θ, can you construct new sets of estimating functions for θ by replacing V_{1i} and $\widetilde{V_{2i}}$ respectively with the covariance matrices for the Y_{ij}^{**} and the Y_{ijk}^{**} in (8.57)?

(c) Instead of using the indictors R_{ij} to describe the pairwise association for the components of Y_i^* in §8.7.1, can you directly use components Y_{ij}^* to describe modeling of the misclassification process by following the discussion of modeling for the response components Y_{ij}?

(d) How does the development of (b) and (c) differ from that of §8.7.1?

(e) Can you apply the expectation correction strategy, described in §2.5.2, to develop an estimation procedure for θ that is associated with the models in §8.7.1?

(Chen, Yi and Wu 2011)

8.11. When there is no gold standard of a diagnostic test for a disease, repeated measurements may be used to assess the reliability of the test. Let Y_i be the true binary status for subject i, taking value 1 if subject i is diseased and 0 otherwise. Let Y_{ij}^* be the binary result of the jth test for individual i, where $Y_{ij}^* = 1$ for a positive result and $Y_{ij}^* = 0$ for a negative result, $j = 1, \ldots, m_i$, and $i = 1, \ldots, n$. Assume that each test is independently applied and the probability of having a false-positive or false-negative is constant. Let

$$\gamma_{01} = P(Y_{ij}^* = 1 | Y_i = 0),\ \gamma_{10} = P(Y_{ij}^* = 0 | Y_i = 1),$$

and $\widetilde{\pi} = P(Y_i = 1)$. Let $\theta = (\gamma_{01}, \gamma_{10}, \widetilde{\pi})^{\mathrm{T}}$.

(a) Construct the likelihood for parameter θ.
(b) Show that parameter θ is not identifiable in (a).
(c) If we assume that $\gamma_{01} + \gamma_{10} < 1$ and $m_i \geq 3$ for some i, then θ in (a) is identifiable.
(d) We wish to test the hypothesis $H_o : \gamma_{01} = 0$. Can the likelihood ratio test be applied for this purpose? What might be the problem?
(e) To get rid of associated constraints for θ, we reparameterize θ as:

$$\alpha_0 = \text{logit}\ \gamma_{01};\ \alpha_1 = \text{logit}\ \gamma_{10};\ \beta = \text{logit}\ \widetilde{\pi};$$

and let $\vartheta = (\alpha_1, \alpha_0, \beta)^{\mathrm{T}}$. With the conditions in (c), can you apply the likelihood method to conduct inference about ϑ?
(f) Fujisawa and Izumi (2000) discussed a serological data set which was obtained from Hiroshima and Nagasaki city residents. Table 8.3 displays the frequency of outcomes observed in repeated serological tests for the MNSs blood system by location of laboratory. Analyze the data by incorporating that misclassification may be affected by the laboratory equipment at different locations and different occasions for the MNSs system.

Table 8.3. *Frequency of Observed Positive Responses ($\sum_{j=1}^n Y_{ij}^*$) among Repeated Serological Tests (m_i) for the MNSs Blood System by Location of Laboratory (Fujisawa and Izumi 2000)*

		$\sum_{j=1}^n Y_{ij}^* (m_i = 2)$			$\sum_{j=1}^n Y_{ij}^* (m_i = 3)$				$\sum_{j=1}^n Y_{ij}^* (m_i = 4)$				
Antigen	City	0	1	2	0	1	2	3	0	1	2	3	4
M	Hiroshima	419	8	1918	77	4	1	279	4	1	0	0	29
	Nagasaki	257	13	958	26	2	1	127	3	0	0	0	13
N	Hiroshima	714	23	1587	117	5	10	225	13	0	0	2	19
	Nagasaki	324	70	799	40	3	27	85	4	1	0	4	7
S	Hiroshima	1823	29	208	269	1	10	33	24	1	0	2	1
	Nagasaki	868	52	43	83	1	7	4	8	0	0	0	0
s	Hiroshima	19	1	2316	9	0	0	349	0	0	0	1	33
	Nagasaki	5	5	1065	1	1	3	133	0	0	0	0	15

(Fujisawa and Izumi 2000)

8.12.

(a) Suppose there are K covariate patterns $\{Z_k : k = 1, \ldots, K\}$. For each Z_k with $k = 1, \ldots, K$, run a Bernoulli trial independently n_k times, and let Y_{ki} and Y_{ki}^*, respectively, be the unobserved true outcome and the observed outcome of the ith trial where $i = 1, \ldots, n_k$. Define $N_{k+}^* = \sum_{i=1}^{n_k} Y_{ki}^*$ for $k = 1, \ldots, K$.

For $k = 1, \ldots, K$ and $i = 1, \ldots, n_k$, assume that the conditional probabilities $P(Y_{ki} = 1|Z_k)$ are free of i, and let $\mu_k = P(Y_{ki} = 1|Z_k)$. Consider a generalized linear model

$$g(\mu_k) = \beta^{\mathrm{T}} Z_k,$$

where $g(\cdot)$ is a link function, β is the parameter vector, and $k = 1, \ldots, K$.

For $k = 1, \ldots, K$ and $i = 1, \ldots, n_k$, assume that the misclassification probabilities $P(Y_{ki}^* = y_{ki}^*|Y_{ki}, Z_k)$ are free of Z_k and i, and then define

$$\gamma_{01} = P(Y_{ki}^* = 1|Y_{ki} = 0) \text{ and } \gamma_{10} = P(Y_{ki}^* = 0|Y_{ki} = 1).$$

Let $\theta = (\beta^{\mathrm{T}}, \gamma_{01}, \gamma_{10})^{\mathrm{T}}$.

(i) Find the distribution of N_{k+}^* for $k = 1, \ldots, K$.
(ii) Construct the likelihood function of θ.
(iii) Discuss the identifiability of model parameter θ.

(b) Paulino, Soares and Neuhaus (2003) analyzed the data on a study of human papilloma virus (HPV) infection. The study screened 104 women. The data recorded for each woman her infection status (HPVS) at the end of the study, whether she had a history of vulvar warts (VW), whether she had any new sexual partner in the last 2 months at baseline (NSP), and whether she had a history of herpes simplex (HS). HPV is a family of viruses responsible for various epithelial lesions of which over 90 subtypes have been described. However, any test for HPV infection is limited to one subtype or a group of subtypes, thus, the response variable HPV is bound to be affected by misclassification.

Let Z_k be the covariate vector (VW, NSP, HS) with the kth pattern, and n_k be the number of women with covariate vector Z_k. Let Y_{ki} be the true HPV infection status of woman i with Z_k, Y_{ki}^* be the corresponding observed infection status, and N_{k+}^* be defined as in (a). The data are presented in Table 8.4.

Table 8.4. *HPV Infection Data (Paulino, Soares and Neuhaus 2003)*

z_k	N^*_{k+}	n_k
(0,0,0)	12	44
(0,0,1)	1	2
(0,1,0)	29	40
(0,1,1)	3	3
(1,0,0)	6	9
(1,1,0)	1	4
(1,1,1)	2	2
Total	54	104

Conduct sensitivity analyses for this data set using the results in (a) where γ_{01} and γ_{10} are specified as various values. Compare the results by choosing different link functions:

(i) the logit link $g(v) = \log\left(\frac{v}{1-v}\right)$;
(ii) the probit link $g(v) = \Phi^{-1}(v)$;
(iii) the complementary log-log link $g(v) = \log\{-\log(1-v)\}$.

9

Miscellaneous Topics

Many methods discussed in this book are motivated by research problems arising from various fields, including nutrition studies, cancer research and environmental studies. Methods and application of measurement error models are vast in the epidemiology literature. Although the book discusses some research in this field, the coverage is far from complete. Measurement error and misclassification have been a long-standing concern in many other fields such as econometrics and have attracted extensive research. This book has, however, not looked into the details in those areas.

The book focuses on the development of measurement error models in the statistics literature. While the methods developed for other fields are of equal importance and usefulness, it is difficult to summarize all the available work in this book; even for the research appearing in the statistical journals, many methods have not been touched upon in this book. For example, measurement error is a common issue in survey science but this book does not cover this topic. Research of measurement error in surveys has been extensive in the literature. A document in this area was provided by Biemer et al. (1991).

The inference objective of this book centers around estimation of model parameters, which intrinsically position us in the frequentist framework. Placing measurement error and misclassification problems in the Bayesian paradigm, many authors explored methods and strategies for dealing with effects arising from mismeasurement. A book treatment on this topic is available in Gustafson (2004) and Carroll et al. (2006, Ch. 9).

To close the book, in this chapter we outline several topics that are available in the literature but are not described in the book. Interested readers may find the details from the references mentioned and the references therein.

G. Y. Yi, *Statistical Analysis with Measurement Error or Misclassification*,
Springer Series in Statistics, DOI 10.1007/978-1-4939-6640-0_9

9.1 General Issues on Measurement Error Models

In this book, we concentrate on discussing models and methods for handling mismeasurement in variables for a number of application areas. The development is derived under the assumption that the assumed models used for inferences are feasible. Although a variety of inferential methods, especially estimation procedures, are described to account for effects induced from measurement error and misclassification, many questions and issues remain unanswered or untouched upon in this book. These questions include

- For given models, if there are multiple ways to develop inference methods to account for measurement error or misclassification effects, how do we choose the most suitable or the best method among those candidates?
- With error-contaminated data, how do we even start with a model building? How do we decide what variables should be included in the model and what variables should not?
- When reasonable candidate models are available, how do we ensure the model parameters to be identifiable and estimable?
- In the presence of measurement error or misclassification in the variables, how do we perform goodness-of-fit to assess the feasibility of the response model, the measurement error or misclassification model, and even the model for the covariates?
- What is the impact on inferential procedures if model misspecification arises?
- To reduce the risk of model misspecification, how do we proceed with semiparametric or nonparametric approaches? Compared with parametric modeling, what may be the loss of using semiparametric or nonparametric approaches?
- Do measurement error and misclassification always have to be taken into account? Are there situations where attempting to account for mismeasurement effects is not worthy but ignoring mismeasurement is more beneficial than taking care of it?
- We concentrate on developing estimation procedures to incorporate measurement error and misclassification effects. How does measurement error effects influence hypothesis testing and prediction?
- How does the featrue of measurement error affect the design of a study?

While these questions do not exhaust all the problems on measurement error models, they are important to study. However, we are unable to provide precise answers to them to uncover all possible circumstances. To give the readers a brief idea, here we skim on these issues by mentioning some work in the literature.

Use of a Plausible Method

In §2.5 we present general strategies, although incomprehensive, for dealing with error-contaminated data. Applications, modifications, and extensions of those strategies are developed throughout Chapters 3–8 for a broad range of problems. A natural question arises: with the given data and the same model assumptions, if there are multiple methods to accommodate mismeasurement effects, is there a best method among them? If yes, how do we know which method is the best?

While some authors studied and compared the performance of certain methods of adjusting measurement error effects (see Freedman et al. (2008) for instance), it is generally difficult to provide analytical comparisons among different candidate methods for general situations. Numerical experiences, however, may sometimes help us understand the performance of various methods. For instance, in nutrition and physical activity epidemiology, measurement error in covariates may be dominant and the failure time outcome may occur for only a small fraction of the study cohort. In this context, with a biomarker subsample that plausibly adheres to a classical measurement model, Shaw and Prentice (2012) found that simple regression calibration tends to be much more efficient than nonparametric correction procedures and produces negligible bias in analysis results. In a personal correspondence, Ross Prentice suggested that nonparametric correction procedures that simply replace the elements of an estimating function by unbiased estimates thereof may be too ad hoc to have good efficiency in such settings. Stated another way, these nonparametric procedures may be too far from any suitable likelihood.

In other simulation settings, Ross Prentice and his collaborators noted that the conditional scores procedure lacks robustness to departures from normality for measurement error. This phenomenon has also been observed for other methods, such as the SIMEX method. Yi and He (2012) demonstrated, using simulation studies, that the performance of the SIMEX approach is sensitive to misspecification of the normality assumption for the measurement error model.

It is difficult to offer universal guidance for the readers as to what measurement error approaches are to be preferred over others. This depends on many factors, including, but not limited to, the form of the response and measurement error/misclassification models, the association structures among the variables, the magnitude of mismeasurement in variables, and the availability of computing facilities. Even for a very simple case where an error-prone covariate is binary, the answer is not obvious. Yi et al. (2016) provided a detailed discussion on this issue.

Measurement Error Models

Models for delineating mismeasurement processes are outlined in §2.6. However, they are far from complete for dealing with various practical problems. Many types of measurement error models have been considered in the literature. To name a few, see Rosner (1996), Carroll et al. (1998), Black, Berger and Scott (2000), Arellano-Valle, Bolfarine and Gasco (2002), Kukush, Markovsky and Huffel (2002), Arellano-Valle et al. (2005), and Midthune et al. (2016), among others.

Much of the development in this book is directed to measurement error and misclassification for time-invariant variables. For example, the regression calibration method, presented in §2.5.2 and §3.3.1, is for error-prone covariates which are time-independent. However, time-varying covariates may also be error-contaminated; in this case, proper modifications should be introduced to factor in temporal effects. Xie, Wang and Prentice (2001), Liao et al. (2011) and Shaw and Prentice (2012) developed the *risk set calibration* approaches which extend the standard regression calibration method with the time factor taken into account.

Measurement error in time-varying covariates is an important and practical topic. Although we discuss this aspect at various places, such as §4.3, §4.4, and Chapters 5 and 6, new issues on time-evolving covariates with mismeasurement emerge and need to be substantially addressed for individual applications.

Identification and Estimation

As discussed throughout the book, in the presence of measurement error, non-identifiability becomes a concern which is primarily caused by additional modeling of the measurement error process. Many authors studied the issues concerning identification and estimation under individual circumstances (e.g., Paulino and de Bragança Pereira 1994). For instance, under linear regression models with a binary covariate subject to misclassification, Bollinger (1996) established lower and upper bounds for the model parameters. The approach by Bollinger (1996) reveals maximum amount of misclassification which may feasibly be present in order to make meaningful inferences. Klepper (1988) examined the same problem but considered different models where multiple dichotomous variables are subject to misclassification and multiple continuous variables are subject to classical measurement error. Klepper and Leamer (1984) and Krasker and Pratt (1986) considered the situation where mismeasured covariates are continuous variables. Hu (2006) discussed a linear regression model with a mismeasured regressor where the measurement error is correlated with both the latent variable and the regression error. He showed that if the mismeasured regressor contains enough information on the latent variable, the finite bounds on the parameters can be found using the variance of the latent variable, regardless of the correlation between the measurement error and the regression error. While unidentification arises frequently from linear measurement error models, this feature is not necessarily retained by models for repeated observation data. This point was discussed by Griliches and Hausman (1986) and Wansbeek and Koning (1991).

In the presence of measurement error in continuous covariates under nonlinear models, Hausman et al. (1991) considered identification and estimation of the coefficients of a polynomial regression function. Lewbel (1998) discussed conditions for semiparametric identification for general latent variable models using instruments uncorrelated with measurement errors. Carroll, Chen and Hu (2010) considered the setting with two samples which share the same conditional distribution of the response given the true covariates, but the distributions of the latent true covariates are different. Their discussion concerns issues of identification and estimation in the absence of knowledge about the measurement error distribution, of an instrumental variable and of validation data as well as of replicated surrogate measurements. Assuming that the conditional distribution of the response given the true covariates is modeled parametrically, they developed a sieve quasi-MLE approach to estimation, with the measurement error distribution and the distribution of the latent variable featured nonparametrically.

Most methods for correcting for measurement error effects require additional information, such as validation data, measurement error distributions to be known, repeated measurements, or instrumental variables. In contrast, Schennach and Hu (2013) established that the fully nonparametric classical errors-in-variables model is identifiable from data on the regressor and the dependent variable alone. Their result basically relies on regularity conditions taking the form of smoothness constraints and nonvanishing characteristic functions. Their discussion offers a new perspective on handling measurement error in nonlinear and nonparametric models.

Instrumental Variables

Wang (2004) suggested that a nonlinear model with Berkson error is usually identifiable without extra information under certain model assumptions. However, in order for a classical measurement error model to be identifiable, extra information, such as validation data or replicate data, is often needed, as discussed throughout the book. In the event that validation data or replicate data are unavailable, information from instrumental data may be useful to undertake inferences under measurement error models. Many authors studied estimation for measurement error models using instrumental variables, and much work may be found in the econometrics literature. To give the readers an idea, we briefly review several methods, bearing in mind this is far from complete.

Feldstein (1974) proposed an estimation method using a weighted average of the instrumental variable estimator and the ordinary least squares estimator. Carter and Fuller (1980) discussed alternative instrumental variable estimators for the slope in the simple errors-in-variables model using the likelihood-based method. For linear measurement error models, Fuller (1987, Ch. 2) discussed estimation methods using instrumental variables, among many other authors.

Amemiya (1985, 1990) studied instrumental methods for general nonlinear regression models. Stefanski and Buzas (1995) considered generalized linear measurement error models with instrumental variables. Buzas and Stefanski (1996a) discussed estimation for a parametric structural probit model with measurement error, while Buzas and Stefanski (1996b) exploited functional methods for generalized linear measurement error models with instrumental variables which are assumed to follow a conditional normal distribution. Using the information from instrumental variables, Abarin and Wang (2012) explored a method of moments for estimation of parameters associated with generalized linear measurement error models.

Carroll et al. (2004) discussed the use of instrumental variables for covariate measurement error problems for a general class of regression models in which regression functions may be modeled linearly, nonlinearly, and nonparametrically. They showed that the regression function and all parameters in the measurement error model are identified under weak conditions. Their results extend the applicability of instrumental variable estimation to many interesting situations.

With the availability of instrumental variables, Hu and Schennach (2008) established the identification for a class of nonclassical nonlinear errors-in-variables models with continuously distributed variables. They showed that the identification problem may be cast into the form of an operator diagonalization problem in which the operator to be diagonalized is defined in terms of observable densities, while the resulting eigenvalues and eigenfunctions provide the unobserved joint densities of the variables of interest.

Under the Bayesian inference framework, Gustafson (2007) considered measurement error modeling using an approximate instrumental variable. He contrasted inferences arising from the approximate instrumental variable assumption with their exact instrumental variable counterparts and uncovered the benefit of basing inferences on a more realistic model versus the cost of basing inferences on an unidentified model.

Model Selection and Dimension Reduction

In application, we may collect a large number of covariates, and some of them have no predictive value on the response variable. Including such covariates in modelling and inferential procedures would greatly degrade the quality of the results. Variable selection thus becomes necessary and critical for valid inferences. There is a large body of variable selection methods for settings which are free of measurement error (e.g., Tibshirani 1996; Fan and Li 2001; Miller 2002). In the presence of measurement error, however, research on this topic is relatively limited but not unavailable.

For linear measurement error models, Huang and Zhang (2013) proposed variable selection procedures based on penalized score functions. With cross-sectional error-contaminated data, Liang and Li (2009) and Ma and Li (2010) exploited variable selection methods based on the SCAD penalty function (Fan and Li 2001). In contrast, for longitudinal data with covariate measurement error, Shen and Chen (2015) considered marginal regression analysis and proposed a model selection criterion. Their method is based on the expected quadratic error measuring the discrepancy between the true and the considered model for the marginal mean. Yi, Tan and Li (2015) developed a simulation-based procedure to conduct model selection and parameter estimation simultaneously; they also considered the feature of missing data in the development. Other relevant work includes Wang, Zou and Wan (2012) and the references therein.

From a different but closely related perspective, measurement error effects have been investigated for *dimension reduction* in regression models. Dimension reduction has attracted extensive interest for settings without mismeasurement. (e.g., Cook 2007). In the presence of measurement error, research is sparse but suggestive. With covariate measurement error, Carroll and Li (1992) and Lue (2004) discovered that the usual dimension reduction techniques, such as ordinary least squares, sliced inverse regression and principle Hessian directions methods, still apply to the observed surrogate measurements with a suitable adjustment; and the modified methods can produce consistent estimates for the original regression problem involving the unobserved true covariates. More generally, Li and Yin (2007) established a general invariance law between the surrogate and the original dimension reduction spaces, which implies that at the population level, the two dimension reduction problems are in fact equivalent.

Model Checking and Semiparametric Methods

In this book, our discussion focuses on the parametric and semiparametric settings, where the measurement error process is typically modeled parametrically, and the response process is modulated by a parametric or semiparametric regression model. With this setup, concerns of model misspecification naturally arise. The discussion on model misspecification in the presence of measurement error may be classified into three categories: (1) only the response model $f(y|x,z)$ is misspecified, (2) only the nuisance models, including measurement error model $f(x,x^*|z)$ and the covariate model $f(x|z)$, are misspecified, and (3) both the response and nuisance models are misspecified.

It is well demonstrated that biased results are often derived if model misspecification is present. For example, with scenario (2), Reddy (1992) illustrated the impact of ignoring correlated measurement error under some simple structural equation models. Schneeweiss and Cheng (2006) studied the bias of structural quasi-score estimators when the distribution of X is misspecified.

Model diagnosing is thus very important for assessing the validity of the results obtained from the assumed models. Huang, Stefanski and Davidian (2006) proposed methods for diagnosing misspecification of the distribution of the true covariates for structural measurement error models. For group testing data which involve covariate measurement error, Huang (2009) proposed a method for detecting latent-variable model misspecification in structural measurement error models. Regarding fitting a parametric mean regression model, Koul and Song (2008) discussed test procedures for covariate measurement error which follows the Berkson measurement error model.

To reduce the impact induced from model misspecification, it is tempting to make minimal model assumptions. Regarding the treatment of the true covariates, the functional modeling strategy, discussed in §2.4, is desirable to invoke and many methods have been available in the literature. On the other hand, if the structural modeling strategy has to be struck, it is useful to develop inference methods that are robust or less insensitive to misspecification of the distribution of the true covariates. Many authors explored in this direction. For instance, Lachos et al. (2009) used skew-normal distributions to model the unobserved error-prone covariates. For nonlinear errors-in-variables models, Li (2002) developed a two-stage estimation procedure by assuming randomness for the true, unobserved regressors but making no parametric assumption for the distribution of these regressors. The first stage involves nonparametric estimation of the conditional density of these regressors, given the measurements; and at the second stage, a semiparametric nonlinear least-squares estimator is developed for the response model parameters.

Using the semiparametric efficient score derived under a possibly incorrect distributional assumption for the unobserved error-prone covariates, Tsiatis and Ma (2004) developed estimating equations methods and proposed a class of locally efficient semiparametric estimators. Implementing the technique of Tsiatis and Ma (2004) to generalized linear models with normal measurement error, Ma and Tsiatis (2006) showed the equivalence of the resulting estimator to the efficient score estimator derived by Stefanski and Carroll (1987).

Ma and Carroll (2006) constructed locally efficient estimators under semiparametric measurement error models where the error-free variables Z are nonparametrically modeled through the local kernel and a parametric specification is assumed for the measurement error and error-prone covariate X. They established semiparametric efficiency for the resulting estimators. Using repeated surrogate measurements of the unobserved true covariates, Sinha and Ma (2014) applied a semiparametric approach to fitting a linear transformation model for analysis of right censored data with error-prone covariates.

To address the consequences of model misspecification, another strategy is to relax assumptions on modeling the measurement error process. Flexible parametric models are developed to characterize measurement error, see Carroll, Roeder and Wasserman (1999), for instance. Semiparametric or nonparametric modeling may also be applied to handle the measurement error process. For example, using the technique by Li (2002), Li and Hsiao (2004) developed robust estimation for generalized linear models without specifying distributional assumptions on measurement errors and the true covariate X. Carroll, Knickerbocker and Wang (1995) considered a semiparametric estimation method for general regression model when some covariates are measured with error. Using the dimension reduction techniques, they assumed that the true covariates depend only on a linear combination of the observed covariates and surrogates, which allows them to avoid using higher-order kernels for estimation.

Other robust inference methods for measurement error models are available as well. For example, Wang and Rao (2002) and Cui and Chen (2003) employed the empirical likelihood method to account for measurement error effects. Huang (2011) considered the application of the empirical likelihood method to a partially linear single-index measure error model with right censored data. Sinha et al. (2010) developed a Bayesian method where semiparametric modeling is employed to describe the relationship between the disease and exposure variables as well as the relationship between the surrogate and the true exposure measurements. Sarkar, Mallick and Carroll (2014) described a Bayesian semiparametric method based on mixtures of B-splines and mixtures induced by Dirichlet processes.

Influential Observations and Robust Inference

In contrast to robustness to model misspecification, it is also useful to develop methods which are robust to influential observations, or outliers. In the absence of measurement error, research on this topic has received a great deal of attention since the paper by Cook (1977). In the context with measurement error, many authors studied the problems of identifying outliers or influential observations. For instance, with linear regression models with measurement error in both response and covariate variables, Kelly (1984) proposed diagnostic procedures for the detection of influential observations. Wellman and Gunst (1991) developed influence diagnostics to assess the influence of extreme observations on estimators of linear measurement error models. Zhao, Lee and Hui (1994) derived influence functions and case-deletion diagnostics for generalized linear measurement error models while Zhao and Lee (1995) considered the problem for nonlinear measurement error models. For the simple linear regression model with an additive error in the covariate, Abdullah (1995) explored the detection of influential observations using influence diagnostics based on leverage values, influence curve, and case-deletion methods. For linear and generalized linear models with measurement error, Lee and Zhao (1996) performed local influence analysis, which extends the development of Cook (1986) and Thomas and Cook (1989) that are only applicable to settings without measurement error.

For the simple structural errors-in-variables model, Kim (2000) considered the outlier detection problem using the likelihood displacement approach. Assuming that the observed variables follow a bivariate Student-t distribution, Galea, Bolgarine and Vilcalabra (2002) discussed local influence and diagnostics for the structural errors-in-variables models. Discussion on this topic can also be found in Fuller (1987, Ch. 3).

Using the corrected likelihood of Nakamura (1990), Zare and Rasekh (2011) developed case-deletion diagnostics for detecting influential points for linear mixed measurement error models. Lachos, Montenegro and Bolfarine (2008) considered issues concerning inference and influence diagnostic for measurement error regression models; they adopted the structural modeling scheme with the true covariate X assumed a univariate skew-normal distribution. Taking the Bayesian perspective, Vidal, Iglesias and Galea (2007) discussed detection of influential observations for the simple linear regression model with an additive error in the covariate.

Nonparametric Inference and Measurement Error

Research on nonparametric estimation in the presence of measurement error has attracted much attention in the literature. Many authors studied nonparametric methods from multiple angles. Delaigle (2014) provided a review on this topic and summarized the main techniques related to kernel estimators, which are the most popular nonparametric errors-in-variables methods. Here we briefly mention a few papers in this direction to give the readers a brief idea.

Density estimation from a sample contaminated with classical errors, often referred to as a *deconvolution problem*, has been extensively studied in the literature, see, for example, Fan and Truong (1993), Li and Vuong (1998), and Meister (2006). Among many nonparametric density estimators, the deconvolution kernel estimator, developed by Carroll and Hall (1988) and Stefanski and Carroll (1990b), is the one that has perhaps received the most attention.

In contrast to the extensive study of density estimation from a sample contaminated with classical measurement error, Delaigle, Hall and Qiu (2006) discussed nonparametric techniques for analyzing data that are generated by the Berkson measurement error model. Delaigle (2007) discussed density estimation for the situation where the data contain two types of measurement error: incurred before and after the experiment. She proposed two nonparametric estimators of a density function that account for classical errors, Berkson errors, or a mixture of the two. Carroll, Delaigle and Hall (2007) explored nonparametric estimation of a regression function when the covariate is observed with a mixture of Berkson and classical measurement errors. They established consistency of the resulting estimator, derived rates of convergence, and described a data-driven implementation procedure.

With sample units being measured with error, Stefanski and Bay (1996) studied estimation of a cumulative distribution function and proposed a bias-adjusted estimator. Carroll, Maca and Ruppert (1999) considered the problem of nonparametric regression function estimation in the presence of measurement error in the predictor. They used the SIMEX method and established asymptotic results for kernel regression, which requires no assumption about the distribution of the unobserved error-prone predictor. They also developed an approach using regression spline under the assumption that the error-prone predictor has a distribution of a mixture of normals with an unknown number of components. Delaigle and Gijbels (2002) proposed kernel estimators for integrated squared density derivatives from a sample that is contaminated with random noise. They derived asymptotic expressions for the bias and the variance of the estimator. Staudenmayer, Ruppert and Buonaccorsi (2008) considered density estimation when the variable is subject to heteroscedastic measurement error. They studied the effects of heteroscedastic measurement error and presented an equivalent kernel for a spline-based density estimator.

Contrasting to the broad use of local polynomial estimators for nonparametric regression estimation for error-free settings, Delaigle, Fan and Carroll (2009) proposed a local polynomial estimator of any order in the errors-in-variables context and derived its design-adaptive asymptotic properties. For nonparametric inference, Carroll and Hall (2004) suggested kernel and orthogonal series methods that are applicable to both deconvolution and regression with errors in explanatory variables.

Within the Bayesian framework, Berry, Carroll and Ruppert (2002) considered the problem of nonparametric regression when the independent variables are measured with error, where the regression function is modeled with smoothing splines and regression P-splines. Sarkar et al. (2014) proposed Bayesian semiparametric approaches for estimating the density of a random variable when precise measurements on the variable are not available but replicated proxies contaminated with measurement error are available.

Hypothesis Test

Research on measurement error models largely concentrates on estimation rather than hypothesis testing, as reflected by the contents of this book. It is known that ignoring measurement error can cause misleading results, such as bias in point estimates and variance estimates for parameter estimation. The impact of mismeasurement on hypothesis testing, however, has been much less studied (Carroll et al. 2006, Ch. 10). As briefly discussed in §2.2, hypothesis testing may be less sensitive to mismeasurement, or may even remain unchanged in some situations. Under linear regression models, Cheng and Tsai (2004) investigated the invariance property of score tests for assessing heteroscedasticity, first-order autoregressive disturbance, and the need for a Box–Cox power transformation. Under certain constraints, they showed that the score tests for measurement error models are identical to the corresponding well-established tests derived from standard regression models.

Kim and Goldberg (2001) studied the effects of outcome misclassification and measurement error on the type I error rate and the power of equivalence trials. Lagakos (1988) and Begg and Lagakos (1992, 1993) studied the consequences of measurement error for different test procedures. Brunner and Austin (2009) focused on how the Type I error rate may be inflated for multiple regression with error-prone covariates.

Under generalized linear models with covariate measurement error, Stefanski and Carroll (1990a) and Sepanski (1992) investigated score tests, and Stefanski and Carroll (1991) discussed deconvolution-based score tests. For generalized linear models with covariate measurement error, Tosteson and Tsiatis (1988) derived a score test for association in the presence of nuisance parameters.

Hanfelt and Liang (1997) studied an approximate likelihood test based on the conditional score method of Stefanski and Carroll (1987). Gimenez, Colosimo and Bolfarine (2000) and Gimenez, Bolfarine and Colosimo (2000) examined test procedures based on a corrected score method proposed by Nakamura (1990). Using the score tests for the variance components in random effects models, Li and Lin (2003b) proposed procedures for testing the within-cluster correlation and extended the results to clustered censored discrete failure time data. With logistic measurement error models, Thoresen and Laake (2007) conducted simulation studies to compare the performance of the likelihood ratio test, a Wald-type test and the score test. Using the maximum likelihood approach and the method of moments, Galea and Giménez (2010) discussed test procedures for linear regression models with an additive error in covariates.

de Castro, Galea and Bolfarine (2008) proposed test statistics for the case where the observations follow a bivariate normal distribution and the measurement errors are normally distributed. With functional measurement error models, Ma et al. (2011) studied a score-type local test and an orthogonal series-based goodness-of-fit test for the semiparametric framework where no likelihood function is available.

Commented by Murad and Freedman (2007), analysis of models with interaction effects in the presence of measurement error was initially investigated by behavioral researchers, such as Kenny and Judd (1984), Jaccard and Wan (1995) and Joreskog and Yang (1996), who considered structural equation models with nonlinear effects such as interaction and quadratic terms. Kenny and Judd (1984) proposed a method for removing the bias from the interaction effect based on latent variable modelling. Using the method of moments and the regression calibration approach, Murad and Freedman (2007) discussed procedures for testing interactions in a linear regression model when normally distributed explanatory variables are subject to classical measurement error. With both continuous and categorical variables involved in linear measurement error models, Huang, Wang and Cox (2005) discussed issues concerning the assessment of slope-by-factor interactions.

Prediction

Mismeasurement may or may not have effects on prediction (e.g., Schaalje and Butts 1993). Lindley (1947) showed that in the presence of measurement error in covariate X, the simple regression of response Y on X is still appropriate for prediction of Y from X, provided that the population parameters from which the new X is drawn are identical to those of the data to which the regression was fitted. Ganse, Amemiya and Fuller (1983) presented the prediction equation for the situation where the parameters of the estimation population differ from those of the prediction population.

Under the linear measurement error model, if the objective is prediction, it is generally not necessary to adjust for measurement errors (Fuller 1987, §1.6) in many cases. Buonaccorsi (1995) discussed when correction of measurement error effects is needed for predication, and proposed a method of estimating the prediction standard deviation. Carroll, Delaigle and Hall (2009) considered nonparametric prediction in measurement error models. They showed how to predict in errors-in-variables regression by combining the information from different sources for the setting where the errors have different distributions.

In contrast to estimation in the presence of measurement error, which often requires additional information in order to overcome model nonidentifiability issues, unidentifiable measurement error models can even be useful if the goal is prediction, and in some situations additional information is not needed for prediction. Huwang and Hwang (2002) identified such cases with two nonlinear measurement error models: exponential and log-linear models. They applied pseudo-likelihood estimation of variance functions involved with the weighted least squares method and constructed prediction and confidence intervals for these two models.

Design

In §7.6, we discuss two-phase designs with an exposure variable subject to misclassification. There has been limited investigation on optimal designs of collecting data for providing the necessary information to conduct valid inferences when some variables are anticipated to be inevitably error-prone, though some work has been available (Spiegelman 1994). Tosteson and Ware (1990) considered designing a logistic regression study using surrogate measurements for the exposure and outcome variables. Spiegelman and Gary (1991) discussed reasonably inexpensive but statistically powerful cohort study designs for epidemiologic research when a single continuous covariate is measured with error. Carroll, Freedman and Pee (1997) investigated design and analysis aspects for linear measurement error models with missing surrogate data. Lyles, Lin and Williamson (2004) proposed a study design for repeated binary outcomes which are subject to misclassification. Under the estimating functions framework, Spiegelman, Zhao and Kim (2005) proposed several study designs with correlated measurement errors taken into account. Covariate measurement error has the impact on the calculation of the power and sample sizes. Ignoring covariate measurement error tends to overestimate the power and underestimate the actual sample size required to achieve the desired power. Using a generalized score test, Tosteson et al. (2003) discussed the power and sample size calculations for generalized linear measurement error models. With differential measurement error considered, White (2003) provided an approximate expression to characterize measurement error effects on the odds ratio arising from a continuous error-prone exposure and discussed how to design a validity/reliability study in order to address measurement error effects.

9.2 Causal Inference with Measurement Error

This book focuses on addressing measurement error effects for association studies where relationships between response variables and covariates are described in the manner of *association* rather than *causal-effects*. This is mainly driven by the abundance of the literature on measurement error models on association studies. Research on measurement error is quite sparse in the framework of causal inference, although the interest in this topic has been growing in recent years.

In this section, we outline limited work on causal inference with measurement error problems. Causal inferences about the effect of an exposure on an outcome can be seriously biased by errors in the measurement of the exposure, the outcome, and confounders. For instance, Zidek et al. (1996) illustrated that measurement error may conspire with multicollinearity among confounders to mislead the investigator, and a causal variable measured with error may be overlooked. Goetghebeur and Vansteelandt (2005) reviewed the literature on structural mean models for the analysis of exposures resulting from partial compliance in randomized clinical trials and discussed the impact of measurement error on inferences. Regier, Moodie and Platt (2014) conducted simulation studies to assess the effect of mismeasured continuous confounders on the estimation of the causal parameter when using marginal structural models and inverse probability-of-treatment weighting (IPTW). They observed counterintuitive effects of confounder measurement error on the estimation of the causal parameter.

Hernán and Cole (2009) described the use of causal diagrams to represent various types of measurement error, which are classified as *independent nondifferential*, *dependent nondifferential*, *independent differential*, and *dependent differential* errors. Assuming the nondifferential measurement error mechanism, Pierce and VanderWeele (2012) studied the effects of exposure and outcome measurement error for Mendelian randomization (Bochud and Rousson 2010), a useful approach for determining whether or not there is a causal relationship between an exposure and a disease.

With treatment or exposure being subject to misclassification, Lewbel (2007) provided conditions for identification and estimation of the average effect in nonparametric and semiparametric regression. Assuming there are no unmeasured confounders, Babanezhad, Vansteelandt and Goetghebeur (2010) investigated asymptotic biases of causal effect estimators that are induced from misclassification in exposure. They considered various estimators of the average causal effect of exposure on the outcome, including the IPTW estimators, doubly robust estimators for the exposure effect in linear marginal structural mean models, and G-estimators. With classical additive measurement error in covariates, McCaffrey, Lockwood and Setodji (2013) and Shu and Yi (2017a) developed inverse-probability-weighted estimation approaches for estimation of causal effects from observational studies with error-prone covariates. When the outcome is subject to measurement error or misclassification, Shu and Yi (2017b) examined bias analysis and developed valid estimation methods for the average treatment effect.

For causal inference with differential measurement error, Imai and Yamamoto (2010) investigated identification issues of the average treatment effect when a binary treatment variable is subject to misclassification and offered a sensitivity analysis to assess the robustness of the results to different magnitudes of misclassification. In circumstances where model parameters are unidentifiable or not estimable from the observed data, Díaz and van der Laan (2013) explored a sensitivity analysis for inferences about causal parameters.

In the context of graph-based causal inference, Pearl (2010) discussed computational and representational problems related to estimation of causal effects when confounders are mismeasured or misclassified.

With mediation analysis, several authors, including VanderWeele, Valeri and Ogburn (2012), Ogburn and VanderWeele (2012), and Blakely, McKenzie and Carter (2013), studied the impact of mismeasurement and investigated how measurement error may bias estimates of direct and indirect effects.

9.3 Statistical Software on Measurement Error and Misclassification Models

This section includes the information on statistical software and implementation algorithms of measurement error and misclassification models.

R Software

R packages *simex* and *mcsimex*, developed by W. Ledere and H. Küchenhoff, implement the SIMEX algorithm initiated by Cook and Stefanski (1994) and the MCSIMEX algorithm proposed by Küchenhoff, Mwalili and Lesaffre (2006). Jackknife and asymptotic variance estimation are implemented. Details were documented by Lederer and Küchenhoff (2006) and the packages were posted at R-CRAN at the link:

https://cran.r-project.org/web/packages/simex/index.html.

simexaft, developed by J. Xiong, W. He and G. Y. Yi, is an R package which implements the SIMEX method for accelerated failure time models with covariates subject to additive measurement error. Detailed procedures were documented by He, Xiong and Yi (2012) and the package was posted at R-CRAN at the link:

https://cran.r-project.org/web/packages/simexaft/index.html.

NPsimex is an R software package for performing nonparametric estimation for error-contaminated data using the SIMEX method. This package contains a collection of functions to perform nonparametric deconvolution. The estimator adopts the SIMEX idea but bypasses the simulation step in the original SIMEX algorithm. The package was posted at R-CRAN by X.-F. Wang at the link:

https://cran.r-project.org/web/packages/NPsimex/index.html.

GLSME, developed by K. Bartoszek, is an R package which fits the general linear model with correlated data and observation error in both dependent and independent variables. The package was discussed by Hansen and Bartoszek (2012) and posted at R-CRAN at the link:

https://cran.r-project.org/web/packages/GLSME/index.html.

eivi, developed by M. H. Satman and E. Diyarbakirliogl, is an R package which implements an algorithm for reducing errors-in-variables bias in simple linear regression. The function was posted at R-CRAN at the link:

https://cran.r-project.org/web/packages/eive/index.html.

msm, developed by C. Jackson, is an R package which deals with multi-state Markov and hidden Markov models. It is designed for processes observed at arbitrary times in the continuous-time scale. Both Markov transition rates and the hidden Markov output process may be modelled in terms of covariates, which may be constant or piecewise-constant in time (Jackson 2011). This package was posted at R-CRAN at the link:

https://cran.r-project.org/web/packages/msm/index.html.

decon is an R software package for nonparametric measurement error problems. This package contains a collection of functions for dealing with nonparametric measurement error problems using deconvolution kernel methods. The details were documented by Wang and Wang (2011) and discussed by Delaigle (2014) who pointed out some issues of the package. The package was posted at R-CRAN by X.-F. Wang and B. Wang at the link:

https://cran.r-project.org/web/packages/decon/index.html.

deamer, developed by J. Stirnemann, A. Samson and F. Comte (with contribution from Claire Lacou), provides deconvolution algorithms for nonparametric estimation of the density of an error-prone variable with an additive error. Estimation may be performed for one of the situations with (1) a known density of the error, (2) an auxiliary sample of pure noise, and (3) an auxiliary sample of replicate measurements. Estimation is performed using adaptive model selection and penalized contrasts. The package was posted at R-CRAN at the link:

https://cran.r-project.org/web/packages/deamer/index.html.

Pérez et al. (2012) developed an R function, called *Intake_epis_food*, to implement a bivariate nonlinear measurement error model in order to estimate usual and energy intake for episodically consumed foods. They considered a Bayesian analysis using WinBUGS to estimate the distribution of usual intake for episodically consumed foods and energy.

Muff et al. (2013) discussed a Bayesian approach to account for measurement error in covariates. They extended the *integrated nested Laplace approximation* approach to formulating generalized linear mixed models with Gaussian measurement error models. An R code of the implementation was provided by Muff et al. (2013).

Other implementation R packages on error-prone data may be found at R-CRAN at the following links:

https://cran.r-project.org/web/packages/svapls/index.html
https://cran.r-project.org/web/packages/detect/index.html
https://cran.r-project.org/web/packages/obs.agree/index.html
https://cran.r-project.org/web/packages/hsmm/index.html
https://cran.r-project.org/web/packages/obsSens/index.html
https://cran.r-project.org/web/packages/CVcalibration/index.html.

STATA Software

A general purpose STATA software package for the implementation of the regression calibration and the SIMEX methods was developed by R. J. Carroll, J. Hardin, and H. Schmiediche. The package, including STATA commands *qvf*, *rcal*, *simex*, and *simexplot*, deals with generalized linear models with one or more covariates which are measured with error. The use of the software and related measurement error issues were documented by Hardin, Schmiediche and Carroll (2003a,b). Details are available at the link:

http://www.stata.com/merror/.

Rabe-Hesketh, Skrondal and Pickles (2003) described a command, *cme*, that calls *gllamm* for estimation associated with generalized linear measurement error models. A single covariate is subject to measurement error and a classical measurement model is assumed.

Other Information

Other than the foregoing packages, other software packages and implementation procedures on measurement error models were developed by different people and research groups for various settings. For example, S. Mwalili prepared a program for fitting a Bayesian ordinal logistic regression model to correct for inter-observer measurement error in a geographical oral health study, which is available at the link:

https://ibiostat.be/online-resources/online-resources/measurement.

D. Spiegelman and her research group, and R. Carroll and his research group posted software information, respectively, at

http://www.hsph.harvard.edu/faculty/donna-spiegelman/software
http://www.stat.tamu.edu/~carroll/matlab_programs/software.php.

Other software packages concerning measurement error models include *ODRPACK*, a software package for *weighted orthogonal distance regression*. *ODRPACK* is to find the parameters that minimize the sum of the squared weighted orthogonal distances from a set of observations to the curve or surface determined by the parameters; this package may be used to handle measurement error models (Boggs et al. 1992).

Appendix

This appendix includes some basic mathematics and statistics material that is used in the book, along with some computational techniques or algorithms which are often used in the standard statistical analysis when measurement error is not present. The material in this appendix may have dispersed in various reference books. The purpose of including this appendix is to provide readers a quick access to the material used throughout the book.

A.1 Matrix Algebra: Some Notation and Facts

Notation Related to Vectors and Matrices

In the book, we use the following format to present an operation of a vector or a matrix. Let $\theta = (\theta_1, \ldots, \theta_p)^{\mathrm{T}}$ be a $p \times 1$ vector where p is a positive integer. Suppose $k(\theta)$ is a differentiable function of θ and $U(\theta) = (U_1(\theta), \ldots, U_q(\theta))^{\mathrm{T}}$ is a $q \times 1$ vector, where $U_j(\theta)$ is a differentiable function of θ for $j = 1, \ldots, q$, and q is a positive integer greater than 1. Then the derivatives of $k(\theta)$ and $U(\theta)$ with respect to θ are defined to be

$$\frac{\partial k(\theta)}{\partial \theta} = \left(\frac{\partial k(\theta)}{\partial \theta_1} \quad \frac{\partial k(\theta)}{\partial \theta_p}\right)^{\mathrm{T}}$$

and

$$\frac{\partial U(\theta)}{\partial \theta^{\mathrm{T}}} = \begin{pmatrix} \frac{\partial U_1(\theta)}{\partial \theta_1} & \cdots & \frac{\partial U_1(\theta)}{\partial \theta_p} \\ \frac{\partial U_2(\theta)}{\partial \theta_1} & \cdots & \frac{\partial U_2(\theta)}{\partial \theta_p} \\ \vdots & & \vdots \\ \frac{\partial U_q(\theta)}{\partial \theta_1} & \cdots & \frac{\partial U_q(\theta)}{\partial \theta_p} \end{pmatrix},$$

respectively.

G. Y. Yi, *Statistical Analysis with Measurement Error or Misclassification*, Springer Series in Statistics, DOI 10.1007/978-1-4939-6640-0

If $k(\theta)$ is also a function of a random variable (or vector), and $U(\theta)$ is also a vector of a random variable (or vector), then the expectation of $\partial k(\theta)/\partial\theta$ is defined as

$$E\left(\frac{\partial k(\theta)}{\partial\theta}\right) = \left(E\left(\frac{\partial k(\theta)}{\partial\theta_1}\right)\dots E\left(\frac{\partial k(\theta)}{\partial\theta_p}\right)\right)^{\mathrm{T}},$$

and the expectation of $\partial U(\theta)/\partial\theta^{\mathrm{T}}$ is defined as a $q\times p$ matrix whose (j,k) element is

$$E\left(\frac{\partial U_j(\theta)}{\partial\theta_k}\right)$$

for $j = 1,\dots,q$ and $k = 1,\dots,p$.

If $A(v) = (A_1(v),\dots,A_q(v))^{\mathrm{T}}$ is a $q\times 1$ vector where $A_j(v)$ is an integrable function for $j = 1,\dots,q$, then notation $\int A(v)dv$ represents the $q\times 1$ vector whose jth component is $\int A_j(v)dv$ for $j = 1,\dots,q$.

Inverse Block Matrix

Suppose that A is an invertible block matrix

$$A = \begin{pmatrix} A_{11} & A_{12} \\ A_{21} & A_{22} \end{pmatrix},$$

where A_{11} is a $p\times p$ matrix, A_{22} is a $q\times q$ matrix, A_{12} is a $p\times q$ matrix, and A_{21} is a $q\times p$ matrix. Assume that the following inverse matrices exist, then the inverse matrix of A is given by

$$A^{-1} = \begin{pmatrix} A^{11} & A^{12} \\ A^{21} & A^{22} \end{pmatrix},$$

where

$$\begin{aligned} A^{11} &= (A_{11} - A_{12}A_{22}^{-1}A_{21})^{-1}; \\ A^{21} &= -A_{22}^{-1}A_{21}(A_{11} - A_{12}A_{22}^{-1}A_{21})^{-1}; \\ A^{12} &= -A_{11}^{-1}A_{12}(A_{22} - A_{21}A_{11}^{-1}A_{12})^{-1}; \\ A^{22} &= (A_{22} - A_{21}A_{11}^{-1}A_{12})^{-1}. \end{aligned}$$

In particular, if

$$A = \begin{pmatrix} A_{11} & A_{12} \\ 0_{q\times p} & A_{22} \end{pmatrix}, \text{ then } A^{-1} = \begin{pmatrix} A_{11}^{-1} & -A_{11}^{-1}A_{12}A_{22}^{-1} \\ 0_{q\times p} & A_{22}^{-1} \end{pmatrix};$$

if

$$A = \begin{pmatrix} A_{11} & 0_{p\times q} \\ A_{21} & A_{22} \end{pmatrix}, \text{ then } A^{-1} = \begin{pmatrix} A_{11}^{-1} & 0_{p\times q} \\ -A_{22}^{-1}A_{21}A_{11}^{-1} & A_{22}^{-1} \end{pmatrix}.$$

Positive Definite and Nonnegative Definite Matrices

Let A be an $m \times m$ symmetric matrix. If

$$x^{\mathrm{T}}Ax > 0 \text{ for any } m \times 1 \text{ nonzero vector } x,$$

then A is called *positive definite*. If

$$x^{\mathrm{T}}Ax \geq 0 \text{ for any } m \times 1 \text{ vector } x,$$

then A is called *nonnegative definite*.

Properties:

(a) Suppose A an $n \times m$ matrix, then AA^{T} and $A^{\mathrm{T}}A$ are nonnegative definite.
(b) Suppose $m \times m$ matrix A is positive definite and $m \times m$ matrix B is nonnegative definite. Then $A + B$ is positive definite and $A^{-1} - (A + B)^{-1}$ is nonnegative definite.
(c) If matrix A is positive definite, then A is nonsingular and A^{-1} is positive definite.
(d) If $m \times m$ matrices A and B both are positive definite. Then $A - B$ is positive definite if and only if $B^{-1} - A^{-1}$ is positive definite.

A.2 Definitions and Facts

This appendix records some basic definitions, notation, and the properties which are frequently used in the book.

Convergence Rate of Real-Valued Functions

When dealing with two real-valued functions, we may be interested in comparing their growth rate as the argument approaches infinity or a given constant. It is convenient to use big $O(\cdot)$ or small $o(\cdot)$ to express their relationship. Suppose $g(v)$ and $k(v)$ are two real-valued functions defined on a set of real numbers. We write

$$g(v) = O(k(v)) \quad \text{as} \quad v \to \infty \tag{A.1}$$

if and only if there exists real numbers $\widetilde{v}$ and $M > 0$ such that

$$|g(v)| \leq M|k(v)| \quad \text{for all } v \text{ with } v \geq \widetilde{v}. \tag{A.2}$$

We write

$$g(v) = O(k(v)) \quad \text{as} \quad v \to v_0$$

if and only if there exist positive numbers ω and M such that

$$|g(v)| \leq M|k(v)| \quad \text{for all } v \text{ with } |v - v_0| < \omega,$$

where v_0 is a value of interest. In many cases where the limit of the argument is clear by the context, we use a simpler way

$$g(v) = O(k(v))$$

to express (A.1) or (A.2).

If $k(v)$ is nonzero or at least becomes nonzero beyond a certain point or in a neighborhood of a point v_o, then we write

$$g(v) = o(k(v))$$

if

$$\lim_{v \to \infty} \frac{g(v)}{k(v)} = 0$$

or

$$\lim_{v \to v_0} \frac{g(v)}{k(v)} = 0.$$

Convergence Rate in Probability Sense

The *order in probability* notation is useful in establishing asymptotic results. Let $\{X_n : n = 1, 2, \ldots\}$ be a sequence of random variables and $\{a_n : n = 1, 2, \ldots\}$ be a sequence of constants. If X_n/a_n converges to zero in probability as $n \to \infty$, we write

$$X_n = o_p(a_n) \text{ or } X_n/a_n = o_p(1).$$

Precisely, $X_n/a_n = o_p(1)$ is defined as

$$\lim_{n \to \infty} P(|X_n/a_n| \geq \epsilon) = 0 \text{ for every } \epsilon > 0.$$

If for any $\epsilon > 0$, there exists a finite positive number M such that for any n,

$$P(|X_n/a_n| > M) < \epsilon,$$

i.e., the X_n/a_n are stochastically bounded, then we write

$$X_n = O_p(a_n).$$

Conditional Moments and Moment Generating Function

Suppose U and V are random variables. Let $k(V)$ be a function of V and $g(U, V)$ be a function of U and V. Then

$$\begin{aligned}
E[E\{g(U,V)|V\}] &= E\{g(U,V)\}; \\
E\{k(V)g(U,V)|V\} &= k(V)E\{g(U,V)|V\}; \\
\text{var}(U) &= E\{\text{var}(U|V)\} + \text{var}\{E(U|V)\}.
\end{aligned}$$

Suppose V follows a multivariate normal distribution with mean μ and covariance matrix Σ. Then the moment generating function of V is

$$M(v) = \exp(v^{\mathrm{T}}\mu + v^{\mathrm{T}}\Sigma v/2),$$

where v is a vector of any real numbers.

A.3 Newton–Raphson and Fisher–Scoring Algorithms

Suppose random variable Y has a probability density or mass function $f(y;\theta)$ and $y(n) = \{y_1, \ldots, y_n\}$ are the measurements of a random sample chosen from $f(y;\theta)$. Let

$$L(\theta) = \sum_{i=1}^{n} \log f(y_i;\theta) \quad \text{and} \quad \ell(\theta) = \log L(\theta)$$

be the likelihood and log-likelihood functions of θ for the given sample measurements $y(n)$, respectively.

Suppose that the likelihood is differentiable, unimodal and bounded above, and the maximum likelihood estimate, denoted by $\widehat{\theta}$, of θ is unique. Then the maximum likelihood estimate $\widehat{\theta}$ can be found by solving the likelihood equations

$$\frac{\partial \ell(\theta)}{\partial \theta} = 0 \tag{A.3}$$

for θ.

For the distributions whose score functions are linear or quadratic in θ, the solutions to (A.3) are readily found with analytic forms. In general situations, finding a solution of (A.3) has to call for a numerical approximation approach which often requires iterations. The *Newton–Raphson* algorithm is a useful procedure for this purpose.

The idea is to first approximate the log-likelihood $\ell(\theta)$ with a quadratic function using the Taylor series expansion and then iteratively update an estimate of θ until convergence. Specifically, let $\theta^{(0)}$ denote an initial guess of θ and $\theta^{(k)}$ be the updated estimate of θ at the kth iteration. At iteration $(k+1)$, for the given sample measurements $y(n)$, applying the Taylor series expansion to $\ell(\theta)$ about $\theta^{(k)}$ gives

$$\begin{aligned}\ell(\theta) = \ell(\theta^{(k)}) &+ \left(\left.\frac{\partial \ell(\theta)}{\partial \theta^{\mathrm{T}}}\right|_{\theta=\theta^{(k)}} \right)(\theta - \theta^{(k)}) \\ &+ \frac{1}{2}(\theta - \theta^{(k)})^{\mathrm{T}} \left(\left.\frac{\partial^2 \ell(\theta)}{\partial \theta \partial \theta^{\mathrm{T}}}\right|_{\theta=\theta^{(k)}} \right)(\theta - \theta^{(k)}) + \text{remainder}.\end{aligned}$$

When θ is close to $\theta^{(k)}$ in the sense that the norm of $(\theta - \theta^{(k)})$ is small, the remainder is negligible. In this case, we approximate $\ell(\theta)$ using the quadratic function

$$\begin{aligned}\ell(\theta) \approx \ell(\theta^{(k)}) &+ \left(\left.\frac{\partial \ell(\theta)}{\partial \theta^{\mathrm{T}}}\right|_{\theta=\theta^{(k)}} \right)(\theta - \theta^{(k)}) \\ &+ \frac{1}{2}(\theta - \theta^{(k)})^{\mathrm{T}} \left(\left.\frac{\partial^2 \ell(\theta)}{\partial \theta \partial \theta^{\mathrm{T}}}\right|_{\theta=\theta^{(k)}} \right)(\theta - \theta^{(k)}).\end{aligned} \tag{A.4}$$

As a result, finding the maximizer of $\ell(\theta)$ becomes finding the stationary point of the quadratic approximation. Calculating the derivative of the right-hand side of (A.4) with respective to θ and setting it to be zero gives

$$\left(\frac{\partial \ell(\theta)}{\partial \theta}\bigg|_{\theta=\theta^{(k)}}\right) + \left(\frac{\partial^2 \ell(\theta)}{\partial \theta \partial \theta^{\mathrm{T}}}\bigg|_{\theta=\theta^{(k)}}\right)(\theta - \theta^{(k)}) = 0,$$

or equivalently,

$$\theta = \theta^{(k)} + \left(-\frac{\partial^2 \ell(\theta)}{\partial \theta \partial \theta^{\mathrm{T}}}\bigg|_{\theta=\theta^{(k)}}\right)^{-1} \left(\frac{\partial \ell(\theta)}{\partial \theta}\bigg|_{\theta=\theta^{(k)}}\right), \tag{A.5}$$

assuming the existence of the inverse matrix.

Motivated by (A.5), we apply the following iterative equation to find the estimate of θ for iteration $(k+1)$:

$$\theta^{(k+1)} = \theta^{(k)} + \left(-\frac{\partial^2 \ell(\theta)}{\partial \theta \partial \theta^{\mathrm{T}}}\bigg|_{\theta=\theta^{(k)}}\right)^{-1} \left(\frac{\partial \ell(\theta)}{\partial \theta}\bigg|_{\theta=\theta^{(k)}}\right), \tag{A.6}$$

where $k = 1, 2, \ldots$.

If the log-likelihood $\ell(\theta)$ is a quadratic function of θ, then convergence is reached after one iteration. If the log-likelihood $\ell(\theta)$ is concave and unimodal, then with a good starting value $\theta^{(0)}$, $\{\theta^{(k)} : k = 0, 1, 2, \ldots\}$ converge to the maximum likelihood estimate $\widehat{\theta}$ of θ as $k \to \infty$ (Tanner 1996).

The Fisher–scoring method is an alternative algorithm which replaces the observed information matrix in (A.6) with the expected information matrix evaluated at $\theta^{(k)}$. That is, the iterative equation is given by

$$\theta^{(k+1)} = \theta^{(k)} + \left(E\left[-\frac{\partial^2 \{\sum_{i=1}^n \log f(Y_i;\theta)\}}{\partial \theta \partial \theta^{\mathrm{T}}}\right]\bigg|_{\theta=\theta^{(k)}}\right)^{-1} \left(\frac{\partial \ell(\theta)}{\partial \theta}\bigg|_{\theta=\theta^{(k)}}\right)$$

for $k = 0, 1, 2, \ldots$, where $Y_1, \ldots, Y_n$ are independent and identically distributed random variables having the same distribution as Y.

The Newton–Raphson and Fisher–scoring algorithms are not just restricted to finding the maximum likelihood estimates. They are also applicable to general situations of solving estimating equations. For example, the Newton–Raphson algorithm may be modified with $\partial \ell(\theta)/\partial \theta$ and $\partial^2 \ell(\theta)/\partial \theta \partial \theta^{\mathrm{T}}$ in (A.6), respectively, replaced by estimating functions and their partial derivatives which are applied to the sample measurements. Specifically, let $U(\theta; y)$ be an estimating function of θ and $y(n) = \{y_1, \ldots, y_n\}$ be the measurements of a random sample chosen from $f(y;\theta)$. To solve

$$\sum_{i=1}^n U(\theta; y_i) = 0 \tag{A.7}$$

for θ, we apply the iterative equation

$$\theta^{(k+1)} = \theta^{(k)} - \left\{ \sum_{i=1}^{n} \frac{\partial U(\theta; y_i)}{\partial \theta^{\mathrm{T}}} \bigg|_{\theta=\theta^{(k)}} \right\}^{-1} \left\{ \sum_{i=1}^{n} U(\theta^{(k)}; y_i) \right\}$$

to obtain a sequence of estimates $\{\theta^{(k)} : k = 0, 1, 2, \ldots\}$ until convergence. The limit is taken as the estimate, denoted by $\widehat{\theta}$, of θ obtained from solving the estimating equation (A.7).

A.4 The Bootstrap and Jackknife Methods

The *bootstrap* algorithm was introduced by Efron (1979) as a computer-based method for estimating the standard error of an estimator for a model parameter. This algorithm is easy to implement and applicable to broad settings no matter how mathematically complicated the estimator is.

Suppose $y(n) = \{y_1, \ldots, y_n\}$ are the observed measurements of a random sample chosen from an unknown probability distribution F and θ is a parameter related to F which is to be estimated. Suppose $\widehat{\theta} = \widehat{\theta}(y(n))$ is an estimate of θ obtained from applying a method to data $y(n)$. To assess the accuracy of $\widehat{\theta}$, the bootstrap algorithm may be used to estimate the standard error of $\widehat{\theta}$ following the three steps (Efron and Tibshirani 1993):

Step 1: Choose a positive integer B. For $b = 1, \ldots, B$, independently generate a *bootstrap sample* $y^{(b)}(n) = \{y_1^{(b)}, \ldots, y_n^{(b)}\}$ whose elements are drawn *with replacement* from the population of n objects $y(n) = \{y_1, \ldots, y_n\}$.

Step 2: For each bootstrap sample $y^{(b)}(n)$, calculate the corresponding estimate $\widehat{\theta}^{(b)} = \widehat{\theta}(y^{(b)}(n))$ of θ for $b = 1, \ldots, B$.

Step 3: Calculate the sample standard deviation of the B replications:

$$\widehat{\text{se}}_{\text{B}} = \left[\frac{1}{B-1} \sum_{b=1}^{B} \{\widehat{\theta}^{(b)} - \widehat{\theta}^{(\cdot)}\}^2 \right]^{1/2}, \tag{A.8}$$

which is an estimate of the standard error of $\widehat{\theta}$, where $\widehat{\theta}^{(\cdot)} = B^{-1} \sum_{b=1}^{B} \widehat{\theta}^{(b)}$. Sometimes, $\widehat{\text{se}}_{\text{B}}$ is called a *nonparametric bootstrap estimate.*

Estimates of the standard error of $\widehat{\theta}$ depend on the choice of bootstrap samples as well as the number of bootstrap samples, B. By the factor $1/(B-1)$ in (A.8), one might expect that a larger B may yield a better estimate of the standard error of $\widehat{\theta}$.

Since there are only $\binom{2n-1}{n}$ different bootstrap samples for given n distinct measurements in $y(n)$ (Efron and Tibshirani 1993, p. 49), it is tempting to take $B = \binom{2n-1}{n}$ and let $y^{(b)}(n)$ exhaust those different bootstrap samples by setting $b = 1, \ldots, B$. This idea works if n is quite small, such as $n \leq 5$. Even for small size n, this approach requires intensive computation. For example, if $n = 10$, this approach requires the evaluation of $B = 92{,}378$ estimates $\widehat{\theta}^{(b)}$ in Step 2 in order to obtain $\widehat{\mathrm{se}}_{\mathrm{B}}$; if $n = 20$, there are 68,923,264,410 different bootstrap samples. When $n = 50$, the number of distinct bootstrap samples is of the scale 5.045×10^{28}, which is practically impossible to be exhausted in order to obtain an accurate estimate of the standard error of $\widehat{\theta}$.

Numerical experiences, however, suggest that even a small number of bootstrap replications is usually sufficient for producing a good estimate of the standard error of $\widehat{\theta}$. Often, $B = 50$ is taken; it is seldom to take B greater than 200 (although much larger values of B are needed for constructing bootstrap confidence intervals) (Efron and Tibshirani 1993, p. 52). More refined versions of the bootstrap algorithm for different settings were discussed by Efron and Tibshirani (1993).

In contrast, the *jackknife* is a technique for estimating the bias and standard error of an estimate which shares similarities to the bootstrap algorithm. Instead of forming B bootstrap samples based on random draws, we form a *jackknife sample* by *leaving out one observation at a time*. For $i = 1, \ldots, n$, let

$$y_{(i)}(n) = \{y_1, \ldots, y_{i-1}, y_{i+1}, \ldots, y_n\}$$

be the ith jackknife sample which is a subset of $y(n)$ with the ith observation removed.

Apply the estimation method to the ith jackknife sample and obtain the ith *jackknife replication* of $\widehat{\theta}$:

$$\widehat{\theta}_{(i)} = \widehat{\theta}(y_{(i)}(n)).$$

Let $\widehat{\theta}_{(\cdot)} = n^{-1} \sum_{i=1}^{n} \widehat{\theta}_{(i)}$. Then the jackknife estimate of bias is defined as

$$\widehat{\mathrm{bias}}_{\mathrm{J}} = (n-1)(\widehat{\theta}_{(\cdot)} - \theta),$$

and the jackknife estimate of standard error is defined as

$$\widehat{\mathrm{se}}_{\mathrm{J}} = \left\{ \frac{n-1}{n} \sum_{i=1}^{n} (\widehat{\theta}_{(i)} - \widehat{\theta}_{(\cdot)})^2 \right\}^{1/2}.$$

The jackknife was proposed by Quenouille (1949) for estimation of bias and by Tukey (1958) for estimating standard errors. The jackknife is closely related to the bootstrap; Efron and Tibshirani (1993, Ch. 11) illustrated that the jackknife can be viewed as an approximation to the bootstrap. The jackknife is easier to implement than the bootstrap for the standard error estimation if n is less than B which is set as a number between 100 and 200 for the bootstrap method, but it may be less efficient than the bootstrap otherwise. When the estimator $\widehat{\theta}$ is not "smooth", the jackknife may fail to provide reasonable results. Efron and Tibshirani (1993, Ch. 11) discussed these issues and described a remedy which forms a jackknife sample by leaving out more than one observations at a time.

A.5 Monte Carlo Method and MCEM Algorithm

We outline the *Monte Carlo* method and the *Monte Carlo EM* (MCEM) algorithm. The description here is based on Tanner (1996, §3.3, §4.4, §4.5) with modifications.

The Monte Carlo method is useful for approximating integrals or expectations. Suppose U is a continuous random variable (or vector) and $h(u)$ is its probability density function. For a given function $g(\cdot)$, we want to evaluate the expectation

$$E\{g(U)\} = \int g(u)h(u)du,$$

where the expectation exists and has no analytic form.

The Monte Carlo method may be applied to approximate the integral. Choose a positive integer B and independently generate a sequence of values, $\{u^{(1)}, \ldots, u^{(B)}\}$, from the distribution $h(u)$. Then we approximate $E\{g(U)\}$ using

$$\widehat{E\{g(U)\}} = \frac{1}{B}\sum_{b=1}^{B} g(u^{(b)}).$$

The Monte Carlo method has applied widely in practice. For instance, it can be used in combination with the EM algorithm (discussed in §2.5.1), and the resulting algorithm is called the *Monte Carlo EM* algorithm. Specifically, at iteration k of the E-step, the expectations in function $Q(\theta; \theta^{(k)})$, determined by (2.14), are approximated by applying the Monte Carlo method. For a specified positive integer B, we independently generate a sequence of values, $x_i^{(1)}, \ldots, x_i^{(B)}$, from the distribution $f(x_i|y_i, x_i^*, z_i; \theta^{(k)})$ for each given $i = 1, \ldots, n$. Let

$$\widehat{Q}(\theta; \theta^{(k)}) = \sum_{i=1}^{n} \frac{1}{B}\left\{\sum_{b=1}^{B} \log f(y_i, x_i^{(b)}, x_i^*|z_i; \theta)\right\}.$$

At the M-step, $\widehat{Q}(\theta; \theta^{(k)})$ is maximized with respect to θ to obtain $\theta^{(k+1)}$.

It is important to specify a large enough number B and monitor convergence of the updated values $\{\theta^{(k)} : k = 0, 1, 2, \ldots\}$. One may use different values of B for different iterations. In early iterations, B can be taken as small numbers and then be increased to larger numbers as the iteration number gets larger. Convergence of $\{\theta^{(k)} : k = 0, 1, \ldots\}$ may be monitored by plotting $\theta^{(k)}$ versus iteration number k.

Let $\widehat{\theta}$ denote the convergence value of $\theta^{(k)}$ as k approaches infinity. The precision of $\widehat{\theta}$ can be obtained using the formula of Louis (1982) by calculating the Hessian matrix of $\ell_o(\theta)$ evaluated at $\hat{\theta}$ (Tanner 1996, §4.4). Specifically, the Hessian matrix of $\ell_o(\theta)$ is given by

$$-\frac{\partial^2 \ell_o(\theta)}{\partial\theta\partial\theta^{\mathrm{T}}} = -\sum_{i=1}^{n} E_{X_i|(Y_i,X_i^*,Z_i)}\left\{\frac{\partial^2 \log f(Y_i,X_i,X_i^*|Z_i;\theta)}{\partial\theta\partial\theta^{\mathrm{T}}}\right\}$$
$$-\sum_{i=1}^{n} \mathrm{var}_{X_i|(Y_i,X_i^*,Z_i)}\left\{\frac{\partial \log f(Y_i,X_i,X_i^*|Z_i;\theta)}{\partial\theta}\right\}, \qquad \text{(A.9)}$$

where the expectation and the variance are evaluated with respect to the model $f(x_i|y_i,x_i^*,z_i;\theta)$. In most situations, it is difficult to analytically compute the integrals on the right-hand side of (A.9). Monte Carlo methods may then be used to approximate those integrals, thus leading to an approximation of the Hessian matrix of $\ell_o(\theta)$.

For a given positive integer B and $i = 1,\ldots,n$, independently generate a sequence of values, $\{x_i^{(b)} : b = 1,\ldots,B\}$, from the distribution $f(x_i|y_i,x_i^*,z_i;\widehat{\theta})$. Then the Hessian matrix (A.9) is approximated by

$$-\sum_{i=1}^{n}\left\{\frac{1}{B}\sum_{b=1}^{B}\frac{\partial^2 \log f(y_i,x_i^{(b)},x_i^*|z_i;\theta)}{\partial\theta\partial\theta^{\mathrm{T}}}\right\}$$
$$-\sum_{i=1}^{n}\left[\frac{1}{B}\sum_{b=1}^{B}\left\{\frac{\partial \log f(y_i,x_i^{(b)},x_i^*|z_i;\theta)}{\partial\theta}\right\}\left\{\frac{\partial \log f(y_i,x_i^{(b)},x_i^*|z_i;\theta)}{\partial\theta}\right\}^{\mathrm{T}}\right]$$
$$+\sum_{i=1}^{n}\left[\left\{\frac{1}{B}\sum_{b=1}^{B}\frac{\partial \log f(y_i,x_i^{(b)},x_i^*|z_i;\theta)}{\partial\theta}\right\}\left\{\frac{1}{B}\sum_{b=1}^{B}\frac{\partial \log f(y_i,x_i^{(b)},x_i^*|z_i;\theta)}{\partial\theta}\right\}^{\mathrm{T}}\right].$$

References

Abarin, T. and Wang, L. (2012). Instrumental variable approach to covariate measurement error in generalized linear models. *Annals of the Institute of Statistical Mathematics*, 64, 475–493.

Abdullah, M. B. (1995). Detection of influential observations in functional errors-in-variables model. *Communications in Statistics – Theory and Methods*, 24, 1585–1595.

Adcock, R. J. (1878). A problem in least squares. *Analyst*, 5, 53–54.

Aguirre-Hernández, R. and Farewell, V. T. (2002). A Pearson-type goodness-of-fit test for stationary and time-continuous Markov regression models. *Statistics in Medicine*, 21, 1899–1911.

Aigner, D. J. (1973). Regression with a binary independent variable subject to errors of observation. *Journal of Econometrics*, 1, 49–60.

Akazawa, K., Kinukawa, N., and Nakamura, T. (1998). A note on the corrected score function corrected for misclassification. *Journal of the Japan Statistical Society*, 28, 115–123.

Albert, P. S. (1999). A mover-stayer model for longitudinal marker data. *Biometrics*, 55, 1252–1257.

Albert, P. S., Hunsberger, S. A., and Biro, F. M. (1997). Modeling repeated measures with monotonic ordinal responses and misclassification, with applications to studying maturation. *Journal of the American Statistical Association*, 92, 1304–1311.

Allman, E. S., Matias, C., and Rhodes, J. A. (2009). Identifiability of parameters in latent structure models with many observed variables. *The Annals of Statistics*, 37, 3099–3132.

Amemiya, Y. (1985). Instrumental variable estimator for the nonlinear errors-in-variables model. *Journal of Econometrics*, 28, 273–289.

Amemiya, Y. (1990). Two-stage instrumental variable estimators for the nonlinear errors-in-variables model. *Journal of Econometrics*, 44, 311–332.

G. Y. Yi, *Statistical Analysis with Measurement Error or Misclassification*,
Springer Series in Statistics, DOI 10.1007/978-1-4939-6640-0

Andersen, E. W. (2005). Two-stage estimation in copula models used in family studies. *Lifetime Data Analysis*, 11, 333–350.

Andersen, P. K. and Gill, R. D. (1982). Cox regression model for counting processes: A large sample study. *The Annals of Statistics*, 10, 1100–1120.

Anderson, T. W. and Hsiao, C. (1982). Formulation and estimation of dynamic models using panel data. *Journal of Econometrics*, 18, 47–82.

Andersen, P. K. and Keiding, N. (2002). Multi-state models for event history analysis. *Statistical Methods in Mdeical Research*, 11, 91–115.

Andersen, P. K., Borgan, O., Gill, R. D., and Keiding, N. (1993). *Statistical Models Based on Counting Processes*. Springer-Verlag, New York.

Apanasovich, T. V., Carroll, R. J., and Maity, A. (2009). SIMEX and standard error estimation in semiparametric measurement error models. *Electronic Journal of Statistics*, 3, 318–348.

Arellano-Valle, R. B., Bolfarine, H., and Gasco, L. (2002). Measurement error models with nonconstant covariance matrices. *Journal of Multivariate Analysis*, 82, 395–415.

Arellano-Valle, R. B., Ozan, S., Bolfarine, H., and Lachos, V. H. (2005). Skew normal measurement error models. *Journal of Multivariate Analysis*, 96, 265–281.

Armstrong, B. G., Whittemore, A. S., and Howe, G. R. (1989). Analysis of case–control data with covariate measurement error: Application to diet and colon cancer. *Statistics in Medicine*, 8, 1151–1163.

Augustin, T. (2004). An exact corrected log-likelihood function for Cox's proportional hazards model under measurement error and some extensions. *Scandinavian Journal of Statistics*, 31, 43–50.

Augustin, T. and Schwarz, R. (2002). Cox's proportional hazards model under covariate measurement error — A review and comparison of methods. In: S. Van Huffel and P. Lemmerling (eds.). *Total Least Squares and Errors-in-Variables Modeling: Analysis, Algorithms and Applications*. Kluwer, Dordrecht, 179–188.

Azzalini, A. (1994). Logistic regression for autocorrelated data with application to repeated measures. *Biometrika*, 81, 767–775.

Babanezhad, M., Vansteelandt, S., and Goetghebeur, E. (2010). Comparison of causal effect estimators under exposure misclassification. *Journal of Statistical Planning and Inference*, 140, 1306–1319.

Bai, Z. D. and Fu, J. C. (1987). On the maximum-likelihood estimator for the location parameter of a Cauchy distribution. *The Canadian Journal of Statistics*, 15, 137–146.

Barndorff-Nielsen, O. (1983). On a formula for the distribution of the maximum likelihood estimator. *Biometrika*, 70, 343–365.

Barndorff-Nielsen, O. E. (1986). Inference on full or partial parameters based on the standardized signed log likelihood ratio. *Biometrika*, 73, 307–322.

Barron, B. A. (1977). The effects of misclassification on the estimation of relative risk. *Biometrics*, 33, 414–418.

Begg, M. D. and Lagakos, S. (1992). Effects of mismodeling on tests of association based on logistic regression models. *The Annals of Statistics*, 20, 1929–1952.

Begg, M. D. and Lagakos, S. (1993). Loss in efficiency caused by omitting covariates and misspecifying exposure in logistic regression models. *Journal of the American Statistical Association*, 88, 166–170.

Berkson, J. (1950). Are there two regressions? *Journal of the American Statistical Association*, 45, 164–180.

Berry, S. M., Carroll, R. J., and Ruppert, D. (2002). Bayesian smoothing and regression splines for measurement error problems. *Journal of the American Statistical Association*, 97, 160–169.

Bhapkar, V. P. (1972). On a measure of efficiency of an estimating equation. *Sankhyā: The Indian Journal of Statistics, Series A*, 34, 467–472.

Bickel, P. J. and Doksum, K. A. (1977). *Mathematical Statistics*. Holden-Day, Inc. San Francisco.

Biemer, P. P., Groves, R. M., Lyberg, L. E., Mathiowetz, N. A., and Sudman, S. (1991). *Measurement Error in Surveys*. John Wiley & Sons, Inc., Hoboken, New Jersey.

Black, D. A., Berger, M. C., and Scott, F. A. (2000). Bounding parameter estimates with non-classical measurement error. *Journal of the American Statistical Association*, 95, 739–748.

Blakely, T., McKenzie, S., and Carter, K. (2013). Misclassification of the mediator matters when estimating indirect effects. *Journal of Epidemiology & Community Health*, 67, 458–466.

Bochud, M. and Rousson, V. (2010). Usefulness of Mendelian randomization in observational epidemiology. *International Journal of Environmental Research and Public Health*, 7, 711–728.

Boggs, P. T., Byrd, R. H., Rogers, J. E., and Schnabel, R. B. (1992). User's reference guide for ODRPACK version 2.01 software for weighted orthogonal distance regression. *Applied and Computational Mathematics Division. National Institute of Standards and Technology, Gaithersburg, MD 20899.*

Bollinger, C. R. (1996). Bounding mean regressions when a binary regressor is mismeasured. *Journal of Econometrics*, 73, 387–399.

Bollinger, C. R. and David, M. H. (1997). Modeling discrete choice with response error: Food stamp participation. *Journal of the American Statistical Association*, 92, 827–835.

Bollinger, C. R. and David, M. H. (2001). Estimation with response error and nonresponse: Food-stamp participation in the SIPP. *Journal of Business & Economic Statistics*, 19, 129–141.

Booth, J. G. and Hobert, J. P. (1999). Maximizing generalized linear mixed models likelihoods with an automated Monte Carlo EM algorithm. *Journal of the Royal Statistical Society, Series B*, 61, 265–285.

Box, G. E. P. (1979). Some problems of statistics and everyday life. *Journal of the American Statistical Association*, 74, 1–4.

Breslow, N. (1974). Covariance analysis of censored survival data. *Biometrics*, 30, 89–99.

Breslow, N. E. and Cain, K. C. (1988). Logistic regression for two-stage case–control data. *Biometrika*, 75, 11–20.

Breslow, N. E. and Day, N. E. (1980). *Statistical Methods in Cancer Research, Volume 1–The Analysis of Case–Control Studies*. Lyon, International Agency for Research on Cancer.

Breslow, N. E., Day, N. E., Halvorsen, K. T., Prentice, R. L., and Sabai, C. (1978). Estimation of multiple relative risk functions in matched case–control studies. *American Journal of Epidemiology*, 108, 299–307.

Broders, A. C. (1920). Squamous-cell epithelioma of the lip. *Journal of the American Medical Association*, 74, 656–664.

Bross, I. (1954). Misclassification in 2 × 2 tables. *Biometrics*, 10, 478–486.

Brunner, J. and Austin, P. C. (2009). Inflation of Type I error rate in multiple regression when independent variables are measured with error. *The Canadian Journal of Statistics*, 37, 33–46.

Buonaccorsi, J. P. (1995). Prediction in the presence of measurement error: General discussion and an example predicting defoliation. *Biometrics*, 51, 1562–1569.

Buonaccorsi, J. P. (1996). Measurement error in the response in the general linear model. *Journal of the American Statistical Association*, 91, 633–642.

Buonaccorsi, J. P. (2010). *Measurement Error: Models, Methods, and Applications*. Chapman & Hall/CRC.

Buonaccorsi, J. P., Demidenko, E., and Tosteson, T. (2000). Estimation in longitudinal random effects models with measurement error. *Statistica Sinica*, 10, 885–903.

Buonaccorsi, J. P., Laake, P., and Veierød, M. B. (2005). On the effect of misclassification on bias of perfectly measured covariates in regression. *Biometrics*, 61, 831–836.

Bureau, A., Hughes, J. P., and Shiboski, S. C. (2000) An S-Plus implementation of hidden Markov models in continuous time. *Journal of Computational and Graphical Statistics*, 9, 621–632.

Bureau, A., Shiboski, S., and Hughes, J. P. (2003). Applications of continuous time hidden Markov models to the study of misclassified disease outcomes. *Statistics in Medicine*, 22, 441–462.

Burr, D. (1988). On errors-in-variables in binary regression-Berkson case. *Journal of the American Statistical Association*, 83, 739–743.

Buzas, J. S. (1998). Unbiased scores in proportional hazards regression with covariate measurement error. *Journal of Statistical Planning and Inference*, 67, 247–257.

Buzas, J. S. and Stefanski, L. A. (1996a). Instrumental variable estimation in a probit measurement error model. *Journal of Statistical Planning and Inference*, 55, 47–62.

Buzas, J. S. and Stefanski, L. A. (1996b). Instrumental variable estimation in generalized linear measurement error models. *Journal of the American Statistical Association*, 91, 999–1006.

Buzas, J. S., Stefanski, L. A., and Tosteson, T. D. (2007). Measurement Error. *Handbook of Epidemiology*, 729–765. Edited by W. Ahrens and I. Pigeot. Berlin: Springer.

Cai, J. and Prentice, R. L. (1995). Estimating equations for hazard ratio parameters based on correlated failure time data. *Biometrika*, 82, 151–164.

Cappé, O., Moulines, E., and Rydén, T. (2005). *Inference in Hidden Markov Models*. New York: Springer.

Carpenter, J. R., Kenward, M. G., and Vansteelandt, S. (2006). A comparison of multiple imputation and doubly robust estimation for analyses with missing data. *Journal of the Royal Statistical Society, Series A*, 169, 571–584.

Carroll, R. J. (1989). Covariance analysis in generalized linear measurement error models. *Statistics in Medicine*, 8, 1075–1093.

Carroll, R. J. (1997). Surprising effects of measurement error on an aggregate data estimator. *Biometrika*, 84, 231–234.

Carroll, R. J. and Gallo, P. P. (1982). Some aspects of robustness in the functional errors-in-variables regression model. *Communications in Statistics – Theory and Methods*, 11, 2573–2585.

Carroll, R. J. and Hall, P. (1988). Optimal rates of convergence for deconvolving a density. *Journal of the American Statistical Association*, 83, 1184–1186.

Carroll, R. J. and Hall, P. (2004). Low order approximations in deconvolution and regression with errors in variables. *Journal of the Royal Statistical Society, Series B*, 66, 31–46.

Carroll, R. J. and Li, K.-C. (1992). Measurement error regression with unknown link: Dimension reduction and data visualization. *Journal of the American Statistical Association*, 87, 1040–1050.

Carroll, R. J. and Ruppert, D. (1996). The use and misuse of orthogonal regression in linear errors-in-variables models. *The American Statistician*, 50, 1–6.

Carroll, R. J. and Stefanski, L. A. (1985). Covariate measurement error in logistic regression. *The Annals of Statistics*, 13, 1335–1351.

Carroll, R. J. and Stefanski, L. A. (1990). Approximate quasi-likelihood estimation in models with surrogate predictors. *Journal of the American Statistical Association*, 85, 652–663.

Carroll, R. J. and Stefanski, L. A. (1994). Meta-analysis, measurement error and corrections for attenuation. *Statistics in Medicine*, 13, 1265–1282.

Carroll, R. J. and Wand, M. P. (1991). Semiparametric estimation in logistic measurement error models. *Journal of the Royal Statistical Society, Series B*, 53, 573–585.

Carroll, R. J. and Wang, Y. (2008). Nonparametric variance estimation in analysis of microarray data: A measurement error approach. *Biometrika*, 95, 437–449.

Carroll, R. J., Chen, X., and Hu, Y. (2010). Identification and estimation of nonlinear models using two samples with nonclassical measurement errors. *Journal of Nonparametric Statistics*, 22, 379–399. Rejoinder to discussion pages 419–423.

Carroll, R. J., Delaigle, A., and Hall, P. (2007). Nonparametric regression estimation from data contaminated by a mixture of Berkson and classical errors. *Journal of the Royal Statistical Society, Series B*, 69, 859–878.

Carroll, R. J., Delaigle, A., and Hall, P. (2009). Nonparametric prediction in measurement error models (with discussion). *Journal of the American Statistical Association*, 104, 993–1014.

Carroll, R. J., Freedman, L., and Pee, D. (1997). Design aspects of calibration studies in nutrition, with analysis of missing data in linear measurement error models. *Biometrics*, 53, 1440–1457.

Carroll, R. J., Gail, M. H., and Lubin, J. H. (1993). Case–control studies with errors in covariates. *Journal of the American Statistical Association*, 88, 185–199.

Carroll, R. J., Gallo, P., and Gleser, L. J. (1985). Comparison of least squares and errors-in-variables regression, with special reference to randomized analysis of covariance. *Journal of the American Statistical Association*, 80, 929–932.

Carroll, R. J., Knickerbocker, R. K., and Wang, C. Y. (1995). Dimension reduction in a semiparametric regression model with errors in covariates. *The Annals of Statistics*, 23, 161–181.

Carroll, R. J., Maca, J. D., and Ruppert, D. (1999). Nonparametric regression in the presence of measurement error. *Biometrika*, 86, 541–554.

Carroll, J. C., Roeder, K., and Wasserman, L. (1999). Flexible parametric measurement error models. *Biometrics*, 55, 44–54.

Carroll, R. J., Ruppert, D., and Stefanski, L. A. (1995). *Measurement Error in Nonlinear Models*. Chapman & Hall/CRC.

Carroll, R. J., Wang, S., and Wang, C. Y. (1995). Prospective analysis of logistic case–control studies. *Journal of the American Statistical Association*, 90, 157–169.

Carroll, R. J., Freedman, L. S., Kipnis, V., and Li, L. (1998). A new class of measurement error models, with applications to dietary data. *The Canadian Journal of Statistics*, 26, 467–477.

Carroll, R. J., Küchenhoff, H., Lombard, F., and Stefanski, L. A. (1996). Asymptotics for the SIMEX estimator in nonlinear measurement error models. *Journal of the American Statistical Association*, 91, 242–250.

Carroll, R. J., Ruppert, D., Crainiceanu, C. M., Tosteson, T. D., and Karagas, M. R. (2004). Nonlinear and nonparametric regression and instrumental variables. *Journal of the American Statistical Association*, 99, 736–750.

Carroll, R. J., Ruppert, D., Stefanski, L. A., and Crainiceanu, C. M. (2006). *Measurement Error in Nonlinear Models*. 2nd ed., Chapman & Hall/CRC.

Carroll, R. J., Spiegelman, C. H., Lan, K. K. G., Bailey, K. T., and Abbott, R. D. (1984). On errors-in-variables for binary regression models. *Biometrika*, 71, 19–25.

Carter, R. L. and Fuller, W. A. (1980). Instrumental variable estimation of the simple errors-in-variables model. *Journal of the American Statistical Association*, 75, 687–692.

Chen, Z. (2010). *Analysis of Correlated Data with Measurement Error in Responses or Covariates*. Ph.D. Thesis, The University of Waterloo, Canada.

Chen, H. Y. (2011). A unified framework for studying parameter identifiability and estimation in biased sampling designs. *Biometrika*, 98, 163–175.

Chen, J. and Huang, Y. (2015). A Bayesian mixture of semiparametric mixed-effects joint models for skewed-longitudinal and time-to-event data. *Statistics in Medicine*, 34, 2820–2843.

Chen, P.-L. and Sen, P. K. (2007). Markov chain model selection by misclassified model probabilities. *Communications in Statistics – Theory and Methods*, 36, 143–153.

Chen, B., Yi, G. Y., and Cook, R. J. (2009). Likelihood analysis of joint marginal and conditional models for longitudinal categorical data. *The Canadian Journal of Statistics*, 37, 182–205.

Chen, B., Yi, G. Y., and Cook, R. J. (2010a). Analysis of interval-censored disease progression data via multi-state models under a nonignorable inspection process. *Statistics in Medicine*, 29, 1175–1189.

Chen, B., Yi, G. Y., and Cook, R. J. (2010b). Weighted generalized estimating functions for longitudinal response and covariate data that are missing at random. *Journal of the American Statistical Association*, 105, 336–353.

Chen, B., Yi, G. Y., and Cook, R. J. (2011). Progressive multi-state models for informatively incomplete longitudinal data. *Journal of Statistical Planning and Inference*, 141, 80–93.

Chen, Z., Yi, G. Y., and Wu, C. (2011). Marginal methods for correlated binary data with misclassified responses. *Biometrika*, 98, 647–662.

Chen, Z., Yi, G. Y., and Wu, C. (2014). Marginal analysis of longitudinal ordinal data with misclassification in both response and covariates. *Biometrical Journal*, 56, 69–85.

Chen, B., Yi, G. Y., Cook, R. J., and Zhou, X. (2012). Marginal methods for clustered longitudinal binary data with incomplete covariates. *Journal of Statistical Planning and Inference*, 142, 2819–2831.

Cheng, Y.-J. and Crainiceanu, C. M. (2009). Cox models with smooth functional effect of covariates measured with error. *Journal of the American Statistical Association*, 104, 1144–1154.

Cheng, K. F. and Hsueh, H. M. (2003). Estimation of a logistic regression model with mismeasured observations. *Statistica Sinica*, 13, 111–127.

Cheng, C.-L. and Tsai, C.-L. (2004). The invariance of some score tests in the linear model with classical measurement error. *Journal of the American Statistical Association*, 99, 805–809.

Cheng, C.-L. and Van Ness, J. W. (1994). On estimating linear relationships when both variables are subject to errors. *Journal of the Royal Statistical Society, Series B*, 56, 167–183.

Cheng, C.-L. and Van Ness, J.W. (1999). *Statistical Regression with Measurement Error*. Edward Arnold Publishers Ltd., London and Baltimore.

Cheng, S.-C. and Wang, N. (2001). Linear transformation models for failure time data with covariate measurement error. *Journal of the American Statistical Association*, 96, 706–716.

Cheng, C.-L., Schneeweiss, H., and Thamerus, M. (2000). A small sample estimator for a polynomial regression with errors in the variables. *Journal of the Royal Statistical Society, Series B*, 62, 699–709.

Cheng, S. C., Wei, L. J., and Ying, Z. (1995). Analysis of transformation models with censored data. *Biometrika*, 82, 835–845.

Chesher, A. (1991). The effect of measurement error. *Biometrika*, 78, 451–462.

Choi, Y.-H., Yi, G. Y., and Matthews, D. E. (2006). A simulation-extrapolation method for bivariate survival data with covariates subject to measurement error. *Journal of Applied Probability and Statistics*, 1, 49–66.

Chu, R., Gustafson, P., and Le, N. (2010). Bayesian adjustment for exposure misclassification in case–control studies. *Statistics in Medicine*, 29, 994–1003.

Chu, H., Cole, S. R., Wei, Y., and Ibrahim, J. G. (2009). Estimation and inference for case–control studies with multiple non-gold standard exposure assessments: with an occupational health application. *Biostatistics*, 10, 591–602.

Chua, T. C. and Fuller, W. A. (1987). A model for multinomial response error applied to labor flows. *Journal of the American Statistical Association*, 82, 46–51.

Clayton, D. G. (1978). A model for association in bivariate life tables and its application in epidemiological studies of familial tendency in chronic disease incidence. *Biometrika*, 65, 141–151.

Clayton, D. and Cuzick, J. (1985). Multivariate generalizations of the proportional hazards model (with discussion). *Journal of the Royal Statistical Society, Series A*, 148, 82–117.

Cochran, W. G. (1977). *Sampling Techniques*, 3rd edition. New York: Wiley.

Coffin, M. and Sukhatme, S. (1997). Receiver operating characteristic studies and measurement errors. *Biometrics*, 53, 823–837.

Cook, R. D. (1977). Detection of influential observation in linear regression. *Technometrics*, 19, 15–18.

Cook, R. D. (1986). Assessment of local influence (with discussion). *Journal of the Royal Statistical Society B*, 48, 133–169.

Cook, R. D. (2007). Fisher lecture: Dimension reduction in regression. *Statistical Science*, 22, 1–26.

Cook, R. J. and Lawless, J. F. (2007). *The Statistical Analysis of Recurrent Events*. Springer Science + Business Media, LLC.

Cook, R. J. and Lawless, J. F. (2014). Statistical issues in modeling chronic disease in cohort studies. *Statistics in Biosciences*, 6, 127–161.

Cook, J. R. and Stefanski, L. A. (1994). Simulation-extrapolation estimation in parametric measurement error models. *Journal of the American Statistical Association*, 89, 1314–1328.

Cook, R. J., Kalbfleisch, J. D., and Yi, G. Y. (2002). A generalized mover-stayer model for panel data. *Biostatistics*, 3, 407–420.

Cook, R. J., Yi, G. Y., Lee, K.-A., and Gladman, D. D. (2004). A conditional Markov model for clustered progressive multistate processes under incomplete observation. *Biometrics*, 60, 436–443.

Cornfield, J. (1951). A method of estimating comparative rates from clinical data. Applications to cancer of the lung, breast and cervix. *Journal of the National Cancer Institute*, 11, 1269–1275.

Cox, D. R. (1972). Regression models and life tables (with discussion). *Journal of the Royal Statistical Society, Series B*, 34, 187–220.

Cox, D. R. (1975). Partial likelihood. *Biometrika*, 62, 269–276.

Cox, D. R. (2006). *Principles of Statistical Inference*. Cambridge University Press, Cambridge.

Cox, D. R. and Hinkley, D. V. (1974). *Theoretical Statistics*. Chapman & Hall/CRC, Boca Raton, Florida.

Cox, D. R. and Lewis, P. A. W. (1966). *The Statistical Analysis of Series of Events*. Chapman & Hall/CRC, London.

Cox, D. R. and Miller, H. D. (1965). *The Theory of Stochastic Processes*. Methuen & Co Ltd.

Cox, D. R. and Oakes, D. (1984). *Analysis of Survival Data*. Chapman & Hall/CRC, Boca Raton, Florida.

Cox, D. R. and Reid, N. (1987). Parameter orthogonality and approximate conditional inference. *Journal of the Royal Statistical Society, Series B*, 49, 1–39.

Crowder, M. (1995). On the use of a working correlation matrix in using generalized linear models for repeated measures, *Biometrika*, 82, 407–410.

Cui, H. and Chen, S. X. (2003). Empirical likelihood confidence region for parameters in the errors-in-variables models. *Journal of Multivariate Analysis*, 84, 101–115.

Dabrowska, D. M. and Doksum, K. A. (1988). Partial likelihood in transformation models with censored data. *Scandinavian Journal of Statistics*, 15, 1–23.

Dagenais, M. G. and Dagenais, D. L. (1997). Higher moment estimators for linear regression models with errors in the variables. *Journal of Econometrics*, 76, 193–221.

Daniels, M. J. and Hogan, J. W. (2008). *Missing Data in Longitudinal Studies: Strategies for Bayesian Modeling and Sensitivity Analysis*. Chapman & Hall/CRC, Boca Raton, Florida.

Davidian, M. and Giltinan, D. M. (1995). *Nonlinear Models for Repeated Measurement Data*. London: Chapman & Hall/CRC, Boca Raton, Florida.

de Castro, M. Galea, M., and Bolfarine, H. (2008). Hypothesis testing in an errors-in-variables model with heteroscedastic measurement errors. *Statistics in Medicine*, 27, 5217–5234.

Delaigle, A. (2007). Nonparametric density estimation from data with a mixture of Berkson and classical errors. *The Canadian Journal of Statistics*, 35, 89–104.

Delaigle, A. (2014). Nonparametric kernel methods with errors-in-variables: Constructing estimators, computing them, and avoiding common mistakes. *Australian & New Zealand Journal of Statistics*, 56, 105–124.

Delaigle, A. and Gijbels, I. (2002). Estimation of integrated squared density derivatives from a contaminated sample. *Journal of the Royal Statistical Society, Series B*, 64, 869–886.

Delaigle, A. and Hall, P. (2008). Using SIMEX for smoothing-parameter choice in errors-in-variables problems. *Journal of the American Statistical Association*, 103, 280–287.

Delaigle, A., Fan, J., and Carroll, R. J. (2009). A design-adaptive local polynomial estimator for the errors-in-variables problem. *Journal of the American Statistical Association*, 104, 348–359.

Delaigle, A., Hall, P., and Qiu, P. (2006). Nonparametric methods for solving the Berkson errors-in-variables problem. *Journal of the Royal Statistical Society, Series B*, 68, 201–220.

Dempster, A. P., Laird, N. M., and Rubin, D. B. (1977). Maximum likelihood from incomplete data via the EM algorithm. *Journal of the Royal Statistical Society: Series B*, 39, 1–38.

Devanarayan,V. and Stefanski, L. A. (2002). Empirical simulation extrapolation for measurement error models with replicate measurements. *Statistics & Probability Letters*, 59, 219–225.

Díaz, I. and van der Laan, M. J. (2013). Sensitivity analysis for causal inference under unmeasured confounding and measurement error problems. *The International Journal of Biostatistics*, 9, 149–160.

Diggle, P. and Kenward, M. G. (1994). Informative drop-out in longitudinal data analysis (with discussion). *Applied Statistics*, 43, 49–93.

Diggle, P. J., Liang, K.-Y., Heagerty, P., and Zeger, S. L. (2002). *Analysis of Longitudinal Data*. Oxford, England: Oxford University Press.

Ding, J. and Wang, J.-L. (2008). Modeling longitudinal data with nonparametric multiplicative random effects jointly with survival data. *Biometrics*, 64, 546–556.

Draper, D. (1995). Assessment and propagation of model uncertainty. *Journal of the Royal Statistical Society, Series B*, 57, 45–97.

Drews, C. D., Flanders, W. D., and Kosinski, A. S. (1993). Use of two data sources to estimate odds ratios in case–control studies. *Epidemiology*, 4, 327–335.

Duffy, S. W., Rohan, T. E., and Day, N. E. (1989). Misclassification in more than one factor in a case–control study: A combination of Mantel-Haenszel and maximum likelihood approaches. *Statistics in Medicine*, 8, 1529–1536.

Dunn, G. (2004). *Statistical Evaluation of Measurement Errors: Design and Analysis of Reliability Studies*. 2nd ed., Oxford University Press Inc., New York.

Dupuy, J.-F. (2005). The proportional hazards model with covariate measurement error. *Journal of Statistical Planning and Inference*, 135, 260–275.

Durbin, J. (1960). Estimation of parameters in time-series regression models. *Journal of the Royal Statistical Society, Series B*, 22, 139–153.

Eckert, R. S., Carroll, R. J., and Wang, N. (1997). Transformations to additivity in measurement error models. *Biometrics*, 53, 262–272.

Efron, B. (1979). Bootstrap method: Another look at the jackknife. *The Annals of Statistics*, 7, 1–26.

Efron, B. (1994). Missing data, imputation, and bootstrap (with discussion). *Journal of the American Statistical Association*, 89, 463–475.

Efron, B. and Tibshirani, R. J. (1993). *An Introduction to the Bootstrap*. Chapman & Hall, New York.

Elton, R. A. and Duffy, S. W. (1983). Correcting for the effect of misclassification bias in a case–control study using data from two different questionnaires. *Biometrics*, 39, 659–663.

Fan, J. and Li, R. (2001). Variable selection via nonconcave penalized likelihood and its oracle properties. *Journal of the American Statistical Association*, 96, 1348–1360.

Fan, J. and Truong, Y. K. (1993). Nonparametric regression with errors in variables. *The Annals of Statistics*, 21, 1900–1925.

Feldstein, M. (1974). Errors in variables: A consistent estimator with smaller MSE in finite samples. *Journal of the American Statistical Association*, 69, 990–996.

Ferguson, T. S. (1978). Maximum likelihood estimates of the parameters of the Cauchy distribution for samples of size 3 and 4. *Journal of the American Statistical Association*, 73, 211–213.

Ferguson, H., Reid, N., and Cox, D. R. (1991). Estimating equations from modified profile likelihood. In *Estimating Functions*, Edited by V. P. Godambe, 279–293. Oxford University Press, Oxford.

Fisher, R. A. (1922). On the mathematical foundations of theoretical statistics. *Philosophical Transactions of the Royal Society of London, Series A*, 222, 309–368.

Fitzmaurice, G., Davidian, M., Verbeke, G., and Molenberghs, G. (2009). *Longitudinal Data Analysis*, Chapman & Hall /CRC, Boca Raton, Florida.

Forbes, A. B. and Santner, T. J. (1995). Estimators of odds ratio regression parameters in matched case–control studies with covariate measurement error. *Journal of the American Statistical Association*, 90, 1075–1084.

Freedman, D. A. (2009). *Statistical Models: Theory and Practice*. Cambridge University Press, New York.

Freedman, L. S., Fainberg, V., Kipnis, V., Midthune, D., and Carroll, R. J. (2004). A new method for dealing with measurement error in explanatory variables of regression models. *Biometrics*, 60, 172–181.

Freedman, L. S., Midthune, D., Carroll, R. J., and Kipnis, V. (2008). A comparison of regression calibration, moment reconstruction and imputation for adjusting for covariate measurement error in regression. *Statistics in Medicine*, 27, 5195–5216.

Frydman, H. (1984). Maximum likelihood estimation in the mover-stayer model. *Journal of the American Statistical Association*, 79, 632–638.

Fuchs, H. J., Borowitz, D. S., Christiansen, D. H., Morris, E. M., Nash, M. L., Ramsey, B.W., Rosenstein, B. J., Smith, A. L., and Wohl, M. E. for The Pulmozyme Study Group. (1994). Effect of aerosolized recombinant human DNase on exacerbations of respiratory symptoms and on pulmonary function in patients with cystic fibrosis. *New England Journal of Medicine*, 331, 637–642.

Fujisawa, H. and Izumi, S. (2000). Inference about misclassification probabilities from repeated binary responses. *Biometrics*, 56, 706–711.

Fuller, W. A. (1987). *Measurement Error Models*. Wiley, New York.

Fung, K. Y. and Krewski, D. (1999). On measurement error adjustment methods in Poisson regression. *Environmetrics*, 10, 213–224.

Gabrielsen, A. (1978). Consistency and identifiability. *Journal of Econometrics*, 8, 261–263.

Galea, M. and Giménez, P. (2010). Estimation and testing in elliptical functional measurement error models. *Communications in Statistics – Theory and Methods*, 39, 2031–2045.

Galea, M., Bolgarine, H., and Vilcalabra, F. (2002). Influence diagnostics for the structural errors-in-variables model under the Student-t distribution. *Journal of Applied Statistics*, 29, 1191–1204.

Ganse, R. A., Amemiya, Y., and Fuller, W. A. (1983). Prediction when both variables are subject to error, with application to earthquake magnitudes. *Journal of the American Statistical Association*, 78, 761–765.

Gimenez, P., Bolfarine, H., and Colosimo, E. A. (2000). Hypotheses testing for error-in-variables models. *Annals of the Institute of Statistical Mathematics*, 52, 698–711.

Gimenez, P., Colosimo, E. A., and Bolfarine, H. (2000). Asymptotic relative efficiency of Wald tests in measurement error models. *Communications in Statistics – Theory and Methods*, 29, 549–564.

Gleser, L. J., Carroll, R. J. and Gallo, P. P. (1987). The limiting distribution of least squares in an errors-in-variables linear regression model. *The Annals of Statistics*, 15, 220–233.

Glidden, D. V. (2000). A two-stage estimation of the dependence parameter for the Clayton-Oakes model. *Lifetime Data Analysis*, 6, 141–156.

Godambe, V. P. (1960). An optimum property of regular maximum likelihood estimation. *The Annals of Mathematical Statistics*, 31, 1208–1212.

Godambe, V. P. (1991). *Estimating Functions*. Oxford University Press, USA.

Goetghebeur, E. and Vansteelandt, S. (2005). Structural mean models for compliance analysis in randomized clinical trials and the impact of errors on measures of exposure. *Statistical Methods in Medical Research*, 14, 397–415.

Goldberg, J. D. (1975). The effects of misclassification on the bias in the differences between two proportions and the relative odds in the fourfold table. *Journal of the American Statistical Association*, 70, 561–567.

Gong, G., Whittemore, A. S., and Grosser, S. (1990). Censored survival data with misclassified covariates: A case study of breast-cancer mortality. *Journal of the American Statistical Association*, 85, 20–28.

Gorfine, M., Hsu, L., and Prentice, R. L. (2003). Estimation of dependence between paired correlated failure times in the presence of covariate measurement error. *Journal of the Royal Statistical Society, Series B*, 65, 643–661.

Gorfine, M., Hsu, L., and Prentice, R. L. (2004). Nonparametric correction for covariate measurement error in a stratified Cox model. *Biostatistics*, 5, 75–87.

Gorfine, M., Lipshtat, N., Freedman, L. S., and Prentice, R. L. (2007). Linear measurement error models with restricted sampling. *Biometrics*, 63, 137–142.

Gould, A. L., Boye, M. E., Crowther, M. J., Ibrahim, J. G., Quartey, G., Micallef, S., and Bois, F. Y. (2015). Joint modeling of survival and longitudinal non-survival data: Current methods and issues. Report of the DIA Bayesian joint modeling working group. *Statistics in Medicine*, 34, 2181–2195.

Gourieroux, C., Monfort, A., and Trognon, A. (1984). Pseudo maximum likelihood methods: Theory. *Econometrica*, 52, 681-700.

Green, M. S. (1983). Use of predictive value to adjust relative risk estimates biased by misclassification of outcome status. *American Journal of Epidemiology*, 117, 98–105.

Greene, W. F. and Cai, J. (2004). Measurement error in covariates in the marginal hazards model for multivariate failure time data. *Biometrics*, 60, 987–996.

Greenland, S. (2000). An introduction to instrumental variables for epidemiologists. *International Journal of Epidemiology*, 29, 722–729.

Griliches, Z. and Hausman, J. A. (1986). Errors in variables in panel data. *Journal of Econometrics*, 31, 93–118.

Gruger, J., Kay, R., and Schumacher, M. (1991). The validity of inferences based on incomplete observations in disease state models. *Biometrics*, 47, 595–605.

Guo, J. Q. and Li, T. (2002). Poisson regression models with errors-in-variables: implication and treatment. *Journal of Statistical Planning and Inference*, 104, 391–401.

Guolo, A. (2008a). A flexible approach to measurement error correction in case–control studies. *Biometrics*, 64, 1207–1214.

Guolo, A. (2008b). Robust techniques for measurement error correction: A review. *Statistical Methods in Medical Research*, 17, 555–580.

Gustafson, P. (2002). On the simultaneous effects of model misspecification and errors in variables. *The Canadian Journal of Statistics*, 30, 463–474.

Gustafson, P. (2004). *Measurement Error and Misclassification in Statistics and Epidemiology*. Chapman & Hall/CRC, Boca Raton, Florida.

Gustafson, P. (2005). On model expansion, model contraction, identifiability and prior information: Two illustrative scenarios involving mismeasured variables. *Statistical Science*, 20, 111–140.

Gustafson, P. (2007). Measurement error modelling with an approximate instrumental variable. *Journal of the Royal Statistical Society, Series B*, 69, 797–815.

Gustafson, P., Le, N. D., and Saskin, R. (2001). Case–control analysis with partial knowledge of exposure misclassification probabilities. *Biometrics*, 57, 598–609.

Halimi, R. E. (2009). *Nonlinear Mixed-Effects Models and Bootstrap Resampling*. VDM Verlag.

Hammer, S. M., Katzenstein, D. A., Hughes, M. D., Gundaker, H., Schooley, R. T., Haubrich, R. H., Henry, W. K., Lederman, M. M., Phair, J. P., Niu, M., Hirsch, M. S., and Merigan, T. C., for the Aids Clinical Trials Group Study 175 Study Team (1996). A trial comparing nucleoside monotherapy with combination therapy in HIV-infected adults with CD4 cell counts from 200 to 500 per cubic millimeter. *New England Journal of Medicine*, 335, 1081–1090.

Hanfelt, J. J. and Liang, K.-Y. (1995). Approximate likelihood ratios for general estimating functions. *Biometrika*, 82, 461–477.

Hanfelt, J. J. and Liang, K. Y. (1997). Approximate likelihoods for generalized linear errors-in-variables models. *Journal of the Royal Statistical Society, Series B*, 59, 627–637.

Hansen, L. P. (1982). Large sample properties of generalized method of moments estimators. *Econometrica*, 50, 1029–1054.

Hansen, T. F. and Bartoszek, K. (2012). Interpreting the evolutionary regression: The interplay between observational and biological errors in phylogenetic comparative studies. *Systematic Biology* 61, 413–425.

Hardin, J. W. and Hilbe, J. M. (2012). *Generalized Estimating Equations*. Second edition, Chapman and Hall/CRC, Boca Raton, Florida.

Hardin, J. W., Schmiediche, H., and Carroll, R. J. (2003a). The regression-calibration method for fitting generalized linear models with additive measurement error. *The Stata Journal*, 3, 361–372.

Hardin, J. W., Schmiediche, H., and Carroll, R. J. (2003b). The simulation extrapolation method for fitting generalized linear models with additive measurement error. *The Stata Journal*, 3, 373–385.

Härdle, W. and Linton, O. (1994). Nonparametric regression. In *Handbook of Econometrics*, Vol. 4, edited by R. Engle and D. McFadden. Amsterdam: North-Holland.

Hauck, W. W. (1979). The large sample variance of the Mantel-Haenszel estimator of a common odds ratio. *Biometrics*, 35, 817–819.

Hausman, J. A., Abrevaya, J., and Scott-Morton, F. M. (1998). Misclassification of the dependent variable in a discrete-response setting. *Journal of Econometrics*, 87, 239–269.

Hausman, J. A., Newey, W. K., Ichimura, H., and Powell, J. L. (1991). Identification and estimation of polynomial errors-in-variables models. *Journal of Econometrics*, 50, 273–295.

He, W. (2014). Analysis of multivariate survival data with Clayton regression models under conditional and marginal formulations. *Computational Statistics & Data Analysis*, 74, 52–63.

He, F. (2015). *Analysis of Multi-State Models with Mismeasured Covariates or Misclassified States*. Ph.D. Thesis, The University of Waterloo, Canada.

He, W. and Lawless, J. F. (2003). Flexible maximum likelihood methods for bivariate proportional hazards models. *Biometrics*, 59, 837–848.

He, X. and Liang, H. (2000). Quantile regression estimates for a class of linear and partially linear errors-in-variables models. *Statistica Sinica*, 10, 129–140.

He, W. and Yi, G. Y. (2011). A pairwise likelihood method for correlated binary data with/without missing observations under generalized partially linear single-index models. *Statistica Sinica*, 21, 207–229.

He, W., Xiong, J., and Yi, G. Y. (2011). Analysis of error-contaminated survival data under the proportional odds model. *Journal of Statistical Research*, 45, 111–130.

He, W., Xiong, J., and Yi, G. Y. (2012). SIMEX R package for accelerated failure time models with covariate measurement error. *Journal of Statistical Software*, 46, Code Snippet 1, 1–14.

He, W., Yi, G. Y., and Xiong, J. (2007). Accelerated failure time models with covariates subject to measurement error. *Statistics in Medicine*, 26, 4817–4832.

Heagerty, P. J. (2002). Marginalized transition models and likelihood inference for longitudinal categorical data. *Biometrics*, 58, 342–351.

Heagerty, P. J. and Zeger, S. L. (2000). Marginalized multilevel models and likelihood inference. *Statistical Science*, 15, 1–19.

Henmi, M. and Eguchi, S. (2004). A paradox concerning nuisance parameters and projected estimating functions. *Biometrika*, 91, 929–941.

Hernán, M. A. and Cole, S. R. (2009). Invited commentary: Causal diagrams and measurement bias. *American Journal of Epidemiology*, 170, 959–962.

Heyde, C. C. (1997). *Quasi-Likelihood and its Application: A General Approach to Optimal Parameter Estimation*. Springer-Verlag New York, Inc.

Heyde, C. C. and Morton, R. (1998). Multiple roots in general estimating equations. *Biometrika*, 85, 954–959.

Higgins, K. M., Davidian, M., and Giltinan, D. M. (1997). A two-step approach to measurement error in time-dependent covariates in nonlinear mixed-effects models, with application to IGF-I pharmacokinetics. *Journal of the American Statistical Association*, 92, 436–448.

Hildesheim, A., Mann, V., Brinton, L. A., Szklo, M., Reeves, W. C., and Rawls, W. E. (1991). Herpes simplex virus type 2: A possible interaction with human papillomavirus types 16/18 in the development of invasive cervical cancer. *International Journal of Cancer*, 49, 335–340.

Hilton, J. F., Alves, M., Anastos, K., Canchola, A. J., Cohen, M., Delapenha, R., Greenspan, D., Levine, A., MacPhail, L. A., Micci, S. J., Mulligan, R., Navazesh, M., Phelan, J., and Tsaknis, P. (2001). Accuracy of diagnoses of HIV-related oral lesions by medical clinicians. Findings from the Women's Interagency HIV Study. *Community Dentistry and Oral Epidemiology*, 29, 362–372.

Hong, H. and Tamer, E. (2003). A simple estimator for nonlinear error in variable models. *Journal of Econometrics*, 117, 1–19.

Hougaard, P. (1986). A class of multivariate failure time distributions. *Biometrika*, 73, 671–678.

Hougaard, P. (1999). Multi-state models: A review. *Lifetime Data Analysis*, 5, 239–264.

Hougaard, P. (2000). *Analysis of Multivariate Survival Data*. Springer-Verlag, New York.

Hu, Y. (2006). Bounding parameters in a linear regression model with a mismeasured regressor using additional information. *Journal of Econometrics*, 133, 51–70.

Hu, C. and de Gruttola, V. (2007). Joint modeling of progression of HIV resistance mutations measured with uncertainty and failure time data. *Biometrics*, 63, 60–68.

Hu, C. and Lin, D. Y. (2002). Cox regression with covariate measurement error. *The Scandinavian Journal of Statistics*, 29, 637–655.

Hu, C. and Lin, D. Y. (2004). Semiparametric failure time regression with replicates of mismeasured covariates. *Journal of the American Statistical Association*, 99, 105–118.

Hu, Y. and Schennach, S. M. (2008). Instrumental variable treatment of nonclassical measurement error models. *Econometrika*, 76, 195–216.

Hu, P., Tsiatis, A. A., and Davidian, M. (1998). Estimating the parameters in the Cox model when covariate variables are measured with error. *Biometrics*, 54, 1407–1419.

Huang, X. (2009). An improved test of latent-variable model misspecification in structural measurement error models for group testing data. *Statistics in Medicine*, 28, 3316–3327.

Huang, Z. (2011). Empirical likelihood for a partially linear single-index measurement error model with right-censored data. *Communications in Statistics – Theory and Methods*, 40, 1015–1029.

Huang, X. and Tebbs, J. M. (2009). On latent-variable model misspecification in structural measurement error models for binary response. *Biometrics*, 65, 710–718.

Huang, Y. and Wang, C. Y. (2000). Cox regression with accurate covariates unascertainable: A nonparametric-correction approach. *Journal of the American Statistical Association*, 95, 1209–1219.

Huang, Y. and Wang, C. Y. (2001). Consistent functional methods for logistic regression with error in covariates. *Journal of the American Statistical Association*, 96, 1469–1482.

Huang, Y. and Wang, C. Y. (2006). Error-in-covariates effect on estimating functions: Additivity in limit and nonparametric correction. *Statistica Sinica*, 16, 861–881.

Huang, X. and Zhang, H. (2013). Variable selection in linear measurement error models via penalized score functions. *Journal of Statistical Planning and Inference*, 143, 2101–2111.

Huang, X., Stefanski, L. A., and Davidian, M. (2006). Latent-model robustness in structural measurement error models. *Biometrika*, 93, 53–64.

Huang, L-S., Wang, H., and Cox, C. (2005). Assessing interaction effects in linear measurement error models. *Applied Statistics*, 54, 21–30.

Huber, P. J. (1967). The behavior of maximum likelihood estimates under nonstandard conditions. In *Proceedings of the Fifth Berkeley Symposium on Mathematical Statistics and Probability*, University of California Press, Berkeley, 221–233.

Hughes, M. D. (1993). Regression dilution in the proportional hazards model. *Biometrics*, 49, 1056–1066.

Hui, S. L. and Zhou, X. H. (1998). Evaluation of diagnostic tests without gold standards. *Statistical Methods in Medical Research*, 7, 354–370.

Huwang, L. and Hwang, J. T. G. (2002). Prediction and confidence intervals for nonlinear measurement error models without identifiability information. *Statistics & Probability Letters*, 58, 355–362.

Hwang, J. T. (1986). Multiplicative errors-in-variables models with applications to recent data released by the U.S. Department of Energy. *Journal of the American Statistical Association*, 81, 680–688.

Imai, K. and Yamamoto, T. (2010). Causal inference with differential measurement error: Nonparametric identification and sensitivity analysis. *American Journal of Political Science*, 54, 543–560.

Iturria, S. J., Carroll, R. J., and Firth, D. (1999). Polynomial regression and estimating functions in the presence of multiplicative measurement error. *Journal of the Royal Statistical Society, Series B*, 61, 547–561.

Jaccard, J. and Wan, C. K. (1995). Measurement error in the analysis of interaction effects between continuous predictors using multiple regression: Multiple indicator and structural equation approaches. *Psychological Bulletin*, 117, 348–357.

Jackson, C. H. (2011). Multi-state models for panel data: The msm package for R. *Journal of Statistical Software*, 38, Issue 8, 1–28.

Jackson, C. H., Sharples, L. D., Thompson, S. G., Duffy, S. W., and Couto, E. (2003). Multi-state Markov models for disease progression with classification error. *The Statistician*, 52, 193–209.

Jiang, J. (2007). *Linear and Generalized Linear Mixed Models and Their Applications.* Springer Science + Business Media, LLC.

Jiang, W. and Turnbull, B. W. (2004). The indirect method: Inference based on intermediate statistics – A synthesis and examples. *Statistical Science*, 19, 239–263.

Jiang, W., Turnbull, B. W., and Clark, L. C. (1999). Semiparametric regression models for repeated events with random effects and measurement error. *Journal of the American Statistical Association*, 94, 111–124.

Joreskog, K. G. and Yang, F. (1996). Nonlinear structural equation models: The Kenny–Judd model with interaction effects. In *Advanced Structural Equation Modeling*, Marcoulides, G. A. and Schumacker, R. E. (eds). Lawrence Erlbaum: Hillsadle, NJ, 57–88.

Kalbfleisch, J. D. and Lawless, J. F. (1985). The analysis of panel data under a Markov assumption. *Journal of the American Statistical Association*, 80, 863–871.

Kalbfleisch, J. D. and Lawless, J. F. (1989). Inference based on retrospective ascertainment. An analysis of the data on transfusion-related AIDS. *Journal of the American Statistical Association*, 84, 360–372.

Kalbfleisch, J. D. and Prentice, R. L. (2002). *The Statistical Analysis of Failure Time Data*, 2nd ed., John Wiley & Sons, New York.

Kalbfleisch, J. D. and Sprott, D. A. (1970). Application of likelihood methods to models involving large numbers of parameters (with discussion). *Journal of the Royal Statistical Society, Series B*, 32, 175–208.

Kannel, W. B., Neaton, J. D., Wentworth, D., Thomas, H. E., Stamler, J., Hulley, S. B., and Kjelsberg, M. O. (1986). Overall and coronary heart disease mortality rates in relation to major risk factors in 325,348 men screened for the MRFIT. *American Heart Journal*, 112, 825–836.

Kelly, G. (1984). The influence function in the errors in variables problem. *The Annals of Statistics*, 12, 87–100.

Kenny, D. and Judd, C. M. (1984). Estimating the nonlinear and interactive effects of latent variables. *Psychological Bulletin*, 96, 201–210.

Kent, J. T. (1982). Robust properties of likelihood ratio tests. *Biometrika*, 69, 19–27.

Kim, M. G. (2000). Outliers and influential observations in the structural errors-in-variables model. *Journal of Applied Statistics*, 27, 451–460.

Kim, Y.-J. (2007). Analysis of panel count data with measurement errors in the covariates. *Journal of Statistical Computation and Simulation*, 77, 109–117.

Kim, J. and Gleser, L. J. (2000). SIMEX approaches to measurement error in ROC studies. *Communications in Statistics - Theory and Methods*, 29, 2473–2491.

Kim, M. Y. and Goldberg, J. D. (2001). The effects of outcome misclassification and measurement error on the design and analysis of therapeutic equivalence trials. *Statistics in Medicine*, 20, 2065–2078.

Kim, H. M. and Saleh, A. K. Md. E. (2005). Improved estimation of regression parameters in measurement error models. *Journal of Multivariate Analysis*, 95, 273–300.

Kim, S., Li, Y., and Spiegelman, D. (2016). A semiparametric copula method for Cox models with covariate measurement error. *Lifetime Data Analysis*, 22, 1–16.

Kipnis, V., Midthune, D., Freedman, L. S., and Carroll, R. J. (2012). Regression calibration with more surrogates than mismeasured variables. *Statistics in Medicine*, 31, 2713–2732.

Kipnis, V., Freedman, L. S., Carroll, R. J., and Midthune, D. (2016). A bivariate measurement error model for semicontinuous and continuous variables: Application to nutritional epidemiology. *Biometrics*, 72, 106–115.

Klepper, S. (1988). Bounding the effects of measurement error in regressions involving dichotomous variables. *Journal of Econometrics*, 37, 343–359.

Klepper, S. and Leamer, E. E. (1984). Consistent sets of estimates for regressions with errors in all variables. *Econometrica*, 52, 163–184.

Knuiman, M. W., Cullent, K. J., Bulsara, M. K., Welborn, T. A., and Hobbs, M. S. T. (1994). Mortality trends, 1965 to 1989, in Busselton, the site of repeated health surveys and interventions. *Australian Journal of Public Health*, 18, 129–135.

Ko, H. and Davidian, M. (2000). Correcting for measurement error in individual-level covariates in nonlinear mixed effects models. *Biometrics*, 56, 368–375.

Kong, F. H. (1999). Adjusting regression attenuation in the Cox proportional hazards model. *Journal of Statistical Planning and Inference*, 79, 31–44.

Kong, F. H. and Gu, M. (1999). Consistent estimation in Cox proportional hazards model with covariate measurement errors. *Statistica Sinica*, 9, 953–969.

Koopmans, T. C. (1949). Identification problems in economic model construction. *Econometrica*, 17, 125–144.

Koopmans, T. C. and Reiersøl, O. (1950). The identification of structural characteristics. *The Annals of Mathematical Statistics*, 21, 165–181.

Koul, H. L. and Song, W. (2008). Regression model checking with Berkson measurement errors. *Journal of Statistical Planning and Inference*, 138, 1615–1628.

Krasker, W. S. and Pratt, J. W. (1986). Bounding the effects of proxy variables on regression coefficients. *Econometrica*, 54, 641–655.

Küchenhoff, H., Bender, R., and Langner, I. (2007). Effect of Berkson measurement error on parameter estimates in Cox regression models. *Lifetime Data Analysis*, 13, 261–272.

Küchenhoff, H., Mwalili, S. M., and Lesaffre, E. (2006). A general method for dealing with misclassification in regression: The misclassification SIMEX. *Biometrics*, 62, 85–96.

Kuha, J. and Temple, J. (2003). Covariate measurement error in quadratic regression. *International Statistical Review*, 71, 131–150.

Kukush, A., Markovsky, I., and Huffel, S. V. (2002). Consistent fundamental matrix estimation in a quadratic measurement error model arising in motion analysis. *Computational Statistics and Data Analysis*, 41, 3–18.

Kulich, M. and Lin, D. Y. (2000). Additive hazards regression with covariate measurement error. *Journal of the American Statistical Association*, 95, 238–248.

Lachos, V. H., Montenegro, L. C., and Bolfarine, H. (2008). Inference and local influence assessment in skew-normal null intercept measurement error model. *Journal of Statistical Computation and Simulation*, 78, 395–419.

Lachos, V. H., Garibay, V., Labra, F. V., and Aoki, R. (2009). A robust multivariate measurement error model with skew-normal/independent distributions and Bayesian MCMC implementation. *Statistical Methodology*, 6, 527–541.

Lagakos, S. W. (1988). Effects of mismodelling and mismeasuring explanatory variables on tests of their association with a response variable. *Statistics in Medicine*, 7, 257–274.

Lai, T. L. and Small, D. (2007). Marginal regression analysis of longitudinal data with time-dependent covariates: A generalized method of moments approach. *Journal of the Royal Statistical Society, Series B*, 69, 79–99.

Lakshminarayanan, M. Y. and Gunst, R. F. (1984). Estimation of parameters in linear structural relationships: Sensitivity to the choice of the ratio of error variances. *Biometrika*, 71, 569–573.

Lane-Claypon, J. E. (1926). A further report on cancer of the breast. *Reports on Public Health and Medical Subjects 32: Ministry of Health*, H. M. S. O., London.

Lawless, J. F. (1987). Regression methods for Poisson process data. *Journal of the American Statistical Association*, 82, 808–815.

Lawless, J. F. (2003). *Statistical Models and Methods for Lifetime Data*. 2nd ed., John Wiley & Sons, Inc., Hoboken, New Jersey.

Lawless, J. F. and Zhan, M. (1998). Analysis of interval-grouped recurrent-event data using piecewise constant rate functions. *The Canadian Journal of Statistics*, 26, 549–565.

Lederer, W. and Küchenhoff, H. (2006). A short introduction to the SIMEX and MCSIMEX. *R News*, 6(4), 26–31.

Lee, L.-F. and Sepanski, J. H. (1995). Estimation of linear and nonlinear errors-in-variables models using validation data. *Journal of the American Statistical Association*, 90, 130–140.

Lee, A. H. and Zhao, Y. (1996). Assessing local influence in measurement error models. *Biometrical Journal*, 38, 829–841.

Lehmann, E. L. (1999). *Elements of Large-Sample Theory.* Springer-Verlag New York, LLC.

Lehmann, E. L. and Casella, G. (1998). *Theory of Point Estimation.* 2nd edition, Springer-Verlag New York, Inc.

Lewbel, A. (1998). Semiparametric latent variable model estimation with endogenous or mismeasured regressors. *Econometrica*, 66, 105–121.

Lewbel, A. (2007). Estimation of average treatment effects with misclassification. *Econometrica*, 75, 537–551.

Li, T. (2002). Robust and consistent estimation in nonlinear errors-in-variables models. *Journal of Econometrics*, 110, 1–26.

Li, L. and Greene, T. (2008). Varying coefficients model with measurement error. *Biometrics*, 64, 519–526.

Li, T. and Hsiao, C. (2004). Robust estimation of generalized linear models with measurement errors. *Journal of Econometrics*, 118, 51–65.

Li, Y. and Lin, X. (2000). Covariate measurement errors in frailty models for clustered survival data. *Biometrika*, 87, 849–866.

Li, Y. and Lin, X. (2003a). Functional inference in frailty measurement error models for clustered survival data using the SIMEX approach. *Journal of the American Statistical Association*, 98, 191–203.

Li, Y. and Lin, X. (2003b). Testing the correlation for clustered categorical and censored discrete time-to-event data when covariates are measured without/with errors. *Biometrics*, 59, 25–35.

Li, Y. and Ryan, L. (2004). Survival analysis with heterogeneous covariate measurement error. *Journal of the American Statistical Association*, 99, 724–735.

Li, Y. and Ryan, L. (2006). Inference on survival data with covariate measurement error – An imputation-based approach. *Scandinavian Journal of Statistics*, 33, 169–190.

Li, T. and Vuong, Q. (1998). Nonparametric estimation of the measurement error model using multiple indicators. *Journal of Multivariate Analysis*, 65, 139–165.

Li, H. and Yi, G. Y. (2013a). Estimation methods for marginal and association parameters for longitudinal binary data with nonignorable missing observations. *Statistics in Medicine*, 32, 833–848.

Li, H. and Yi, G. Y. (2013b). A pairwise likelihood approach for longitudinal data with missing observations in both response and covariates. *Computational Statistics & Data Analysis*, 68, 66–81.

Li, H. and Yi, G. Y. (2016). Missing data mechanisms for analysing longitudinal data with incomplete observations in both responses and covariates. *Australian & New Zealand Journal of Statistics*, 58, 377–396.

Li, B. and Yin, X. (2007). On surrogate dimension reduction for measurement error regression: An invariance law. *The Annals of Statistics*, 35, 2143–2172.

Li, L., Hu, B., and Greene. T. (2009). A semiparametric joint model for longitudinal and survival data with application to hemodialysis study. *Biometrics*, 65, 737–745.

Li, L., Shao, J., and Palta, M. (2005). A longitudinal measurement error model with a semicontinuous covariate. *Biometrics*, 61, 824–830.

Li, L., Lin, X., Brown, M. B., Gupta, S., and Lee, K.-H. (2004). A population pharmacokinetic model with time-dependent covariates measured with errors. *Biometrics*, 60, 451–460.

Liang, K.-Y. (1987). Estimating functions and approximate conditional likelihood. *Biometrika*, 74, 695–702.

Liang, H. (2009). Generalized partially linear mixed-effects models incorporating mismeasured covariates. *Annals of the Institute of Statistical Mathematics*, 61, 27–46.

Liang, H. and Li, R. (2009). Variable selection for partially linear models with measurement errors. *Journal of the American Statistical Association*, 104, 234–248.

Liang, K.-Y. and Zeger, S. L. (1986). Longitudinal data analysis using generalized linear models. *Biometrika*, 73, 13–22.

Liang, K.-Y. and Zeger, S. L. (1995). Inference based on estimating functions in the presence of nuisance parameters. *Statistical Science*, 10, 158–173.

Liang, H., Wang, S., and Carroll, R. J. (2007). Partially linear models with missing response variables and error-prone covariates. *Biometrika*, 94, 185–198.

Liang, K.-Y., Zeger, S. L., and Qaqish, B. (1992). Multivariate regression analyses for categorical data (with discussion). *Journal of the Royal Statistical Society, Series B*, 54, 3–40.

Liao, X., Zucker, D. M., Li, Y., and Spiegelman, D. (2011). Survival analysis with error-prone time-varying covariates: A risk set calibration approach. *Biometrics*, 67, 50–58.

Lin, X. and Carroll, R. J. (1999). SIMEX variance component tests in generalized linear mixed measurement error models. *Biometrics*, 55, 613–619.

Lin, X. and Carroll, R. J. (2000). Nonparametric function estimation for clustered data when the predictor is measured without/with error. *Journal of the American Statistical Association*, 95, 520–534.

Lin, D. Y. and Ying, Z. (1994). Semiparametric analysis of the additive risk model. *Biometrika*, 81, 61–71.

Lin, H., Scharfstein, D. O., and Rosenheck, R. A. (2004). Analysis of longitudinal data with irregular, outcome-dependent follow-up. *Journal of the Royal Statistical Society, Series B*, 66, 791–813.

Lindley, D. V. (1947). Regression lines and the linear functional relationship. *Journal of the Royal Statistical Society (Suppl.)*, 9, 218–244.

Lindsay, B. G. (1982). Conditional score functions: Some optimality results. *Biometrika*, 69, 503–512.

Lindsay, B. G. (1988). Composite likelihood methods. *Contemporary Mathematics*, 80, 221–239.

Lindsay, B. G., Yi, G., Y., and Sun, J. (2011). Issues and strategies in the selection of composite likelihoods. *Statistica Sinica*, 21, 71–105.

Lipsitz, S. R., Laird, N. M., and Harrington, D. P. (1991). Generalized estimating equations for correlated binary data: Using the odds ratio as a measure of association. *Biometrika*, 78, 153–160.

Little, R. J. A. (1993). Pattern-mixture models for multivariate incomplete data. *Journal of the American Statistical Association*, 88, 125–134.

Little, R. J. A. (1995). Modeling the drop-out mechanism in repeated-measures studies. *Journal of the American Statistical Association*, 90, 1112–1121.

Little, R. J. A. and Rubin, D. B. (2002). *Statistical Analysis with Missing Data*. 2nd ed., John Wiley & Sons, Inc., New Jersey.

Liu, C. and Rubin, D. B. (1994). The ECME algorithm: A simple extension of EM and ECM with faster monotone convergence. *Biometrika*, 81, 633–648.

Liu, W. and Wu, L. (2007). Simultaneous inference for semiparametric nonlinear mixed-effects models with covariate measurement errors and missing responses. *Biometrics*, 63, 342–350.

Lobach, I., Carroll, R. J., Spinka, C., Gail, M. H., and Chatterjee, N. (2008). Haplotype-based regression analysis and inference of case–control studies with unphased genotypes and measurement errors in environmental exposures. *Biometrics*, 64, 673–684.

Longini, I. M., Clark, W. S., Haber, M., and Horsburgh, R. (1989). The stages of HIV infection: Waiting times and infection transmission probabilities. In *Mathematical and Statistical Approaches to AIDS Epidemiology*, Lecture Notes in Biomathematics, 83, C. Castillo-Chavez (ed), 111–137. New York: Springer-Verlag.

Louis, T. A. (1982). Finding the observed information matrix when using the EM algorithm. *Journal of the Royal Statistical Society, Series B*, 44, 226–233.

Luan, X., Pan, W., Gerberich, S. G., and Carlin, B. P. (2005). Does it always help to adjust for misclassification of a binary outcome in logistic regression? *Statistics in Medicine*, 24, 2221–2234.

Lue, H.-H. (2004). Principal Hessian directions for regression with measurement error. *Biometrika*, 91, 409–423.

Luo, X., Stefanski, L. A., and Boos, D. D. (2006). Tuning variable selection procedures by adding noise. *Technometrics*, 48, 165–175.

Lyles, R. H. (2002). A note on estimating crude odds ratios in case–control studies with differentially misclassified exposure. *Biometrics*, 58, 1034–1036.

Lyles, R. H., Lin, H.-M., and Williamson, J. M. (2004). Design and analytic considerations for single-armed studies with misclassification of a repeated binary outcome. *Journal of Biopharmaceutical Statistics*, 14, 229–247.

Ma, Y. and Carroll, R. J. (2006). Locally efficient estimators for semiparametric models with measurement error. *Journal of the American Statistical Association*, 101, 1465–1474.

Ma, Y. and Li, R. (2010). Variable selection in measurement error models. *Bernoulli*, 16, 274–300.

Ma, Y. and Tsiatis, A. A. (2006). On closed form semiparametric estimators for measurement error models. *Statistica Sinica*, 16, 183–193.

Ma, Y. and Yin, G. (2008). Cure rate model with mismeasured covariates under transformation. *Journal of the American Statistical Association*, 103, 743–756.

Ma, Y., Hart, J. D., Janicki, R., and Carroll, R. J. (2011). Local and omnibus goodness-of-fit tests in classical measurement error models. *Journal of the Royal Statistical Society, Series B*, 73, 81–98.

MacDonald, I. L. and Zucchini, W. (1997). *Hidden Markov and Other Models for Discrete-valued Time Series*. New York: Chapman & Hall/CRC.

Madansky, A. (1959). The fitting of straight lines when both variables are subject to error. *Journal of the American Statistical Association*, 54, 173–205.

Mak, T. S. H., Best, N., and Rushton, L. (2015). Robust Bayesian sensitivity analysis for case–control studies with uncertain exposure misclassification probabilities. *The International Journal of Biostatistics*, 11, 135–149.

Mallick, B., Hoffman, F. O., and Carroll, R. J. (2002). Semiparametric regression modeling with mixtures of Berkson and classical error, with application to fallout from the Nevada test site. *Biometrics*, 58, 13–20.

Mantel, N. and Haenszel, W. (1959). Statistical aspects of the analysis of data from retrospective studies of disease. *Journal of the National Cancer Institute*, 22, 719–748.

Marinos, A. T., Tzonou, A. J., and Karantzas, M. E. (1995). Experimental quantiles of epidemiological indices in case–control studies with non-differential misclassification. *Statistics in Medicine*, 14, 1291–1306.

Martinussen, T. and Scheike, T. H. (2006). *Dynamic Regression Models for Survival Data*. Springer, New York.

McCaffrey, D. F., Lockwood, J. R., and Setodji, C. M. (2013). Inverse probability weighting with error-prone covariates. *Biometrika*, 100, 671–680.

McCullagh, P. (1983). Quasi-likelihood functions. *The Annals of Statistics*, 11, 59–67.

McCullagh, P. and Nelder, J. A. (1989). *Generalized Linear Models*. 2nd edition. London: Chapman & Hall/CRC.

McCullagh, P. and Tibshirani, R. (1990). A simple method for the adjustment of profile likelihoods. *Journal of the Royal Statistical Society, Series B*, 52, 325–344.

McGilchrist, C. A. and Aisbett, C. W. (1991). Regression with frailty in survival analysis. *Biometrics*, 47, 461–466.

McGlothlin, A., Stamey, J. D., and Seaman, J. W., Jr. (2008). Binary regression with misclassified response and covariate subject to measurement error: A Bayesian approach. *Biometrical Journal*, 50, 123–134.

McLachlan, G. J. and Krishnan, T. (1997). *The EM Algorithm and Extensions*. John Wiley & Sons, New York.

McNamee, R. (2005). Optimal design and efficiency of two-phase case–control studies with error-prone and error-free exposure measures. *Biostatistics*, 6, 590–603.

McShane, L. M., Midthune, D. N., Dorgan, J. F., Freedman, L. S., and Carroll, R. J. (2001). Covariate measurement error adjustment for matched case–control studies. *Biometrics*, 57, 62–73.

Meier, A. S., Richardson, B. A., and Hughes, J. P. (2003). Discrete proportional hazards models for mismeasured outcomes. *Biometrics*, 59, 947–954.

Meira-Machado, L., de Uña-Álvarez, J., Cadarso-Suárez, C., and Andersen, P. K. (2009). Multi-state models for the analysis of time-to-event data. *Statistical Methods in Medical Research*, 18, 195–222.

Meister, A. (2006). Density estimation with normal measurement error with unknown variance. *Statistica Sinica*, 16, 195–211.

Meng, X. L. and Van Dyk, D. (1998). Fast EM-type implementations for mixed effects models. *Journal of the Royal Statistical Society, Series B*, 60, 559–578.

Midthune, D., Carroll, R. J., Freedman, L. S., and Kipnis, V. (2016). Measurement error models with interactions. *Biostatistics*, 17, 277–290.

Miller, A. (2002). *Subset Selection in Regression*. 2nd ed. Chapman & Hall/CRC, Boca Raton, Florida.

Molenberghs, G. and Verbeke, G. (2005). *Models for Discrete Longitudinal Data*. New York: Springer.

Morrissey, M. and Spiegelman, D. (1999). Matrix methods for estimating odds ratios with misclassified exposure data: Extensions and comparisons. *Biometrics*, 55, 338–344.

Morton, R. (1981). Efficiency of estimating equations and the use of pivots. *Biometrika*, 68, 227–233.

Muff, S., Riebler, A., Rue, H., Saner, P., and Held, L. (2013). Bayesian analysis of measurement error models using INLA. *arXiv:1302.3065 [stat.ME]*.

Müller, P. and Roeder, K. (1997). A Bayesian semiparametric model for case–control studies with errors in variables. *Biometrika*, 84, 523–537.

Murad, H. and Freedman, L. S. (2007). Estimating and testing interactions in linear regression models when explanatory variables are subject to classical measurement error. *Statistics in Medicine*, 26, 4293–4310.

Nakamura, T. (1990). Corrected score functions for errors-in-variables models: Methodology and application to generalized linear models. *Biometrika*, 77, 127–137.

Nakamura, T. (1992). Proportional hazards model with covariates subject to measurement error. *Biometrics*, 48, 829–838.

Nelsen, R. B. (2006). *An Introduction to Copulas*. 2nd ed., New York: Springer.

Neuhaus, J. M. (1999). Bias and efficiency loss due to misclassified responses in binary regression. *Biometrika*, 86, 843–855.

Neuhaus, J. M. (2002). Analysis of clustered and longitudinal binary data subject to response misclassification. *Biometrics*, 58, 675–683.

Newey, W. K. and McFadden, D. (1994). Large sample estimation and hypothesis testing. In *Handbook of Econometrics*, Vol. 4, 2111–2245, eds. R.F. Engle and D. L. McFadden, Amsterdam: North-Holland.

Neyman. J. and Scott, E. L. (1948). Consistent estimates based on partially consistent observations. *Econometrica*, 16, 1–32.

Ning, Y., Yi, G. Y., and Reid, N. (2017). A class of weighted estimating equations for semiparametric transformation models with missing covariates. *Scandinavian Journal of Statistics* (to appear).

Novick, S. J. and Stefanski, L. A. (2002). Corrected score estimation via complex variable simulation extrapolation. *Journal of the American Statistical Association*, 97, 472–481.

Nummi, T. (2000). Analysis of growth curves under measurement errors. *Journal of Applied Statistics*, 27, 235–243.

Ogburn, E. L. and VanderWeele, T. J. (2012). Analytic results on the bias due to nondifferential misclassification of a binary mediator. *American Journal of Epidemiology*, 176, 555–561.

Pakes, A. and D. Pollard (1989). Simulation and the asymptotics of optimization estimators. *Econometrica*, 57, 1027–1057.

Palta, M. and Lin, C.-Y. (1999). Latent variables, measurement error and methods for analysing longitudinal binary and ordinal data. *Statistics in Medicine*, 18, 385–396.

Pan, W., Lin, X., and Zeng, D. (2006). Structural inference in transition measurement error models for longitudinal data. *Biometrics*, 62, 402–412.

Pan, W., Zeng, D., and Lin, X. (2009). Estimation in semiparametric transition measurement error models for longitudinal data. *Biometrics*, 65, 728–736.

Paulino, C. D. M. and de Bragança Pereira, C. A. (1994). On identifiability of parametric statistical models. *Journal of the Italian Statistical Society*, 1, 125–151.

Paulino, C. D., Soares, P., and Neuhaus, J. (2003). Binomial regression with misclassification. *Biometrics*, 59, 670–675.

Pearl, J. (2010). On measurement bias in causal inference. In *Proceedings of the 26th Conference on Uncertainty in Artificial Intelligence (UAI 2010)*. Corvallis, Oregon: AUAI Press.

Pepe, M. S. (1992). Inference using surrogate outcome data and a validation sample. *Biometrika*, 79, 355–365.

Pepe, M. S. and Anderson, G. L. (1994). A cautionary note on inference for marginal regression models with longitudinal data and general correlated response data. *Communications in Statistics – Simulation and Computation*, 23, 939–951.

Pepe, M. S. and Couper, D. (1997). Modeling partly conditional means with longitudinal data. *Journal of the American Statistical Association*, 92, 991–998.

Pepe, M. S. and Fleming, T. R. (1991). A nonparametric method for dealing with mismeasured covariate data. *Journal of the American Statistical Association*, 86, 108–113.

Pepe, M. S., Reilly, M., and Fleming, T. R. (1994). Auxiliary outcome data and the mean score method. *Journal of Statistical Planning and Inference*, 42, 137–160.

Pepe, M. S., Self, S. G., and Prentice, R. L. (1989). Further results on covariate measurement errors in cohort studies with time to response data. *Statistics in Medicine*, 8, 1167–1178.

Pérez, A., Zhang, S., Kipins, V., Midthune, D., Freedman, L. S., and Carroll, R. J. (2012). Intake_epis_food(): An R function for fitting a bivariate nonlinear measurement error model to estimate usual and energy intake for episodically consumed foods. *The Journal of Statistical Software*, 46, 1–17.

Pfeffermann, D., Skinner, C., and Humphreys, K. (1998). The estimation of gross flows in the presence of measurement error using auxiliary variables. *Journal of the Royal Statistical Society, Series A*, 161, 13–32.

Pierce, D. A. and Kellerer, A. M. (2004). Adjusting for covariate errors with nonparamtric assessment of the true covariate distribution. *Biometrika*, 91, 863–876.

Pierce, B. L. and VanderWeele, T. J. (2012). The effect of non-differential measurement error on bias, precision and power in Mendelian randomization studies. *International Journal of Epidemiology*, 41, 1383–1393.

Pierce, D. A., Stram, D. O., Vaeth, M., and Schafer, D. W. (1992). The errors-in-variables problem: considerations provided by radiation dose-response analyses for the A-bomb survivor data. *Journal of the American Statistical Association*, 87, 351–359.

Pollard, D. (1985). New ways to prove central limit theorems. *Econometric Theory*, 1, 295–313.

Prentice, R. L. (1982). Covariate measurement errors and parameter estimation in a failure time regression model. *Biometrika*, 69, 331–342.

Prentice, R. L. (1986). Binary regression using an extended beta-binomial distribution, with discussion of correlation induced by covariate measurement errors. *Journal of the American Statistical Association*, 81, 321–327.

Prentice, R. L. (1988). Correlated binary regression with covariates specific to each binary observation. *Biometrics*, 44, 1033–1048.

Prentice, R. L. (1989). Surrogate endpoints in clinical trials: definition and operational criteria. *Statistics in Medicine*, 8, 431–440.

Prentice, R. L. and Breslow, N. E. (1978). Retrospective studies and failure time models. *Biometrika*, 65, 153–158.

Prentice, R. L. and Huang, Y. (2011). Measurement error modeling and nutritional epidemiology association analyses. *The Canadian Journal of Statistics*, 39, 498–509.

Prentice, R. L. and Pyke, R. (1979). Logistic disease incidence models and case–control studies. *Biometrika*, 66, 403–411.

Prentice, R. L., Sugar, E., Wang, C. Y., Neuhouser, M., and Patterson, R. (2002). Research strategies and the use of nutrient biomarkers in studies of diet and chronic disease. *Public Health Nutrition*, 5, 977–984.

Prescott, G. J. and Garthwaite, P. H. (2005). Bayesian analysis of misclassified binary data from a matched case–control study with a validation sub-study. *Statistics in Medicine*, 24, 379–401.

Putter, H., Fiocco, M., and Geskus, R. B. (2007). Tutorial in biostatistics: Competing risks and multi-state models. *Statistics in Medicine*, 26, 2389–2430.

Qu, A., Lindsay, B. G., and Li, B. (2000). Improving generalised estimating equations using quadratic inference functions. *Biometrika*, 87, 823–836.

Qu, A., Yi, G. Y., Song, P. X.-K., and Wang, P. (2011). Assessing the validity of weighted generalized estimating equations. *Biometrika*, 98, 215–224.

Quenouille, M. H. (1949). Approximate tests of correlation in time-series. *Journal of the Royal Statistical Society, Series B*, 11, 68–84.

Rabe-Hesketh, S., Skrondal, A., and Pickles, A. (2003). Maximum likelihood estimation of generalized linear models with covariate measurement error. *The Stata Journal*, 3, 386–411.

Rao, B. L. S. P. (1992). *Identifiability in Stochastic Models: Characterization of Probability Distributions*. Boston Academic Press.

Reddy, S. K. (1992). Effects of ignoring correlated measurement error in structural equation models. *Educational and Psychological Measurement*, 52, 549–570.

Reeves, G. K., Cox, D. R., Darby, S. C., and Whitley, E. (1998). Some aspects of measurement error in explanatory variables for continuous and binary regression models. *Statistics in Medicine*, 17, 2157–2177.

Regier, M. D., Moodie, E. E. M., and Platt, R. W. (2014). The effect of error-in-confounders on the estimation of the causal parameter when using marginal structural models and inverse probability-of-treatment weights: A simulation study. *The International Journal of Biostatistics*, 10, 1–15.

Reiersøl, O. (1950). Identifiability of a linear relation between variables which are subject to error. *Econometrica*, 18, 375–389.

Reilman, M. A. and Gunst, R. F. (1985). Structural model estimation with correlated measurement errors. *Biometrika*, 72, 669–672.

Reilman, M. A., Gunst, R. F., and Lakshminarayanan, M. Y. (1986). Stochastic regression with errors in both variables. *Journal of Quality Technology*, 18, 162–169.

Rice, K. (2003). Full-likelihood approaches to misclassification of a binary exposure in matched case–control studies. *Statistics in Medicine*, 22, 3177–3194.

Richardson, D. H. and Wu, D.-M. (1970). Least squares and grouping method estimators in the errors in variables model. *Journal of the American Statistical Association*, 65, 724–748.

Rizopoulos, D. (2012). *Joint Models for Longitudinal and Time-to-Event Data: with Applications in R*. Chapman & Hall/CRC.

Robins, J. M. and Rotnitzky, A. (2001). Comment on "Inference for semiparametric models: Some questions and an answer", by P. J. Bickel and J. Kwon, *Statistica Sinica*, 11, 920–936.

Robins, J. M., Rotnitzky, A., and Zhao, L. P. (1994). Estimation of regression coefficients when some regressors are not always observed. *Journal of the American Statistical Association*, 89, 846–866.

Robins, J. M., Rotnitzky, A., and Zhao, L. P. (1995). Analysis of semiparametric regression models for repeated outcomes in the presence of missing data. *Journal of the American Statistical Association*, 90, 106–121.

Roeder, K., Carroll, R. J., and Lindsay, B. G. (1996). A semiparametric mixture approach to case–control studies with errors in covariables. *Journal of the American Statistical Association*, 91, 722–732.

Roehrig, C. S. (1988). Conditions for identification in nonparametric and parametric models. *Econometrica*, 56, 433–447.

Rosner, B. A. (1996). Measurement error models for ordinal exposure variables measured with error. *Statistics in Medicine*, 15, 293–303.

Rosner, B. and Munoz, A. (1992). Conditional linear models for longitudinal data. *Statistical Models for Longitudinal Studies of Health*, eds. J. Dwyer, M. Feinleib, P. Lippert, and H. Hoffmeister, New York: Oxford University Press.

Rosner, B., Willett, W. C., and Spiegelman, D. (1989). Correction of logistic regression relative risk estimates and confidence intervals for systematic within-person measurement error. *Statistics in Medicine*, 8, 1051–1069.

Rosner, B., Muñoz, A., Tager, I., Speizer, F., and Weiss, S. (1985). The use of an autoregressive model for the analysis of longitudinal data in epidemiologic studies. *Statistics in Medicine*, 4, 457–467.

Rosychuk, R. J. and Islam, S. (2009). Parameter estimation in a model for misclassified Markov data - a Bayesian approach. *Computational Statistics & Data Analysis*, 53, 3805–3816.

Rosychuk, R. J. and Thompson, M. E. (2003). Bias correction of two-state latent Markov process parameter estimates under misclassification. *Statistics in Medicine*, 22, 2035–2055.

Rosychuk, R. J. and Thompson, M. E. (2004). Parameter identifiability issues in a latent Markov model for misclassified binary responses. *Journal of Iranian Statistical Society*, 3, 39–57.

Rothenberg, T. J. (1971). Identification in parametric Models. *Econometrica*, 39, 577–591.

Roy, S. and Banerjee, T. (2009). Analysis of misclassified correlated binary data using a multivariate probit model when covariates are subject to measurement error. *Biometrical Journal*, 51, 420–432.

Roy, S., Banerjee, T., and Maiti, T. (2005). Measurement error model for misclassified binary responses. *Statistics in Medicine*, 24, 269–283.

Royall, R. M. (1986). Model robust confidence intervals using maximum likelihood estimators. *International Statistical Review*, 54, 221–226.

Sarkar, A., Mallick, B. K., and Carroll, R. J. (2014). Bayesian semiparametric regression in the presence of conditionally heteroscedastic measurement and regression errors. *Biometrics*, 70, 823–834.

Sarkar, A., Mallick, B. K., Staudenmayer, J., Pati, D., and Carroll, R. J. (2014). Bayesian semiparametric density deconvolution in the presence of conditionally heteroscedastic measurement errors. *Journal of Computational and Graphical Statistics*, 23, 1101–1125.

Satten G. A. (1999). Estimating the extent of tracking in interval-censored chain-of-events data. *Biometrics*, 55, 1228–1231.

Satten G. A. and Longini, I. M. (1996). Markov chains with measurement error: Estimating the "true" course of a marker of the progression of human immunodeficiency virus disease. *Journal of the Royal Statistical Society, Series C*, 45, 275–309.

Schaalje, G. B. and Butts, R. A. (1993). Some effects of ignoring correlated measurement errors in straight line regression and prediction. *Biometrics*, 49, 1262–1267.

Schafer, D. W. (2001). Semiparametric maximum likelihood for measurement error model regression. *Biometrics*, 57, 53–61.

Schennach, S. M. and Hu, Y. (2013). Nonparametric identification and semiparametric estimation of classical measurement error models without side information. *Journal of the American Statistical Association*, 108, 177–186.

Schill, W., Jöckel, K.-H., Drescher, K., and Timm, J. (1993). Logistic analysis in case–control studies under validation sampling. *Biometrika*, 80, 339–352.

Schlesselman, J. J. (1982). *Case–Control Studies: Design, Conduct, Analysis*. Oxford University Press, Inc.

Schmid, C. H. (1996). An EM algorithm fitting first-order conditional autoregressive models to longitudinal data. *Journal of the American Statistical Association*, 91, 1322–1330.

Schmid, C. H. and Rosner, B. (1993). A Bayesian approach to logistic regression models having measurement error following a mixture distribution. *Statistics in Medicine*, 12, 1141–1153.

Schmid, C. H., Segal, M. R., and Rosner, B. (1994). Incorporating measurement error in the estimation of autoregressive models for longitudinal data. *Journal of Statistical Planning and Inference*, 42, 1–18.

Schneeweiss, H. and Cheng, C.-L. (2006). Bias of the structural quasi-score estimator of a measurement error model under misspecification of the regressor distribution. *Journal of Multivariate Analysis*, 97, 455–473.

Selén, J. (1986). Adjusting for errors in classification and measurement in the analysis of partly and purely categorical data. *Journal of the American Statistical Association*, 81, 75–81.

Self, S. G. and Liang, K.-Y. (1987). Asymptotic properties of maximum likelihood estimators and likelihood ratio tests under nonstandard conditions. *Journal of the American Statistical Association*, 82, 605–610.

Sepanski, J. H. (1992). Score tests in a generalized linear model with surrogate covariates. *Statistics & Probability Letters*, 15, 1–10.

Sepanski, J. H. (2001). On a repeated-measurement model with errors in dependent variable. *Statistics*, 35, 97–112.

Sepanski, J. H. and Carroll, R. J. (1993). Semiparametric quasilikelihood and variance function estimation in measurement error models. *Journal of Econometrics*, 58, 223–256.

Sepanski, J. H., Knickerbocker, R. K., and Carroll, R. J. (1994). A semiparametric correction for attenuation. *Journal of the American Statistical Association*, 89, 1366–1373.

Serfling, R. J. (1980). *Approximation Theorems of Mathematical Statistics*. New York: Wiley.

Shao, J. (2003). *Mathematical Statistics*. 2nd edition, Springer-Verlag New York, Inc.

Shardell, M. and Miller, R. R. (2008). Weighted estimating equations for longitudinal studies with death and non-monotone missing time-dependent covariates and outcomes. *Statistics in Medicine*, 27, 1008–1025.

Shaw, P. A. and Prentice, R. L. (2012). Hazard ratio estimation for biomarker-calibrated dietary exposures. *Biometrics*, 68, 397–407.

Shen, C.-W. and Chen, Y.-H. (2015). Model selection for marginal regression analysis of longitudinal data with missing observations and covariate measurement error. *Biostatistics*, 16, 740–753.

Shih, J. H. and Albert, P. S. (1999). Latent model for correlated binary data with diagnostic error. *Biometrics*, 55, 1232–1235.

Shih, J. H. and Louis, T. A. (1995) Inference on the association parameter in copula models for bivariate survival data. *Biometrics*, 51, 1384–1399.

Shu, D. and Yi, G. Y. (2017a). Inverse-probability-of-treatment weighted estimation of causal parameters in the presence of error-contaminated and time-dependent confounders. Submitted for publication.

Shu, D. and Yi, G. Y. (2017b). Causal inference with measurement error in outcomes: Bias analysis and estimation methods. Submitted for publication.

Sinha, S. and Ma, Y. (2014). Semiparametric analysis of linear transformation models with covariate measurement errors. *Biometrics*, 70, 21–32.

Sinha, S., Mallick, B. K., Kipnis, V., and Carroll, R. J. (2010). Semiparametric Bayesian analysis of nutritional epidemiology data in the presence of measurement error. *Biometrics*, 66, 444–454.

Skrondal, A. and Rabe-Hesketh, S. (2004). *Generalized Latent Variable Modeling: Multilevel, Longitudinal, and Structural Equation Models*. Boca Raton, Florida: Chapman & Hall/CRC.

Smith, T. and Vounatsou, P. (2003). Estimation of infection and recovery rates for highly polymorphic parasites when detectability is imperfect, using hidden Markov models. *Statistics in Medicine*, 22, 1709–1724.

Solomon, P. J. and Cox, D. R. (1992). Nonlinear component of variance models. *Biometrika*, 79, 1–11.

Song, X. and Huang, Y. (2005). On corrected score approach for proportional hazards model with covariate measurement error. *Biometrics*, 61, 702–714.

Song, X., Davidian, M., and Tsiatis, A. A. (2002). An estimator for the proportional hazards model with multiple longitudinal covariates measured with error. *Biostatistics*, 3, 511–528.

Spiegelman, C. H. (1986). Two pitfalls of using standard regression diagnostics when both x and y have measurement error. *The American Statistician*, 40, 245–248.

Spiegelman, D. (1994). Cost-efficient study designs for relative risk modeling with covariate measurement error. *Journal of Statistical Planning and Inference*, 42, 187–208.

Spiegelman, D. and Gary, R. (1991). Cost-efficient study designs for binary response data with Gaussian covariate measurement error. *Biometrics*, 47, 851–869.

Spiegelman, D., Rosner, B., and Logan, R. (2000). Estimation and inference for logistic regression with covariate misclassification and measurement error in main study/validation study designs. *Journal of the American Statistical Association*, 95, 51–61.

Spiegelman, D., Zhao, B., and Kim, J. (2005). Correlated errors in biased surrogates: study designs and methods for measurement error correction. *Statistics in Medicine*, 24, 1657–1682.

Sposto, R., Preston, D. L., Shimizu, Y., and Mabuchi, K. (1992). The effect of diagnostic misclassification on non-cancer and cancer mortality dose response in A-bomb survivors. *Biometrics*, 48, 605–617.

Stamey, J. and Gerlach, R. (2007). Bayesian sample size determination for case–control studies with misclassification. *Computational Statistics & Data Analysis*, 51, 2982–2992.

Staudenmayer, J. and Buonaccorsi, J. P. (2005). Measurement error in linear autoregressive models. *Journal of the American Statistical Association*, 100, 841–852.

Staudenmayer, J. and Ruppert, D. (2004). Local polynomial regression and simulation-extrapolation. *Journal of the Royal Statistical Society, Series B*, 66, 17–30.

Staudenmayer, J., Ruppert, D., and Buonaccorsi, J. P. (2008). Density estimation in the presence of heteroscedastic measurement error. *Journal of the American Statistical Association*, 103, 726–736.

Stefanski, L. A. (1985). The effects of measurement error on parameter estimation. *Biometrika*, 72, 583–592.

Stefanski, L. A. (1989). Unbiased estimation of a nonlinear function of a normal mean with application to measurement error models. *Communications in Statistics – Theory and Methods*, 18, 4335–4358.

Stefanski, L. A. and Bay, J. M. (1996). Simulation extrapolation deconvolution of finite population cumulative distribution function estimators. *Biometrika*, 83, 407–417.

Stefanski, L. A. and Buzas, J. S. (1995). Instrumental variable estimation in binary measurement error models. *Journal of the American Statistical Association*, 90, 541–550.

Stefanski, L. A. and Carroll, R. J. (1985). Covariate measurement error in logistic regression. *The Annals of Statistics*, 13, 1335–1351.

Stefanski, L. A. and Carroll, R. J. (1987). Conditional scores and optimal scores for generalized linear measurement-error models. *Biometrika*, 74, 703–716.

Stefanski, L. A. and Carroll, R. J. (1990a). Score tests in generalized linear measurement error models. *Journal of the Royal Statistical Society, Series B*, 52, 345–359.

Stefanski, L. A. and Carroll, R. J. (1990b). Deconvoluting kernel density estimators. *Statistics*, 21, 169–184.

Stefanski, L. A. and Carroll, R. J. (1991). Deconvolution-based score tests in measurement error models. *The Annals of Statistics*, 19, 249–259.

Stefanski, L. A. and Cook, J. R. (1995). Simulation-extrapolation: The measurement error jackknife. *Journal of the American Statistical Association*, 90, 1247–1256.

Stouffer, S. A. (1936). Evaluating the effect of inadequately measured variables in partial correlation analysis. *Journal of the American Statistical Association*, 31, 348–360.

Stroup, W. W. (2012). *Generalized Linear Mixed Models: Modern Concepts, Methods and Applications*. CRC Press.

Stubbendick, A. L. and Ibrahim, J. G. (2003). Maximum likelihood methods for nonignorable missing responses and covariates in random effects models. *Biometrics*, 59, 1140–1150.

Stürmer, T., Thürigen, D., Spiegelman, D., Blettner, M., and Brenner, H. (2002). The performance of methods for correcting measurement error in case–control studies. *Epidemiology*, 13, 507–516.

Sun, J. (2006). *The Statistical Analysis of Interval-Censored Failure Time Data*. Springer, New York.

Sun, J. and Wei, L. J. (2000). Regression analysis of panel count data with covariate-dependent observation and censoring times. *Journal of the Royal Statistical Society, Series B*, 62, 293–302

Sun, L., and Zhou, X. (2008). Inference in the additive risk model with time-varying covariates subject to measurement errors. *Statistics & Probability Letters*, 78, 2559–2566.

Sun, L., Song, X., and Mu, X. (2012). Regression analysis for the additive hazards model with covariate errors. *Communications in Statistics – Theory and Methods*, 41, 1911–1932.

Sun, L., Zhang, Z., and Sun, J. (2006). Additive hazards regression of failure time data with covariate measurement errors. *Statistica Neerlandica*, 60, 497–509.

Sypsa, V., Touloumi, G., Kenward, M., Karafoulidou, A., and Hatzakis, A. (2001). Comparison of smoothing techniques for CD4 data in a Markov model with states defined by CD4: An example on the estimation of the HIV incubation time distribution. *Statistics in Medicine*, 20, 3667–3676.

Tanner, M. A. (1996). *Tools for Statistical Inference*. Third Edition. Springer-Verlag New York, Inc.

Therneau, T. M. and Grambsch, P. M. (2000). *Modeling Survival Data: Extending the Cox Model*. Springer, New York.

Thiébaut, A. C. M., Freedman, L. S., Carroll, R. J., and Kipnis, V. (2007). Is it necessary to correct for measurement error in nutritional epidemiology? *Annals of Internal Medicine*, 146, 65–67.

Thomas, W. and Cook, R .D. (1989). Assessing influence on regression coefficients in generalized linear models. *Biometrika*, 76, 741–749.

Thomas, L., Stefanski, L., and Davidian, M. (2011). A moment-adjusted imputation method for measurement error models. *Biometrics*, 67, 1461–1470.

Thompson, J. R. and Carter, R. L. (2007). An overview of normal theory structural measurement error models. *International Statistical Review*, 75, 183–198.

Thoresen, M. and Laake, P. (2003). The use of replicates in logistic measurement error modelling. *Scandinavian Journal of Statistics*, 30, 625–636.

Thoresen, M. and Laake, P. (2007). A simulation study of statistical tests in logistic measurement error models. *Journal of Statistical Computation and Simulation*, 77, 683–694.

Thürigen, D., Spiegelman, D., Blettner, M., Heuer, C., and Brenner, H. (2000). Measurement error correction using validation data: A review of methods and their applicability in case–control studies. *Statistical Methods in Medical Research*, 9, 447–474.

Thurston, S. W., Spiegelman, D., and Ruppert, D. (2003). Equivalence of regression calibration methods in main study/external validation study designs. *Journal of Statistical Planning and Inference*, 113, 527–539.

Thurston, S. W., Williams, P. L., Hauser, R., Hu, H., Hernandez-Avila, M., and Spiegelmana, D. (2005). A comparison of regression calibration approaches for designs with internal validation data. *Journal of Statistical Planning and Inference*, 131, 175–190.

Tibshirani, R. (1996). Regression shrinkage and selection via the lasso. *Journal of the Royal Statistical Society, Series B*, 58, 267–288.

Titman, A. C. and Sharples, L. D. (2008). A general goodness-of-fit test for Markov and hidden Markov models. *Statistics in Medicine*, 27, 2177–2195.

Titman, A. C. and Sharples, L. D. (2010a). Model diagnostics for multi-state models. *Statistical Methods in Medical Research*, 19, 621–651.

Titman, A. C. and Sharples, L. D. (2010b). Semi-Markov models with phase-type sojourn distributions. *Biometrics*, 66, 742–752.

Torrance-Rynard, V. L. and Walter, S. D. (1997). Effects of dependent errors in the assessment of diagnostic test performance. *Statistics in Medicine*, 16, 2157–2175.

Tosteson, T. D. and Tsiatis, A. A. (1988). The asymptotic relative efficiency of score tests in a generalized linear model with surrogate covariates. *Biometrika*, 75, 507–514.

Tosteson, T. D. and Ware, J. H. (1990). Designing a logistic regression study using surrogate measures for exposure and outcome. *Biometrika*, 77, 11–21.

Tosteson, T. D., Buonaccorsi, J. P., and Demidenko, E. (1998). Covariate measurement error and the estimation of random effect parameters in a mixed model for longitudinal data. *Statistics in Medicine*, 17, 1959–1971.

Tosteson, T.D., Buzas, J. S., Demidenko, E., and Karagas, M. (2003). Power and sample size calculations for generalized regression models with covariate measurement error. *Statistics in Medicine*, 22, 1069–1082.

Tseng, Y.-K., Hsieh, F., and Wang, J.-L. (2005). Joint modelling of accelerated failure time and longitudinal data. *Biometrika*, 92, 587–603.

Tsiatis, A. A. (2006). *Semiparametric Theory and Missing Data*. Springer, New York.

Tsiatis, A. A. and Davidian, M. (2001). A semiparametric estimator for the proportional hazards model with longitudinal covariates measured with error. *Biometrika*, 88, 447–458.

Tsiatis, A. A. and Davidian, M. (2004). Joint modeling of longitudinal and time-to-event data: An overview. *Statistica Sinica*, 14, 809–834.

Tsiatis, A. A. and Ma, Y. (2004). Locally efficient semiparametric estimators for functional measurement error models. *Biometrika*, 91, 835–848.

Tsiatis, A. A., Degruttola, V., and Wulfsohn, M. S. (1995). Modeling the relationship of survival to longitudinal data measured with error. Applications to survival and CD4 counts in patients with AIDS. *Journal of the American Statistical Association*, 90, 27–37.

Tukey, J. W. (1958). Bias and confidence in not-quite large samples (Abstract). *The Annals of Mathematical Statistics*, 29, 614.

Turnbull, B. W., Jiang, W., and Clark, L. C. (1997). Regression models for recurrent event data: Parametric random effects models with measurement error. *Statistics in Medicine*, 16, 853–864.

Ury, H. K. (1975). Efficiency of case–control studies with multiple controls per case: Continuous or dichotomous data. *Biometrics*, 31, 643–649.

Vandenhende, F. and Lambert, P. (2002). On the joint analysis of longitudinal responses and early discontinuation in randomized trials. *Journal of Biopharmaceutical Statistics*, 12, 425–440.

van der Vaart, A. W. (1998). *Asymptotic Statistics*. Cambridge University Press, Cambridge.

VanderWeele, T. J., Valeri, L., and Ogburn, E. L. (2012). The role of measurement error and misclassification in mediation analysis. *Epidemiology*, 23, 561–564.

Varin, C., Reid, N., and Firth, D. (2011). An overview of composite likelihood methods. *Statistica Sinica*, 21, 5–42.

Veierød, M. and Laake, P. (2001). Exposure misclassification: Bias in category specific Poisson regression coefficients. *Statistics in Medicine*, 20, 771–784.

Verbeke, G. and Molenberghs, G. (2000). *Linear Mixed Models for Longitudinal Data*. New York: Springer-Verlag.

Vidal, I., Iglesias, P., and Galea, M. (2007). Influential observations in the functional measurement error model. *Journal of Applied Statistics*, 34, 1165–1183.

Wald, A. (1940). The fitting of straight lines if both variables are subject to error. *The Annals of Mathematical Statistics*, 11, 284–300.

Wang, L. (2003). Estimation of nonlinear Berkson-type measurement error models. *Statistica Sinica*, 13, 1201–1210.

Wang, L. (2004). Estimation of nonlinear models with Berkson measurement errors. *The Annals of Statistics*, 32, 2559–2579.

Wang, L. (2007). A unified approach to estimation of nonlinear mixed effects and Berkson measurement error models. *The Canadian Journal of Statistics*, 35, 233–248.

Wang, C. Y. (2008). Non-parametric maximum likelihood estimation for Cox regression with subject-specific measurement error. *Scandinavian Journal of Statistics*, 35, 613–628.

Wang, C. Y. and Carroll, R. J. (1994). On robust estimation in case–control studies with errors in covariates. In *Statistical Decision Theory and Related Topics*, Volume 5, J. O. Berger and S. S. Gupta (eds), 107–120. New York: Springer-Verlag.

Wang, N. and Davidian, M. (1996). A note on covariate measurement error in nonlinear mixed effects models. *Biometrika*, 83, 801–812.

Wang, C. Y., and Pepe, M. S. (2000). Expected estimating equations to accommodate covariate measurement error. *Journal of the Royal Statistical Society, Series B*, 62, 509–524.

Wang, Q. and Rao, J. N. K. (2002). Empirical likelihood-based inference in linear errors-in-covariables models with validation data. *Biometrika*, 89, 345–358.

Wang, C. Y. and Song, X. (2013). Expected estimating equations via EM for proportional hazards regression with covariate misclassification. *Biostatistics*, 14, 351–365.

Wang, X.-F. and Wang, B. (2011). Deconvolution estimation in measurement error models: The R package decon. *Journal of Statistical Software*, 39(10), 1–24.

Wang, N., Carroll, R. J., and Liang, K.-Y. (1996). Quasilikelihood estimation in measurement error models with correlated replicates. *Biometrics*, 52, 401–411.

Wang, M. C., Qin, J., and Chiang, C.-T. (2001). Analyzing recurrent event data with informative censoring. *Journal of the American Statistical Association*, 96, 1057–1065.

Wang, C. Y., Wang, N., and Wang, S. (2000). Regression analysis when covariates are regression parameters of a random effects model for observed longitudinal measurements. *Biometrics*, 56, 487–495.

Wang, H., Zou, G., and Wan, A. T. K. (2012). Model averaging for varying-coefficient partially linear measurement error models. *Electronic Journal of Statistics*, 6, 1017–1039.

Wang, C. Y., Hsu, L., Feng, Z. D., and Prentice, R. L. (1997). Regression calibration in failure time regression. *Biometrics*, 53, 131–145.

Wang, C. Y., Huang, Y., Chao, E. C., and Jeffcoat, M. K. (2008). Expected estimating equations for missing data, measurement error, and misclassification, with application to longitudinal nonignorable missing data. *Biometrics*, 64, 85–95.

Wang, N., Lin, X., Gutierrez, R. G., and Carroll, R. J. (1998). Bias analysis and SIMEX approach in generalized linear mixed measurement error models. *Journal of the American Statistical Association*, 93, 249–261.

Wansbeek, T. J. and Koning, R. H. (1991). Measurement error and panel data. *Statistica Neerlandica*, 45, 85–92.

Wansbeek, T. and Meijer, E. (2000). *Measurement Error and Latent Variables in Econometrics*, North-Holland.

Wedderburn, R. W. M. (1974). Quasi-likelihood, generalized linear models, and the Gauss-Newton method. *Biometrika*, 61, 439–447.

Wen, C. C. (2010). Semiparametric maximum likelihood estimation in Cox proportional hazards model with covariate measurement errors. *Metrika*, 72, 199–217.

Wei, Y. and Carroll, R. J. (2009). Quantile regression with measurement error. *Journal of the American Statistical Association*, 104, 1129–1143.

Wei, L. J., Lin, D. Y., and Weissfeld, L. (1989). Regression analysis of multivariate incomplete failure time data by modeling marginal distributions. *Journal of the American Statistical Association*, 84, 1065–1073.

Wellman, J. M. and Gunst, R. F. (1991). Influence diagnostics for linear measurement error models. *Biometrika*, 78, 373–380.

White, H. (1982). Maximum likelihood estimation of misspecified models. *Econometrica*, 50, 1–25.

White, E. (2003). Design and interpretation of studies of differential exposure measurement error. *American Journal of Epidemiology*, 157, 380–387.

Whittemore, A. S. and Keller, J. B. (1988). Approximations for regression with covariate measurement error. *Journal of the American Statistical Association*, 83, 1057–1066.

Wolfe, R., Carlin, J. B., and Patton, G. C. (2003). Transitions in an imperfectly observed binary variable: Depressive symptomatology in adolescents. *Statistics in Medicine*, 22, 427–440.

Wolfinger, R. (1993). Laplace's approximation for nonlinear mixed models. *Biometrika*, 80, 791–795.

Wolfinger, R. D. and Lin, X. (1997). Two Taylor-series approximations methods for nonlinear mixed models. *Computational Statistics & Data Analysis*, 25, 465–490.

Wong, M. Y. (1989). Likelihood estimation of a simple linear regression model when both variables have error. *Biometrika*, 76, 141–148.

Woodhouse, G., Yang, M., Goldstein, H., and Rasbash, J. (1996). Adjusting for measurement error in multilevel analysis. *Journal of the Royal Statistical Society*, Series A., 159, 201–212.

Woolf, B. (1955). On estimating the relation between blood group and disease. *Annals of Human Genetics*, 19, 251–253.

Wu, L. (2002). A joint model for nonlinear mixed-effects models with censoring and covariates measured with error, with application to AIDS studies. *Journal of the American Statistical Association*, 97, 955–964.

Wu, L. (2009). *Mixed Effects Models for Complex Data*. Chapman and Hall/CRC, Boca Raton, Florida.

Wu, M. C. and Carroll, R. J. (1988). Estimation and comparison of changes in the presence of informative right censoring by modelling the censoring process. *Biometrics*, 44, 175–188.

Wu, L., Liu, W., Yi, G. Y., and Huang, Y. (2012). Analysis of longitudinal and survival data: Joint modeling, inference methods, and issues. *Journal of Probability and Statistics*, Article ID 640153.

Wulfsohn, M. S. and Tsiatis, A. A. (1997). A joint model for survival and longitudinal data measured with error. *Biometrics*, 53, 330–339.

Xiao, Z., Shao, J., and Palta, M. (2010). GMM in linear regression for longitudinal data with multiple covariates measured with error. *Journal of Applied Statistics*, 37, 791–805.

Xie, S. X., Wang, C. Y., and Prentice, R. L. (2001). A risk set calibration method for failure time regression by using a covariate reliability sample. *Journal of the Royal Statistical Society, Series B*, 63, 855–870.

Xiong, J., He, W., and Yi, G. Y. (2014). Joint modeling of survival data and mismeasured longitudinal data using the proportional odds model. *Statistics and Its Interface*, 7, 241–250.

Yan, Y. (2014). *Statistical Methods on Survival Data with Measurement Error*. Ph.D. Thesis, The University of Waterloo, Canada.

Yan, Y. and Yi, G. Y. (2015). A corrected profile likelihood method for survival data with covariate measurement error under the Cox model. *The Canadian Journal of Statistics*, 43, 454–480.

Yan, Y. and Yi, G. Y. (2016a). Analysis of error-prone survival data under additive hazards models: Measurement error effects and adjustments. *Lifetime Data Analysis*, 22, 321–342.

Yan, Y. and Yi, G. Y. (2016b). A class of functional methods for error-contaminated survival data under additive hazards models with replicate measurements. *Journal of the American Statistical Association*, 111, 684–695.

Yanagimoto, T. and Yamamoto, E. (1991). The role of unbiasedness in estimating equations. In *Estimating Functions*, Edited by V. P. Godambe, 89–101. Oxford University Press, Oxford.

Yanez, N. D., Kronmal, R. A., and Shemanski, L. R. (1998). The effects of measurement error in response variables and tests of association of explanatory variables in change models. *Statistics in Medicine*, 17, 2597–2606.

Ye, W., Lin, X., and Taylor, J. M. G. (2008). Semiparametric modeling of longitudinal measurements and time-to-event data: A two-stage regression calibration approach. *Biometrics*, 64, 1238–1246.

Yi, G. Y. (2005). Robust methods for incomplete longitudinal data with mismeasured covariates. *The Far East Journal of Theoretical Statistics*, 16, 205–234.

Yi, G. Y. (2008). A simulation-based marginal method for longitudinal data with dropout and mismeasured covariates. *Biostatistics*, 9, 501–512.

Yi, G. Y. (2009). Measurement error in life history data. *International Journal of Statistical Sciences*, 9, 177–197.

Yi, G. Y. and Cook, R. J. (2002). Marginal methods for incomplete longitudinal data arising in clusters. *Journal of the American Statistical Association*, 97, 1071–1080.

Yi, G. Y. and Cook, R. J. (2005). Errors in the measurement of covariates. *The Encyclopedia of Biostatistics*, 2nd ed., Vol. 3. Ed. by P. Armitage and T. Colton, John Wiley & Sons Ltd., 1741–1748.

Yi, G. Y. and He, W. (2006). Methods for bivariate survival data with mismeasured covariates under an accelerated failure time model. *Communications in Statistics – Theory and Methods*, 35, 1539–1554.

Yi, G. Y. and He, W. (2009). Median regression models for longitudinal data with dropouts. *Biometrics*, 65, 618–625.

Yi, G. Y. and He, W. (2012). Bias analysis and the simulation-extrapolation method for survival data with covariate measurement error under parametric proportional odds models. *Biometrical Journal*, 54, 343–360.

Yi, G. Y. and He, W. (2017). Analysis of case–control data with interacting misclassified covariates. Submitted for publication.

Yi, G. Y. and Lawless, J. F. (2007). A corrected likelihood method for the proportional hazards model with covariates subject to measurement error. *Journal of Statistical Planning and Inference*, 137, 1816–1828.

Yi, G. Y. and Lawless, J. F. (2012). Likelihood-based and marginal inference methods for recurrent event data with covariate measurement error. *The Canadian Journal of Statistics*, 40, 530–549.

Yi, G. Y. and Reid, N. (2010). A note on mis-specified estimating functions. *Statistica Sinica*, 20, 1749–1769.

Yi, G. Y., Cook, R. J., and Chen, B. (2010). Estimating functions for evaluating treatment effects in cluster-randomized longitudinal studies in the presence of drop-out and non-compliance. *The Canadian Journal of Statistics*, 38, 232–255.

Yi, G. Y., Chen, Z., and Wu, C. (2017). Analysis of correlated data with error-prone response under generalized linear mixed models. Springer Edited Refereed Volume *Big and Complex Data Analysis: Methodologies and Applications*, Edited by S. Ejaz Ahmed. Springer, Cham Heidelberg New York.

Yi, G. Y., He, W., and He, F. (2017). Analysis of panel data under hidden mover-stayer models. *Statistics in Medicine* (to appear).

Yi, G. Y., Liu, W., and Wu, L. (2011). Simultaneous inference and bias analysis for longitudinal data with covariate measurement error and missing responses. *Biometrics*, 67, 67–75.

Yi, G. Y., Ma, Y., and Carroll, R. J. (2012). A functional generalized method of moments approach for longitudinal studies with missing responses and covariate measurement error. *Biometrika*, 99, 151–165.

Yi, G. Y., Tan, X., and Li, R. (2015). Variable selection and inference procedures for marginal analysis of longitudinal data with missing observations and measurement error. *The Canadian Journal of Statistics*, 43, 498–518.

Yi, G. Y., Zeng, L., and Cook, R. J. (2011). A robust pairwise likelihood method for incomplete longitudinal binary data arising in clusters. *The Canadian Journal of Statistics*, 39, 34–51.

Yi, G. Y, Ma, Y., Spiegelman, D., and Carroll R. J. (2015). Functional and structural methods with mixed measurement error and misclassification in covariates. *Journal of the American Statistical Association*, 110, 681–696.

Yi, G. Y., Yan, Y., Liao, X., and Spielgeman, D. (2016). Estimating functions with covariate misclassification in main study/validation study designs: Applications to nutritional epidemiology. Submitted for publication.

Young, G. A. and Smith, R. L. (2005). *Essentials of Statistical Inference*. Cambridge University Press, New York.

Yucel, R. M. and Zaslavsky, A. M. (2005). Imputation of binary treatment variables with measurement error in administrative data. *Journal of the American Statistical Association*, 100, 1123–1132.

Zare, K. and Rasekh, A. (2011). Diagnostic measures for linear mixed measurement error models. *SORT*, 35, 125–144.

Zeger, S. L. and Edelstein, S. L. (1989). Poisson regression with a surrogate X; An analysis of Vitamin A and Indonesian children's mortality. *Applied Statistics*, 38, 309–318.

Zeng, D. and Cai, J. (2010). A semiparametric additive rate model for recurrent events with an informative terminal event. *Biometrika*, 97, 699–712.

Zhang, J., He, W., and Li, H. (2014). A semi-parametric approach for accelerated failure time models with covariates subject to measurement error. *Communications in Statistics – Simulation and Computation*, 43, 329–341.

Zhang, L., Mukherjee, B., Ghosh, M., Gruber, S., and Moreno, V. (2008). Accounting for error due to misclassification of exposures in case–control studies of gene-environment interaction. *Statistics in Medicine*, 27, 2756–2783.

Zhao, Y. and Lee, A. H. (1995). Assessment of influence in nonlinear measurement error models. *Journal of Applied Statistics*, 22, 215–225.

Zhao, Y., Lee, A. H., and Hui, Y. V. (1994). Influence diagnostics for generalized linear measurement error models. *Biometrics*, 50, 1117–1128.

Zheng, G. and Tian, X. (2005). The impact of diagnostic error on testing genetic association in case–control studies. *Statistics in Medicine*, 24, 869–882.

Zhou, Y. and Liang, H. (2009). Statistical inference for semiparametric varying-coefficient partially linear models with error-prone linear covariates. *The Annals of Statistics*, 37, 427–458.

Zhou, H. and Pepe, M. S. (1995). Auxiliary covariate data in failure time regression. *Biometrika*, 82, 139–149.

Zhou, H. and Wang, C.-Y. (2000). Failure time regression with continuous covariates measured with error. *Journal of the Royal Statistical Society, Series B*, 62, 657–665.

Zidek, J. V., Le, N. D., Wong, H., and Burnett, R. T. (1998). Including structural measurement errors in the nonlinear regression analysis of clustered data. *The Canadian Journal of Statistics*, 26, 537–548.

Zidek, J. V., Wong, H., Le, N. D., and Burnett, R. (1996). Causality, measurement error and multicollinearity in epidemiology. *Environmetrics*, 7, 441–451.

Zucker, D. M. (2005). A pseudo-partial likelihood method for semiparametric survival regression with covariate errors. *Journal of the American Statistical Association*, 100, 1264–1277.

Zucker, D. M. and Spiegelman, D. (2004). Inference for the proportional hazards model with misclassified discrete-valued covariates. *Biometrics*, 60, 324–334.

Zucker, D. M. and Spiegelman, D. (2008). Corrected score estimation in the proportional hazards model with misclassified discrete covariates. *Statistics in Medicine*, 27, 1911–1933.

Author Index

G. Y. Yi, *Statistical Analysis with Measurement Error or Misclassification*, Springer Series in Statistics, DOI 10.1007/978-1-4939-6640-0

Subject Index

G. Y. Yi, *Statistical Analysis with Measurement Error or Misclassification*, Springer Series in Statistics, DOI 10.1007/978-1-4939-6640-0

D

CPSIA information can be obtained
at www.ICGtesting.com
Printed in the USA
LVOW02*2214060817
544058LV00005B/50/P